Law *for* Fitness Managers *and* Exercise Professionals

MINIMIZING LIABILITY *and* MAXIMIZING SAFETY

JoAnn M. Eickhoff-Shemek, PhD
Founder and President
Fitness Law Academy, LLC
Parrish, FL
and
Professor Emeritus, Exercise Science
University of South Florida
Tampa, FL

Barbara J. Zabawa, JD, MPH
Founder and President
Center for Health & Wellness Law, LLC
McFarland, WI
and
Clinical Assistant Professor, College of Health Sciences
University of Wisconsin Milwaukee
Milwaukee, WI

Paul R. Fenaroli, JD
Associate Attorney
Ishimbayev Law Firm, P.C.
New York, NY

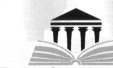

Fitness Law Academy
Fitness Law Academy, LLC
Parrish, Florida
www.fitnesslawacademy.com

Printed in the United States of America.

Library of Congress Cataloging-in-Publication Data

International Standard Book Number (ISBN): 9798669120771 (paperback)
Library of Congress Control Number (LCCN): 2020916687 (print)

Title: *Law for Fitness Managers and Exercise Professionals*
Authors: Eickhoff-Shemek, JoAnn M., Zabawa, Barbara J., and Fenaroli, Paul R.
Description: 516 pages; includes bibliographic references and index

DISCLAIMER: See page iv.

Additional copies of this book can be purchased on Amazon's website (www.amazon.com). Visit the Fitness Law Academy, LLC website at https://www.fitnesslawacademy.com for more information about this textbook and related educational programs.

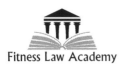

Fitness Law Academy

BRIEF CONTENTS

DISCLAIMER

This book is for your general education. Care has been taken to confirm the accuracy of the information presented and to describe generally accepted practices. However, the material presented is not exhaustive, and the authors and publisher are not responsible for errors or omissions or for any consequences from application of the information in this book.

THE INFORMATION IN THIS BOOK IS PROVIDED "AS-IS", AND THE AUTHORS MAKE NO EXPRESS OR IMPLIED REPRESENTATIONS OR WARRANTIES, INCLUDING WARRANTIES OF PERFORMANCE, MERCHANTABILITY, OR FITNESS FOR A PARTICULAR PURPOSE, REGARDING THE INFORMATION. THE AUTHORS DO NOT GUARANTEE THE COMPLETENESS, ACCURACY, OR TIMELINESS OF THIS INFORMATION. YOUR USE OF THIS INFORMATION IS AT YOUR OWN RISK.

Application of this information in a particular situation remains the professional responsibility of the practitioner; the risk management strategies described and recommended may not be considered absolute and universal recommendations.

The information contained in this book is not offered as, nor should it be construed as, legal, medical, or other advice. This book does not create an attorney-client relationship between you and any author or any of their associates. If legal, medical, or other advice is required, the services of a competent professional should be obtained, and you should not act on or rely on any of the information in this book without seeking such guidance. Moreover, in the field of physical activity and exercise (or health/fitness, fitness/wellness), the services of such competent professionals must be obtained. Some of the principles mentioned may be subject to exceptions and qualifications that may not be noted in the text. Furthermore, case law and statutes are subject to revision and may not apply in every state. Because of the quick pace of technological change, some of the information in this book may be outdated by the time you read it. Readers should be aware that business practices and legislation continue to evolve in these rapidly changing professions and industries.

Publisher: Fitness Law Academy, LLC
Authors: JoAnn M. Eickhoff-Shemek, Barbara J. Zabawa, Paul. R. Fenaroli

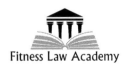
Fitness Law Academy

ABOUT THE AUTHORS

JoAnn M. Eickhoff-Shemek, PhD, FACSM, FAWHP

Dr. JoAnn Eickhoff-Shemek is the Founder and President of the Fitness Law Academy, LLC and Professor Emeritus, Exercise Science, at the University of South Florida. She has 45+ years of experience in the exercise profession. Prior to becoming an academician in 1994, Dr. Eickhoff-Shemek worked as a fitness manager/educator in community and clinical settings for nearly 20 years. She served as the Coordinator of the graduate program in Fitness and Wellness Management at the University of Nebraska at Omaha and the Founding Coordinator of the undergraduate program in Exercise Science at the University of South Florida. She received outstanding teaching awards at both institutions.

Dr. Eickhoff-Shemek is an internationally known researcher, author, and speaker in the areas of legal liability, risk management, and fitness safety. She has authored or co-authored numerous publications including three textbooks—*Law for Fitness Managers and Exercise Professionals* (lead author), *Risk Management for Health/Fitness Professionals: Legal Issues and Strategies* (lead author) and *Rule the Rules of Worksite Wellness Programs* (co-author)—and over 90 journal articles and book chapters. Dr. Eickhoff-Shemek was also a contributing author to *The Australia Fitness Industry Risk Management Manual*. She has presented her research at more than100 professional conferences and meetings including several, invited keynote presentations.

Dr. Eickhoff-Shemek has been elected and appointed to many leadership positions, serving several fitness and wellness professional organizations. She was the Legal Columnist and an Associate Editor of *ACSM's Health & Fitness Journal* for 10 years (2000-2010) and, as of January 2020, is serving as the Fitness Safety Columnist for this same *Journal*. Dr. Eickhoff-Shemek also serves as the Editor of the Fitness Law Academy's quarterly newsletter that began in January 2018. During her active career, she possessed several professional certifications in Health/Fitness Management, Clinical Exercise, Exercise Physiology, Worksite Wellness Management, and Health Education. Dr. Eickhoff-Shemek is a Fellow (Emeritus) of ACSM and a Fellow of the former Association for Worksite Health Promotion (AWHP). She received her PhD from the University of Nebraska-Lincoln in 1995.

Barbara J. Zabawa, JD, MPH

Barbara J. Zabawa, JD is the Founder and President of the Center for Health and Wellness Law, LLC, a law firm dedicated to improving legal access and compliance for the health and wellness industries. She is also lead author of the book *Rule the Rules of Workplace Wellness Programs,* published by the American Bar Association. She is a frequent writer and speaker on health and wellness law topics, having presented for national organizations such as

WELCOA, National Wellness Conference, HPLive, Healthstat University, and HERO. Barbara is also a Clinical Assistant Professor for the University of Wisconsin Milwaukee College of Health Sciences, Department of Health Services Administration where she teaches graduate and undergraduate courses in health law and compliance, U.S. health care delivery, and health professions career development.

Before graduating with honors from the University of Wisconsin Law School in 2001, Barbara obtained a Master of Public Health (MPH) degree from the University of Michigan. Immediately prior to starting her own firm, she was Associate General Counsel and HIPAA Privacy Officer for a large health insurer where she advised on Affordable Care Act matters. She was also a shareholder and Health Law Team Leader at a large Wisconsin law firm.

Barbara serves health and wellness professionals and organizations across the country as an advocate, a transactional lawyer, and a compliance resource. Her commitment to improving health and wellness also shows through her community service. Barbara founded the Wellness Compliance Institute, a nonprofit organization that seeks to improve wellness program and activity compliance. She has started a new podcast called LemonSpark, where she seeks stories that offer hope, inspiration and a sense of belonging for people experiencing trauma. She has also served on the Board of Directors for the National Wellness Institute and Rogers Behavioral Health System. Barbara is licensed to practice law in both Wisconsin and New York.

Paul R. Fenaroli, JD

Paul R. Fenaroli, JD, is an associate attorney with Ishimbayev Law Firm, P.C., a law firm committed to supporting small businesses and startups. Paul is licensed to practice law in Connecticut and counsels health and wellness ventures throughout the state. Paul graduated from Villanova University Charles Widger School of Law in May 2019. While earning his Juris Doctorate, he participated in Villanova's Health Law Clinic and served as a legal apprentice at Kendall, P.C., a boutique life sciences firm which represents global pharmaceutical and medical device manufacturers. Prior to embarking on his legal career, Paul was an offensive lineman for the Atlanta Falcons, Green Bay Packers, and New York Giants, and operated a personal training business in Monroe, CT. Prior to organizing his business, Paul was credentialed as a Certified Strength and Conditioning Specialist by the NSCA.

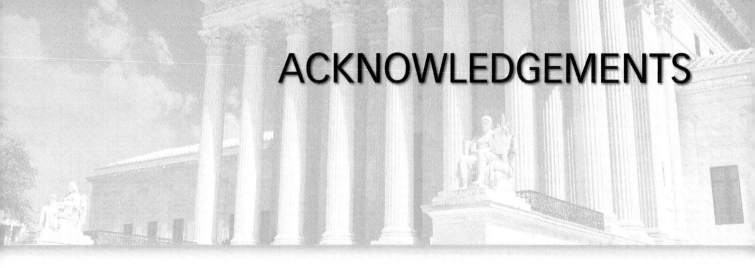

ACKNOWLEDGEMENTS

In the almost three years it took to prepare this textbook, there are many people I would like to acknowledge and thank for their assistance and contributions. First and foremost is my husband, Patrick Shemek. As with many former academic endeavors, he provided much love, support, assistance, and amazing patience throughout the completion of this textbook.

A special thanks to my co-authors, Barbara J. Zabawa, JD, MPH who took the lead with Chapter 3 and Paul R. Fenaroli, JD who took the lead with Chapter 11. It was a distinct pleasure to work with such gifted legal experts and scholars. I would also like to thank the outstanding group of expert peer reviewers who are listed below. Their feedback and suggestions were instrumental in the final preparations of this textbook and enhanced its content and organization.

Thank you, also, to the many graduate exercise science students who enrolled in my Legal/Risk Management course that I taught for 20 years prior to my retirement from academia. Their positive feedback regarding the importance of education in this area is a major reason for preparing this new textbook. One of these students, Taylor Locke, MS, assisted me in the preparation of the spotlight cases and other content in this textbook. She is recognized as a contributing author below.

In addition, I would like to acknowledge those who granted permissions to include their materials that appear throughout the textbook. They include American Bar Association, American Law Institute Publishers, American Physical Therapy Association, ASTM International, David Herbert (PRC Publishing, Inc.), Technogym, Kris Berg, Thomas Bowler, Daniel Connaughton, Jeannie Hannan, Aaron Keese, Ken Reinig, and Susan Selde.

Finally, I would like to give special thanks and recognition to Mary Francis McGavic, owner of "the Creative Spark"—a book production studio. She created and designed this entire textbook. Her work and professionalism is stellar! I highly recommend her to anyone who is looking for an experienced professional to produce a book or other similar creative work. For more information, email mary@creativespark.com.

Dr. JoAnn Eickhoff-Shemek
Founder and President,
Fitness Law Academy, LLC

Peer Reviewers

Daniel P. Connaughton, EdD
Joe Forward, JD
Lisa Giblin, MS
Savanna Jackson Mapelli, JD

Teresa Merrick, PhD
James H. (Jim) Moss, JD
Zoe Morris, PhD
Yasmin Timm, MS

Suzanne Wambold, PhD, RN
Carrie J. White, JD, EdD

Contributing Author: Taylor Locke, MS

Taylor Locke works as an Exercise Physiologist and Health Coach focusing on chronic disease prevention, management, and treatment. She received her bachelor's degree in Exercise Science at Slippery Rock University and a master's degree in Exercise Science (Health and Wellness concentration) from the University of South Florida. Taylor is an American College of Sports Medicine (ACSM) Certified Exercise Physiologist and also possesses the Exercise is Medicine® (EIM) Level 2 Credential. She has several years of professional experience working in workplace wellness and other settings.

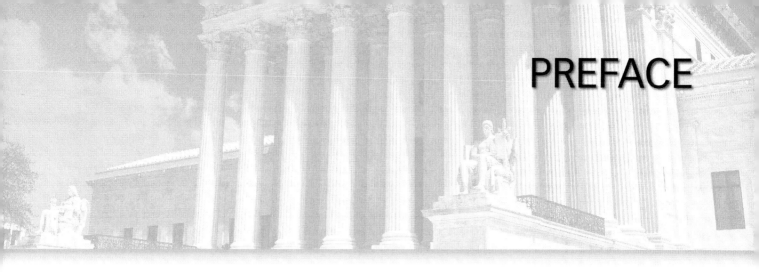

The Preface contains two parts:
Part I: The Need for Legal and Risk Management Education
Part II: Textbook Organization, Special Features, Definitions, and Website

Part I The Need for Legal and Risk Management Education:

Personal Perspectives from Lead Author, Dr. JoAnn Eickhoff-Shemek

During my 45+ years in the exercise profession, I have observed many advances and tremendous growth. When I began my career as a fitness manager and exercise professional back in the 70s, few educational opportunities were available. Today, fitness managers and exercise professionals have a plethora of educational opportunities – undergraduate and graduate academic programs in exercise science (or related areas), certifications, professional conferences, and journals such as *ACSM's Health & Fitness Journal*. These opportunities have changed and improved the profession significantly. Today, fitness managers and exercise professionals have access to many quality resources that can be used to help ensure the safety of their participants. **So, why are a high number of injuries continuing to occur and, unfortunately, many subsequent negligence claims and lawsuits?** One major reason is the lack of legal and risk management education. To fully understand what is meant by *fitness safety,* fitness managers and exercise professionals need to obtain a basic knowledge of the law, legal liability, and risk management. This textbook provides this education by addressing the: what, why, and how.

▶ **WHAT:** What laws do fitness managers and exercise professional need to know?
▶ **WHY:** Why do fitness managers and exercise professionals need to know the laws?
▶ **HOW:** How do fitness managers and exercise professionals apply the laws?

The Need to Focus on Fitness Safety

As the fitness safety columnist for *ACSM's Health & Fitness Journal,* the title of my first column was, "Top Five Reasons to Make Fitness Safety Priority No. 1" (1). Fitness managers and exercise professionals have many responsibilities, but participant safety is their most important responsibility. Three of these top five reasons are briefly summarized:

▶ **Significant increase in the number of exercise/exercise equipment injuries.**
Based on National Electronic Injury Surveillance System (NEISS) data, a nearly

90% increase in the number of injuries in the exercise/exercise equipment category occurred between 2007 and 2018. NEISS data only track visits to hospital emergency rooms. Additional NEISS data and other studies describing increases in the number of exercise injuries in various programs are presented throughout this textbook.

▶ **Litigation avoidance.** Given our litigious society, lawsuits are common. Negligence lawsuits have many negative consequences for fitness managers and exercise professionals. The costs, negative publicity, and the emotional distress can be significant. A negligence lawsuit may take years before the case is settled or goes to trial. Fitness managers and exercise professionals will have many time-consuming tasks to complete during the discovery phase that takes place prior to a settlement or trial. See Chapter 1 that describes the discovery phase.

▶ **Harm beyond the victim.** As demonstrated in many of the lawsuits described in this textbook, injuries can be severe resulting in life-long disabilities and even death. The victim is, obviously, of utmost concern. However, such tragedies are devasting to the victim's family and, thus, they desire monetary compensation by filing negligence or wrongful death lawsuits. Serious injuries and deaths can also be emotionally distressful for fitness managers and exercise professionals when they happen under their watch, especially if the injuries or deaths were preventable or foreseeable.

The Need to Understand the Causes of Injuries

There are many causes of injuries that occur in physical activity programs. This textbook focuses on the injuries due to the negligence of fitness managers and exercise professionals, demonstrating their need for legal/risk management education. Negligence cases described throughout the textbook have shown:

▶ Fitness managers failed to properly (a) maintain their exercise equipment and facility (b) manage and supervise the facility's programs/services, and (c) hire, train, and supervise personnel who lead exercise programs and/or work with individual clients.

▶ Exercise professionals failed to teach in a reasonably safe manner and/or prescribed an exercise or exercise routine that was unsafe or too intense, given the individual's health and fitness status.

Increase in Risky Exercise Programs

In recent years, many types of risky exercise programs have increased in popularity. Consequently, injuries in these high intensity, advanced, and/or complex exercise programs are quite common. See Chapters 7, 8, and 9. As evident from the cases described in the textbook, the exercise professionals leading these programs did not appear to have the knowledge and practical skills to take necessary safety precautions. They had individuals participate in these programs who were not physically able or ready (e.g., they did not have the endurance, strength, balance, and coordination to safely perform the activities) or had medical conditions that likely would have restricted or limited such activities.

The Need to Educate Exercise Professionals

Degree and certification programs help prepare exercise professionals for their many job-related responsibilities. However, often missing in these programs is adequate preparation related to their many legal and risk management responsibilities.

Degree Preparation Programs

Research, both formal and informal, has shown that legal/risk management content is not being adequately covered in undergraduate and graduate academic programs that prepare exercise professionals. The lack of preparation of undergraduates was evident in the Legal/Risk Management graduate courses that I taught for 20 years (1997–2017) at two universities. For example, in the last class I taught in the year prior to my retirement from University of South Florida (USF) in 2017, I had 21 graduate students in this class. Four of these students graduated from our USF undergraduate program in exercise science. They had exposure to legal/risk management content in the undergraduate Fitness Management course that I taught. The remaining 17 students, all from different universities throughout the country, had little or no exposure to legal/risk management content in their undergraduate exercise science (or related) programs. Feedback from the graduate students in this course, provided on the anonymous, end-of-class, course evaluations, included comments such as:

> *"The course gave me a ton of insight that I never considered beforehand as far as legal matters are concerned. I can safely say that I can use much of what I have learned in this course with risk management."*

> *"I am very glad I took this class as it has taught me a lot of legal situations that can arise within the Exercise Science field. I believe this class is really important and should be a requirement for all students…It is important that as professionals entering the field we are aware of different legal scenarios that can occur, how to avoid them and handle them if they do arise."*

Certification Programs

Many certification programs, including accredited certifications, for personal fitness trainers and group exercise leaders do not require any formal education such as classroom education and practical training. Requirements to sit for these examinations are minimal (e.g., 18 years old, high school diploma, and CPR/AED certification). It is essential that employers understand that "certified" does not necessarily mean an exercise professional is "competent", as demonstrated in several of the negligence cases described in this textbook. I believe the lack of practical training led to many of the injuries in these cases. The **lack of practical skills** was also evident in a negligence lawsuit in which I served as an expert witness. When reviewing the testimony of the defendants, an exercise instructor and fitness manager each with several fitness certifications, it was obvious they did not understand safe principles of exercise and they certainly did not possess basic practical skills to apply safe principles in the design and delivery of an exercise program. The link between the lack of practical skills and a breach of a legal duty (negligence) is described in Chapter 5.

Most certification programs that require a degree to sit for the examination, also, only require passing a written examination. There is no formal assessment of practical skills. If important practical skills are not developed and assessed in their academic program, these professionals may also lack important practical skills. As the Founding Coordinator of the undergraduate exercise science program at USF, we required our students to take several courses to help them develop important practical and job-related skills, such as the courses listed in Exhibit 5-1 in Chapter 5. In addition, they completed typical courses offered in exercise science programs (see Table 5-2 in Chapter 5). Our internship site supervisors often commented on how our students were well-prepared.

Employing Certified Fitness Professionals: A Trend or Legal Duty?

Given the issues related to certifications, a major concern is employers believing that a certified professional has obtained the competence to properly perform the job. A "certified" professional may or may not be competent. As described in Chapter 5, employers need to take a deep dive into the credentials and competence of exercise professionals prior to hiring them. If they are inadequate, employers should require candidates to obtain education and practical training or provide on-the-job education/training to minimize their liability.

"Employing certified fitness professionals" is a trend listed in the Worldwide Survey of Fitness Trends (2). It was ranked #6 in 2019 and #10 in 2020. A trend is defined as "a general development or change in a situation or in the way people are behaving" (2, p. 11). In prior surveys, this trend was stated as "employing educated, certified, and experienced fitness professionals" (2, p. 16). No matter how the trend is stated, it really is not a trend but, rather, a **potential legal duty.** See Chapter 5 for information on how employers can be vicariously and directly liable if they do not hire credentialed and competent exercise professionals. All of the other trends listed in the survey make sense as "trends" and the results of this annual survey are always quite interesting to review.

As a health/fitness manager starting back in the 1970s, I only hired degreed and competent full-time exercise professionals. All of our part-time group exercise leaders had to successfully complete a 12-week classroom course and practical training *before* they could teach an exercise class. Practical training included working as a "student teacher" under the supervision of one of our competent and experienced group exercise leaders. There were no certifications back then. If there had been, and if they only required passing a written examination as they do now, I would still require the classroom and practical training—a must to help ensure the safety of participants. More than 40 years ago, I only employed credentialed and competent employees and I know many of my colleagues (true professionals) back then did the same. So, employing qualified professionals has been going on for a long time. It is not anything new or trending.

The Need to Follow Litigation Trends

In addition to litigation involving injuries due to negligence, fitness managers and exercise professionals need to be aware of litigation trends so they can develop and implement risk management strategies to help prevent civil lawsuits and statutory violations. For example, discrimination lawsuits against fitness facilities appear to be increasing. Cases involving religious, sexual, and disability **discrimination** are described in Chapter 3.

Litigations regarding violations of data privacy, security, and breach notification laws have occurred and will likely continue as more **technological applications** will be created and utilized. Fitness managers and exercise professionals need be aware of federal and state privacy laws (described in Chapter 3) and state statutes addressing the collection and use of biometric data. Biometric Information Privacy Acts, described in Chapter 10, have been enacted in some states and are being considered in other states. Virtual exercise programs (live and on-demand) are additional technology platforms that may create litigation concerns. See Chapters 8 and 10 on recommended risk management strategies related to these programs. Virtual exercise programs have increased significantly since the COVID-19 pandemic forced many fitness facilities to close. Litigations related to COVID-19 will be another topic to follow. See Chapter 10 for recommendations to help minimize liability when re-opening a facility after a pandemic.

Physical activity has become an important component of medical care through initiatives such as Exercise is Medicine®. The **integration of exercise and health care** has created opportunities for fitness managers and exercise professionals to collaborate and/or partner with health care professionals (see Chapter 7). Legal liability issues have been raised by health care professionals regarding these arrangements, especially since the exercise profession is not a licensed profession. To minimize their legal liability, health care professionals will expect managers/professionals to provide evidence that they are compliant with applicable laws, safety standards, and employ exercise professionals with advanced credentials who have the expertise and competence to properly design and deliver programs for clinical populations. A comprehensive risk management plan, as described in Chapter 2, can help provide such evidence.

1) Eickhoff-Shemek J. Top Five Reasons to Make Fitness Safety Priority No. 1. *ACSM's Health & Fitness Journal*, 24(1), 37-38, 2020.
2) Thompson WR. Worldwide Survey of Fitness Trends for 2020. *ACSM's Health & Fitness Journal*, 23(6), 10-18, 2019.

Part II Textbook Organization, Special Features, Definitions, and Website

This textbook is **the** "comprehensive" resource covering the law, legal liability and risk management for fitness managers and exercise professionals. It was specifically written for a "lay" audience by organizing and describing applicable laws so they could be easily understood by fitness managers and exercise professionals. Also described are risk management strategies that can be effective in complying with applicable laws. The major goals of this textbook are to:

- Help fitness managers and exercise professionals minimize legal liability
- Promote and enhance the safety of fitness participants
- Advance the reputation of the exercise profession

The information will provide fitness managers and exercise professionals with background knowledge to discuss legal/risk management issues with their legal, insurance, and medical advisors.

ORGANIZATION

The 11 chapters in this textbook are organized into two parts:

- Part I: Overview of the Law, Legal Liability, and Risk Management (Chapters 1-4)

▶ Part II: Legal Liability Exposures and Risk Management Strategies (Chapters 5-11). Content covered in Part I is essential to understand before proceeding to the Chapters in Part II. See "Contents" to review the major topics covered in all 11 chapters.

SPECIAL FEATURES

The special features throughout the textbook are designed to enrich the learning experiences and outcomes for the reader. These include:

Spotlight Cases: There are 30 spotlight cases prepared as a case brief (a legal case summary that includes the facts, issue, court's ruling, and court's reasoning). The majority of these cases are appellate court cases. At the end of each spotlight case are "lessons learned" (legal and risk management) from that case. Also, there are more than 80 additional cases described throughout the textbook. Reviewing case law is one of the best ways to learn the law. These cases reflect "real" situations that occurred and could happen in any fitness facility or program. See the Case Index for a listing of the spotlight and additional cases included in each chapter.

Key Points: Several key points are provided in each chapter. Their purpose is to highlight and emphasize important legal and risk management principles and concepts.

Tables, Figures, Exhibits, and Photos: There are over 100 tables, figures, exhibits, and photos included throughout the textbook. They provide: (a) additional, relevant information, (b) sample forms and documents, and (c) illustrations of textual content.

Risk Management Audits: Toward the end of Chapters 5-11 is a Risk Management Audit that provides a list of the recommended risk management strategies described in each of these chapters. Fitness managers and exercise professionals can use each Risk Management Audit to assess whether or not they have developed and implemented the strategies recommended.

Appendices: Chapters 3, 6, 8, 9 and 11 include an appendix. These appendices provide supplemental information to assist fitness managers and exercise professionals with their risk management efforts.

Additional Features: Along with the Case Index, the following are provided in the back of the textbook: List of Abbreviations, Glossary, and Index.

DEFINITIONS

Several terms frequently used throughout the textbook are defined as follows:

Exercise Professionals: Professionals who design and deliver all types of physical activity and exercise programs for fitness participants. See Figure 5-1 in Chapter 5 that describes five levels of exercise professionals (e.g., those with little or no formal education to those with master degrees).

Fitness Facilities: Facilities that offer physical activity and exercise programs/services in all types of settings: (a) corporate, (b) college/university, (c) commercial, for-profit, (d) community, non-profit, (e) government, (f) hospitals/medical clinics, (g) retirement centers, and (h) home gyms. See Exhibit 2-1 in Chapter 2 for specific examples in each of these settings.

Fitness Managers: Owners, managers, and directors of fitness facilities and those who are in supervisory roles such as: (a) assistant managers or directors, (b) program coordinators such as personal fitness training, group exercise, and strength and conditioning coordinators, and (c) others who have oversight of programs such as youth physical activity programs.

Fitness Participants: Members and guests of fitness facilities, clients of personal fitness trainers, participants in group exercise classes, children in youth physical activity programs, athletes in strength and conditioning programs, patients in cardiac rehabilitation or other clinical exercise programs, and first responders/military personnel in fitness training programs.

Legal Liability Exposures: Situations that create a risk of an injury or reflect noncompliance to federal, state, and/or local laws.

Risk Management: A proactive administrative process that will help minimize legal liability exposures facing fitness facilities and exercise professionals.

Risk Management Strategies: Recommended policies and procedures that can help minimize legal liability exposures.

WEBSITE

Textbook resources can be found on the Fitness Law Academy's website (www.fitnesslawacademy.com) such as certain forms/documents presented in the text, study questions for each chapter, and descriptions of educational programs that accompany the textbook for academicians, fitness managers, exercise professionals, and others such as health care professionals, lawyers, and insurance providers involved in the exercise profession. **TEXTBOOK UPDATES:** Updated information, listed by chapter, can also be found on the website. See Textbook Updates.

CONTENTS

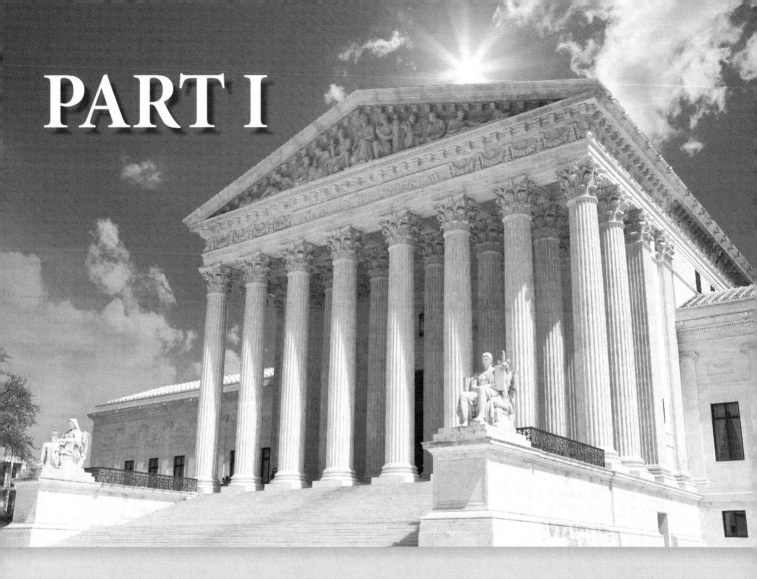

PART I

Overview of the Law, Legal Liability, and Risk Management

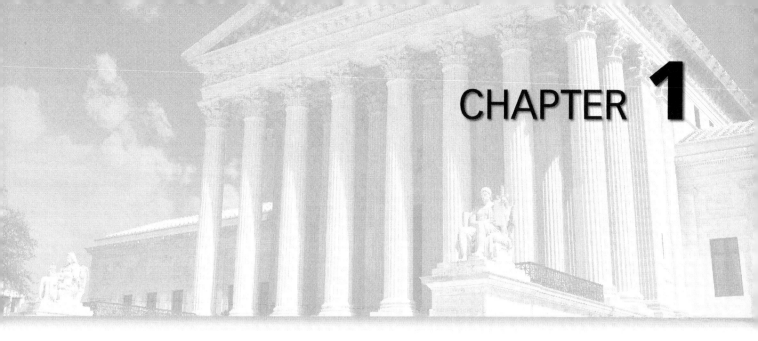

U.S. Law and Legal System

LEARNING OBJECTIVES

After reading this chapter, fitness managers and exercise professionals will be able to:

1. Define legal terms introduced in this chapter and used throughout the textbook.

2. Identify the three branches of the federal government and explain the functions of each.

3. Distinguish between primary sources of law and secondary sources of law.

4. Define substantive law and procedural law and provide examples of each.

5. Compare and contrast civil law and criminal law.

6. Describe the U.S. court system and the functions of trial courts and appellate courts.

7. Explain the legal process or phases that occur in a civil lawsuit.

8. Define tort and summarize the fault basis of tort law.

9. Describe how intentional tort, negligence, and strict liability apply to the exercise profession.

10. Identify and explain the four essential elements that the plaintiff must prove in a negligence lawsuit.

11. Distinguish between ordinary negligence and gross negligence.

12. Describe defenses to negligence that are legally effective and legally ineffective.

13. Explain respondeat superior, a common law doctrine that imposes vicarious liability upon an employer.

14. List and describe the four elements of a valid contract.

15. Discuss examples of contracts used in the exercise profession.

16. Explain why contracts need to be prepared by a competent lawyer.

17. Describe federal employment laws and other employment laws that are applicable to the exercise profession.

18. Explain how workers' compensation may apply in employer-sponsored fitness programs.

19. Identity Internet resources to find legal and risk management information.

20. Describe why reading case law is one of the best ways to learn the law and its application to the exercise profession.

INTRODUCTION

This chapter provides fitness managers and exercise professionals with an overview of U.S. law and legal system. Obtaining an understanding and appreciation of the content in this chapter is essential. It serves as the foundation for the remaining chapters. Major topics include primary sources of law, the legal process of a civil lawsuit, the function of trial and appellate courts, and areas of law that are especially relevant in the exercise profession—tort, contract, and employment law. Many legal terms used throughout this textbook are defined in this chapter. Legal research and resources are discussed toward the end of the chapter as well as why reviewing case law is one of the best ways to learn the law and how to apply it to the daily operations of fitness facilities and programs.

Editorial Note: *The content in this chapter, up to the Employment Law section, reflects content from Chapter 2 in Risk Management for Health/Fitness Professionals: Legal Issues and Strategies (1). The publisher transferred the rights to this textbook to the authors in 2017. Permission to reprint and revise/update this content was granted by the author of Chapter 2, Daniel P. Connaughton, Ed.D.*

PRIMARY SOURCES OF LAW

In addition to federal and state constitutional law, **primary sources of law** also include statutory, administrative, and case law. The description of each of these is provided, primarily, in the context of the federal branches. Keep in mind that these primary sources of law include state and local branches of government. Because primary sources represent the actual law, they are the only sources fitness managers and exercise professionals should rely upon to determine what the law requires (1). **Secondary sources of law**, on the other hand, are sources that may help explain or summarize laws. They are published by various individuals, organizations, or businesses. Examples include books, restatements (e.g., *Restatement of the Law Third, Torts*), treatises, law review journal articles, legal dictionaries, and a plethora of sources available on the Internet. Secondary sources can help provide insight and understanding of primary sources that may be helpful for fitness managers and exercise professionals. Both primary and secondary sources of law are cited throughout this textbook.

Constitutional Law

On September 17, 1787, the U.S. Constitution became the supreme law of the land. As shown in Figure 1-1, it created the national government and its three branches: (a) legislative, (b) executive, and (c) judicial. The legislative branch makes laws, the executive branch carries out laws, and the judicial branch interprets laws. The Constitution allocated a **separation of powers** based on the functions of each branch. This allows each branch to check on the other two branches to help prevent any one branch from, illegally, exercising power (2).

The U.S. Constitution protects individual rights (2). Many of these rights are found in the Bill of Rights, the first 10 amendments to the Constitution, as well as other amendments. For example, the First Amendment protects rights such as the freedom of religion, speech, and press. In *Cooksey v. Futrell*, described in Chapter 7, an individual claimed his First Amendment speech rights were violated when the North Carolina State Board required him to remove certain content from his website because it constituted practicing dietetics without a license. Also, see *Jalal v. Lucille Roberts Health Clubs, Inc.* in Chapter 3—a case involving religious discrimination.

In addition, the U.S. Constitution guarantees that individual states retain powers not delegated to the federal government (1, 2). These state powers are reflected in the state constitutions that serve as the supreme law of each state. Like the U.S. Constitution, each state's constitution creates the state government and its three branches—legislative, executive, and judicial. States cannot enact laws that conflict with federal laws but they have numerous powers to create their own laws. For example, as described in Chapter 3, states have passed their own occupational and safety laws/regulations that need to be followed, in addition to those specified in the federal Occupational Safety and Health Act. States have passed laws that are not reflected in federal laws such as waiver statutes (discussed in Chapter

Figure 1-1: U.S. Constitution and Three Branches of Government*

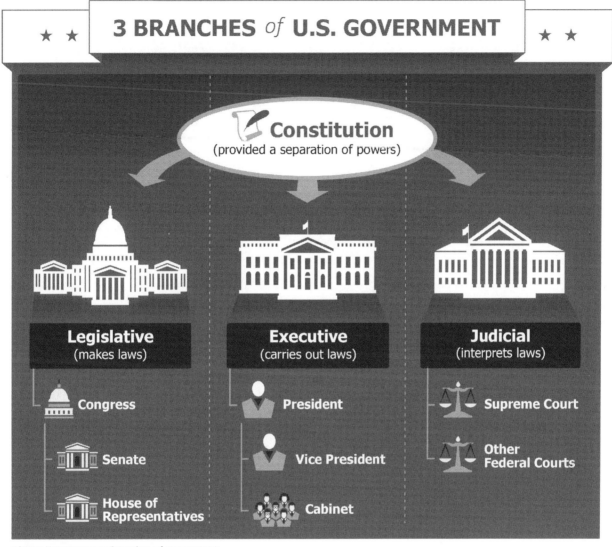

* https://www.usa.gov/branches-of-government

4) and statutes that require fitness facilities to have an Automated External Defibrillator (AED). These AED statutes are described in Chapter 11. In addition, criminal law and civil law, described later, are primarily regulated by state law (1).

Statutory Law—Legislative Branch

As shown in Figure 1-1, Congress is the legislative branch of the federal government that makes laws for the nation. This body of law, enacted through the legislative process, is referred to as **statutory law**. Congress has two legislative chambers: the Senate and House

of Representatives. Members of the Senate (100—two from every state) and the House of Representatives (435—number is based on each state's population) are elected by popular vote (1). Anyone elected to either chamber can submit a bill—a proposal for a new law (3). See Figure 1-2 that describes five steps on how a legislative bill becomes a law.

The laws enacted through the legislative process are referred to as **statutes** at both the federal and state level. Federal statutes, organized by Titles and Chapters, can be found at: http://uscode.house.gov/ (Office of the Law Revision Counsel, United State Code). Laws passed by local governments (e.g., municipalities and

Figure 1-2: How a Legislative Bill Becomes Law*

HOW DOES A BILL BECOME A LAW?

① EVERY LAW STARTS WITH AN IDEA

That idea can come from anyone, even you! Contact your elected officials to share your idea. If they want to try to make it a law, they will write a bill.

② THE BILL IS INTRODUCED

A bill can start in either house of Congress when it's introduced by its primary sponsor, a Senator or a Representative. In the House of Representatives, bills are placed in a wooden box called "the hopper."

③ THE BILL GOES TO COMMITTEE

Representatives or Senators meet in a small group to research, talk about, and make changes to the bill. They vote to accept or reject the bill and its changes before sending it to:

the House or Senate floor for debate or to a subcommittee for further research.

Here, the bill is assigned a legislative number before the Speaker of the House sends it to a committee.

④ CONGRESS DEBATES AND VOTES

Members of the House or Senate can now debate the bill and propose changes or amendments before voting. If the majority vote for and pass the bill, it moves to the other house to go through a similar process of committees, debate, and voting. Both houses have to agree on the same version of the final bill before it goes to the President.

DID YOU KNOW?

The House uses an electronic voting system while the Senate typically votes by voice, saying "yay" or "nay."

HOUSE MAJORITY → **SENATE** MAJORITY

⑤ PRESIDENTIAL ACTION

When the bill reaches the President, he or she can:

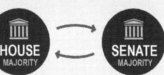
✓ APPROVE and PASS
The President signs and approves the bill. The bill is law.

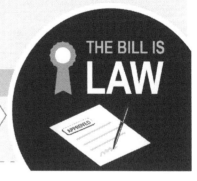
THE BILL IS LAW

The President can also:

Veto

The President rejects the bill and returns it to Congress with the reasons for the veto. Congress can override the veto with 2/3 vote of those present in both the House and the Senate and the bill will become law.

Choose no action

The President can decide to do nothing. If Congress is in session, after 10 days of no answer from the President, the bill then automatically becomes law.

Pocket veto

If Congress adjourns (goes out of session) within the 10 day period after giving the President the bill, the President can choose not to sign it and the bill will not become law.

* https://www.usa.gov/how-laws-are-made#item-35837

counties) are often referred to as **ordinances** and include rules such as parking regulations, zoning regulations, and leash laws (1). Collectively, statutes and ordinances are referred to as the **written law**. It is important to realize that the written law is limited to matters of jurisdiction. "Federal statutory law is limited to matters of federal jurisdiction; similar limitations hold for state statutes and local ordinances" (1, p. 24). If jurisdictions overlap, federal law prevails over state law, as does state law over local law (1, 2). Several federal laws enacted by Congress are described in this textbook including:

- Americans with Disabilities Act (ADA)
- Affordable Care Act (ACA)
- Title VII of the Civil Rights Act of 1964
- Health Insurance Portability and Accountability Act (HIPAA)
- Federal Trade Commission Act (FTCA)
- Fair Labor Standards Act (FLSA)
- Equal Pay Act (EPA)
- Occupational Safety and Health Act
- Volunteer Protection Act

Several state laws are also described in this textbook and include (a) waiver statutes, (b) state licensing statutes, (c) consumer protection laws such as unfair and/or deceptive acts or practices and statutes that regulate health club membership contracts, (d) data privacy statutes such as Biometric Information Privacy Acts, and (e) AED statutes.

Administrative Law—Executive Branch

The executive branch carries out the laws passed by the legislature. As shown in Figure 1-1, it is made up of the President, Vice-President, and Cabinet. Cabinet members are heads or secretaries of 15 departmental agencies including Education, Health and Human Services (HHS), Defense, and Homeland Security (4). This branch of government, also, includes regulatory agencies such as the Food and Drug Administration (FDA), Occupational Health and Safety Administration (OSHA), Internal Revenue Services (IRS), Equal Employment Opportunity Commission (EEOC), and the Consumer Product Safety Commission (CPSC).

These regulatory agencies have a great deal of power. They enact **regulations,** referred to as **administrative**

law. For example, after Congress passed the Occupational Safety and Health Act in 1970, the OSHA was formed which enacted many regulations that employers need to follow. As described in several chapters in this textbook, fitness managers/owners need to comply with many OSHA regulations as well as other agency regulations. The EEOC enforces federal discrimination claims that are alleged to have occurred in the workplace. See Chapter 3 for several discrimination cases that have occurred in fitness facilities. The IRS determines if a worker has been properly classified as an employee or independent contractor as described in Chapter 5. These agencies have the power to investigate violations of their regulations and resolve disputes. In addition, they can impose sanctions when violations have occurred. Large financial penalties have been levied as sanctions for violations of administrative agency regulations (5). For example, fitness facilities have had to pay large financial penalties for violations of OSHA regulations and for misclassifying independent contractors as described in Chapters 3 and 5, respectively.

Case Law—Judicial Branch

As shown in Figure 1-1, the judicial branch interprets laws. This branch of government resolves disputes through the court system which is described later. U.S. **case law** is primarily based on English **common law,** a system that originated in medieval England when opinions and court rulings began to be recorded. This system was adopted by the U.S. at the time of the American Revolution (2). U.S. common law is often referred to as judge-made law (1, 2). Judges began to follow previously decided court rulings referred to as **precedent**. Judges were eventually obligated to follow previous court rulings or precedent, which is termed **stare decisis**—meaning "it stands decided" (1).

There are many cases described in this textbook where courts have relied on previous court rulings. For example, in a 1992 Supreme Court case in Virginia, the Court "ruled that waivers protecting against liability for personal injury due to negligence are against public policy and are unenforceable" (6, p. 216). Subsequent Virginia courts have followed this ruling when the same type of factual dispute was raised. Fitness managers/owners in Virginia need to realize that a waiver will not provide protection for personal injuries due to negligent conduct. Waiver law is covered in Chapter 4.

"Precedence makes the law more efficient and predictable" (1, p. 24). It is based on decisions of appellate courts (appellate courts are described below) in which judges write their opinions and rulings (i.e., a written judicial opinion). These written opinions are then published so that others can access them and be informed of important court rulings or precedent. Many of the cases described in this textbook are appellate court cases at the federal and/or state level. Fitness managers and exercise professionals can learn from these cases to help develop policies and procedures for their fitness facility and programs that reflect these court rulings.

As described above, **jurisdiction** is based on federal and state statutes. Jurisdiction refers to "the geographic area in which the court has authority and types of cases it has the power to hear" (2, p. 759). The types of cases that courts will hear will depend on **subject matter jurisdiction** (e.g., limited jurisdiction meaning a court is limited to the types of cases it can hear). A court with **general jurisdiction** can hear and decide almost any type of case (2) Some of the cases described in this textbook have addressed jurisdiction issues, such as *Tynes v. Buccaneers Limited Partnership* in Chapter 10.

KEY POINT

Fitness managers and exercise professionals have an important responsibility to be familiar with statutory, administrative, and case law. The failure to follow applicable statutory, administrative, and case law increases legal liability. Knowledge of these laws is essential to develop and implement effective risk management strategies that reflect the laws and to minimize legal liability.

CATEGORIES OF LAW

In addition to federal and state law, additional categories of law include (a) private and public law, (b) substantive and procedural law, and (d) civil and criminal law. **Private law** "defines, regulates, enforces, and administers relationships among individuals, associations, and corporations" (7, p. 830). **Public law** "defines rights and duties with either the operation of government or relationships between the government and individuals, associations, and corporations" (7, p. 857). Most of the cases described in this textbook deal with private law (e.g., private parties such as a fitness participant who has filed a negligence lawsuit against his/her personal trainer and/or fitness facility). However, other cases described in this textbook have involved public law. Examples include individuals who have filed negligence lawsuits against a government agency such as a public university, a police/fire department, or the military. *UCF Athletics Association v. Plancher* and *Hajdusek v. United States* are cases described in Chapter 8 involving a collegiate athlete and Marine Corps recruit, respectively. Sovereign immunity, which provides protection for governmental or public agencies, was addressed in both of these cases. Sovereign immunity does not apply in cases involving private parties—a major difference between private and public law.

Substantive and Procedural Law

The law can also be categorized into substantive and procedural law. **Substantive law** creates, defines, and regulates the duties of parties and includes tort, contract, employment, and criminal law (7). **Procedural law** prescribes methods of enforcing substantive law, such as the law of jurisdiction and law of evidence (7). Procedural law sets forth rules that need to be followed once a case arises such as "the dates and time limits when certain papers must be filed, what information legal papers must contain, how witnesses can be examined prior to trial, how the jury may be selected, when and where the trial will be held, and so on" (1, p. 26). Both substantive and procedural law apply in civil and criminal court cases. If a filed claim does not address an area of substantive law, the court is not obligated to provide any legal remedy to that party and can dismiss the case. If a party does not follow the procedural rules, the court is not obligated to provide any legal remedy to that party. For example, in *Abston v. Fitness Co.* (216 F.R.D. 143, 2003), the defendant failed to respond to numerous interrogatories (defined later) from the plaintiff. Instead of entering a default judgment against the defendant for failing to follow Federal Rules of Civil Procedure, the DC District Court issued significant and costly sanctions against the defendant. Fitness managers and exercise professionals facing litigation need to work with their legal counsel so that substantive and procedural laws are properly followed.

Civil and Criminal Law

It is essential that fitness managers and exercise professionals understand differences between **civil law** and **criminal law**. The major differences are presented in Table 1-1. Civil law deals with disputes between two parties and criminal law deals with crimes against society. Most of the cases described in this textbook deal with civil law involving tort (e.g., negligence), contract (e.g., waivers), and employment law (e.g., discrimination). However, some of the cases included in this textbook have involved criminal acts such as sexual sexual assault. See *Jessica H. v. Equinox* and *Elena Myers Court v. Loews Philadelphia Hotel, Inc.* described in Chapter 5 as well as the Penn State University and Michigan State University cases also described in Chapter 5.

A civil lawsuit involves two parties—the **plaintiff** (e.g., an injured fitness participant who claims his/her injury was due to the negligent conduct of an exercise professional) and the **defendant** (e.g., the party or parties the plaintiff is suing such as the exercise professional and/or the fitness facility). Often, there are multiple defendants in a civil lawsuit as demonstrated in many of the negligence cases described in this textbook. For example, see *Jacob v. Grant Life Choices* in Chapter 5. In that case, there were four defendants: (a) employee, Robert Getz, (b) Club Management, Inc. (CMI)—the management company (vendor) who managed Grant Life Choices Center, (c) Grant Life Choices Center (the fitness facility), and (d) Grant Medical Center (hospital affiliated with the fitness center). The standard of proof that must be demonstrated in a civil lawsuit is the **preponderance of the evidence**—meaning more likely than not (51% or greater) the defendant's conduct

Table 1-1	Differences Between Civil Law and Criminal Law*	
	CIVIL LAW	**CRIMINAL LAW**
General Description	Deals with disputes between two parties (e.g., individuals, organizations, and businesses). Party #1 (plaintiff) hires a lawyer who files a lawsuit claiming that Party #2 (defendant) failed to carry out a legal duty that resulted in some type of harm to Party #1.	Deals with crimes against society (e.g., conduct that reflects a violation of a federal or state statute) and the punishment of the crime. The government files the case against the defendant accused of committing the crime.
Examples	Negligent conduct (e.g., an exercise professional who provides improper instruction to a client that results in harm to the client), breach of contract, noncriminal statutory violations, and civil rights violations.	Criminal conduct such as practicing medicine or dietetics without a license (e.g., violation of a state licensing statute), theft, and sexual assault.
Standard of Proof	Preponderance of the evidence, meaning more likely than not (51% or greater) the defendant's conduct caused the harm.	Beyond a reasonable doubt, meaning the defendant's guilt is fully demonstrated (100% certainty, no doubt) based on the evidence.
Burden of Proof	The plaintiff has the burden of proof, so must provide evidence that a legal duty existed and that the duty was breached.	The prosecution (government) must prove that the defendant was guilty; the defendant is innocent until proven guilty.
Type of Punishment	If the court rules the defendant liable for the harm, the defendant must compensate the plaintiff (usually financial compensation for injuries or damages) and may be ordered to stop the practice causing the harm.	If the court rules the defendant guilty of the crime, he/she is subject to fines, community service, probation, imprisonment or any combination of these.

caused the harm to the plaintiff. The plaintiff has the burden of proof as shown in Table 1-1. If the court rules the defendant **liable** for the harm, the defendant must compensate the plaintiff (usually financial compensation) for injuries or damages.

A criminal case also involves two parties—the **defendant** who is the individual accused of a crime against society (the people), and *the people* who are represented by the government—a district attorney. Crimes reflect violations of federal and/or state statutes as well as local ordinances. The standard of proof is **beyond a reasonable doubt**—meaning the defendant's guilt is fully (100%) demonstrated, based on the evidence. If the court finds the defendant **guilty**, he/she is subject to fines, community service, probation, imprisonment or any combination of these. Exercise professionals need to understand that they can face criminal charges for conduct such as sexual assault as well as a civil lawsuit. Sexual assault, in addition to a crime, is an intentional tort (civil wrong) described later under tort law.

CIVIL LAWSUITS: THE LEGAL PROCESS

All cases must follow a well-established legal process. Because this textbook focuses on civil procedures (e.g., civil lawsuits involving negligence) more so than criminal procedures, the following discussion will describe the legal process based on a civil lawsuit. First, it is important to review the U.S. trial and appellate court system.

Trial and Appellate Courts

Trial courts—the lowest level of courts—conduct the initial proceedings in a civil lawsuit. The next level of courts are the intermediate appellate courts and the highest level of courts are supreme courts. This hierarchy of courts exists in both federal and state court systems as shown in Table 1-2. Courts at the state level deal with state matters and courts at the federal level deal with federal matters. Federal courts also hear cases when parties are from different states (1).

The purposes of the trial proceedings are "(1) to determine the facts of dispute... (2) to determine what

Table 1-2	Hierarchy of Federal and State Courts	
FEDERAL (RULE ON FEDERAL LAW ISSUES)	**TYPE OF COURT**	**STATE—FLORIDA EXAMPLE** (RULE ON STATE LAW ISSUES)
United States Supreme Court	**Supreme Court (Appellate Court)**	Supreme Court of Florida
United States Courts of Appeals (13 in the U.S.)	**Intermediate Courts of Appeal (Appellate Courts)**	District Courts of Appeals (Florida has five)
United States District Courts (Florida has three)	**General or Limited Jurisdiction Courts (Trial Courts)**	Circuit and County Courts in Florida

rules of law should be applied to the facts, and (3) to apply those rules to the facts" (2, p. 91). Judges preside over the trial court proceedings. At the end of the trial, the judge or jury renders a judgment or ruling in favor of one of the parties. If either party believes the trial court erred in its ruling, substantively or procedurally, the party can appeal to a higher court (i.e., an intermediate court of appeals, requesting a different ruling). Most trial court cases are not appealed (1). However, many of the cases described in this textbook are appellate court cases including cases appealed to state Supreme Courts and U.S. Courts of Appeal.

At the federal level, there are 94 district courts. The number of these trial courts vary by state. For example, Nebraska has one federal district court and Florida has three (Southern, Northern, and Middle). The number of trial courts at the state level also vary. For example, Florida has 67 county courts, one in each county, and 20 circuit courts (8).

Regarding federal intermediate courts of appeal, there are 13 circuit courts (12 regional and one federal). For example, Florida, Georgia and Alabama make up one of the 12 regions—the 11th Circuit. See Figure 1-3. As shown in this figure, the DC Circuit (12th Circuit) and the Federal District are located in Washington, D.C. A U.S. Court of Appeals hears appeals from the district courts within its circuit. The number of state intermediate courts of appeal vary by state. Florida has five as shown in Figure 1-4.

Figure 1-3: Intermediate Courts of Appeal—Federal Level*

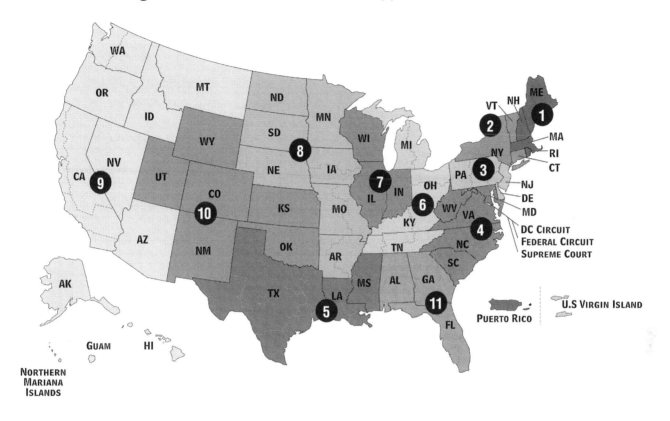

* United States Courts. Court Role and Structure. Available at: https://www.uscourts.gov/about-federal-courts/court-role-and-structure.

Figure 1-4: Intermediate Courts of Appeal— State Level (Florida example)*

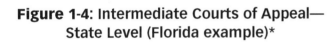

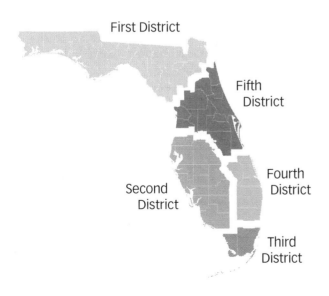

First District

Fifth District

Fourth District

Second District

Third District

*Florida Courts. District Courts of Appeal. Available at: https://www.flcourts.org/Florida-Courts/District-Courts-of-Appeal.

The highest appellate court at the federal level is the U.S. Supreme Court. Each state also has a Supreme Court. Some states may use a name other than Supreme Court for its highest court such as New York in which the highest court is the New York Court of Appeals. All appellate courts are made up of judges only. For example, the U.S. Supreme Court has nine justices and the Florida Supreme Court has seven justices. An odd number is used so that a majority ruling can be made. For example, 5-4 decisions of the U.S. Supreme Court are quite common. The U.S Supreme Court decides which cases it will hear. Four of the nine justices need to agree to hear a case. The case needs to address an important federal question such as a constitutional issue. The Court then issues a **writ of certiorari** to the court of appeals or highest state court requesting the case records (2). The Court receives approximately 7,000-8,000 petitions for a writ of certiorari each year and grants and hears oral argument in about 80 cases (9).

When the Court decides not to review a case, the decision of the lower court stands.

Civil Lawsuit—Pre-Trial and Trial Court Phases

Once the plaintiff's lawyer determines his/her client has a **cause of action** (an appropriate legal basis for suing) and has identified the appropriate jurisdiction to file the lawsuit, the plaintiff's lawyer files a **complaint**—a document that initiates the lawsuit (1, 2). The complaint may include the allegations related to the plaintiff's harm such as the negligent conduct of the defendant, and claims or theories of relief the plaintiff is seeking (e.g., monetary damages). For example, in a negligence lawsuit, the negligence claims are often listed in the complaint. See *Baldi-Perry v. Kaifas and 360 Fitness Center, Inc.* (Exhibit 2-3 in Chapter 2) in which the complaint listed 26 negligence claims against a personal fitness trainer and 16 negligence claims against the fitness facility. The complaint may also list several counts. For example, in *Miller v. The YMCA of Central Massachusetts, et al.* (spotlight case in Chapter 10), three counts were listed in the complaint as follows: Count I - a violation of the wrongful death statute on behalf of Mr. Miller's beneficiaries, Count II—conscious pain and suffering, and Count III—gross negligence.

The complaint needs to be filed within the state's **statute of limitations**—the maximum time the plaintiff's lawyer has to file the complaint. For personal injury cases, this time period in most states is two-three years, but in some states it can be one year (e.g., Louisiana and Tennessee), four-five years, or even six years as in Maine and North Dakota (10). In *D'Amico v. LA Fitness*, spotlight case in Chapter 5, the first two counts in the complaint that dealt with negligence were not filed within the state's statute of limitation.

After the complaint is filed, a **summons** is then delivered by an officer of the court to the defendant(s). The summons informs the defendant(s) of the lawsuit and the timeframe in which a response is needed such as 30 days (1, 2). Failure to respond may result in the plaintiff winning the case by default (2). The defendant(s), at this point, needs to have a lawyer to prepare an **answer**—a response to the summons within the specified timeframe. Instead of an answer, the defendant(s) may file a **motion to dismiss** (or demurrer)

claiming the complaint is legally insufficient on substantive grounds or that the action is barred, procedurally, such as not being filed within the jurisdiction's statute of limitations (2). Together, the summons and the answer are referred to as the **pleadings** (1).

The next pre-trial phase of a civil lawsuit is referred to as **discovery.** This, often lengthy, phase continues until the case goes to trial or is settled out-of-court. Discovery involves various methods to learn about the facts in the dispute (2) such as:

- **Interrogatories**—written questions that are directed to either party (e.g., a set of written questions sent by the plaintiff's lawyer to the other party). The questions must be answered by the other party under oath, with the guidance of legal counsel, and within a given time period. The questions and answers can serve as evidence at trial (1).
- **Depositions**—oral questioning of a witnesses or an adverse party by the opposing attorney, under oath and in the presence of a court stenographer and the other party's attorney (1, 2). Transcripts of depositions can serve as evidence at trial.
- **Motions to Produce**—requests by legal counsel to a judge to order the opposing party to provide certain evidence that may be relevant in the case (2). For example, in negligence cases involving fitness facilities these requested items may include membership contracts, pre-activity screening forms, waivers, informed consents, injury reports, employee handbook, emergency action plan, staff training and/or certification records, personal fitness training agreements or records, exercise equipment inspections/maintenance records, and the exercise equipment the plaintiff was using when allegedly harmed.

If there are no factual disputes that need to be resolved after the discovery phase, the case may be decided without going to trial. Either party can file a motion for **summary judgment.** The party filing this motion needs to establish that there is no genuine issue of material fact and that he/she is entitled to judgment as a matter of law (11). The judge then reviews the motion and renders a judgment. If the judge grants the motion,

KEY POINT

#1 — It is emphasized throughout this textbook that fitness managers and exercise professionals need to have and keep documents to help demonstrate legal duties were properly carried out. For example, evidence of proper exercise equipment maintenance can be effective in defending negligence claims. See *Chavez v. 24 Hour Fitness* and *Grebing v. 24 Hour Fitness* in Chapter 9. In *Chavez,* the facility was liable for gross negligence for not following exercise equipment maintenance specifications, whereas in *Grebing,* the facility was not liable because it had evidence (documents) that regular inspections and preventative maintenance were conducted by a trained technician.

#2 — In addition to the high costs and negative publicity associated with negligence lawsuits, fitness managers and exercise professionals need to realize the many other negative aspects of a lawsuit, such as the time, effort and stress often required during discovery. See *Jessica H. v. Equinox* in Chapter 5 in which Equinox produced 750 pages of documents in response to all of the discovery requests.

no trial takes place (2). As demonstrated in many of the cases described in this textbook, motions for summary judgment are very common in the legal process. For example, courts have granted defendants their motion for summary judgment based on the waiver the plaintiff signed, if the waiver was legally enforceable. On occasion, the other party will disagree with the judge's decision to grant the motion for summary judgment and then file an appeal claiming the judge made an error.

Also, after the discovery phase, either party can request a pretrial conference or hearing in which the judge and the attorneys discuss the matters in the case and plans for trial (2). The judge may encourage the parties to reach an **out-of-court settlement** to avoid going to trial. As described in Chapter 5, about 95% of personal injury cases end in a pre-trial settlement meaning that, approximately, one in 20 cases go to trial to be resolved by a judge or jury (12). The data also show that personal injury trials favor the plaintiff in over 90% of the cases (12). Therefore, pre-trial settlements may be best for defendants who lack strong

evidence to defend themselves (12). Some of the cases described in this textbook ended with out-of-court settlements. See *National Music Publishers' Association v. Peloton* (13, 14), a music copyright infringement case in Chapter 3 and *Tynes v. Buccaneers Limited Partnership,* a personal injury case in Chapter 10. The terms of the settlement, such as the monetary damages awarded, most often are not made public as in these two cases. The plaintiffs in these cases were seeking $150 million (Peloton) and $20 million (Buccaneers) in damages.

If the case goes to trial, the plaintiff in a civil case has the choice to have the case heard by a judge or jury. Having a jury is a legal right specified in the U.S. Constitution (7th amendment) and in state constitutions (2). At the beginning of a trial, the plaintiff's attorney gives his/her opening remarks and the defendant's attorney may also make an opening statement. The statements inform the **triers of fact** (judge or jury) what each party expects to prove in the trial and the evidence they will be presenting (1, 2). **Evidence** is everything the judge or jury is entitled to consider in order to determine the facts in the case (2). It must be relevant to the case. Evidence not related to the facts is inadmissible. After the opening statements, the attorney for the plaintiff calls and examines the witnesses representing the plaintiff. These witnesses are then cross-examined by the defendant's attorney, often redirected by the plaintiff's attorney, and then re-crossed by the defendant's attorney (1). The defendant's attorney then calls and examines the witnesses representing the defendant followed by the same cross-examination process. Note: Prior to trial, attorneys on both sides can ask the court for a **subpoena**—a writ ordering a person to appear in court and testify as a witness (2).

There are two types of witnesses—**fact witnesses** and **expert witnesses**. Fact witnesses, for example in a personal injury case, are individuals who have information about the plaintiff's injury. They were present when the plaintiff was injured and, thus, observed, heard, or felt something regarding the injury (1). They testify as to the facts only. Expert witnesses have specialized knowledge and/or training in a field. They are recognized by the court as such and are allowed to provide their expert opinions regarding the plaintiff's injury and its causes. For example, in a negligence lawsuit, they educate the court as to the **standard of care** (or duty) that the defendant owed to the plaintiff and if, in their opinion, the defendant breached that duty. Duty and breach of duty are described later under tort law. There are several negligence cases presented in this textbook in which expert witnesses provided testimony. For example, in *Vaid v. Equinox,* spotlight case in Chapter 8, the plaintiff's expert witnesses included medical and exercise professionals.

Once the questioning of witnesses has finished and all evidence has been offered, the plaintiff's attorney gives his/her closing statement followed by the closing statement of the defendant's attorney (2). The plaintiff's attorney then concludes. If there is a jury, the judge then gives **jury instructions** instructing the jury on applicable laws. The jury deliberates and returns with a verdict (the jury's decision). When there is no jury, the judge renders a decision after the closing statements. If the losing party disagrees with the court's decision, they can appeal within a certain timeframe.

Civil Lawsuit—Appellate Court Phase

Appellate courts are made up of three or more judges—always an odd number as stated earlier. There are no attorneys, juries, or witnesses involved. All of the judges, or a panel of judges, review the trial court transcripts and evidence as well as written briefs prepared by attorneys including their legal arguments on how the law was mistakenly applied, substantively or procedurally (1). After the appellate court completes its review, it decides as to whether or not the trial court correctly applied the law. If the trial court made an error, the appellate court "may *modify* or *reverse* the lower's court's decision, and either enter a new judgment or **remand** (send back) the case to the trial court for a new trial in compliance with the appellate court's instructions" (1, p. 27). The error made by the trial court must be significant for the appellate court to overturn the trial court's decision. If the trial court did not make an error, the appellate court *affirms* the trial court's ruling.

As stated previously, many of the cases described in this textbook are appellate court cases so there are several examples of these courts modifying, reversing, remanding, or affirming the trial court's decision. Based on precedent or stare decisis, described earlier, lower courts are obligated to follow and apply decisions and interpretations of higher courts in similar cases. Appellate courts prepare a written opinion for each case they review, which is published so that lower courts and others are informed of their decisions and interpretations. If all the appellate judges agree, it is called a **unanimous opinion**. If it is not unanimous, a **majority opinion** is written (2). In some cases, a judge, who disagrees with the majority, may write a **dissenting opinion** that explains his/her arguments for disagreeing with the majority. Dissenting opinions may be relevant because they may provide the basis of arguments for overruling a majority opinion in the future (2). Some dissenting opinions are summarized in the cases described in this textbook. For example, see Exhibit 4-5 in Chapter 4 for the dissenting opinion written by two judges in *Stelluti v. Casapenn Enterprises, LLC, dba Powerhouse Gym.* This opinion helps explain why courts disfavor waivers and why several courts have ruled that waivers for personal injury are against public policy. Statutes in some states also prohibit waivers based on public policy. More information on waivers and public policy is discussed in Chapter 4.

TORT LAW

A **tort** can be defined as conduct that reflects a legal wrong that causes harm (1)—physical harm, emotional harm, or both. Conduct that causes harm can impose **civil liability** (e.g., a defendant can be liable for his/her conduct that causes harm to the plaintiff). A plaintiff is awarded damages (money) when courts find the defendant(s) liable for such conduct. The defendant is responsible for the monetary damages awarded to the plaintiff, which helps the plaintiff pay for his/her medical and other expenses as well as help make the plaintiff whole again. Almost every civil lawsuit falls under tort law with the exception of contractual disputes that fall under contract law—discussed later in this chapter. Tort law is primarily based on common law (case law) but sometimes is derived from noncriminal statutory violations and civil rights violations as described in Table 1-1. For example, see *D'Amico v. LA Fitness*, spotlight case in Chapter 5, in which the plaintiff claimed her injury was, in part, due to the fitness facility's false advertising of the credentials of their fitness personnel. In this case, it was a violation of the Connecticut Unfair Trade Practices Act. The court agreed with the plaintiff.

THE FAULT BASIS OF TORT LIABILITY

All tort claims are not the same. As shown in Figure 1-5, there are three levels or categories of fault under tort liability—intentional, negligence, and strict liability. Each of these are described.

Figure 1-5: Fault Basis of Tort Liability

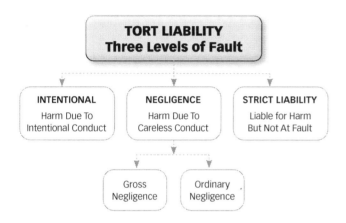

Intentional Torts

If an individual acts with the intent to cause harm or acts knowingly that his/her conduct is substantially certain to cause harm, it would be considered an **intentional tort** (15). Many criminal acts are also considered intentional torts because they are committed with the intent to cause harm. For example, there are several cases described in this textbook involving sexual assault. Victims of sexual assault can sue the wrongdoer in civil court for a *private wrong*—an intentional tort. In intentional tort cases, plaintiffs can receive monetary damages as they do in other civil cases. Victims of sexual assault can also file criminal charges (e.g., file a report with the local police department) against the wrongdoer. Then, the government may prosecute the wrongdoer in criminal court for his/her criminal act—a *public wrong* to society (1). There are various types of intentional torts. Some of these are briefly summarized in Table 1-3.

Table 1-3	Examples of Intentional Torts
INTENTIONAL TORT	**BRIEF DESCRIPTION**
Battery	Intentional bodily contact to cause harm or offensive touching against an individual's will or wishes; Contact does not have to result in a physical injury (1, 15).
Assault	Intentional act to cause harmful or offensive contact (e.g., battery) or imminent apprehension of such contact; Threatening behavior; No contact is involved (1, 15).
False Imprisonment	Intentional confinement of an individual against his/her will; Confinement can be a physical barrier, physical force, and/or threat of physical force (1).
Emotional Harm	Intentional infliction of emotional harm; Extreme and outrageous conduct that intentionally or recklessly causes severe emotional harm to another (15).
Invasion of Privacy	Intentional act that is an unjustified exploitation of one's personal activity, personality, or name/likeness; Unreasonable intrusion on the privacy of another (1, 2).
Defamation	Intentional act that injures another person's good reputation through false and harmful statements made to another; Such statements can be made orally (slander) or in writing (libel) (2).

Case Examples—Invasion of Privacy and Defamation

Invasion of Privacy. Given the increased use of technology such as cell phone/mobile device cameras and small easy-to-hide cameras, there has been an apparent increase in allegations/criminal arrests/convictions and civil liability involving privacy violations. In 2019, the Athletic Business E-Newsletter published several articles describing fitness facility employees or participants who committed privacy violations. Three of these articles are listed in Chapter 10, but the following is a list of additional, similar articles published in this newsletter:

◆ Club Employee Arrested for Photographing Women, March 2019 (16)

(Club Fitness employee posted 175 cell phone photos of women in various stages of undress at the Club)

◗ Ex-Gym Owner Sentenced in Hidden Camera Case, April 2019 (17)
(Gym owner of a Michigan CrossFit location filmed 13 adults and one juvenile with a hidden camera)

◗ Ex-Planet Fitness Staffer Sentenced for Filming Women, May 2019 (18)
(Employee at Planet Fitness, using a cell phone, filmed five women while they were in tanning beds at the facility)

In addition to the intentional tort of invasion of privacy, fitness managers and exercise professionals need to be aware of federal and state privacy laws. These laws are described in Chapter 3 as well as in the spotlight case, *Cormier v. PF Fitness-Midland, LLC*, involving a transgender locker room issue. The plaintiff, Yvette Cormier, sued Planet Fitness in Michigan state court for invasion of privacy, sexual harassment and retaliation in violation of Michigan law, breach of contract, intentional infliction of emotional distress and violation of the Michigan Consumer Protection Act (MCPA). The Michigan Supreme Court stated that the plaintiff's MCPA rights may have been violated when Planet Fitness failed to inform her of its policy that men, who self-identify as women, were allowed to use the women's locker room and restrooms.

Defamation. Steven Hammond, a lawyer and former partner of a law firm, filed a $10 million defamation suit against Equinox and one of its employees, Michael Alexander, in May 2019 (19). In Hammond's complaint, he alleged that a hyper-sexualized Equinox campaign emboldened Alexander to make a false misconduct allegation against him (lewd conduct in the facility's steam room). Hammond alleged that Alexander had been threatened with termination and that he "maliciously fabricated his defamatory allegation" to enhance his bargaining position with Equinox. The charges of lewd conduct in 2018 generated local headlines. However, prosecutors dropped the case after finding some credibility issues. In his complaint, Hammond claims he suffered "immense financial and emotional harm as well as irreparable public embarrassment" after the allegations became public. His lawsuit claims defamation, negligence, breach of contract, negligent hiring and supervision, and infliction of emotional distress. This lawsuit was pending at the time this chapter was written.

Fitness managers/owners need to establish policies and procedures that address privacy and defamation issues. Training all employees regarding these policies and procedures is essential. Staff training is discussed in Chapters 2 and 5. In addition, as described in Chapter 10, fitness participants need to be informed of the facility's policies such as use of cell phones. Marketing strategies need to portray professional messages and images. In Hammond's complaint, as an example of the hyper-sexualized marketing, he alleged that Equinox had an ad campaign—Equinox Made Me Do It—that featured people "in various stages of undress…" that could be interpreted as inappropriate sexual activity.

Negligence

Fitness managers and exercise professionals need to realize that negligence lawsuits are the most common type of lawsuit they may face. The vast majority of cases described in this textbook involve negligence. Therefore, it is essential that fitness managers and exercise professionals acquire a good understanding of negligence and how to help prevent these types of claims and lawsuits. An entire chapter in this textbook (Chapter 4) is devoted to this topic. The following focuses on the elements of negligence and defenses that fitness managers and exercise professionals have to help refute negligence claims.

Negligence is not intentional conduct but is unintentional or *careless conduct* that causes harm as shown in Figure 1-4. It can be defined as failing to do something that a reasonable prudent person would have done (omission) or doing something that a reasonable prudent person would not have done (commission) given the same or similar circumstances (20) as shown in Figure 1-6. The negligence lawsuits described in this textbook provide many examples of claims of *omission* such as the failure to conduct pre-activity health screening, failure to maintain exercise equipment, and *commission* such as improper instruction or improper emergency care.

As depicted in Figure 1-5, there are two categories of negligence—ordinary and gross. Ordinary negligence is "careless" conduct but **gross negligence** goes beyond careless and is often referred to as reckless or willful/wanton conduct in which there is a conscious

Figure 1-6: Negligent Conduct: Omission and Commission*

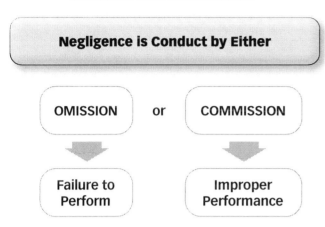

Negligence is Conduct by Either

OMISSION   or   COMMISSION

Failure to Perform   Improper Performance

disregard of a legal duty and the consequences of such disregard toward another. The *Restatement of the Law Third, Torts* states that reckless conduct occurs when "(a) the person knows of the risk of harm created by the conduct or knows facts that make the risk obvious to another in the person's situation, and (b) the precaution that would eliminate or reduce the risk involves burdens that are so slight relative to the magnitude of the risk…" (15, p. 13). Often, plaintiffs make both ordinary and gross negligence claims against the defendant(s) in their complaint. Sometimes, plaintiffs can prove the defendant(s) was grossly negligent.

There are several cases described in this textbook in which the court found the defendant(s) grossly negligent. Courts often refer to gross negligence as the defendant's failure to exercise even slight care/diligence or an extreme departure from the standard of care. For example, in *Bartlett v. Push to Walk* (21), spotlight case in Chapter 7, the court found the defendant (exercise professional) grossly negligent for improper instruction that caused the plaintiff's injury. The court referred to gross negligence as "a person's conduct where an act or failure to act creates an unreasonable risk of harm to another person because of the person's failure to exercise slight care or diligence" (p. 9). Courts often use the terms gross negligence and reckless conduct interchangeably. However, some courts may distinguish

gross negligence from reckless conduct as did the court in *Bartlett*. The court in this jurisdiction (New Jersey) provided the following distinctions:

> …*negligence is the failure to exercise ordinary or reasonable care that leads to a natural and probable injury, gross negligence is the failure to exercise slight care or diligence. Although gross negligence is something more than inattention or mistaken judgment, it does not require willful or wanton misconduct or recklessness (p. 8).*

After its analysis, the court indicated that the defendant's conduct was not reckless or willful/wanton, but it was considered gross negligence.

In *Jimenez v. 24 Hour Fitness* (22), spotlight case in Chapter 9, the appellate court ruled that 24 Hour Fitness was grossly negligent because they did not provide a six-foot safety zone behind the treadmill—a standard practice in the industry. The court stated that their "failure to provide the *minimum* safety zone was an extreme departure from the ordinary standard of conduct…" (p. 237). The court stated, "24 Hour knew it was violating the manufacturer's express safety directions when it deliberately arranged the gym equipment without providing a six-foot safety zone for the treadmills…" (p. 238). Generally, if a defendant knows (has actual or constructive knowledge) or should have known, of a situation that caused, or could cause, an injury and then chooses not to correct it, it could be considered gross negligence, willful/wanton, or reckless conduct. For example, if managers/exercise professionals know that injuries have occurred due to slip and falls in the locker/shower areas, they need to take precautions to help minimize/reduce these injuries from occurring in the future. Documenting that such precautions were taken may help refute any future ordinary and gross negligence claims that might occur.

Elements of Negligence

In a negligence lawsuit, the plaintiff has the burden of proof. This means that the plaintiff must show four essential elements—duty, breach of duty, causation, and harm/damages—in order for a defendant to be liable for negligence. See Figure 1-7. In addition, the standard of proof for the plaintiff is the preponderance of the evidence, meaning that it was more likely than not (51% or greater) that the defendant's conduct caused the harm.

Figure 1-7: Four Essential Elements of Negligence

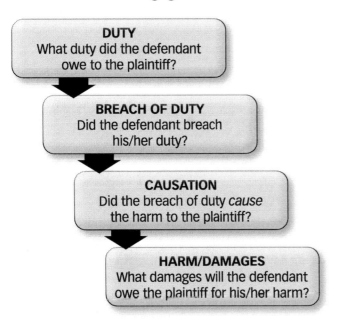

DUTY
What duty did the defendant owe to the plaintiff?

BREACH OF DUTY
Did the defendant breach his/her duty?

CAUSATION
Did the breach of duty *cause* the harm to the plaintiff?

HARM/DAMAGES
What damages will the defendant owe the plaintiff for his/her harm?

Duty

Courts determine duty—not attorneys, juries, plaintiffs, or defendants. Betty van der Smissen (23) states that duty is formed from three primary origins: (a) inherent in the situation, (b) voluntary assumption, and (c) mandated by statute. Each of these is described in Chapter 4. As demonstrated in many of the negligence lawsuits presented in this textbook, courts examine the relationships that are formed such as those inherent in the situation. Examples of these relationships include fitness managers and the members they serve, personal fitness trainers and their clients, group exercise leaders and their class participants, health/wellness coaches and their clients, strength and conditioning coaches and their athletes, and clinical exercise physiologists and their patients in a cardiac rehabilitation program.

Because of these naturally-formed relationships, fitness managers and exercise professionals have a **duty** to provide *reasonably safe* programs and facilities for their participants. "Reasonably safe" means

taking precautions (i.e., developing and implementing risk management strategies) to help prevent *foreseeable* risks of injuries. Many of the plaintiffs' injuries in the cases described in this textbook occurred because fitness managers/exercise professionals did not take necessary precautions to prevent foreseeable risks of injuries. Consequently, plaintiffs experienced all types of injures such as fractures, herniated discs, exertional rhabdomyolysis, stroke, heart attack, and even death. Many of these injuries and subsequent lawsuits could have been prevented if the defendants had not breached their duties. Generally, if the risk of injury is not foreseeable, the defendant does not have a duty (1).

Breach of Duty

A **breach of duty** is an act (i.e., the behavior or conduct that reflects negligent omission or commission, that caused the harm to the plaintiff). The complaint filed by the plaintiff often includes a list of negligent claims, which are, in essence, a list of the alleged breach of duties committed by the defendant(s) that caused the injury to the plaintiff. In determining if the defendant breached any duties, the court decides if a certain **standard of care** was met. The reasonable person standard of care and the standard of care of a professional are discussed in Chapter 4. The professional standard is applicable to fitness managers and exercise professionals. For example, the question for the court is, did the exercise professional (defendant) act like a prudent exercise professional, given the circumstances. In other words, the standard of care describes the level of care that an exercise professional owed to a plaintiff to help protect the plaintiff from harm.

Standards of care can be set by law (statutory, administrative, and case law) but also by standards of practice published by independent and professional organizations, often referred to as best practices. Examples of these published standards of practice are described in Chapters 4 through 11. Often, expert witnesses, in their testimony, refer to published standards of practice that are applicable to the case to help provide evidence of duty. These published standards of practice can be relevant factors to help the court determine if a breach of duty occurred. See Figure 1-8.

Figure 1-8: Potential Legal Impact of Published Standards of Practice

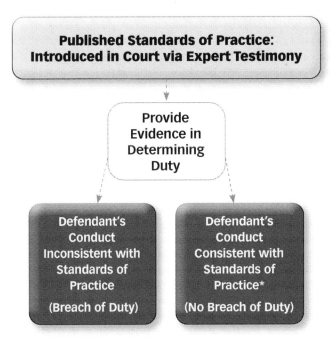

*Even if the exercise professional's conduct is consistent with published standards of practice, it does not necessarily mean the professional did not breach a duty. Courts also consider other factors regarding duty or the standard of care as described in Chapter 4.

Courts also consider other factors, as described in Chapter 4, to determine if there was a breach of duty or the standard of care. However, to help minimize legal liability, it is essential that fitness managers and exercise professionals are aware of, understand, and follow published standards of practice.

The Connection Between the Lack of Practical Skills and Breach of Duties. This connection is described in Chapter 5. As demonstrated in most of the negligence cases in this textbook, the defendants (e.g., exercise professionals such as personal fitness trainers, group exercise leaders, strength and conditioning coaches), did not appear to have the necessary practical skills to train/teach/coach in a reasonably safe manner. If they had possessed these skills, the injuries to the plaintiffs and subsequent litigations would, likely, not have occurred. Too often, these important "practical" skills are not addressed in the exercise profession as they are in almost all other professions and vocations. For example, to become a certified personal fitness trainer or fitness

instructor, passing a written examination is often the only requirement. There is no requirement to obtain practical skills nor demonstrate assessment of practical skills. In addition, academic programs in exercise science may fall short in providing coursework that helps students acquire practical skills in training/teaching/coaching. For more information regarding credentials and competence of exercise professionals, see Chapter 5.

Causation

Causation, or factual cause, is an important element in proving negligence. It is essential that the negligent conduct was the *substantial cause* of the injury. Sometimes, negligence lawsuits are filed when the injury was not due to a negligent act of the defendant (e.g., the injury was due to risks inherent in the activity). Generally, courts do not allow for legal remedies when an injury is due to these types of risks. This topic is covered in more detail in Chapter 4. Lawsuits filed, in which there is no legal remedy, may be classified by some as frivolous. However, certain factors are required if an attorney's conduct is considered frivolous. See *Jafri v. Equinox Holdings* in Chapter 9.

In determining causation, the "but for" standard is used, which states "an act is a factual cause of an outcome if, in the absence of the act, the outcome would not have occurred" (15, p. 116). Many of the negligent cases in this textbook involve exercise professionals who have prescribed a contraindicated exercise such as an unsafe exercise or an exercise program that was too intense, given the individual's health/fitness status. The "but for" test is pretty straight forward in these cases (i.e., if the contraindicated exercise had not been prescribed, the injury would not have happened). When the "but for" test is not applicable, courts will use the "substantial factor" test. "If the negligence act was a substantial factor in causing the injury, then the requirement of causation is satisfied" (1, p. 33).

Courts will use terms such as **actual cause** (or cause in fact) and **proximate cause**. Actual cause is determined by the "but for" test (2). Proximate cause is "that which, in a natural and continuous sequence, unbroken by any efficient intervening cause, produces injury, and without which the result would not have occurred" (7, p. 852). In other words, the injury to the plaintiff must be reasonably related to the negligent act of the defendant (2).

Harm/Damages

The plaintiff must prove that he/she suffered a legally recognized harm to receive monetary damages. The harm can be physical injury and/or emotional injury as well as damage to the plaintiff's property. Examples of the **damages** awarded to plaintiffs for their physical and emotional injuries are described in several of the cases in this textbook as well as cases involving damages awarded to the victim's family for **wrongful death.** Wrongful death lawsuits due to the negligence or gross negligence of the defendant(s) include *Miller v. The YMCA of Central Massachusetts, et al.* and *Angelo v. USA Triathlon* in Chapter 10 and *Locke v. Life Time Fitness, Inc.* in Chapter 11.

There are various types of damages. **Compensatory damages** are actual damages (i.e., money awarded to the plaintiff for a real loss or injury). Compensatory damages may include two types: (a) special or economic, and (b) general or non-economic (2) as shown in Table 1-4. **Punitive damages**, also shown in Table 4-1, are damages awarded to the plaintiff in addition to compensatory damages.

Table 1-4	Types of Monetary Damages (1, 2)
TYPE	**DESCRIPTION**
Special Damages (Economic damages)	Damages that include past, present, and future medical expenses and lost wages, and the repair or replacement of property.
General Damages (Non-economic damages)	Damages that include pain and suffering, loss of consortium, emotional distress, and, in defamation cases, loss of reputation.
Punitive Damages (Exemplary damages)	Damages that are awarded, in addition to special and general damages, to punish the wrongdoer for gross negligence, reckless, or willful/wanton conduct.

Several negligence cases, described in this textbook, have included special, general, and punitive damages awarded to the plaintiffs such as:

- *Assaf Blecher v. 24 Hour Fitness Inc. and David Stevens* (Chapter 9)—the plaintiff was awarded $892,650 in damages ($142,650 for medical expenses and $750,000 for pain and suffering).
- *Waller v. Blast Fitness Group* (Chapter 3)—the plaintiff requested a judgment totaling more than $2.5 million including (a) economic damages of $28,435, (b) compensatory damages for pain and suffering of approximately $1 million, (c) punitive damages of $1.5 million, (d) $94,728 in attorney's fees, and (d) $2,338 in court costs. The court granted Waller's request for economic damages but significantly reduced the compensatory and punitive damages.

In some cases, the plaintiffs have been awarded damages for future expenses. For example, the jury in *Lee v. Louisiana Board of Trustees for State Colleges* (24), described in Chapter 8, awarded the plaintiff (a collegiate athlete) $2,529,229 in damages as follows:

1. Past and future physical pain and suffering $200,000
2. Past and future mental pain and suffering $1,000,000
3. Past medical expenses. $15,229
4. Future medical expenses $24,000
5. Past lost wages $90,000
6. Loss of earning capacity $600,000
7. Loss of enjoyment of life $600,000

The damages in the *Lee* case were reduced to $659,227 based on sovereign immunity.

Plaintiffs have also requested damages for claims such as "negligent infliction of emotional distress" (see *Angleo v. USA Triathlon* in Chapter 10) and **loss of consortium.** *Note:* Negligent infliction of emotional distress is different that "intentional" infliction of emotional distress. As stated above, "intentional" requires extreme and outrageous conduct that intentionally or recklessly causes severe emotional harm. Loss of

> ### KEY POINT
>
> Negligence lawsuits are the most common type of lawsuit that fitness managers and exercise professionals may face. The vast majority of cases described in this textbook involve negligence. Therefore, it is essential that fitness managers and exercise professionals acquire a good understanding of negligence and how to prevent these types of claims and lawsuits. An entire chapter in this textbook (Chapter 4) is devoted to this topic.

consortium refers to a loss of (or interference with) a relationship such as a spouse, parent, or child and is often a claim when there is a wrongful death or serious injury. For example, plaintiffs in the following cases made loss of consortium claims: (a) *Chavez v. 24 Hour Fitness* in Chapter 9—the husband (plaintiff) whose wife was seriously injured, and (b) *Zihlman v. Wichita Falls YMCA* in Chapter 11—the children (plaintiffs) whose mother died.

Defenses Against Negligence Claims—Legally Effective

The best defense defendants have against negligence is not to breach their legal duties. If duties are carried out properly, the likelihood of an injury is minimized. If there is no injury, then there is no lawsuit. However, if a participant is injured and files a lawsuit, he/she needs to prove that the injury was due to the defendant's breach of duty. If the defendant(s) can show (e.g., has documented evidence that no breach of duty was committed), it will be very difficult for the plaintiff to prevail or produce a **prima facie case** against the defendant, despite the injury. Remember, all four essential elements are needed to prove negligence.

As demonstrated in cases described in this textbook, defendants have effectively used various types of defenses to counter claims of negligence. Therefore, they were either not held liable for the plaintiff's injury or were held only partially liable for damages. These defenses include contributory and comparative negligence, assumption of risk, procedural defenses, immunity defenses, and defenses based on contract law.

Contributory and Comparative Negligence

Plaintiffs are sometimes injured due to their own fault, such as misusing exercise equipment. In cases like this, defendants have defenses such as **contributory negligence** and **comparative negligence.** States apply certain systems for allocating fault and damages such as (a) pure contributory negligence, (b) pure comparative fault, and (c) modified comparative fault (25). The pure contributory negligence defense does not allow a plaintiff to recover any damages if he/she was even 1% at fault and the defendant was 99% at fault. Because this is a harsh rule, only a minority of states (Alabama, Maryland, North Carolina, and Virginia) have adopted it. Most states have adopted one of the comparative fault systems. With the pure comparative fault defense system, the damages are based on proportionate shares of fault. For example, in the *Baldi-Perry v. Kaifas and 360 Fitness Center* case, described in Chapter 2, the jury returned a verdict of $1.4 million. However, the verdict was reduced to $980,000 due to the jury's finding that the plaintiff was 30% at fault. This case occurred in New York which has the pure comparative rule. If the jury had found the plaintiff 70% at fault, she would have received $420,000 in damages.

In the modified comparative fault system, the damages are still proportioned based on percentages of fault of each party except when the plaintiff's negligence reaches a certain designated percentage, 50% or 51% (25). At that percentage bar, the plaintiff cannot recover any damages. Ten states follow the 50% bar rule and 23 states follow the 51% bar rule (25). In *Vaid v. Equinox*, spotlight case in Chapter 8, the jury returned a verdict of $14,500,000. However, it was reduced to $10,875,000 based on a finding that the plaintiff was 25% at fault. This case occurred in Connecticut which has a modified comparative fault system using the 51% bar rule. Therefore, if the plaintiff had been 51% or more at fault, he would not have recovered any damages. Comparative negligence (and contributory negligence) can be very effective defenses. However, as described in Chapter 11, obtaining evidence (e.g., interviewing witnesses, completing an injury report) immediately following an injury and retaining such evidence is key to strengthening this defense.

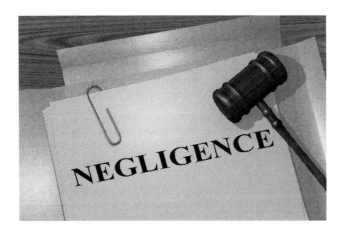

Assumption of Risk

Assumption of risk is a legal doctrine in which a plaintiff cannot recover damages for a personal injury or wrongful death action. When applying this defense, "the defendant claims that no duty whatsoever was owed to the injured party" (1, p. 64), meaning no duty existed to protect the plaintiff from injuries due to risks inherent in the activity. To be an effective defense, the plaintiff must (a) possess full understanding of the risks inherent in the activity, and (b) voluntarily agree to participate in the activity (1). This doctrine is frequently used successfully in sport/recreation activities and in high-risk activities such as race car driving and parachute jumping (1). However, it has also been successfully used when injuries have occurred from participation in exercise activities, but not always. Because this is a common defense used by defendants in exercise injury cases, it is described in more detail in Chapter 4, along with several case examples where this defense was both effective and ineffective in protecting defendants.

Procedural Defenses

As described above, there are several procedural rules that need to be followed in any litigation. If a party does not follow the procedural rules, the court is not obligated to provide any legal remedy to that party. For example, in a negligent lawsuit, the complaint must be filed within a certain amount time as specified in the statute of limitations (2). As previously described in *D'Amico v. LA Fitness*, spotlight case in Chapter 5, the first two counts in the complaint that dealt with

negligent claims were not filed within the state's statute of limitation. Therefore, the court granted the defendant's motion for summary judgment for these two counts.

The statute of limitations for civil lawsuits varies among the states. As stated earlier, it is two to three years in most states (10). Sometimes, the date in which the statute of limitations begin is an issue for the court to decide. Generally, it is from the date the injury occurred or from the date when the injury (cause of action) was discovered. In *D'Amico v. LA Fitness* (26), the plaintiff testified that she sought medical attention four days after the incident on January 25, 2010. The court stated that "the plaintiff knew or should have known that the incident which caused the injuries gave rise to this action occurred on January 25, 2010. The statute of limitations therefore began to run on that date and her action was not timely commenced" (26, p. 4).

Criminal statutes of limitations that provide time limits for when criminal charges must be filed also vary by state (27). Certain crimes have no statute of limitations. For example, murder typically has none and sexual crimes against minors have none in many states (27). There are also federal statutes of limitations for federal crimes (28).

Immunity Defenses

Immunity is an exemption or protection against civil liability under certain circumstances (29). It is used to bar liability claims against governmental entities. However, since the passing of certain federal and state tort claims legislation (e.g., the Federal Torts Claim Act of 1976), injured parties have been able to sue governmental entities under certain circumstances (1, 29). Although there are some distinctions between **sovereign immunity** and **governmental immunity**, they are often used interchangeably (29) when referring to federal, state or local governments. Several cases described in Chapter 8 involve negligence lawsuits against government entities—*Lee, UCF Athletics, Martin, and Hajducek.*

The damages in *Lee v. Louisiana Board of Trustees for State Colleges* were previously described. In this case, and in *UCF Athletics Association v. Plancher*, the damages awarded to the plaintiffs were based on state immunity statutes for state agencies, such as public universities, that limit (e.g., put a cap on) damages, often referred to as limited immunity. These types of state statutes protect the taxpayers in the state. See also *Martin v. Moreau* and *Hajdusek v. United States*. In *Martin*, sovereign immunity did not protect the government from liability but in *Hajdusek* it did.

Another type of immunity applies to volunteers. The federal Volunteer Protection Act (30) provides liability protection for volunteers. The major purpose of this liability protection is to encourage individuals to volunteer their services in nonprofit and government entities. This law provides liability protection only for the volunteer, not for the nonprofit or government entity. For more on the Volunteer Protection Act, see Chapter 5. A minority of states have *charitable immunity* statutes, in which a charitable organization may also have some liability protection. For example, liability is limited by capping the amount that may be awarded, but most states have abolished charitable immunity (31).

Defenses Based on Contract Law

Contracts commonly used by fitness managers and exercise professionals include membership contracts, waivers, and independent contractor contracts. These contracts can provide an effective defense for defendants in negligence cases. Waivers, although technically not a defense (as described in Chapter 4), will be referred to as a defense in this textbook. If enforceable, they absolve the defendant(s) of any "ordinary" negligence. However, they need to be properly written and administered to be enforceable. As stated earlier, some states prohibit the enforceability of waivers based on court rulings or state statutes. More information on waivers is discussed in Chapter 4.

Fitness managers often hire independent contractors for all types of positions such as personal fitness trainers, group exercise leaders and health/wellness coaches. Generally, if a participant is injured due to the negligence of the independent contractor, the liability is shifted from the fitness manager/owner to the independent contractor (1), however, not always. See *Layden v. Plante*, spotlight case in Chapter 7. In order for this defense to be effective, fitness managers/owners need to follow certain regulations such as those established by the Internal Revenue Service (IRS) and be aware of other legal issues when hiring, training, and supervising independent contractors. These regulations and legal issues are described in Chapter 5.

Defenses Against Negligence Claims—Legally Ineffective

Fitness managers and exercise professionals may have reasons they believe are legitimate that will help protect them from liability. However, many of these reasons will not be considered effective defenses in a court of law because they are not legitimate reasons for not following the standard of care. Remember, courts determine duty (or the standard of care) that the defendant owed to the plaintiff. The following are examples of these legally ineffective defenses with a short description. The reference to "it" in the following examples refers to various risk management strategies that reflect the standard of care.

- *Financial Costs*
  "It costs too much"—fitness managers and exercise professionals should not enter into the profession or offer certain services if they do not have the budget to develop and implement proper risk management strategies that reflect the standards of care.

- *Staff Time*
  "It takes too much staff time"—fitness managers and exercise professionals have many responsibilities but ample time needs to be devoted to risk management strategies to help ensure a reasonably safe environment of participants—their #1 legal duty.

- *Misunderstanding of the Law*
  "I did not know the law required that"—fitness managers and exercise professionals need to have adequate legal knowledge in order to have the confidence that they are properly carrying out their legal duties and to, intelligently, discuss such duties with their legal counsel— this is the main purpose of this textbook. Ignorance of the law is not a legal defense.

⬧ *Burden or Barrier for Fitness Participants*
"Our participants do not want to be bothered with …"—fitness managers and exercise professionals need to explain the purposes of important safety procedures/services such as pre-activity health screening and facility orientation. Once new participants understand the purposes, they will likely be more willing to participate and will not perceive certain procedures/services as a burden or barrier.

⬧ *No Need to Inform of Risks*
"Informing participants of risks will scare them"—fitness managers and exercise professionals should inform participants of the risks of injury (minor, major, and life-threatening) and death. The failure to inform of risks is a common negligence claim. Interestingly, a witness for the defense in the *Bursik* case (described in Chapter 9) who had oversight of approximately 185 personal fitness trainers said he would not warn participants of the risk of stroke with heavy resistance training because it would scare them and keep them from exercising.

⬧ *Customary Practice*
"That's how we do things here" or "That's how other professionals or facilities do things"—fitness managers and exercise professionals need to understand that customary practices may not reflect the standard of care and, therefore, will not be an effective defense.

⬧ *Misunderstanding of Credentials*
"My certification lapsed so I no longer have to follow the safety practices of my certifying organization"—in *Baldi-Perry v. Kaifus and 360 Fitness Center, Inc.* (described in Chapter 2), the defendant trainer testified that he did not obtain medical clearance as recommended by the National Strength and Conditioning Association (NSCA). He believed that, because he did not keep his NSCA certification current, he no longer had to follow the NSCA

recommendations. Fitness managers and exercise professionals need to be sure their employees keep their certifications current. However, courts will consider the "conduct" (actions/inactions) of the employee more so than his/her credentials to determine if there was a breach of duty.

⬧ *Poor Advice From Legal Counsel*
"Our legal counsel told us not to do that"—fitness managers and exercise professionals sometimes receive poor advice from their legal counsel. See national pre-activity screening study, described in Chapter 6, in which some American College of Sports Medicine (ACSM) certified exercise professionals indicated that their facility did not conduct screening procedures based on legal counsel advice. If following or relying on any legal advice leads to the facility being liable for injuries, the facility could then file a legal malpractice lawsuit against the lawyer/law firm.

Strict Liability

Intentional torts (intentional conduct) and negligence (careless conduct) are based on fault. However, **strict liability** is not based on the concept of fault but rather on *public policy*—meaning that the law requires certain business to compensate individuals who are injured by their products, services, or activities (1, 2). In these situations, the plaintiff does not have to prove intent or negligence—the defendant is liable even when not at fault. For example, businesses that engage in ultrahazardous activities (e.g., explosives, dangerous chemicals, keeps dangerous animals, operates a nuclear reactor) in which the risk of injury to the general public is very high, would likely always be liable for the harm they caused (2). Areas of strict liability applicable to the exercise profession are (a) product liability, (b) vicarious liability, and (c) workers' compensation.

Product Liability

Product liability only arises if an injured party can prove that his/her injury was due to a defective product, such as a defect in a piece of exercise equipment. The *Restatement of the Law Third, Torts* (15) describes three types of defects: (a) manufacturing defect, (b) design defect, and (c) marketing defect. Fitness managers/owners are not liable for exercise equipment defects as demonstrated in *Grebing v. 24 Hour Fitness*, spotlight case described in Chapter 9. As stated by this appellate court, fitness facilities are not in the business of designing, manufacturing, distributing, or selling exercise equipment and, therefore, are not subject to strict product liability. Plaintiffs should file their negligent claims regarding exercise equipment defects against the manufacturer, not the fitness facility.

Product liability not only applies to manufacturers but can also apply to distributors and sellers of exercise equipment even though they had nothing to do with the making of the product. Product liability law is based on state law (32). For example, some states have innocent seller statutes that can protect distributors and sellers from a plaintiff's product liability claims. It is important to realize that product liability not only applies to the person who purchased the product, but also to one who uses the product, or a bystander injured by the product (1).

In a product liability claim involving a piece of exercise equipment, the plaintiff needs to prove that the exercise equipment was defective and that the defect was the cause of his/her injury. For example, in *Thomas v. Sport City*, spotlight case in Chapter 10, the plaintiff was unsuccessful in proving that his injury, while using a hack squat machine, was caused by a design defect. Plaintiffs need to show that they were using the product in a foreseeable manner, but not necessarily in the *intended* manner as demonstrated in *Barnhard v. Cybex International*, described in Chapter 9. Cybex claimed that Barhard was injured as a result of her misuse of the machine. However, the court stated that although the plaintiff was not using the machine for its intended purpose, the use of the machine for stretching was common and thus *foreseeable.* In this case, Cybex was liable for both a design defect and a marketing defect (failed to warn purchasers and users of the machine's potential tipping hazard). More information on product liability is covered in Chapter 10 including additional cases and examples of manufacturer exercise equipment recall cases.

Workers' Compensation

This form of strict liability is imposed on employers without fault (1). If an employee is injured while on the job, state **workers' compensation** statutes are applied—not negligence. These statutes ensure that employees receive payment for their medical expenses and a portion of lost wages, regardless of who is at fault. Although this compensation might not be as much as the damages that an employee might be awarded in a negligence lawsuit, it provides the employee some compensation without having to file a negligence lawsuit, not to mention the risk of losing the lawsuit and receiving no monetary damages. In addition, workers' compensation is an efficient system to provide prompt relief to the injured employee. These statutes also provide protection for employers by precluding the employee from bringing a tort lawsuit (e.g., negligence) against the employer (33). This protection saves the employer a great deal of time and costs associated with negligence lawsuits. In addition, these statutes motivate employers to make workplaces safer. The Federal Employment Compensation Act provides similar workers' compensation benefits for federal employees (33). More information on workers' compensation, including case law examples, is described below under Employment Law.

Vicarious Liability

Respondeat superior is a common law doctrine that imposes **vicarious liability** upon an employer for injuries to third parties caused by the negligent acts of its employees while performing tasks within their scope of employment (2). This doctrine is similar to strict liability in tort because the employer is not at fault but can be held liable for harm. As demonstrated in many of negligence cases in this textbook, the third party (the injured fitness participant) not only sues the employee (e.g., personal fitness trainer) whose negligent conduct caused the injury but also the employee's employer (e.g., business owner). Many employers were found liable for the harm to the plaintiffs in these cases. It is important to realize that employers would not be liable for employees who commit criminal acts while on the job (except in certain situations), because criminal acts are not within the scope of employment. See Chapter 5 for more on this topic.

The doctrine of respondeat superior is based on three theories (2). First, because the employer has the right to control the acts or services provided by employees, the employer should also be responsible for injuries arising out of those services. Second, because the employer profits from such services provided to third parties, the employer should also suffer the losses. The third is based on the *deep-pocket theory* in which the employer is more likely or able to pay for the losses (damages) than the employee. In other words, the employer has "deep pockets" or more money than the employee (2). For more information on employer vicarious liability as well as another form of employer liability referred to as *direct liability*, see Chapter 5.

CONTRACT LAW

A **contract** is "an agreement that can be enforced in a court" (2, p. 349). In other words, it is legally enforceable, unlike a moral agreement such as promising to take a friend to lunch. Generally, contracts involve two or more parties who exchange binding promises. In a promise, each party declares that they will, or will not, take a specified action in the future (2). A **breach of contract** occurs when one party does not fulfill its promises. Generally, a breach of contract is not a criminal or tortious act. However, in some cases it might be (e.g., if the agreement was corrupted by a tort such as fraud). See *Jimenez v. 24 Hour Fitness*, spotlight case in Chapter 9, in which the waiver the plaintiff signed was administered with fraud and misrepresentation. Often, contracting parties can regard a breach as an alternative performance, especially if the victim of the breach is promptly made whole by payment or some other alternative that offsets the loss suffered (2). If litigation is the only alternative, the court will likely require the breaching party to pay compensatory damages to the victim of the breach or require completion of the specific performance as stated in the contract (1, 2).

Contract law is primarily governed by common law except in cases where it has been modified or replaced by statutory law (34). For example, waiver contracts are based on common law (court opinions) in most states, but some states have statutes that govern waiver law. In addition, specialized statutes exist for certain types of contracts such as insurance policies and employment contracts (1). Contracts that involve the sale and/or purchase or lease of goods are governed by the Uniform Commercial Code (UCC). The UCC has been adopted by all 50 states but there are variations among the states (35). It has the effect of law, but only when it is adopted by the different states.

Types of Contracts

There are various types of contracts. An *express* contract is formed in spoken or written words and an *implied* contract is formed by conduct or body language such as waving to a popcorn vendor in a football stadium and then passing down the money to the vender in exchange for a bag of popcorn (1). For many of the contracts used in the exercise profession, it is best for them to be express, written contracts. The written agreement can provide evidence of the terms of the contract without ambiguity, in case there is any future disputes or litigation related to the contract.

Bilateral contracts are the most common in the exercise profession, such as a membership contract or a personal training contract. Both parties exchange promises that benefit each party. Additional examples are described below in Table 1-6. A *unilateral* contract occurs when one party entices another party to complete some act or task in exchange for something of value (1). For example, a fitness facility may have a membership campaign that entices current members to recruit three new members by a certain date. If they do, they receive a "free" one-year membership. Each member can choose or not choose to participate in the campaign—there is no legal obligation to do so.

Four Elements of a Contract

There are four elements that are required for a contract to be legally formed or a valid contract—agreement, consideration, contractual capacity, and legality. Each of these is briefly described in Table 1-5. Because waiver contracts are widely used in fitness facilities, an example of how each of these elements is applied in the context of a waiver contract is included in Table 1-5. If one of the four elements is missing, it is considered a **voidable contract.** In these cases, either party can withdraw from the contract without liability such as a minor, who freely and intentionally entered into a contract, because a minor lacks legal capacity (1).

A contract is **unenforceable** if it violates a statute or is against public policy. For example, the waiver contracts signed by plaintiffs in several of the waiver cases described in Chapter 4 were unenforceable because they were against public policy or for other reasons. To meet the legality requirement, certain contracts must be in writing under the **Statute of Frauds** such as contracts involving the sale of exercise equipment of $500 or more (2). These statutes may vary by state, but all states require certain contracts to be in writing. They have nothing to do with fraud, as implied by the name. Instead, they deny enforceability to certain contracts that do not comply with the statute's

requirements (34). Valid contracts must be made with genuine assent—meaning the apparent assent of both parties is genuine. If a contract was formed under duress, undue influence, result of fraud, or by a mistake, it may be unenforceable.

Contracts Used in the Exercise Profession

There are a variety of contracts used in the exercise profession. Common ones include membership agreements, waivers, independent contractor contracts, and equipment purchasing/leasing agreements. Note that the term "agreement" is often used interchangeably with the term contract. However, not all agreements are established as legally binding contracts. Agreements that are contracts need to satisfy all four elements as shown in Table 1-5. A list and brief description of contracts used in the exercise profession are provided in Table 1-6 along with the chapter that contains more information about that contract. As stated throughout this textbook, fitness managers and exercise professionals need to have contracts prepared by competent legal counsel to help ensure their enforceability in the applicable jurisdiction.

Table 1-5	Four Elements of a Valid Contract	
CONTRACT ELEMENT	**BRIEF DESCRIPTION ***	**EXAMPLE: WAIVER (RELEASE OF LIABILITY) CONTRACT**
Agreement	One party must *offer* to enter in to a legal agreement and another party must *accept* terms of the offer.	Fitness manager offers a new member a waiver contract to read and sign. The new member accepts the offer agreeing to the terms of the waiver contract.
Consideration	Any promise made by the parties to the contract must be supported by legally sufficient and bargained-for *consideration* (something of value received or promised, such as money to convince a person to make a deal).	The consideration (or value) that the new member receives is access to the facility's programs and services. The value the fitness manager and facility receives is the liability protection of waiver.
Contractual Capacity	Both parties entering into the contract must have contractual capacity to do so; the law must recognize them in possessing characteristics that qualify them for competent parties.	A fitness manager who is under the influence of drugs or alcohol at the time of the contract would not be considered competent. A new member, who is a minor, does not have contractual capacity because of his/her age.
Legality	The contract's purpose must be to accomplish some goal that is legal and not against public policy.	In some states, waivers are against public policy and, thus, are unenforceable.

*West's Business Law (34, p. 199).

Table 1-6	Common Contracts Used in the Exercise Profession	
TYPE OF CONTRACT	**BRIEF DESCRIPTION**	**CHAPTER WITH MORE INFORMATION**
Business Associate Contract	Contract between a HIPAA-covered entity and a vendor (business associate); Data privacy and security rules apply.	3
Waiver	Contract signed by fitness participants; Contains exculpatory language that can absolve exercise professionals and fitness facilities of their own ordinary negligence.	4
Employment Contract	Contract signed by a newly hired or current employee.	5
Independent Contractor Contract	Contract for self-employed individuals hired on a contractual basis (non-employees); IRS regulations apply.	5
Vendor Contract	Contract with a seller of goods or services; All types of fitness/wellness vendors, such as companies that manage in-house fitness facilities in corporate and hospital settings.	5
Internship Contract	Contract between an academic institution and the organization or business providing the student internship program.	3, 5
Informed Consent	Contract used in clinical/medical and research settings as well as prior to fitness testing or participation in an exercise program; Contains no exculpatory language.	6
Equipment Purchase or Lease Agreement	Agreement that specifies the details of a purchase or lease transaction.	9
Exercise Equipment Maintenance Contract	Contract with an exercise equipment manufacturer and/or distributor to provide equipment maintenance services.	9
Membership Contract	Contract that a new member signs when joining or renewing at a fitness facility.	10
Technology Provider Contract	Contract with a third-party vendor who collects biometric data (e.g., athlete performance data via wearable technology).	10
Event Sponsor Contract	Contract between an event organizer and an event sponsor (e.g., a community 5K walk/run).	10
Insurance Contract	Contract specifying the terms of an insurance policy and its coverages.	10
Leasing or Renting Space Agreement	Contract between a fitness facility and a party who leases or rents space in the facility.	10

KEY POINT

As stated throughout this textbook, fitness managers and exercise professionals need to have contracts prepared by competent legal counsel to help ensure enforceability in their jurisdiction (state). Sample contracts found on the Internet or elsewhere, including those provided in this textbook, should never be adopted without individualized legal advice and consultation.

EMPLOYMENT LAW

In addition to tort law and contract law, there are many employment laws that are applicable to fitness facilities and programs. Fitness managers and exercise professionals should become familiar with these laws so they can develop policies and procedures to help ensure compliance with them (e.g., have a sexual harassment policy that all employees need to follow). This section describes employment laws in three areas: (a) federal laws, (b) laws regarding hiring, training, and supervising personnel, and (c) workers' compensation laws.

Employment Laws: Examples of Federal Laws

Chapter 3 covers many federal laws including the federal employment laws described below. It is important to realize that many of these federal laws have similar state laws, such as state discrimination and privacy laws, that may have additional rules and regulations to follow.

- *Discrimination Laws*—laws such as Title VII of the Civil Rights Act that prohibit discrimination based on religion, race/color, national origin, and sex as well as laws that prohibit disability and age discrimination such as the Americans with Disabilities Act (ADA) and the Age Discrimination in Employment Act (ADEA). These discrimination laws not only apply to employees, but some of them also apply to fitness participants. For example, Title I of the ADA covers employees and Title III covers fitness participants.
- *Privacy and Communication Laws*—privacy laws that protect employee data such as the Health Insurance Portability and Accountability Act (HIPAA) may be applicable to certain fitness facilities and/or vendors as well as some employer-sponsored fitness/wellness programs. Communication laws such as the Federal Trade Commission Act (FTCA) govern a fitness facility's advertising and social media posts either directly from the fitness facility or the exercise professional—all must be truthful and non-misleading including the credentials of employees.
- *Employee Wage and Hour Laws*—laws such as the Fair Labor Standards Act (FLSA) that guarantee minimum wage and overtime pay for employees. The FLSA includes regulations regarding student interns and volunteers.
- *Employee Safety Laws*—laws such as the Occupational Safety and Health Act that protect the health and safety of employees. The Occupational Safety and Health Administration (OSHA) has many standards and regulations that employers must follow.

Employment Laws: Hiring, Training, and Supervising Personnel

Employment laws focusing on the hiring, training, and supervision of personnel are covered in Chapter 5. Some of the topics regarding these laws are briefly summarized as follows:

- *Types of Credentials*—Self-regulated credentials (certification, accreditation) and government-regulated credentials (licensure); Credentialing issues such as the connection between lack of practical skills and breach of duties (briefly described above); Future directions regarding credentials of exercise professionals.
- *Employer's Vicarious and Direct Liability*—Vicarious liability is covered in more depth than what is described above; Direct liability can occur when an employer does not properly hire, train, and supervise its employees (see Table 5-5 in Chapter 5 that lists cases involving types of direct liability claims against employers); Employers have a vested interest to hire only credentialed and competent employees to help avoid both vicarious and direct liability.
- *Liability Issues Involving Non-Employees*—Specific liability issues related to independent contractors, vendors, interns, and volunteers; Criteria to consider when contracting with a vendor including indemnification (see Exhibit 5-4 in Chapter 5).
- *Criminal Background Checks*—Liability issues that can arise for failing to conduct criminal background checks; Conducting federal and state background checks; Applicable laws such as Fair Credit Reporting Act (FCRA).
- *Employer Liability for Criminal Acts Committed by Employees such as Sexual Misconduct*—Employer liability (e.g., generally, employers are not liable except in cases where they had prior knowledge or foreseeability of employee criminal misconduct and did not address it properly or covered it up); Cases in athletic settings such as Penn State and Michigan State are described; Title IX regulations for athletic programs.

❧ *Liability Insurance*—The importance of purchasing general liability insurance as well as professional liability insurance for exercise professionals who design/deliver exercise programs; Carefully reviewing any exclusions in the policy; Requiring independent contractors to purchase their own professional liability insurance.

Employment Laws: Workers' Compensation

As described earlier, workers' compensation is a form of strict liability in which no fault is attributed to the employer or the employee. If workers' compensation applies when an employee is injured while on the job (meaning arising out of and in the course of employment), the employee cannot bring a negligence claim/lawsuit against the employer. Therefore, workers' compensation protects the employer from potentially high costs associated with negligence claims/lawsuits. The employee also benefits because he/she receives a fixed compensation for the injury without the inconvenience of filing, and the risk of losing, a negligence lawsuit against his/her employer, or suffering the potential consequences of an employee suing an employer. Workers' compensation is based on state laws that establish the fixed compensation which generally includes only economic damages—medical expenses and a portion of lost wages. Workers' compensation benefits also apply to dependents if an employee dies as a result of a job related injury.

In addition to liability insurance, fitness managers/owners need to purchase workers' compensation insurance which is mandated by state laws that vary depending upon the state. For example, in Georgia, employers with three or more employees are required to purchase workers' compensation insurance to cover both full-time and "regular" part-time employees (36). Fitness managers/owners need to consult with their legal counsel regarding these state laws and the workers' compensation insurance coverage needed to comply with these laws.

Workers' compensation benefits apply to fitness facility employees but also may apply to employees who participate in employer-sponsored fitness programs. The two cases described below involve workers'

compensation claims that occurred in these types of programs. There are certain procedures that are carried out when a workers' compensation claim is disputed. These procedures are established by state law, but most state laws suggest arbitration as the first step in resolving such a dispute (37). The parties voluntarily agree to have an independent arbitrator who makes a decision. However, rarely are these decisions binding (37). An employee can appeal an arbitrator's decision to an administrative body such as a state Workers' Compensation Board, an industrialized commission, or a state court (38) as demonstrated in *Stanner v. Compensation Appeal Board* (39).

In *Stanner*, Anthony Stanner died shortly after a workout in his company's fitness center. His wife filed a claim seeking workers' compensation death benefits. The arbitrator dismissed the case. She appealed to the Pennsylvania Workers' Compensation Board but the Board affirmed the arbitrator's dismissal of the claim. Then, she appealed to the Commonwealth Court of Pennsylvania, a state intermediate court of appeals, which reversed the decision of the Board and awarded her the death benefits. Based on expert witness testimony, the court ruled that the death was work-related, given the company owned and operated the company fitness center and encouraged employees to participate in the program.

Workers' Compensation Cases—Employer-Sponsored Fitness Programs

Fitness managers and exercise professionals, who work in employer-sponsored fitness facilities and programs, need to be aware of how worker's compensation laws might apply. In addition, companies that offer recreational activities (e.g., sport leagues or teams) may be subject to specific state worker's compensation statutes such as (a) employer-sponsored teams and exertional activities encouraged by employer—statute in Pennsylvania, and (b) off-duty athletic activity—statute in New York (5). The following two cases describe factors that courts consider when deciding workers' compensation claims.

Editorial Note: *The content describing the following two cases reflects content from Chapter 13 in Risk Management for Health/Fitness Professionals: Legal Issues and Strategies (1). The publisher transferred the rights to this* *textbook to the authors in 2017. Permission to reprint and revise/update this content was granted by the author of Chapter 13.*

Case #1—Price v. Industrial Claim Appeals Office (40)

In this case, the Colorado Supreme Court established the following five factors after analyzing two applicable appellate court cases (41, 42) dealing with employer-sponsored fitness programs. If any one of these factors is present, the injury would be compensable under workers' compensation.

1. whether injury occurred during working hours;
2. whether injury occurred on employer's premises;
3. whether employer initiated employee's exercise program;
4. whether employer exerted any control or direction over employee's exercise program; and
5. whether employer stood to benefit from employee's exercise program (40, pp. 210-211).

In its analysis of both appellate court cases, the Colorado Supreme Court ruled that the employers in these cases did not have sufficient control of the exercise programs and, therefore, the injuries were not compensable under workers' compensation. In both cases, the employees were exercising at off-premise locations.

The plaintiff in *Price v. Industrial Claim Appeals Office* (41), a prison guard at the Colorado Department of Corrections, was injured while exercising at home. He claimed his supervisor informed him that in order to retain his job, he had to lose some weight and, therefore, sought compensation via workers' compensation. The plaintiff in *City of Northglenn v. Eltrich* (42), a police officer, suffered injuries while riding her bicycle in the vicinity of her home. She claimed that she feared losing her job if she could not pass a cardiovascular fitness test and, therefore, began riding her bike during off-duty hours. All police officers were required to pass a battery of fitness tests to demonstrate maintenance of certain physical fitness levels. The Supreme Court concluded that in both cases, the injuries were not compensable under workers' compensation because they did not "arise out of" or were not "in the course of" employment—Factors 1 and 2 above. The court gave greater weight to these

KEY POINT

With more employees working at home, factors such as Factors 1 and 2 in *Price* are relevant. For example, in *Estate of Gregory Sullwold v. Salvation Army* (43), Sullwold was allowed to work at home. One day he took a break at 3:30 to walk on his treadmill. His wife found him unconscious about 30 minutes later. He did not survive. She filed a petition for workers' compensation death benefits claiming that her husband's work-related stress caused his cardiac arrest that led to his death. After several proceedings, the Maine Supreme Court awarded her death benefits stating that "his injury occurred during work hours, in a place that the Salvation Army sanctioned for his work" (p. 26).

The issue of working from and exercising at home during working hours needs to be addressed regarding a potential injury occurring at home and application of state workers' compensation laws. Managers of employer-sponsored fitness programs need to discuss this issue with their legal counsel.

factors "because these indicia of time and place of injury are particularly strong indicators of whether injury arose out of and in course of employee's employment" (40, p. 211).

Case #2—Jones v. Multi-Color Corp. (44)

In this Ohio case, an employer had their employees sign a waiver of workers' compensation benefits prior to participation in activities during an employer-sponsored fitness day. During a foot race that day, Jones suffered a cardiac arrest and died. The family sought death benefits under workers' compensation. Prior to this event, the Ohio legislature enacted statutes allowing employers to have their employees sign a waiver that would waive their workers' compensation benefits for an injury or disability that could occur during voluntary participation in company-sponsored recreation or fitness programs. See Exhibit 1-1 for an Ohio statute regarding injury during employer-sponsored recreational, social, or athletic activities.

The waiver in *Jones* stated "…waives and relinquishes all rights to Workers' Compensation benefits…for injury or disability…" (44, pp. 391-392), but did not specify anything about dependents' death benefits. The appellate court held that Jones could not, based on the state statutes, waive his dependents' death benefits and that the family was free to proceed to make their death benefits claim under workers' compensation laws in Ohio.

An interesting question arises from the *Jones* case: If employers are allowed by a state statute to have employees waive their workers' compensation benefits via a waiver for employer-sponsored fitness programs, would employees then be allowed to sue their employer for negligence? If so, this seems to defeat one of the main purposes of workers' compensation, which is to protect employers from potentially costly, negligence claims and lawsuits. It is important for employers to consult with a knowledgeable lawyer regarding any state laws applicable to workers' compensation and employer-sponsored fitness programs—and to determine what type of protective legal documents would be best for employees to sign prior to participation in employer-sponsored programs.

LEGAL RESEARCH AND RESOURCES

This final section in Chapter 1 briefly describes various tools that are available to conduct basic legal research and provides a "selected" list of Internet legal resources that fitness managers and exercise professionals might find helpful. In addition, there are many spotlight cases in this textbook that are presented in a "case brief" format. Therefore, a description of the key sections of a legal case brief is provided along with why reviewing case law is one of the best ways to learn the law.

Legal Research

Legal databases such as WESTLAW and LEXIS allow researchers to quickly access both primary and secondary sources of law. In order to conduct important legal research, lawyers and/or law firms need to purchase access to these legal databases. However,

---

Exhibit 1-1: Ohio Workers' Compensation Statute*

Under the Workers' Compensation Act requirement that compensable injury be one received in the course of and arising out of the employment, injuries that occur while the employee is engaged in employer-sponsored social or recreational activities, benefiting the employer, are compensable without regard to whether the accident occurs at the workplace, taking due consideration of the time, place, and circumstances of the injury to determine whether the required nexus exists between the employment relationship and the injurious activity, and consideration of a totality of the facts and circumstances analysis to determine whether a sufficient causal relationship exists.

An injury sustained by an employee while attending a picnic that is sponsored, paid for, and supervised by the employer for the purpose of generating friendly relations with the employees is, as a matter of law, sustained in the course of employment. An employee who is injured in a ball game conducted after working hours and from which the employer derives a business-related benefit although intangible and not immediately measurable, is injured in the course of and out of employment, even though the event is not controlled or supervised by the employer.

> ### Reminder:
>
> The Act, in defining the term "injury," specifically excludes injury or disability incurred in voluntary participation in an employer-sponsored recreation or fitness activity if the employee signs a waiver of the employee's right to compensation or benefits prior to engaging in such activity…
>
> ### Caution:
>
> A waiver signed by an employee waiving all rights to workers' compensation benefits for any injury or disability incurred while participating in an employer's sponsored recreation fitness activities does not bar the death benefits claims of the dependents because a worker cannot effectively waive the rights of dependents.

*94 Ohio Jur. 3d Workers' Compensation § 142. Injury during employer-sponsored recreational, social, or athletic activities.

professors of law schools and law students, while they are law students, have "free" access to these databases at their respective schools. Generally, law school libraries do not allow the public access to these databases. Many academic institutions provide versions of these legal databases (e.g., Westlaw or Campus Research and Nexis Uni for professors to access as well as students while they are enrolled). With these databases, exercise science professors and students can access primary sources of law such as federal and state statutes, regulations, and legal cases as well as many secondary sources such as American Jurisprudence 2d, American Law Reports (ALR), and numerous law reviews and journals.

Legal Resources on the Internet

Fitness managers and exercise professionals, who do not have access to these legal databases, can find reliable sources of law on the Internet. The sources listed in Exhibit 1-2 are only a few examples of the many Internet sources available. It is always necessary to check each source to be sure it is credible. For example, government websites (.gov) would be considered credible sites such as the Government Publishing Office website (www.govinfo.gov). Resources on this site include the Code of Federal Regulations, Federal Register, US District and Appellate Court Opinions, US Code, Public and Private Laws, and Congressional Bills.

Exhibit 1-2: Examples of Internet Legal Resources

1. Federal Statutes and Regulations

- Americans with Disabilities Act—www.ada.gov
- Fair Labor Standards Act—www.dol.gov/agencies/whd/flsa
- HIPAA for Professionals—www.hhs.gov/hipaa/for-professionals/index.html
- Title VII of the Civil Rights Act—www.eeoc.gov/laws/statutes/titlevii.cfm
- Occupational Safety and Health Administration—www.osha.gov
- U.S. Equal Employment Opportunity Commission—www.eeoc.gov

2. Organizations

- ACSM—*ACSM's Health & Fitness Journal*—many legal and fitness safety columns are "free" access on the Journal's website: https://journals.lww.com/acsm-healthfitness/pages/default.aspx
- International Health, Racquet & Sportsclub Association (IHRSA)—many legal articles/resources are "free" access on the IHRSA Legal website: www.ihrsa.org/improve-your-club/topic/legal
- Athletic Business—many articles/resources are "free" access on their Law & Policy website: www.athleticbusiness.com/law-policy.html

3. Other—Numerous "Free" Resources on these Websites:

- The Law Dictionary: *Black's Law Dictionary Free Online Legal Dictionary* 2nd Ed.— https://thelawdictionary.org
- Law Firms, e.g., Matthiesen, Wickert & Lehrer, S.C.—www.mwl-law.com
- Legal Information Institute (Cornell Law School)—www.law.cornell.edu
- FindLaw Search Database—www.findlaw.com
- Law.com—www.law.com
- Nolo—www.nolo.com
- LawInfo—https://www.lawinfo.com
- USLegal—https://uslegal.com
- American Law Source On-Line—http://www.lawsource.com/also/
- National Center for State Courts—https://www.ncsc.org

4. Finding an Experienced Lawyer—Ratings/Reviews Provided

- Martindale Hubble—https://www.martindale.com

Searches on the Internet can also locate legal and risk management information such as negligence lawsuits involving fitness facilities and exercise professionals, injury data (e.g., treadmill, yoga, and boot camp injures, etc.), articles published in professional and trade journals, and blogs written by legal experts. *Note: Legal Forms/Contracts on the Internet.* Fitness managers and exercise professionals need to realize that they should never adopt a sample contract found on the Internet, such as a waiver or service agreement, or elsewhere including examples provided in this textbook. Some of the examples in the textbook include the following: "No form should be adopted without individualized legal advice and consultation." Other examples are preceded with an "Editorial Note: Caution" such as the following for Exhibit 4-2 (Express Assumption of Risk) in Chapter 4.

> *No form should be adopted by any program until it has first been reviewed by legal counsel in the state where a form is to be used as well as by the medical director/advisor/risk manager for the program. To be acceptable, each form must be written in accordance with prevailing state laws by knowledgeable legal counsel and should state to the participant the reasons for the procedure(s), the risks and benefits, etc., in a manner specific to the program activities for which consent, or other form of contractual document, is being obtained.*

Legal Case Brief—Key Sections

Preparing a legal case brief of a published court's opinion is similar to preparing an abstract of a published research study. Both have key sections with the goal to provide a summary. An abstract usually includes sections such as purpose, methods, results, discussion, and conclusion. A legal case brief includes sections such as:

- Facts
  - Historical Facts (summary of what happened, such as how the injury occurred, the waiver signed by the plaintiff)
  - Procedural Facts (complaint filed, legal claims made, motions filed by either party, reasons why a party is appealing)

- Issue(s)—The legal issue(s) the court needs to decide
- Court's Ruling—the court's decision regarding the issue(s)
- Court's Reasoning—the court's analysis and explanation for its ruling—how it applied the facts and the law

The 30 spotlight cases in the textbook follow this case brief format. At the top of each case brief is the citation for the case that includes the: (a) title of the case (e.g., names of the plaintiff and defendant) (b) location of the published opinion, and (c) name of the court and date the case was decided. Citations for other cases described in this textbook appear in the References. The following are citations of two spotlight cases (one state and one federal case) with a description of each.

State Court—Top Appellate Court

Limones v. Sch. Dist., 161 So.3d 384 (Fla., 2015)
- Limones is the plaintiff
- School District is the defendant
- So.3d—*Southern Regional Reporter,* third series, where this case was published (this Reporter publishes state cases in Alabama, Florida, Louisiana, and Mississippi)
- 161 is the volume number of the Reporter
- 384 is the first page of the published opinion
- (Fla., 2015) refers to the Supreme Court of Florida and 2015 is the date the case was decided; If this case had been decided by a Florida District Court of Appeals (Intermediate Court of Appeals), the court reference would be: Fla. Dist. Ct. App., 2015.

Federal Court—Intermediate Court of Appeals

Howard v. Missouri Bone and Joint Center, 615 F.3d 991 (8th Cir., 2010)
- Howard is the plaintiff
- Missouri Bone and Joint Center is the defendant
- F.3d—*Federal Reporter,* third series, where this case was published (this Reporter publishes Circuit Court of Appeals cases)
- 615 is the volume number of the Reporter
- 991 is the first page of the published opinion

(8th Cir., 2010) refers to the 8th Circuit Court of Appeals (see Figure 1-3) and 2010 is the date the case was decided; If this case had been decided by a Federal District Court (trial court) the court reference would be: F. Supp., 2010. The *Federal Supplement* publishes these court opinions.

To find cases using the legal databases, the name (e.g., *Limones v. Sch. Dist.*) or the location (e.g., 161 So.3d 384) can be used. Cases sometimes also include a WESTLAW (WL) or LEXIS citation—another way to find a published opinion.

Each of the 30 spotlight cases includes a "lessons learned" section at the end in which both legal and risk management lessons are provided. One of the best ways to learn the law is by reading case law. The 30 spotlight cases, and more than 80 additional cases, described in this textbook have occurred in various fitness settings and programs and reflect "real" situations that led to lawsuits filed by plaintiffs. By reading these cases—the *what, why,* and *how,* as shown in Figure 1-9, will become evident to fitness managers and exercise professionals with the goal to help them increase compliance with many of the laws applicable to the exercise profession. Linking the what, why, and how is the approach this textbook takes.

Figure 1-9: Linking the What, Why, and How

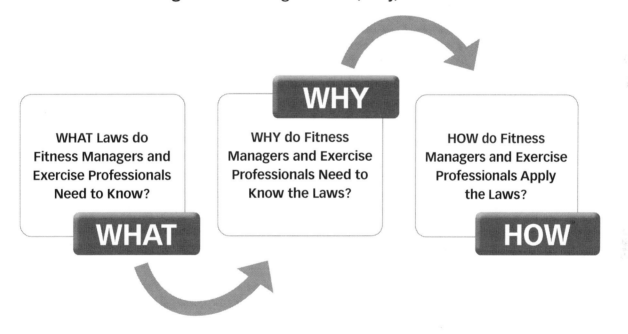

KEY TERMS

- Actual Cause
- Administrative Law
- Answer
- Assumption of Risk
- Beyond a Reasonable Doubt
- Breach of Contract
- Breach of Duty
- Case Law
- Causation
- Cause of Action
- Civil Law
- Civil Liability
- Common Law
- Comparative Negligence
- Compensatory Damages
- Complaint
- Contract
- Contributory Negligence
- Criminal Law
- Damages
- Defendant
- Depositions
- Discovery
- Dissenting Opinion
- Duty
- Evidence
- Expert Witnesses
- Fact Witnesses

- General Jurisdiction
- Governmental Immunity
- Gross Negligence
- Guilty
- Intentional Tort
- Interrogatories
- Jurisdiction
- Jury Instructions
- Liable
- Loss of Consortium
- Majority Opinion
- Motion to Dismiss
- Motions to Produce
- Negligence
- Ordinances
- Out-of-Court Settlement
- Plaintiff
- Pleadings
- Precedent
- Preponderance of the Evidence
- Prima Facie Case
- Primary Sources of Law
- Private Law
- Procedural Law
- Product Liability
- Proximate Cause
- Public Law

- Punitive Damages
- Regulations
- Remand
- Secondary Sources of Law
- Separation of Powers
- Sovereign Immunity
- Standard of Care
- Stare Decisis
- Statute of Frauds
- Statutes
- Statutes of Limitations
- Statutory Law
- Strict Liability
- Subject Matter Jurisdiction
- Subpoena
- Substantive Law
- Summary Judgment
- Summons
- Tort
- Triers of Fact
- Unanimous Opinion
- Unenforceable Contract
- Vicarious Liability
- Voidable Contract
- Workers' Compensation
- Writ of Certiorari
- Written Law
- Wrongful Death

 STUDY QUESTIONS

The Study Questions for Chapter 1 can be found on the Fitness Law Academy website (www.fitnesslawacademy.com) under Textbook. They are provided in a fillable format for convenience.

REFERENCES

1. Eickhoff-Shemek JM, Herbert DL, Connaughton, DP. *Risk Management for Health/Fitness Professionals: Legal Issues and Strategies*. Baltimore, MD: Lippincott Williams & Wilkins, 2009.

2. Carper DL, McKinsey JA. Understanding the Law. 6th Ed. Mason, OH: South-Western, Cengage Learning, 2012.

3. How Laws Are Made and How to Research Them. March 6, 2020. Available at: https://www.usa.gov/how-laws-are-made#item-35837. Accessed March 9, 2020.

4. Our Government. The Executive Branch. Available at: https://www.whitehouse.gov/about-the-white-house/the-executive-branch/. Accessed March 9, 2020.

5. Zabawa BJ, Eickhoff-Shemek JM. *Rule the Rules of Workplace Wellness Programs*. Chicago, IL: American Bar Association, 2017.

6. Cotten DJ, Cotten MB. *Waivers & Releases of Liability*, 9th Ed. Statesboro, GA: Sport Risk Consulting, 2016.

7. Black DC, Nolan JR, Nolan-Haley JM., et al. *Black's Law Dictionary*, 6th Ed. St. Paul, MN: West Publishing Company, 1991.

8. Florida Courts. Trial Courts – Circuit. Available at: https://www.flcourts.org/Florida-Courts/Trial-Courts-Circuit and Florida Courts. Trial Courts – County. Available at: https://www.flcourts.org/Florida-Courts/Trial-Courts-County. Accessed March 11, 2020.

9. Supreme Court of the United States. FAQs - General Information. Available at: https://www.supremecourt.gov/about/faq_general.aspx. Accessed March 12, 2020.

10. Civil Statutes of Limitation by State (2020). PennyGeeks. January 2, 2020. Available at: https://pennygeeks.com/legal-resources/civil-statutes-of-limitations/. Accessed March 12, 2020.

11. Schoepfer Bochicchio KL. The Legal System. In: Cotten DJ, Wolohan JT. (eds). *Law for Recreation and Sport Managers.* 7th Ed. Dubuque, IA: Kendall/Hunt Publishing Company, 2017.

12. Hirby J. What Percentage of Lawsuits Settle Before Trial? What are Some Statistics on Personal Injury Settlements? *The Law Dictionary – Featuring Black's Law Dictionary Free Online Legal Dictionary*, 2nd Ed. Available at: https://thelawdictionary.org/article/what-percentage-of-lawsuits-settle-before-trial-what-are-some-statistics-on-personal-injury-settlements. Accessed March 13, 2020.

13. Durkin H. Why All Gyms Need to Follow the Peloton Music Copyright Case. July 30, 2019. IHRSA. Available at: https://www.ihrsa.org/improve-your-club/why-all-gyms-need-to-follow-the-peloton-music-copyright-case/. Accessed November 25, 2019.

14. Berg A. Peloton Settles with the NMPA Over Music Rights Lawsuit. February 2020. Available at: https://www.athleticbusiness.com/contract-law/peloton-settles-with-nmpa-over-music-rights-lawsuit.html. Accessed March 13, 2020.

15. *A Concise Restatement of TORTS Third Edition*. Compiled by: Bublick EM, Rogers JE. St. Paul, MN: American Law Institute, 2013.

16. Berg A. Club Employee Arrested for Photographing Women. *Athletic Business E-Newsletter*. March 2019. Available at: https://www.athleticbusiness.com/law-policy/fitness-club-employee-arrested-for-photographing-women.html. Accessed March 16, 2020.

17. Scott J. Ex-Gym Owner Sentenced in Hidden Camera Case. *Athletic Business E-Newsletter*. April 2019. Available at: https://www.athleticbusiness.com/law-policy/ex-gym-owner-sentenced-in-hidden-camera-case.html. Accessed March 16, 2020.

18. Berg A. Ex-Planet Fitness Staffer Sentenced for Filming Women. *Athletic Business E-Newsletter*. May 2019. Available at: https://www.athleticbusiness.com/civil-actions/ex-planet-fitness-employee-sentenced-for-filming-women.html. Accessed March 16, 2020.

19. *Hammond v. Equinox Holdings*. Complaint filed on May 20, 2029. Index No. 155061/2019. Supreme Court of the State of New York County of New York. Available at: https://www.documentcloud.org/documents/6024540-Hammond-v-Equinox-complaint.html. Accessed March 16, 2020.

20. Dougherty NJ, Goldberger AS, Carpenter LJ. *Sport, Physical Activity, and the Law*. 3rd Ed. Champaign, IL: Sagamore Publishing, 2007.

21. *Bartlett v. Push to Walk*, No. 2:15-cv-7167-KM-JBC, 2018 WL 1726262 (D. N.J., 2018).

22. *Jimenez v. 24 Hour Fitness*, 188 Cal. Rptr. 3d. 228 (Cal. Ct. App., 2015).

23. van der Smissen B. Elements of Negligence. In: Cotten DJ, Wolohan JT, (eds.) *Law for Recreation and Sport Managers*, 3rd Ed. Dubuque, IA: Kendall/Hunt Publishing Company, 2003.

24. *Lee v. Louisiana Board of Trustees for State Colleges*, 280 So.3d 176, 2019 WL 1198551 (La. Ct. App., 2019).

25. Contributory Negligence/Comparative Fault in All 50 States. Matthiesen, Wickert & Lehrer, S.C., February 19, 2018. Available at: https://www.mwl-law.com/wp-content/uploads/2018/02/COMPARATIVE-FAULT-SYSTEMS-CHART.pdf. Accessed October 10, 2010.

26. *D'Amico v. LA Fitness*, 57 Conn. L. Rptr. 242, 2013 WL 6912912 (Conn. Super. Ct., 2013).

27. Criminal Statutes of Limitations: Time Limits for State Charges. LawInfo. Available at: https://resources.lawinfo.com/criminal-defense/criminal-statute-limitations-time-limits.html. Accessed March 21, 2020.

28. U.S. Federal Statute of Limitations for Federal Crimes. Available at: https://www.statuteoflimitation.info/federal-statute-of-limitations.html. Accessed March 21, 2020.

29. Cotten DJ. Immunity. In: Cotten DJ, Wolohan JT. (eds). *Law for Recreation and Sport Managers*. 7th Ed. Dubuque, IA: Kendall/Hunt Publishing Company, 2017.

30. Volunteer Protection Act. 42 U.S.C.A. § 14503. Limitation on Liability for Volunteers, June 18, 1997.

31. Immunity or Not? Charitable Tort Liability Limits in Modern Times. December 15, 2017. Wagenmaker & Oberly Blog. Available at: https://wagenmakerlaw.com/blog/immunity-or-not-charitable-tort-liability-limits-modern-times. Accessed February 5, 2020.

32. Product Liability in All 50 States. Matthiesen, Wickert & Lehrer, S.C., April 25, 2019. Available at: https://www.mwl-law.com/resources/product-liability-laws-50-states/. Accessed October 11, 2019.

References continued...

33. Workers Compensation. Legal Information Institute. Cornell Law School. Available at: https://www.law.cornell.edu/wex/workers_compensation. Accessed March 30, 2020.

34. Clarkson, KW, Miller RL, Jentz GA, Cross FB. *West's Business Law*. 8th Ed. St. Paul, MN: West Publishing Company, 2001.

35. Uniform Commercial Code. USLegal.com. Available at: https://uniformcommercialcode.uslegal.com/. Accessed March 24, 2020.

36. Workers' Compensation Insurance FAQs. State Board of Workers' Compensation. Available at: https://sbwc.georgia.gov/frequently-asked-questions. Accessed March 26, 2020.

37. What Happens If You Lose a Worker's Comp Case at Arbitration? Nolo. Available at: http://www.disabilitysecrets.com/workmans-comp-question-7.html. Accessed March 30, 2020.

38. Laurence BK. How Do You Start the Workers' Comp Process? Nolo. Available at: http://www.disabilitysecrets.com/workmans-comp-question-18.html. Accessed March 30, 2020.

39. *Stanner v. Compensation Appeal Board (Westinghouse Electric Co.)*, 604 A.2d 1167 (Pa. Commw. Ct., 1992).

40. *Price v. Industrial Claim Appeals Office*, 919 P.2d 207 (Colo., 1996).

41. *Price v. Industrial Claim Appeals Office*, 908 P.2d 136 (Colo. Ct. App., 1995).

42. *City of Northglenn v. Eltrich*, 908 P.2d 139 (Colo. Ct. App., 1995).

43. Herbert DL. Maine Supreme Court Determines Employee's Treadmill Related Death is Compensable. *The Exercise, Sports and Sports Medicine Standards and Malpractice Reporter*, 4(2), 25-25, 2015.

44. *Jones v. Multi-Color Corp.*, 108 Ohio App. 3d. 388 (Ohio Ct. App., 1995).

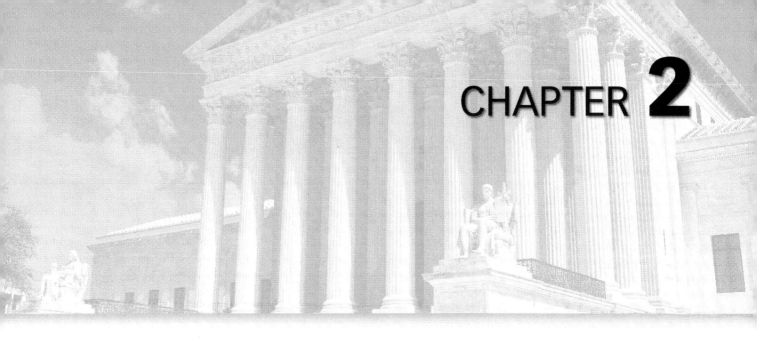

CHAPTER 2

Creating a Safety Culture: Building a Comprehensive Risk Management Plan

 LEARNING OBJECTIVES

After reading this chapter, fitness managers and exercise professionals will be able to:

1. Recognize the increases in the number of "exercise/exercise equipment" injuries as reported by the National Electronic Injury Surveillance System (NEISS).

2. Identify the types of insurance claims that insurance companies have paid out as well as the types of claims that have occurred in recent years.

3. Describe the types of injuries that have occurred in negligence lawsuits against exercise professionals and fitness facilities.

4. List and describe the three major causes of injuries that occur in fitness facilities.

5. Define risk management and related terms such as legal liability

exposures and preventive law (1).

6. Utilize the four steps involved in building a comprehensive risk management plan (1).

7. Explain relevant factors involved in the successful development of a comprehensive risk management plan such as the role of the risk management advisory committee and strategic planning (1).

8. Describe the risk management responsibilities of all fitness facility staff members (1).

9. Explain the differences among the various types of risk management strategies (i.e., exposure avoidance, loss prevention, loss reduction, and contractual transfer of risks).

10. Develop a Risk Management Policies and Procedures Manual (1).

11. Conduct an effective risk management staff training program applying the four Ps of staff training.

12. Conduct both formative and summative evaluations of the fitness facility's comprehensive risk management plan (1).

13. Identify the major benefits (positive outcomes) of a comprehensive risk management plan.

14. Define safety culture and implement strategies to assess and improve safety culture in a fitness facility.

INTRODUCTION

As described in the Preface, there has been tremendous growth of fitness programs and facilities over the past several decades. Access to fitness programs and exercise equipment is no longer available only in health clubs and YMCAs, but in all types of settings such as those listed in Exhibit 2-1. In these settings, fitness managers and exercise professionals need to develop a comprehensive risk management plan to protect themselves and their employers from costly litigation. This chapter begins with background information regarding injuries and litigation to demonstrate the importance of risk management. Next, the four steps involved in the risk management process are described: (a) assessment of legal liability exposures, (b) development of risk management strategies, (c) implementation of the comprehensive risk management plan, and (d) evaluation of the comprehensive risk management plan. Toward the end of the chapter, safety culture is discussed, and a survey is provided that can be used to assess a fitness facility's safety culture.

INJURIES AND LITIGATION

Fitness managers and exercise professionals need to be aware of the types of injuries and lawsuits that occur in exercise programs and fitness facilities. Unfortunately, the number of exercise/exercise equipment injures has significantly increased in recent years (2). When fitness participants experience a personal injury, they often file a negligence lawsuit. This section provides injury and claims data as well as examples of the types of injuries that occur in fitness facilities and the major causes of these injuries.

Injury and Claims Data

The U.S. Consumer Product Safety Commission (CPSC) tracks injury data through its National Electronic Injury Surveillance System (NEISS). Injury data are collected from a sample of hospital emergency departments throughout the country (2). For example, in 2018, 96 hospitals of varying sizes and locations collected and categorized these data. Sport and Recreational

---

Exhibit 2-1: Types of Settings: Fitness Facilities and Programs

⬧ **Corporate**
- employer-sponsored fitness/wellness programs

⬧ **College/University**
- campus recreation for students and employees
- strength and conditioning for athletes

⬧ **Commercial, for-profit**
- health clubs
- boutique fitness studios
- country clubs/resorts
- personal fitness training and group exercise studios
- sports performance centers for youth, adults, and professional athletes

⬧ **Community, non-profit**
- YMCAs/YWCAs,
- JCCs
- public schools
- churches, synagogues, mosques

⬧ **Government**
- military branches
- firefighters/police
- city/county parks and recreation

⬧ **Hospitals/Medical Clinics**
- cardiac and pulmonary rehab
- hospital or clinic-based fitness/wellness
- physical therapy/orthopedic rehab

⬧ **Retirement Centers**
- 55+ communities
- independent living communities
- assisted living communities

⬧ **Home Gyms**
- personal fitness trainer's home
- client's home

Equipment is one of 14 categories. In this category, 28 different sport/recreation activities or products are listed, and Exercise/Exercise Equipment is one of the 28. To help determine the total number of injuries in the U.S., estimates are calculated from the actual data.

Table 2-1 presents these estimates for the number of injuries related to Exercise/Exercise Equipment. There's been a steady and significant increase between 2007 and 2018—almost 90% in 12 years. NEISS also provides a Top 20 Ranking among all its categories and listings, and in 2017 and 2018, Exercise/Exercise Equipment ranked No. 5. These data do not reflect the number of exercise/exercise equipment injuries that did not involve a visit to a hospital emergency room, which would likely be more. These data do not include sport injuries such as hockey and basketball injuries. Given these significant increases in injuries, there is a clear need to focus on injury prevention. According to the Centers for Disease Control and Prevention (CDC), experiencing an injury is a major reason why individuals stop exercising (3). As the exercise profession continues to evolve and as Americans are encouraged to participate in regular physical activity, it will be essential that injury prevention becomes a focus throughout all sectors of the profession including academic preparation, certification preparation, and on-the-job training.

All types of injuries (minor, major, life-threatening) and death can result in negligence claims and lawsuits against exercise professionals and fitness facilities. Insurance companies often settle cases out of court meaning the insurance company and

KEY POINT

Given significant increases in Exercise/Exercise Equipment injuries in the past decade, it is essential that injury prevention becomes a focus throughout the exercise profession including academic preparation, certification preparation, and on-the-job training. Injury prevention begins by recognizing the types of injuries and subsequent liability claims that have occurred in exercise programs and fitness facilities.

the injured party agree on an amount to be paid to the injured party to resolve a claim without trial. It is usually more cost-effective to settle than going to trial and resolve the uncertainties associated with litigation. One company, the former Association Insurance Group, Inc. conducted a study in which they analyzed the type and the number of liability claims that occurred over a 12-year period (1995–2007) for their fitness facility clients. During this period, they received 6,144 incidents of which 2,395 turned into actual claims. The claims were classified into 20 categories and the five categories that were the most frequent are shown in Table 2-2.

As shown in Table 2-2, liability claims can be quite costly. For example, the equipment malfunction claims (N=339), which resulted in an average claim value of $17,063 totaled $5,784,357 over the 12-year period. Equipment malfunction claims included items such as cable failure on selectorized machines, exercise balls that burst, equipment that falls over because it was not installed properly, and seats that fall off spin bikes. Most of these claims were due to poor maintenance of the equipment. Member malfunction is a category of claims where members hurt themselves while working out (e.g., strain a muscle, drop a weight on their foot, and smash their fingers re-racking weights).

It is important to recognize that many of these claims could have been significantly reduced if fitness managers and exercise professionals would have incorporated many of the risk management strategies that are presented throughout this textbook. In addition to reducing the number of injuries and subsequent claims/lawsuits, a comprehensive risk management plan can offer other benefits such as, possibly, lowering liability insurance premiums (4), not having to experience the

Table 2-1	Exercise/Exercise Equipment Injury Data, 2007-2018*
YEAR	**NUMBER OF INJURIES**
2007	264,921
2009	349,962
2011	410,024
2013	472,196
2015	464,346
2016	503,437
2017	526,350
2018	498,498

*NEISS data retrieved July 26, 2019 from: www.cpsc.gov/LIBRARY/neiss.html

Table 2-2	Top Five Most Frequent Health Club Liability Claims Over a 12 Year Period*	
TYPE OF CLAIM	**NUMBER OF CLAIMS**	**AVERAGE CLAIM VALUE****
Member Malfunction	388	$8,902
Premises Liability — Trip and Falls	350	$18,554
Equipment Malfunction	339	$17,063
Slip and Fall — Wet Areas	252	$12,478
Treadmill	233	$8,933

**Claim value includes defense costs, expenses, and reserves.
*Reprinted with permission from Ken Reinig, Former President of the Association Insurance Group, Inc.

stress that is often associated with lawsuits that can go on for a very long time (years in some cases), and not having to prepare answers to discovery requests. See *Jessica H. v. Equinoz Holdings, Inc.*, spotlight case in Chapter 5, in which the defendants prepared 750 pages of such documents.

Update on Claims/Lawsuits

Negligence claims/lawsuits continue to occur in the fitness field as evident from the spotlight and other cases described throughout this textbook. Some trends regarding the types of claims/lawsuits over the past decade are interesting and important. There appears to be an increase in the following types of claims/lawsuits made against exercise professionals and fitness facilities:

a) As described in many of the spotlight and other cases in this textbook, high intensity or extreme conditioning programs, improper instruction, and improper maintenance of exercise equipment have resulted in all types of injuries/lawsuits.

b) An article published by *Club Industry* (5) cited the following types of fitness industry legalities that occurred in 2017: deadly shootings, sexual harassment and rape, locker room policies and transgender individuals, claims involving the violation of the Credit Card Accountability and Disclosure Act, large settlements involving unpaid wages of trainers, and data privacy issues.

c) Litigation regarding violations of data privacy laws (e.g., Health Insurance Portability and Accountability Act, Biometric Information Privacy Acts). See Chapter 3 for more on data privacy as well as Chapters 6, 8, and 10.

d) Discrimination claims/lawsuits (ADA, gender, etc.) appear to be increasing. See Chapter 3 for spotlight and other cases dealing with discrimination in fitness/sport programs. Also, collegiate athletics is experiencing a significant upsurge in Title VII and Title IX discrimination lawsuits that are resulting in million-dollar settlements (6).

Types and Causes of Injuries

There are many physiological and psychological benefits obtained from participation in physical activity and exercise (7). See Exhibit 2-2. However, risks exist that can lead to all types of injuries. Examples of the types of injuries that occurred in selected spotlight cases are described in Table 2-3.

The causes of injuries occurring in fitness programs and facilities are, primarily, due to (a) risks inherent in the activity, (b) negligence, and (c) product defects. Injuries due to **risks inherent in the activity** are inseparable and just happen because of participation. Almost everyone reading this textbook has probably experienced an injury due to these types of risks when participating in physical activity or sports (e.g., an ankle sprain while playing basketball or a muscle strain while lifting weights). They are no one's fault. More information regarding these risks is presented in Chapter 4.

Injuries also can be due to **negligence**—the fault of facility personnel (e.g., improper instruction, improper maintenance of exercise equipment) and/or the fault of the participant (e.g., misusing a piece of exercise equipment). Negligence and a more serious form of negligence called gross negligence are described in more detail in Chapter 4. Most of the case law examples in this textbook involve negligence lawsuits that participants have brought against facility personnel and facilities. In addition, injuries can be caused by **product defects**. In these cases, the manufacturer of the exercise equipment would be liable (product liability) for the participant's injury. More information on product defects and product liability is provided in Chapter 9.

Injuries Often Lead to Negligence Claims/Lawsuits

All the spotlight cases listed in Table 2-3 involved negligence lawsuits against defendants—exercise professionals and/or fitness facilities. In these cases, sometimes the plaintiff won and sometimes the defendant won. In negligence cases, the plaintiff submits a list of negligence claims against the defendants when filing the complaint. For example, in *Baldi-Perry v. Kaifas and 360 Fitness Center, Inc.* (8), there were 26 and 15 such claims against the personal fitness trainer and the facility, respectively. See Exhibit 2-3. As previously described in Chapter 1, employers can be held liable for the negligence acts of their employees based on a legal principle called respondeat superior and, thus, are often named as a defendant in the complaint.

In *Baldi-Perry* (8), the plaintiff had informed her personal fitness trainer that she had back/neck injuries. He told her that he had extensive experience training individuals with such injuries and that he could design a safe program for her. One day, he informed her that he had a new exercise program for her—circuit training with no/little rest periods that was being performed by many others at 360 Fitness Center. She reminded him of her injuries, and he indicated that she needed to trust him and that he was the professional and did this for a living. Relying upon his purported expertise, she performed the new routine as instructed and suffered many severe and permanent injuries including herniated discs, surgery to remove, decompress and fuse discs, ongoing pain/medical care, and future surgery.

Additional information describing this case (9, 10) indicated that the trainer had a college degree in health/wellness/exercise physiology and had

---

Exhibit 2-2: Top 25 Reasons to Exercise*

1. Strengthens heart muscle.
2. Decreases the incidence of heart attack.
3. Reduces risks for heart disease, e.g., reduces bad LDL cholesterol and increases good HDL cholesterol.
4. Improves circulation and oxygen/nutrient transport throughout the body.
5. Helps lose weight and keep it off.
6. Improves breathing efficiency.
7. Strengthens & tones muscles and improves appearance.
8. Helps prevent back problems and back pain.
9. Improves posture.
10. Strengthens bones and helps reduce risk of osteoporosis and falls.
11. Strengthens the tissues around the joints and reduces joint discomfort and arthritis if appropriate exercise is selected and properly performed.
12. Decreases risk for several types of cancer.
13. Improves immune function, which decreases risk for infectious diseases.
14. Maintains physical and mental functions throughout the second half of life.
15. Increases self-confidence and self-esteem.
16. Boosts energy and increases productivity.
17. Improves sleep.
18. Helps create a positive attitude about life.
19. Reduces anxiety and depression.
20. Increases resistance to fatigue.
21. Lengthens lifespan and slows aging.
22. Reduces blood pressure.
23. Decreases the incidence of Type 2 diabetes.
24. Increases resiliency to stress.
25. Slows the loss of cognitive function with aging.

*Reprinted with permission, Eickhoff-Shemek and Berg, 2012 (7).

obtained NSCA certification, but his certification had lapsed at the time he trained the plaintiff. The trainer testified that he did not obtain medical clearance as recommended by NSCA, and because he did not keep his certification current, he no longer had to follow their (NSCA) recommendations. Also, it appeared he did not keep any workout records of the plaintiff. The jury returned a verdict of $1.4 million in favor of the plaintiff, but the plaintiff was 30% at fault so she was awarded $980,000, applying New York's comparative negligence rule. To help avoid negligence lawsuits like this one, fitness managers and exercise professionals need to develop risk management strategies that address the types of negligence claims listed in Exhibit 2-3 as well as the negligent claims made in other cases described throughout this textbook. Development of risk management strategies is discussed later in this chapter.

Table 2-3	Types of Injuries in Selected Spotlight Cases	
TYPE OF INJURY	**HOW THE INJURY OCCURRED**	**SPOTLIGHT CASE (CHAPTER)**
Fractured ankle	Fall off treadmill	*Corrigan v. Musclemakers, Inc.* (4)
Fractured wrists	Fall while performing suicide and backward runs	*Evans v. Fitness & Sports Clubs, LLC* (4)
Back and neck injuries	Fall during an indoor cycling class when handlebars dislodged	*Stelluti v. Casapenn Enterprises, LLC* (4)
Arm and shoulder injury	Intensive, strenuous exercise	*D'Amico v. LA Fitness* (5)
Heart attack	High intensity exercise with little/no rest periods	*Rostai v. Neste Enterprises* (6)
Shattered wrist	Fall during a step test	*Covenant Health System v. Barnett and Barnett* (6)
Herniated disc	Injury while performing a squat exercise	*Howard v. Missouri Bone and Joint Center* (6)
Fractured leg	Kneeling exercise performed by person with spinal cord injury	*Bartlett v. Push to Walk* (7)
Herniated disc	Squat exercise performed by person with known herniated discs	*Layden v. Plante* (7)
Massive stroke	High intensity exercise performed on a rowing machine	*Vaid v. Equinox* (8)
Torn quadriceps	Injury during an indoor cycling class	*Scheck v. Soul Cycle* (8)
Multiple dental injuries	Child's head slammed into a wall after being hit with a ball	*Lotz v. The Claremont Club* (8)
Heat injury resulting in death	Intense exercise training; overexertion of collegiate athlete	*UCF Athletics Association v. Plancher* (8)
Severe head injuries	Fall off treadmill hitting head into an exposed exercise machine	*Jimenez v. 24 Hour Fitness* (9)
Traumatic brain injury	A back panel of an exercise machine struck head	*Chavez v. 24 Hour Fitness* (9)
Wrist and hip fractures requiring surgery	Fall off BOSU ball	*Butler v. Seville et al.* (9)
Hip injury requiring surgery	Trip and fall over a weight belt left on the fitness floor	*Crossing-Lyons v. Town Sport International, Inc.* (10)
Serious injuries in steam room resulting in death	Lack of steam room safety procedures	*Miller v. YMCA of Central Massachusetts et al.* (10)
Cardiac arrest resulting in death	Collapse while playing racquetball	*Miglino v. Bally Total Fitness* (11)

Exhibit 2-3: Negligence Claims in *Baldi-Perry v. Kaifas and 360 Fitness Center, Inc.* (8)

26 Negligence Claims Against the Trainer

- Failing to perform a proper fitness evaluation of the plaintiff before devising an exercise routine;
- Failing to devise a safe and proper exercise routine for the plaintiff;
- Failing to consider the plaintiff's prior injuries and physical condition before preparing an exercise routine;
- Failing to conduct a health risk appraisal;
- Failing to take the necessary and proper steps to minimize the risk of injury to the plaintiff;
- Failing to identify the plaintiff as someone with an increased risk of injury;
- Failing to provide adequate supervision of the plaintiff at Fitness 360;
- Ignoring the plaintiff's concerns about the prescribed exercise routine;
- Failing to provide proper instruction;
- Failing to evaluate the plaintiff's medical condition before preparing an exercise routine;
- Encouraging and instructing the plaintiff to exercise after she expressed concern about the exercise routine;
- Encouraging and instructing the plaintiff to continue to exercise despite complaints of pain;
- Failing to provide a personalized exercise routine as promised;
- Failing to meet the representations made to the plaintiff and to the public at large;
- Failing to follow internal rules, employee manuals, regulations, and operating and training procedures;
- Failing to follow operating and training procedures, and rules and regulations generally accepted in the industry;
- Failing to follow industry standards;
- Encouraging the plaintiff to perform an exercise routine beyond her physical capabilities;
- Failing to properly evaluate the plaintiff's exercise experience before creating an exercise routine;
- Failing to properly train and instruct the plaintiff on the use of equipment and lifting techniques;
- Failing to ensure the plaintiff had adequate rest periods during her exercise routine;
- Holding himself out as a trainer with expertise sufficient to devise a training program that was safe for a person with physical injuries, limitations and a history of surgeries when he did not have adequate education, training and/or experience to do so;
- Failing to warn the plaintiff about the risks of injury associated with her exercise routine;
- Failing to adjust the plaintiff's exercise routine despite the knowledge that such a routine caused injury to others in the past;
- Failing to distinguish those exercises that were safe and appropriate for the plaintiff from those that were dangerous and inappropriate; and
- Being otherwise careless, reckless and negligent (8, pp. 6-8).

16 Negligence Claims Against the Fitness Facility

- Failing to hire properly trained and/or certified personal trainers;
- Failing to have trainers who were certified and/or trained to conduct a proper pre-activity screening;
- Failing to ensure that trainers performed a proper fitness evaluation of clients before devising an exercise routine;
- Failing to have a medical liaison or medical advisory committee to assist in reviewing physical activity screenings and exercise plans;
- Failing to ensure that trainers conducted a health risk appraisal;
- Negligently hiring trainers who were not qualified to design exercise programs for individuals with injuries;
- Failing to have proper pre-activity screening tools in place for its trainers;
- Failing to offer appropriate and necessary training to physical trainers;
- Failing to ensure trainers provided a personalized exercise routine as promised;
- Failing to meet the representations made to the plaintiff and to the public at large;
- Failing to ensure trainers followed internal rules, employee manuals, regulations, and operating and training procedures;
- Failing to follow and/or implement operating and training procedures, and rules and regulations generally accepted in the industry;
- Failing to follow industry standards;
- Failing to have a sufficient number of instructors on the premises;
- Failing to provide proper safety equipment; and
- Being otherwise careless, reckless and negligent (8, pp. 9-10).

KEY POINT

Exercise professionals should always keep their certifications current, but, if they do expire that does not mean that the professional is no longer held to a standard of care of a professional. Courts consider various factors when determining the standard of care of a professional, as described in Chapter 4. The conduct or behavior of an exercise professional is a more important factor than the professional's credentials. The court will determine if the actions or inactions of the professional reflected a breach of duty.

Editorial Note: *Some of the content above and the following reflect content from Chapters 1 and 12 in Risk Management for Health/Fitness Professionals: Legal Issues and Strategies (1). The publisher transferred the rights to this textbook to the authors in 2017. Permission to reprint and revise/update this content was granted by the author of Chapters 1 and 12.*

BUILDING A COMPREHENSIVE RISK MANAGEMENT PLAN

Every fitness facility needs to have a comprehensive risk management plan. This section defines risk management and related terms followed by other relevant factors involved in the risk management process such as strategic planning. Next, each of the four steps involved in the development of a comprehensive plan are described in detail.

Risk Management Defined

The term management can be defined as "the process of planning, organizing, leading, and controlling an organization's or other entity's resources to fulfill its objectives cost-effectively" (11, p. 4). An organization may have several objectives such as growth, profit, and service. In order to prevent a slowing in growth, reduction in profits, or just general interruption of operations, an organization must prevent four types of accidental losses (11): (a) property losses (e.g., property damage due to fire/theft), (b) net income losses (e.g.,

an increase in expenses or a reduction in revenue as result of an accident), (c) liability losses (e.g., claims or lawsuits due to negligence), and (d) personnel losses (e.g., premature death of an employee). Preventing the third type of accidental losses (liability losses) is the focus of this textbook as applied to fitness programs/services and facility operations. The term—**legal liability exposures**—is used throughout this textbook and reflects accidental losses due to liability.

Legal liability exposures are situations that create a risk of an injury (e.g., a personal fitness trainer who does not have the knowledge and skill to teach safe and effective exercise, improper maintenance of exercise equipment) or reflect noncompliance to federal, state, and/or local laws, (e.g., a fitness facility that does not comply with the Americans with Disabilities Act and Automated External Defibrillator state statutes). The failure to minimize legal liability exposures can lead to costly litigation. To minimize litigation, fitness managers and exercise professionals need to first understand and appreciate the many legal liability exposures they face. These legal liability exposures exist in seven major areas as shown in Figure 2-1 and are identified and discussed in the chapters as follows:

#1 **Employment Issues**—*Chapters 3 and 5*
#2 **Pre-Activity Health Screening and Fitness Testing**—*Chapter 6*
#3 **Exercise Prescription and Scope of Practice**—*Chapter 7*
#4 **Instruction and Supervision**—*Chapter 8*
#5 **Exercise Equipment Safety**—*Chapter 9*
#6 **Facility Risks**—*Chapter 3 and 10*
#7 **Emergency Action Plans**—*Chapter 11*

In a broad context to address all four types of accidental losses, Head and Horn define risk management as "the process of making and implementing decisions that will minimize the adverse effects of accidental and business losses on an organization" (11, p. 5). Because this textbook focuses on liability losses, our definition of **risk management** is narrower in focus than the one provided by Head and Horn and is defined as *a proactive administrative process that will help minimize legal liability exposures facing exercise professionals and fitness facilities.* Given this context, risk management is

Figure 2-1: Legal Liability Exposures in Fitness Programs and Facilities Exist in Seven Major Areas

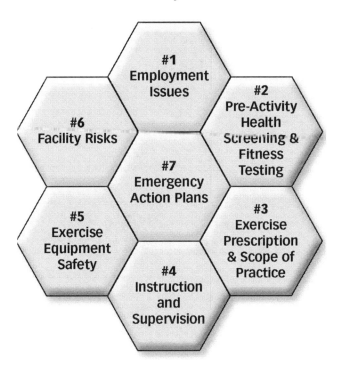

similar to **preventive law** that requires "creative thinking, timely planning, and purposeful execution to minimize legal risks, maximize legal rights, and optimize legal outcomes of transactions (deals), relationships (disputes), and opportunities (challenges)" (12, p. 25). Like preventive medicine that focuses on preventing disease, preventive law focuses on preventing lawsuits. Both preventive medicine and preventive law are *proactive* (preventing problems before they arise) versus *reactive* (responding to problems after they arise).

Head and Horn (11) describe risk management as a decision-making process that includes the following five sequential steps: (a) identify and analyze loss exposure, (b) examine alternative risk management techniques, (c) select risk management techniques, (d) implement techniques, and (e) monitoring results. These five steps can be collapsed into four steps using terms that are familiar to fitness managers and exercise professionals: (a) assessment, (b) development, (c) implementation, and (d) evaluation.

For example, at an individual level when exercise professionals help a participant begin an exercise program, they first *assess* the participant's health risks and fitness levels. The data collected in the assessment are then used to *develop* an exercise prescription tailored for that participant. Exercise professionals then instruct the participant on how to properly *implement* the exercise program. At various times, exercise professionals *evaluate* the progress the participant has made toward his/her fitness goals. At the program planning level, these four steps are used to plan fitness and wellness programs (13). For example, when planning a new program, the needs and interests of the population to be served are assessed. The results of this assessment are then utilized to direct the development of the program. Fitness/wellness program staff members then implement and evaluate the program. These four steps are instrumental in the development of a comprehensive risk management plan and are referred to in this textbook as:

> **Step 1**—*Assessment of Legal Liability Exposures*
> **Step 2**—*Development of Risk Management Strategies*
> **Step 3**—*Implementation of the Comprehensive Risk Management Plan*
> **Step 4**—*Evaluation of the Comprehensive Risk Management Plan*

Figure 2-2 depicts the major components for each of the four risk management steps. These steps and their major components are described in detail later in this chapter. First, relevant factors related to getting started with the development of a comprehensive risk management plan need to be described: (a) risk management responsibilities of staff members, (b) risk management advisory committee, (c) and strategic planning.

KEY POINT

Legal liability exposures are circumstances that create a risk of injury or reflect noncompliance with federal, state, and local laws. Risk management minimizes legal liability exposures and subsequent litigation. Although the fitness manager is ultimately responsible for risk management, all staff members have risk management responsibilities.

Figure 2-2: Major Components for Each of the Four Risk Management Steps

Step 1: Assessment of Legal Liability Exposures

Review Laws
- Statutory Laws
- Administrative Laws
- Case Law, e.g., negligence lawsuits

Review Published Standards of Practice
- Professional Organizations
- Independent Organizations

Step 2: Development of Risk Management Strategies

Exposure Avoidance Strategies
- Eliminate Risk of Injury

Loss Prevention Strategies
- Minimize Risk of Injury
- Reflect Compliance with Laws

Loss Reduction Strategies
- Mitigate an Injury After it Occurs

Contractual Transfer of Risks
- Waiver (Release of Liability)
- Liability Insurance

Step 3: Implementation of the Comprehensive Risk Management Plan

Risk Management Policies and Procedures Manual (RMPPM)

Staff Training
- Initial Training upon Hiring
- Regular In-Service Trainings

Step 4: Evaluation of the Comprehensive Risk Management Plan

Formative
- Ongoing Reveiw of Various Aspects of the Comprehensive Risk Management Plan that may Indicate a Need for Revision of Policies and Procedures

Summative
- Formal Annual Reveiw of the Entire Comprehensive Risk Management Plan to Determine if Revisions are Needed Based on Changes in Laws or Standards

Risk Management Responsibilities of Staff Members

The fitness facility manager has the overall responsibility regarding the development of a comprehensive risk management plan for the facility. He or she may designate a professional staff member to serve or assist in the role as the facility's risk management manager. However, the fitness manager needs to realize that he/she is ultimately responsible and, therefore, should oversee the process. The professional(s) leading this effort should (a) have educational background in legal liability and risk management (e.g., completed the continuing education course (14) that accompanies this textbook), (b) be a respected leader, (c) have superb strategic planning skills, (d) be dedicated and committed to participant safety, and (e) have excellent problem-solving, communication, and teaching skills. It is essential that all staff members realize the many risk management responsibilities they each have when carrying out their jobs. Some of these responsibilities are described in Exhibit 2-4. All staff members should be involved in the development of the comprehensive risk management plan. Not only will their input be valuable, but, they also will feel a sense of ownership by being directly involved and, thus, understand the importance of carrying out the risk management plan.

Risk Management Advisory Committee

Many organizations such as hospitals, corporations, and common carriers such as the airlines have a risk management department that is managed by professionals educated, trained, and certified in risk management. The experts working in these departments develop, implement, and monitor the organization's risk management plan to help minimize losses for the organization. However, fitness facilities, generally, do not have a risk management department or a full-time professional risk management manager. Therefore, to provide guidance and expertise in the development of a comprehensive risk management plan, fitness managers need to form a **risk management advisory committee** (RMAC) made up of experts in the legal, medical, and insurance areas. Fitness managers working for an organization that has a risk management

department should also consider having a representative within this department to serve on the fitness facility's RMAC.

Legal counsel is needed for a variety reasons such as development of risk management strategies that reflect the law, preparing contracts, etc. Having a licensed health care provider such as a physician will be helpful when making decisions regarding pre-activity screening procedures, emergency action plans, etc. It is important to note that (a) some professional organizations have published standards of practice (standards of practice are discussed in Chapter 4) that recommend facilities have a medical advisory committee, medical advisor, or medical liaison, and (b) the failure to have a medical liaison or advisory committee was one of the negligence claims against the facility in the *Baldi-Perry* case. See Exhibit 2-3. An insurance expert can provide guidance regarding the many types of insurance (e.g., general liability, professional liability, cyber security) that is needed given the programs/services provided. It is recommended that fitness facilities employ a clinical exercise physiologist, as discussed in Chapter 7, because many fitness participants have a medical condition or multiple medical conditions (15). Expertise in clinical expertise is needed to safely design/deliver exercise programs for these individuals. For fitness facilities that do not hire a clinical exercise physiologist, it is recommended to have someone with this expertise serve on the RMAC who can, perhaps, provide guidance to fitness staff members working with these populations.

Fitness managers and exercise professionals will learn about the law and how to apply it through risk management by reading this textbook. It will help them acquire a working knowledge of the law to intelligently communicate legal/risk management issues with the experts on their RMAC. However, this textbook does not cover all situations that can arise (e.g., each facility may have legal/risk management situations that pertain to only that facility and, of course, there are local and state laws, in addition to federal laws, that will need to be addressed by each facility). It is recommended that fitness managers and exercise professionals use this textbook with their RMAC as they go through the 4-step risk management, decision-making process and to obtain input and assistance from their RMAC experts when unique or challenging situations arise.

Exhibit 2-4: Key Risk Management Responsibilities of Staff Members

Manager: Has overall responsibility for the facility's risk management plan; Primary liaison with Risk Management Advisory Committee; Ensures that staff members with risk management responsibilities are trained, supervised, and evaluated so that the risk management plan is carried out properly; Ensures staff members are qualified and competent prior to employment

Directors: Working with the Manager, Directors (e.g., fitness director, building supervisor, child care director, marketing/sales director, wellness coordinator) are responsible for the development of the risk management plan in their respective areas; Train, supervise, and evaluate their staff members to help ensure they are properly carrying out the risk management plan; Ensure their staff members are qualified and competent prior to employment

Personal Fitness Coordinator: Working with the Health/Fitness Director, is responsible for the development of the risk management plan involving the personal fitness training program; Trains, supervises, and evaluates personal fitness trainers to help ensure they are properly carrying out the risk management plan; Ensure their personal fitness trainers are qualified and competent prior to employment

Personal Fitness Trainers: Carry out risk management policies and procedures related to client safety, such as proper pre-activity health screening, instruction, and supervision

Group Exercise Coordinator: Working with the Health/Fitness Director, is responsible for the development of the risk management plan involving the group exercise program; Trains, supervises, and evaluates group exercise leaders to help ensure they are properly carrying out the risk management plan; Ensure their group exercise leaders are qualified and competent prior to employment

Group Exercise Leaders: Carry out risk management policies and procedures related to participant safety, such as proper instruction and supervision

Clinical Exercise Physiologist: If the fitness director does not have adequate knowledge, skills, and abilities in clinical exercise then a clinical exercise physiologist should be hired who would work with all fitness staff members to help ensure that risk management strategies are properly carried out, e.g., programs and services for participants who have medical risks and/or certain medical conditions are "safely" designed and meet the current standard of care

Fitness Floor Staff: Carry out risk management policies and procedures properly, e.g., supervise participants to help ensure they are adhering to the facility's safety policies/procedures and utilizing the exercise equipment properly; Report/document incidents that occur, e.g., equipment breaking down, participant non-adherence to safety policies/procedures or misuse of equipment

Nutrition/Weight Management Staff: Carry out risk management policies and procedures properly related to nutrition and weight management programs including proper scope of practice, e.g., provide "general" non-medical nutrition information to participants—only licensed (as required by many state statues) professionals such as Registered Dietitians can provide "individualized" nutritional/dietary advice

Health/Wellness Coaches: Carry out risk management policies and procedures properly related to coaching services provided over the Internet and by phone, e.g., contractual terms including the limitations involved in these services are clearly communicated; Practice within proper scope, e.g., educational and motivational strategies only

Sales Staff: Carry out risk management policies and procedures properly related to sales, e.g., sections within membership contracts such as a waiver of liability are communicated properly

Front Desk Staff: Carry out risk management policies and procedures properly, e.g., certain aspects of the pre-activity health screening process and the medical emergency action plan

Child Care staff: Carry out risk management policies and procedures properly to help ensure safe child care programs and services

Maintenance and Housekeeping Staff: Carry out risk management policies and procedures properly related to the maintenance and cleaning of the facility

For example, it is important for all fitness facilities to conduct pre-activity health screening as discussed in Chapter 6. However, this may be challenging for facilities with very large groups of prospective participants like colleges and universities. Fitness managers and exercise professionals can consult with their RMAC who can help them come up with a screening process that is cost-effective, prudent, and appropriate. At times, fitness managers and exercise professionals will work with individual members of the RMAC and, at other times, the whole committee may need to work together. As the comprehensive risk management plan is being developed, it will be important to maintain good communication with everyone on the RMAC and, of course, proper record-keeping of all communications such as meeting agendas and minutes.

Strategic Planning

As stated above, strategic planning skills are important for the professionals leading the development of a comprehensive risk management plan for the fitness facility. **Strategic planning** is a decision-making process that takes time and effort. The term strategic planning infers that some decisions are more important than others and, therefore, the process can create challenges to prioritize the risk management strategies that need to be developed. Although there are many strategic planning models, a basic strategic model that can be applied to risk management could include the following six steps:

1. **Identify mission.** For example, a mission statement something like the following could be adopted. *It is the mission of _____ (name of facility) to provide a reasonably safe facility and programs/services to our participants. We consider the safety of our participants our most important responsibility. We believe that these efforts also result in the delivery of high-quality programs/services that will lead to increased satisfaction and retention among our valued participants.*

2. **Select goals.** For example, the risk management goals of _____ (name of facility) are:
   - Reduce the frequency and severity of injuries
   - Decrease the number of legal claims and lawsuits
   - Increase the efficiency of daily operations (e.g., staff members know how to properly perform job tasks/carry out risk management policies and procedures)
   - Enhance productivity of staff members (e.g., less time dealing with problems/crises and more time on program improvement/expansion)
   - Improve the quality of programs and services (e.g., staff members know how to design/deliver safe and effective programs)
   - Increase participant satisfaction and retention
   - Increase profits (e.g., higher revenue from increased staff productivity and participant satisfaction/retention and lower expenses such as litigation costs and reduced insurance premiums)
   - Enhance the reputation of the exercise profession especially among healthcare providers

3. **Identify risk management strategies that need to be developed.** For example, once a risk management audit (described later under Step 2) is completed, a list is prepared of the risk management strategies that need to be developed such as (a) written pre-activity screening procedures, (b) written equipment maintenance procedures, and (c) written emergency action plans. The list of "strategies to be developed" then needs to be prioritized by the professional staff and RMAC.

4. **List the action steps needed to develop each risk management strategy.** For example, action steps involved in the development of pre-activity screening procedures would address questions such as (a) how will new participants be informed of the purposes of screening, (b) what screening device(s) will be used, (c) what criteria warrant medical clearance, (d) how will medical clearance be obtained, (e) how will screening data be kept private, confidential, and secure, and (f) what if participants refuse to complete the screening procedures.

5. **Develop a draft of the written risk management strategy.** For example, a designated exercise professional(s) completes the action steps within a certain timeframe and then prepares a draft of the written risk management strategy.

6. **Evaluate/revise and finalize the draft.** The draft is shared with the stakeholders (e.g., professional

staff members and RMAC) for feedback and revisions. Once all feedback is submitted, revisions are made, and a final draft is reviewed again by the stakeholders.

Following these steps will help fitness managers and exercise professionals better manage the complex task of developing a comprehensive risk management plan. It will help to simplify the administrative process for everyone involved by breaking it down into meaningful parts (e.g., first identifying what needs to be done and then listing the steps on how to get it done). No doubt it will take time to address the risk

KEY POINT

Building a comprehensive risk management plan involves strategic planning to carry out four essential steps—(1) assessment, (2) development, (3) implementation, and (4) evaluation—with the assistance and guidance of an expert Risk Management Advisory Committee. Fitness managers and exercise professionals need to possess strategic planning skills to complete these four steps.

management strategies that need to be developed but the many benefits achieved (e.g., accomplishing the goals listed above) will make it worth the effort.

STEP 1—ASSESSEMENT OF LEGAL LIABILITY EXPOSURES

| Assessment of Legal Liability Exposures | | Development of Risk Management Strategies | | Implementation of the Comprehensive Risk Management Plan | | Evaluation of the Comprehensive Risk Management Plan |

As defined above, legal liability exposures are situations that create a risk of an injury or reflect noncompliance to federal, state, and/or local laws. First, it is important to become familiar with federal, state, and local laws that apply to fitness facilities and programs/services. It is impossible for this textbook to cover all these laws. Fitness managers and exercise professionals need to consult with their legal counsel regarding the laws covered, and not covered, in this textbook to help ensure compliance with all applicable laws. Chapter 3 focuses on federal laws such as discrimination laws (e.g., Americans with Disabilities Act, Title VII of the Civil Rights Act), employment laws, and data privacy and security laws such as the Health Insurance Portability and Accountability Act (HIPAA). This textbook also covers some applicable state laws such as waiver law (Chapter 4) and Automated External Defibrillator (AED) statutes (Chapter 11).

The chapters throughout the textbook describe many legal cases, especially negligence lawsuits. Negligence lawsuits involving fitness facilities are interesting to review not only because case law decisions may set **precedent**—a rule that future similar cases will have

to follow, but also because they demonstrate the many types of negligence claims that plaintiffs (injured parties) bring against exercise professionals and fitness facilities. Each one of these claims can reflect a legal liability exposure. See the many claims the plaintiff filed against the defendants in the *Baldi-Perry* case in Exhibit 2-3. Therefore, one of the best ways to assess legal liability exposures is to review the common negligence claims alleged by plaintiffs in these cases.

In addition to federal, state, and local laws, standards of practice published by professional organizations (e.g., standards, guidelines, and position papers) and independent organizations, such as the American Society of Testing and Materials (ASTM) and equipment manufacturers, need to be carefully reviewed. It is essential that fitness managers and exercise professionals incorporate published standards of practice into their daily operations because they can be considered as admissible evidence to help determine the standard of care (legal duty) in negligence claims and lawsuits, as discussed in Chapter 4. Failing to follow industry standards also can be listed as a negligence claim against defendants as it was in the *Baldi-Perry* case. Adherence to published standards of practice decreases legal liability exposures. Failure to adhere to them increases legal liability exposures.

Although Step 1 (assessment) focuses on identifying applicable laws and published standards of practice as depicted in Figure 2-2, fitness managers and exercise professionals should also consider the following when assessing their legal liability exposures:

1. Review injury reports to become familiar with the types of injuries that have occurred at the facility, e.g., a high number of similar injuries may indicate a certain legal liability exposure(s) that exists in that facility.

2. Conduct a facility inspection to determine if there are any situations that are unique to the facility, e.g., an area where participants must step up or down that is not easily visible that may lead to falls and injuries.

3. Evaluate the demographics of the population that is served, e.g., their age, gender, and health history

KEY POINT

Although there are several ways to assess liability exposures, one of the best ways is to review the negligence and other claims in lawsuits against fitness personnel and facilities such as those made by the plaintiff in the *Baldi-Perry* case listed in Exhibit 2-3 as well as in the many other cases described throughout this textbook.

because certain participants may be at increased risk of injury.

It is important to realize that it is impossible to identify all legal liability exposures that exist, but by following the above approaches, fitness managers and exercise professionals can feel confident that they are on the right track with their risk management efforts. Once the assessment of legal liability exposures is completed, the next step is to develop risk management strategies.

STEP 2—DEVELOPMENT OF RISK MANAGEMENT STRATEGIES

| Assessment of Legal Liability Exposures | → | Development of Risk Management Strategies | → | Implementation of the Comprehensive Risk Management Plan | → | Evaluation of the Comprehensive Risk Management Plan |

As shown in Figure 2-2, there are four types of risk management strategies to consider in the development phase (11). These include **exposure avoidance**—strategies that eliminate the risk of injury such as not providing treadmills and not offering extreme conditioning programs, **loss prevention**—strategies that minimize the risk of injury and reflect compliance with laws, **loss reduction**—strategies that mitigate or reduce the severity of an injury after it occurs such as providing appropriate emergency care, and **contractual transfer of risks**—strategies such as waivers signed by participants and liability insurance. Waivers and liability insurance are applicable after a lawsuit is filed and are described in more detail in Chapters 4 and 5, respectively. Loss prevention strategies that lead to compliance with federal laws are addressed primarily in Chapter 3 but

also in other chapters. However, this textbook focuses on loss prevention strategies that minimize injuries (described in Chapters 5-10) and loss reduction strategies that are described in Chapter 11. Toward the end of each of these chapters (Chapters 5 through 11), there is a **risk management audit** (checklist) that fitness managers and exercise professionals can complete to determine what risk management strategies are (a) developed or (b) not developed in their facility. For those not developed, following strategic planning steps #3 – #6, as described previously, will help finalize the development of each risk management strategy.

Many risk management strategies necessitate the development and implementation of various documents. For example, a loss prevention strategy such as conducting pre-activity health screening involves a pre-activity health screening device and a medical clearance form. A loss reduction strategy such as providing emergency care entails completing an injury report form after an injury occurs. A strategy that involves a contractual transfer of risks such as a waiver of liability would entail having participants sign a waiver prior to participation. Examples of these various documents are presented throughout this textbook. Some of them reflect contracts that need to be reviewed by legal counsel prior to using them. Not only is it important to utilize these documents to help demonstrate adherence to the law and/or the standard of care, it is wise to have a second set of these documents (written and/or electronic) stored at another location. **Duplication** of documents serves as a back-up procedure in case the primary documents are ever lost or destroyed (e.g., in a fire).

STEP 3—IMPLEMENTATION OF THE COMPREHENSIVE RISK MANAGEMENT PLAN

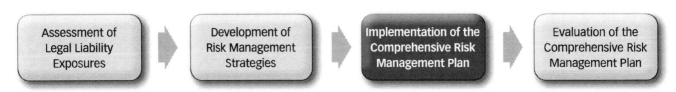

Implementation of the **comprehensive risk management plan** involves two major functions as shown in Figure 2-2: (a) developing a **Risk Management Policies and Procedures Manual**, and (b) conducting staff training. The Risk Management Policies and Procedures Manual should reflect the comprehensive risk management plan of the fitness facility. Comprehensive means that it should contain the written descriptions of the risk management strategies developed in Step 2 that reflect adherence to applicable laws (statutory, administrative, and case law) and standards of practice published by professional and independent organizations. Staff training is essential to help ensure that the policies and procedures in the manual are properly implemented.

Risk Management Policies and Procedures Manual

Various factors need to be addressed in the development of the facility's Risk Management Policies and Procedures Manual (RMPPM). The risk management strategies developed in Step 2 are organized into policies and procedures in the RMPPM. A **policy** is defined as "a definite course or method of action selected from among alternatives and in light of given conditions to guide and determine present and future decisions" and a **procedure** is defined as "a particular way of accomplishing something" or "a series of steps followed in a regular definite order" (16). An example of a policy statement could be something like "It is the policy of this fitness facility to have written Emergency Action Plans (EAPs) that reflect the standard of care and any applicable laws." The procedures related to this policy would be the written action steps that describe what staff members need to do when an evacuation or medical injury occurs as well as inclusion of any related documents (e.g., injury report) and how to properly complete and submit them.

When preparing written risk management procedures that will be inserted into the RMPPM, it is important they are written so they (a) are in a concise sequence that makes sense, (b) are easily understood by staff members, and (c) do not reflect too much detail. Too much detail can result in staff members having to remember more than they may be able to and it can also minimize flexibility given any unique situation that may come up. Therefore, when preparing written risk management procedures, it is important to maintain a balance between being "complete and thorough" and too much written detail that may add confusion or misunderstanding. It may be a good idea, where applicable, to write the risk management procedures using a sequential "step" approach including a brief description below each step.

Once written risk management procedures are finalized and approved by the facility's Risk Management Advisory Committee, they should be inserted into the facility's RMPPM in an organized fashion. See Figure 2-3. For example, the procedures involving the pre-activity health screening process could be inserted behind a tab labeled Pre-Activity Screening and the procedures describing the steps when an evacuation or medical emergency occurs could be inserted behind the tab labeled EAPs, and so on. The policies and procedures in the manual should reflect the major legal liability exposures that exist in the seven areas as shown in Figure 2-1. This manual can then be used as an effective staff training tool and be easily referenced by staff members at any given time. In addition to having hard copies available in the fitness facility, it may also a good idea to have the RMPPM available electronically.

It is wise to have a Preface in the RMPPM that includes the mission statement and goals (as described earlier under strategic planning) of the risk management plan. It is also a good idea to describe the "why" to help convey the importance of the plan. The policies and procedures behind each tab (section) of the RMPPM will describe the "what" and "how" but may not include the "why". To help staff members comply with the risk management policies and procedures, it will be important they understand "why" it is critical they are carried out properly. This section on the "why" would explain how these policies and procedures (a) enhance the safety of participants—the #1 responsibility of staff members and the facility, (b) reflect potential legal duties (standards of care) of staff members and the facility owed to participants, and (c) reflect applicable laws and published standards of practice. It is important that staff members understand that they can be liable for negligent conduct that causes harm to a participant as well as the facility under the legal principle of respondeat superior.

Staff members need to understand and appreciate that once the RMPPM is put into place, it may be discovered and reviewed in litigation involving the facility, which is another reason why the plan be carefully developed, implemented, and followed once adopted. A failure to follow the plan may lead to claims of negligence in the event of a lawsuit. For example, see *Lotz v. The Claremont Club*, spotlight case in Chapter 8. Lastly, it is important to explain to staff members (and to include a statement on the title page in the front of RMPPM) that the RMPPM is an internal, copyrighted document. It should only be used by the staff members within the facility and that no part of it should be reprinted or given to anyone without obtaining appropriate permission. Obviously, staff training is essential in the implementation of the comprehensive risk management plan and is discussed next.

Figure 2-3: Risk Management Policies and Procedures Manual

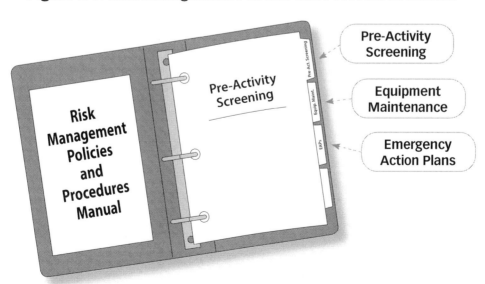

Staff Training

According to Mathis and Jackson, training is a "process whereby people acquire capabilities to aid in the achievement of organizational goals" and it "provides employees with specific, identifiable knowledge and skills for use in their present jobs" (17, p.172). To help achieve the goals of the comprehensive risk management plan and ensure that the policies and procedures in the RMPPM are carried out properly, staff training that focuses on the "what", "how", and "why" is a must. Fitness managers and other supervisors of employees such as assistant directors and program coordinators, should understand that many of their staff members, probably, have had little or no education or training in the law and risk management, Therefore, staff training programs will need to include some basic background in these areas. Fitness managers and other supervisors may first need to obtain the necessary education in the law and risk management before they feel comfortable leading the training efforts for their staff members. Of course, that is the main purpose of this textbook—to provide this education for fitness managers, supervisors, and exercise professionals.

The major cost associated with staff training will be salaries and wages related to the time the fitness manager or other supervisors prepare and present the trainings and paying staff members to attend the trainings. These costs are minimal compared to the costs associated with even one lawsuit, which can be in the hundreds of thousands, if not millions of dollars, not to mention the significant amount of staff time of the defendants (exercise professional, facility manager) to prepare answers to interrogatories and provide testimony. Non-monetary consequences also need to be considered such as the emotional stress of the defendants given that lawsuits may take years before they are finalized and the negative publicity for the facility. Therefore, the benefits of staff training (minimizing legal liability as well as achieving the other goals of risk management listed above under strategic planning) far outweigh the costs. Given the importance of staff training, the (a) types of staff training, (b) timeframe for staff training, and (c) documentation of staff training are presented next.

Types of Staff Training

Three major types of staff training include: (a) internal, (b) external, and (c) e-learning (17). Internal training is, probably, the most common type of training used in fitness facilities and involves both informal training and on-the-job (OTJ) training. Informal training occurs "through interactions and feedback among employees" (17, p. 289). Examples of informal training include: (a) an employee asks his/her supervisor a question regarding a specific risk management procedure and then the supervisor answers that question, and (b) a supervisor notices an employee not carrying out a certain risk management procedure properly then provides some retraining in a timely fashion for the employee.

Unlike informal training, OTJ training (also referred to as in-service training) should be well-planned and follow a logical progression such as the Four P's of Training as shown in Figure 2-4. Because OTJ training is conducted by fitness managers and other supervisors, it is essential that they can effectively teach (e.g., *prepare* and *present* lesson plans) employees how to implement the risk management procedures in the RMPPM. It will be important to make the OTJ training sessions interesting for employees. Just describing all the risk management procedures in the RMPPM they need to follow may be a "boring" approach. Perhaps starting with a relevant legal case that includes the issues (liability exposures) that apply to the risk management procedures presented in the training session will help provide a meaningful and effective experience. There are many cases presented in this textbook to use for this purpose.

When delivering in-service training programs, it is also important to prevent a common training error

Figure 2-4: Four Ps of Staff Training

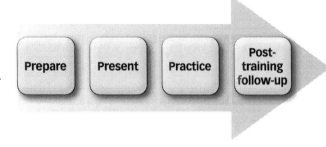

—feeding too much information at one time (18). The entire risk management plan reflected in the RMPPM will be quite complex and will cover a lot of different risk management procedures. It will be necessary to break down the in-service trainings by various risk management topics. For example, a risk management in-service training session on the pre-activity health screening procedures should, perhaps, just cover this area and not attempt to address any other areas at that time.

Having the employees *practice* the tasks related to the risk management procedures will actively engage them in the learning process during the training session. One way to do this is through role-playing. For example, after presenting the procedures on how to carry out the medical emergency EAP, one employee can play the role of the injured party and another employee plays the role of the first responder. The role-playing exercise is then discussed and evaluated by the instructor and other employees in the training. *Post-training follow-up* would involve direct observation of employees as they carry out risk management procedures while on the job and providing positive feedback when performing tasks correctly and constructive feedback and retraining when tasks are performed improperly. Post-training follow-up also involves having staff employees evaluate the training program which will provide feedback on how to improve the training the next time it is offered.

External training (17) may also be an option to consider when providing risk management training. This involves bringing in outside resources (outsourcing) to provide the training. Because the risk management strategies in the RMPPM will be specifically tailored to each individual fitness facility, it will be difficult to, perhaps, outsource the risk management training involving the facility's comprehensive risk management plan. However, fitness facilities may want to have some of the experts on their risk management advisory committee involved, periodically, in risk management training. They should be familiar with most aspects of the RMPPM and may bring in different perspectives that not only help stress the importance of properly carrying out the risk management strategies but will help reinforce what fitness managers and other supervisors are trying to accomplish. External training could also involve officials from federal, state, and local governments. For example, when conducting a training

> **KEY POINT**
>
> Staff training is an essential component of a comprehensive risk management plan. Therefore, it is important that fitness managers and other supervisors providing training programs possess excellent teaching skills and know how to apply the four P's of staff training—prepare, present, practice, and post-training follow-up.

session on the Bloodborne Pathogens Standard, a government official from the Occupational Safety and Health Administration (OSHA) could be invited to kick-off this training session. When appropriate, utilizing outside experts to address the many topic areas covered in the RMPPM can help add interesting and enjoyable dimensions to the educational process.

According to Mathis and Jackson, "e-learning is defined as the use of the Internet or an organizational intranet to conduct training on-line" (17, p. 291). Using the Internet and the facility's intranet should be considered when planning risk management training. The many Internet sites listed as resources in this textbook provide excellent information that can be used when establishing the content of in-service training programs. Employees can be referred to these sites to enhance their own learning or in preparation of an in-service training. The facility's intranet training may be ideal for fitness facilities for their risk management training because it can restrict access to only authorized users such as employees. In addition to posting the RMPPM on the facility's intranet, various on-line training modules could be designed and implemented. For example, a training module could be designed that addresses the procedures related to the facility's medical emergency EAP. Employees would read through the EAP information and then answer questions covering that information that would then be submitted to their supervisor for evaluation and feedback. This type of online training may also be beneficial to help prepare employees for a traditional in-service training session that they will be required to attend.

Finally, when considering the type of staff training, it is important to consider how it will be delivered. Staff training can be done individually, in small groups (e.g., all personal trainers who are newly hired), or large groups (e.g., all staff members). The approach selected (individual, small group, or large group) will be largely determined by the specific risk management training objectives. For example, when providing training related to the facility's pre-activity health screening process, certain staff members need to attend (i.e., those who have direct responsibility for any of the steps involved with these procedures). If this involves only a few (e.g., three to six) staff members, all of them could attend one training session. If this involves a large number of employees, it may be necessary to have two to three training sessions so that there are not too many attendees in any one session. Again, in each training session, the employees should be able to practice the risk management procedures and receive feedback from the instructor regarding their performance. An individual training may be necessary for a newly hired employee that will have responsibilities for pre-activity screening procedures. A different staff training session regarding the facility's pre-activity health screening procedures may also be necessary for those staff members who do not have "direct" responsibilities for pre-activity health screening, but need training to understand and support these procedures, if ever asked by participants. This type of training could be offered to a large number of employees.

Timeframe for Staff Training

There are several times throughout the year that fitness managers and other supervisors should be conducting OTJ or in-service risk management trainings for their staff members. Obviously, when a new staff member is hired, orientation training will be needed regarding his/her risk management responsibilities. Again, because the RMPPM covers a lot of areas, the training needed for a new employee should, perhaps, be divided into several training sessions and prioritized based on the employee's responsibilities. For example, a new fitness floor supervisor will first need to learn his/her risk management responsibilities regarding supervising participants while using exercise equipment as well as the facility's Emergency Action Plans (EAPs). A newly hired personal trainer may need to first learn how to properly implement the pre-activity health screening procedures established by the facility and the facility's EAPs. Once the priority training sessions have been completed, the supervisor of the employee should

establish a plan so that the remaining risk management training sessions are also completed in a timely fashion. Of course, it is the supervisor's responsibility to follow-up by observing the performance of each new employee after training to be sure the facility's risk management procedures are being carried out properly. If they are not being carried out appropriately, re-training would be necessary.

Many of the risk management procedures in the RMPPM reflect things that are done on a daily or regular basis by sstaff members, such as pre-activity health screening, fitness testing and prescription, instruction/supervision, and equipment/facility inspections and maintenance. Therefore, once staff members responsible for these procedures are trained and their supervisors have followed-up to help ensure they are being carried out properly; additional training should not be needed. However, there are some risk management procedures that are not carried out daily, such as the EAPs (evacuation and medical emergency EAPs as described in Chapter 11), which are carried out when needed. Although all staff members should be well trained on how to implement the EAPs upon hiring, it is something that staff members could easily forget because it is not something they do regularly. Therefore, it should be the policy of all health/fitness facilities to provide EAP training on a regular basis, perhaps three-four times throughout the year. These regular trainings should include mock emergency situations, perhaps some announced and some unannounced. In addition, follow-up EAP procedures (e.g., how to properly complete the injury report) need to be reviewed and practiced.

Training may also be necessary after performance appraisals are conducted. Performance appraisals are completed to evaluate employee performance and are usually done during and after an employee's probationary or introductory period, and then annually thereafter. More information on performance appraisals is provided in Chapter 8. How well the employee is carrying out his/her risk management responsibilities should be included in the performance appraisal process. If it is determined that an employee has not adequately performed his/her risk management responsibilities, it will be important that follow-up training be provided and then re-assessment of performance after a given timeframe.

Finally, staff training will be needed if, at any time, changes or revisions are made with the risk management policies and procedures in the RMPPM (see Evaluation of the Risk Management Plan below). For example, if changes are made with the equipment/facility inspection procedures, it will be important that these changes are made in all copies (hard and soft) of the RMPPM first. Then, those staff members directly involved in carrying out these procedures would need to attend a training session to learn and practice the newly changed/revised procedures. In addition, it is likely that some changes with the facility's risk management procedures will occur, at least, annually after the formal evaluation of the entire Comprehensive Risk Management Plan (see Summative Evaluation below). Obviously, when this occurs, staff members will need to be retrained so they are well informed of the changes.

Documentation of Staff Training

As possible future defendants, fitness managers and other supervisors will, likely, need to provide evidence that they did, indeed, provide staff training. The facility's failure to provide staff training is a common negligence claim made by plaintiffs in lawsuits. For example, see the several claims against the facility related to staff training made by the plaintiff in the *Baldi-Perry* case in Exhibit 2-3. Many of the other negligence cases described in this textbook also involved these types of claims.

Documentation is important to prove that proper training did occur. First, it will be important to document the dates when the training sessions were held and the staff members who attended each training session. It is also a good idea to document the content that was covered in each training session—another good reason to have a written lesson plan for each training session. Documentation is also important for internal purposes. As employees attend and participate in staff training sessions, it should be documented in their personnel files. In addition, documentation will help keep track of the staff members who have completed staff training and those who have not, therefore, making it easier to follow-up with those who still need to attend certain training sessions.

STEP 4—EVALUATION OF THE COMPREHENSIVE RISK MANAGEMENT PLAN

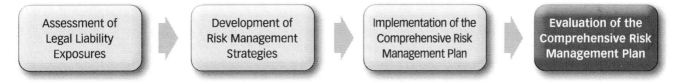

Evaluation of the comprehensive risk management plan involves both **formative evaluation** and **summative evaluation** as shown in Figure 2-2. Many fitness managers and exercise professionals are familiar with these evaluations because they are used to evaluating their fitness/wellness programs. For example, formative evaluations are conducted on an on-going basis throughout the assessment, development, and implementation phases of a program to identify any adjustments, changes, improvements that may be needed. Summative evaluation is conducted at the end of the program to determine if the program should be continued and/or modified before it is offered again as well as to determine if the program was effective. For example,

did participants change their behavior and/or reduce their health risks, was the program cost-effective, and were program goals/objectives met. Although a fitness facility's comprehensive risk management plan is not considered a fitness/wellness program per se, it does reflect a "proactive administrative process" that can be evaluated using both formative and summative approaches as described next.

Formative Evaluation

Formative evaluations of the comprehensive risk management plan should be conducted on an on-going basis. For example, as discussed above regarding staff trainings, staff members should have the opportunity to evaluate the training sessions they attended. This feedback will help determine if any changes/improvements should be made with the training program before it is offered again. Other examples of formative evaluation include:

1. **Risk management procedures in the RMPPM.** At times, it may be necessary to revise or add risk management procedures in the RMPPM (e.g., if a problem arises with a certain procedure such as staff members having difficulty understanding it or carrying it out). It is best to solve the problem in a timely fashion with the guidance/feedback of the facility's RMAC if needed.

2. **After an injury occurs.** The fitness manager and others in supervisory roles need to review what happened and determine if the medical emergency EAP was carried out properly by staff members including proper completion of the injury report form. For example, it will be important to obtain answers to questions such as: (a) could the medical emergency have been prevented, (b) is there a particular risk or danger in the facility that exists that needs to be addressed, (c) are changes needed with any of the EAP risk management procedures, and (d) do staff members need to be retrained on any of their EAP responsibilities? This type of formative evaluation may result in fewer injuries and any subsequent liability in the future.

3. **Observance of improper performance of an employee.** Improper performance can include teaching a client or a fitness class in an unsafe manner, not following the safety policies of the facility, and not adhering to the policies and procedures in the RMPPM. Once the improper performance is observed in an informal manner (e.g., general supervision) or formal manner (e.g., during a performance appraisal), the fitness manager (or the supervisor) needs to meet with the employee and provide constructive feedback and assistance (retraining perhaps) regarding the behavior observed.

Summative Evaluation

Summative evaluation of the risk management plan involves a formal, annual review of the entire Comprehensive Risk Management Plan and includes (a) making revisions with the RMPPM to reflect any changes in laws and/or published standards of practice, and (b) measuring outcomes such as have the goals of the comprehensive risk management plan been met? The law is always evolving, and it is essential to stay abreast of any new laws or changes with current laws. For example, over the past decade, several states have passed legislation that require fitness facilities to have an AED and it is likely this trend will continue to expand to other states. More information on AED legislation is covered in Chapter 11. In addition, professional and independent organizations, periodically, publish updated versions or editions of their standards of practice. The first edition of *ACSM's Health/Fitness Facility Standards and Guidelines* was published in 1992 and the current publication (2019) is in its fifth edition. Changes occurred with each edition of this publication. For the comprehensive risk management plan to remain current, it will be important to revise/update the risk management procedures in the RMPPM to reflect changes/additions with laws and published standards of practice, so it is compliant with the law and the standard of care.

Summative evaluation also involves measuring outcomes of the comprehensive risk management plan (e.g., achievement of the risk management goals such as those listed above under strategic planning). For example, one way to measure if the fitness facility has met the top two goals—a reduction in the frequency and severity of injuries and the number of subsequent legal claims/lawsuits—is to review all the incident report forms in the past year and ask questions such as: (a) have there been fewer and less severe injuries in the past year when compared to the previous year? and (b) have there been fewer legal claims and lawsuits filed against the facility in the past year when compared to the previous year? If the answer is "yes" to these questions, it is likely due to the facility's risk management efforts. It is a good idea to track these types of data and to share it with staff members, risk management advisory committee members, others who have a vested interest in the facility (e.g., owners, CEOs, Board of Directors, etc.), and with the facility's insurance provider. The insurance provider may value positive outcomes and, perhaps, lower the annual liability insurance premium for the facility.

Another risk management goal, to increase efficiency of daily operations, is especially important for fitness managers, supervisors, and exercise professionals. Individuals in these positions have numerous responsibilities including risk management. When the risk management procedures in the RMPPM reflect major legal liability exposures, numerous daily operations automatically become more efficient. For example, well-trained staff members will know how to properly carry out risk management procedures or job tasks such as pre-activity screening, equipment/facility inspections, safe instruction, emergency procedures, etc. Well-trained staff members allow fitness managers and other supervisors to spend less time in a "reactive" mode (e.g., dealing with staff member problems and complaints from participants) and spend more time in a "proactive" mode such as focusing on activities that lead to continued improvement and expansion of programs/services. Spending too much time in a reactive mode is not productive and creates job stress. Mathis and Jackson define productivity as "a measure of the quantity and quality of work done, considering the cost of the resources used" (17, p. 31) and is often evaluated at the time of an annual performance appraisal. Fitness managers, supervisors, and exercise professionals who have taken the time and effort to develop and implement a comprehensive risk management plan, will likely receive a "high" rating in the area of productivity as well as kudos for reductions in the number of injuries/litigations and improvements in the quality of programs/services.

Another goal of risk management—to enhance the quality of programs/services offered to participants—can also be measured. A key component of risk management is to have credentialed, competent, and well-trained employees who make every effort to teach and provide the safest and most effective programs/services possible. The quality of instruction and supervision that participants receive from employees can be evaluated through both informal and formal supervision strategies as described in Chapter 8. High quality programs/services provided to participants will help to keep participants satisfied and help meet another primary goal of most facilities—to retain their participants. The quality of programs and services can be evaluated by obtaining feedback from participants through questionnaires, surveys, etc. The many positive outcomes that result from a comprehensive risk

management plan can lead to increased profits for the fitness facility and perhaps, most importantly, an enhanced reputation of the exercise profession as shown in Figure 2-5. Enhancing the reputation of the exercise profession will be critical as efforts to work with the healthcare profession through initiatives such as Exercise is Medicine® (discussed in Chapter 7) continue to grow.

Figure 2-5: Positive Outcomes of a Comprehensive Risk Management Plan

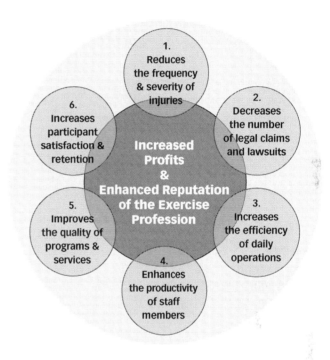

CREATING A SAFETY CULTURE

A **safety culture** can be defined as "a set of core values and behaviors that emphasize safety as an overriding priority" and "expressed through what is said and done—through behavior" (19). Because the safety of participants is the #1 responsibility of fitness managers, supervisors, and exercise professionals, it should be clearly stated in the fitness facility's mission statement and core values. However, core values are only effective if the leadership team ensures that (a) staff members are aware of them and why they are important, (b) they are practiced and upheld when making decisions, and (c) they are integrated into the facility's culture (20).

Building a comprehensive risk management plan using the four steps described in this chapter (assessment, development, implementation, and evaluation) is an important first step in creating a safety culture. But there is more to consider when striving toward a true safety culture. For example, participants of fitness facilities also have safety responsibilities. These responsibilities can be covered in the facility orientation for new participants. Chapter 10 describes six topics that fitness staff members, who provide the instruction for the facility orientations, can cover to help ensure participants understand their safety responsibilities and the facility's safety policies. A facility orientation that focuses on safety sends a positive message to new participants that the facility truly cares about their safety.

A fitness facility's safety culture can be measured by assessing the attitudes and behaviors of employees—a recommendation of safety culture experts. Employees can complete an anonymous survey like the one in Exhibit 2-5. A similar survey could be developed to ask a random sample of fitness participants about their perceptions of the facility's safety culture. The data from the surveys may be helpful for fitness managers, supervisors, and exercise professionals to identify common safety culture issues and steps that can be taken to address the issues. To administer the employee survey, the following steps can be taken: (a) survey is completed by employees anonymously, (b) aggregate results are shared/discussed at employee staff meetings, (c) action steps are developed to make improvements, and (d) survey is completed by employees, again, after 6 -12

KEY POINT

Creating a safety culture involves having all staff members actively engaged in carrying out the facility's comprehensive risk management plan while establishing safety as a "true" core value making it an overriding priority of the fitness facility.

months to evaluate progress. Another resource to help evaluate safety culture is *25 Signs You Have an Awesome Safety Culture* (21). To conclude this section on safety culture, a couple of quotes (22) are provided:

"A health and safety problem can be described by statistics but cannot be understood by statistics. It can only be understood by knowing and feeling the pain, anguish and depression and shattered hopes of the victim and of the wives, husbands, parents, children, grandparents and friends..." (George Robotham, Safety Advocate).

"An incident is just the tip of the iceberg, a sign of a much larger problem below the surface" Don Brown (Owner, Director of Software Products and Services for BasicSafe).

There are many reasons to create a safety culture as described throughout this textbook. Many of these reasons are summarized in a short article titled: Top Five Reasons to Make Fitness Safety Priority No. 1 (23).

Exhibit 2-5: Employee Safety Culture Survey

	YES	NO	DON'T KNOW
1. Safety is emphasized in the fitness facility's mission, vision, or core values.			
2. Fitness facility safety policies and procedures have been established for employees to follow.			
3. New employees receive an orientation or training that focuses on the facility's safety policies and procedures.			
4. The fitness facility managers/supervisors provide in-house safety trainings for employees, e.g., periodic reviews or updates on safety policies/procedures.			
5. Safety issues are placed on the agenda and discussed at scheduled staff meetings.			
6. Employee performance regarding adherence to the facility's safety policies and procedures is formally evaluated by managers/supervisors.			
7. Fitness facility managers/supervisors focus on safety when making decisions.			
8. Employees feel comfortable making suggestions to managers/supervisors when safety issues arise.			
9. When an employee or participant reports a safety issue, managers/supervisors act quickly to investigate the issue.			
10. New members/participants complete pre-activity health screening procedures and obtain medical clearance when needed.			
11. Personal fitness trainers and group exercise leaders are well-educated and trained to help ensure they provide safe instruction and supervision.			
12. Personal fitness trainers who design/deliver programs for individuals with medical conditions possess adequate knowledge and skills in clinical exercise.			
13. Safety inspections of the facility and exercise equipment are conducted daily.			
14. The fitness facility has a sign posted in the facility that lists the safety policies that members/participants are to follow.			
15. New members/participants are informed of the facility's safety policies they are to follow prior to their participation in programs and services.			
16. Employees are well-trained on how to approach members/participants exhibiting an unsafe behavior or non-adherence to safety policies.			
17. Employees are required to attend in-house trainings on how to properly carry out the facility's emergency action plan at least two times/year.			
18. After an injury, managers/supervisors evaluate the possible causes and take steps to minimize the injury in the future.			
19. Managers/supervisors genuinely care about the safety of members/participants.			
20. Please describe any suggestions on how to improve the facility's safety culture.			

KEY TERMS

- Comprehensive Risk Management Plan
- Contractual Transfer of Risks
- Duplication
- Exposure Avoidance
- Formative Evaluation
- Legal Liability Exposures
- Loss Prevention
- Loss Reduction

- Negligence
- Policy
- Precedent
- Preventive Law
- Procedure
- Product Defects
- Risk Management
- Risk Management Advisory Committee

- Risk Management Audit
- Risk Management Policies and Procedures Manual
- Risks Inherent in the Activity
- Safety Culture
- Strategic Planning
- Summative Evaluation

STUDY QUESTIONS

The Study Questions for Chapter 2 can be found on the Fitness Law Academy website (www.fitnesslawacademy.com) under Textbook. They are provided in a fillable format for convenience.

REFERENCES

1. Eickhoff-Shemek JM, Herbert DL, Connaughton, DP. *Risk Management for Health/Fitness Professionals: Legal Issues and Strategies.* Baltimore, MD: Lippincott Williams & Wilkins, 2009.
2. National Electronic Safety Commission (NEISS). U.S. Consumer Product Safety Commission. Available at: www.cpsc.gov/LIBRARY/neiss.html. Accessed July 16, 2018.
3. *Injury Research Agenda 2009-2018.* Centers for Disease Control and Prevention (CDC). Available at: https://stacks.cdc.gov/view/cdc/21769. Accessed October 15, 2018.
4. Appenzeller H. (ed). *Risk Management in Sport. Issues and Strategies,* 2nd Ed. Durham, NC: Carolina Academic Press, 2005.
5. Kufahl P. 2017 in Review: Studio Growth, Health Club Changes, Fitness Industry Legalities. *Club Industry.* December 27, 2017. Available at: https://www.clubindustry.com/insights-resources/2017-review-studio-growth-health-club-changes-fitness-industry-legalities. Accessed October 1, 2018.
6. Schoepfer-Bochicchio K. Discrimination Continues in Collegiate Athletics at High Cost. *Athletic Business,* 24-27, June 2018.
7. Eickhoff-Shemek JM, Berg KE. *Physical Fitness: Guidelines* for Success. 4th ed. 2012. Available at: https://www.fitnesslawacademy.com. Accessed November 18, 2018.
8. *Baldi-Perry v. Kaifas and 360 Fitness Center, Inc.* Complaint. Index No. 2010-1927, Supreme Court, Erie County, New York. February 19, 2010.
9. Herbert DL. Recent Verdict Against Personal Trainer—Lessons to be Learned. CPH & Associates. Available at: https://www.cphins.com/recent-verdict-against-personal-trainer-lessons-to-be-learned/. Accessed August 3, 2018.
10. Herbert DL. New York Case Against Personal Trainer Results in $1.4 Million Verdict. *The Exercise, Sports Medicine, Standards & Malpractice Reporter,* 4(4), 49, 51-55, 2015.
11. Head GL, Horn S. *Essentials of Risk Management* Volume I. 3rd Ed. Malvern PA: Insurance Institute of America, 1997.

12. Zabawa BJ, Eickhoff-Shemek, JM. *Rule the Rules of Workplace Wellness Programs.* Chicago, IL: American Bar Association, 2017.
13. Green LW, Kreuter MW. *Health Program Planning: An Educational and Ecological* Approach. 4th Ed. Boston, MA: McGraw Hill Higher Education, 2005.
14. Educational Courses. Fitness Law Academy, LLC. Available at: https://www.fitnesslawacademy.com. Accessed October 15, 2018.
15. Ward, BW, Schiller JS, Goodman, RA. Multiple Chronic Conditions Among U.S. Adults: A 2012 Update. *Preventing Chronic Disease,* 11:130389, April 2014.
16. Merriam Webster Dictionary. Available at: http://www.m-w.com/dictionary. Accessed on October 12, 2018.
17. Mathis RL, Jackson, JH. *Human Resource Management.* 10th Ed. Mason, OH: Thomson South-Western, 2003.
18. Sawyer TH, Smith O. *The Management of Clubs, Recreation and Sport: Concepts and Applications.* Champaign, IL: Sagamore Publishing, 1999.
19. Agnew J. 7 Keys for Creating a Safety Culture. Aubrey Daniels International. July 3, 2013. Available at: https://www.slideshare.net/AubreyDaniels/7-keys-for-creating-a-safety-culture. Accessed October 15, 2018.
20. Cancialosi C. Two Ways to Ensure Your Corporate Culture and Values Align. *Forbes.* July 20, 2015. Available at: https://www.forbes.com/sites/chriscancialosi/2015/07/20/2-ways-to-ensure-your-corporate-culture-and-values-align/#3fa9fcd46e31. Accessed July 2, 2019.
21. Middlesworth M. 25 Signs You Have an Awesome Safety Culture. ErgoPlus. Available at: https://ergo-plus.com/25-signs-you-have-an-awesome-safety-culture. Accessed October 15, 2018.
22. Brown D. 14 Quotes to Strengthen Your Safety Culture. Safety Management Insights, Basicsafe. August 7, 2014. Available at: http://info.basicsafe.us/safety-management/blog/14-quotes-to-strengthen-your-safety-culture. Accessed October 15, 2018.
23. Eickhoff-Shemek J. Top Five Reasons to Make Fitness Safety Priority No. 1. *ACSM's Health & Fitness Journal, 24(1),* 37-38, 2020.

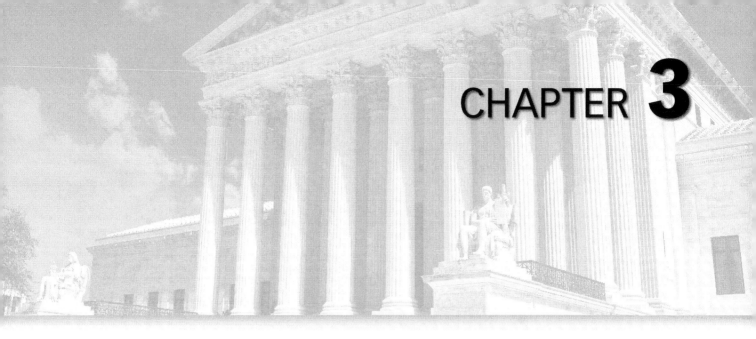

CHAPTER 3

Complying with Federal Laws: Honoring Legal Rights

 LEARNING OBJECTIVES

After reading this chapter fitness managers and exercise professionals will be able to:

1. Identify various federal laws that apply to fitness facilities and exercise professionals.

2. Explain the various forms of discrimination that can occur in fitness facilities and by exercise professionals.

3. Understand that discrimination can occur against both fitness facility employees and participants.

4. Appreciate the importance of complying with data privacy and security laws when collecting employee or fitness participant information.

5. Recognize when HIPAA and other privacy laws apply to fitness facilities and exercise professionals.

6. Describe situations in which fitness facilities could be in violation of the Federal Trade Commission Act (FTCA) or other similar state laws.

7. Know the laws such as the Fair Labor Standards Act (FLSA) and Equal Pay Act (EPA) that pertain to employee wages and hours and how to avoid violating those laws when hiring employees, volunteers and/or interns.

8. Describe the responsibilities of employers and the rights of employees under the OSHA.

9. Explain the importance of complying with the OSHA's General Duty Clause and Hazard Communication Standard.

10. Know how to create a safe workplace in compliance with OSHA and the Clinical Laboratory Improvement Amendments (CLIA).

11. Describe federal laws and agencies that govern wellness products and devices and identify factors that determine a "low-risk" wellness device.

12. Recognize the importance of intellectual property protection and how to avoid intellectual property infringement, such as copyright, patent, or trademark infringement.

13. Explain the importance of purchasing licensing agreements before using music in fitness facilities.

14. Describe the legal mistakes of others through the legal cases presented in this chapter to help learn and appreciate the importance of complying with federal laws.

INTRODUCTION

The law confers legal rights and protections to numerous individuals and organizations involved in the exercise profession. For example, federal and state laws may protect participants or potential participants of fitness facilities from discrimination or privacy violations. The law protects employees from discrimination or harassment, as well as ensures a certain compensation and safe work environment. Federal copyright law protects the rights of those who create content used by fitness facilities and exercise professionals. Finally, certain federal laws such as the Food and Drug Administration (FDA) and the Clinical Laboratory Improvement Act (CLIA) aim to protect users of devices, apps, or supplements as part of a fitness regimen and blood draws as part of a biometric screen.

Fitness managers and exercise professionals must be aware of the state and federal laws that offer these protections to reduce their legal risk and to deliver more effective and inclusive fitness programs. This chapter will highlight federal laws and a number of related state laws in the following six areas:

- Discrimination
- Privacy and Communications
- Employee Wages and Hours
- Employee Safety
- Wellness Products and Devices
- Intellectual Property

To help learn these laws and how to apply them, several spotlight and other case descriptions are provided. In addition, risk management strategies and resources are provided for each of the six areas. It is important to point out that this chapter is not exhaustive. Fitness managers and exercise professionals must be aware of other federal, state, and local laws. For example, employee/supervisor "harassment" training is required by law in some states, but not others. Privacy laws differ from state to state. It is beyond the scope of this textbook to cover all state and local laws. Fitness managers and exercise professionals need to consult with a competent lawyer to become aware of pertinent state and local laws and how to comply with them.

DISCRIMINATION

As described in Chapter 2, discrimination claims against fitness facilities appear to be increasing. Various types of discrimination claims can be made by both fitness facility employees and participants. This is an essential area of law for fitness managers and exercise professionals to understand and to develop risk management strategies to help minimize these claims. This section first provides a general overview of discrimination claims and the laws applicable to these claims. Sections that follow describe discrimination claims that can occur in fitness facilities, including case law examples, as well as resources and risk management strategies to enhance compliance with discrimination laws.

General Overview of Discrimination

Federal discrimination laws, many enforced by the Equal Employment Opportunity Commission (EEOC), exist in several areas as shown in Table 3-1. The EEOC enforces federal discrimination claims that are alleged to have occurred in the workplace. In fiscal year 2018, the most common type of claim brought by an aggrieved employee was a retaliation claim, which made up just over half of the 76,418 charges of discrimination that were filed with the EEOC. An increasingly frequent claim is sexual harassment, which rose by 13.6 percent from 2017. Overall, sexual discrimination claims accounted for just over 30 percent of all charges of discrimination that were filed. The following list shows the distribution of all types of discrimination charges that employees filed with the EEOC in 2018 (1, para. 4). Percentages do not total 100 because some charges allege multiple bases.

- Retaliation: 39,469 (51.6 percent of all charges filed)
- Sex: 24,655 (32.3 percent)
- Disability: 24,605 (32.2 percent)
- Race: 24,600 (32.2 percent)
- Age: 16,911 (22.1 percent)
- National Origin: 7,106 (9.3 percent)
- Color: 3,166 (4.1 percent)
- Religion: 2,859 (3.7 percent)
- Equal Pay Act: 1,066 (1.4 percent)
- Genetic Information: 220 (.3 percent)

Table 3-1	Types of Discrimination Claims and Applicable Federal Law(s)*
DISCRIMINATION CLAIM	**APPLICABLE FEDERAL LAW(S)**
Age	Age Discrimination in Employment Act (ADEA)
Disability	Americans with Disabilities Act (ADA), ADA Amendments Act (ADAAA)
Equal Pay/Compensation	Equal Pay Act (EPA), ADEA, Title VII of the Civil Rights Act of 1964
Genetic Information	Genetic Information Nondiscrimination Act (GINA)
Harassment	Title VII of the Civil Rights Act of 1964, ADEA, ADA
National Origin	Titles II and VII of the Civil Rights Act of 1964, Immigration Reform and Control Act (IRCA) of 1986
Pregnancy	ADA, ADAAA, Family and Medical Leave Act (FMLA) of 1993
Race/Color	Titles II and VII of the Civil Rights Act of 1964
Religion	Titles II and VII of the Civil Rights Act of 1964
Retaliation	Equal Employment Opportunity (EEO) laws
Sex	Title VII of the Civil Rights Act of 1964 (Gender identity, Transgender status, and Sexual orientation)
Sexual Harassment	Title VII of the Civil Rights Act of 1964

*Discrimination by Type. Available at: https://www.eeoc.gov/laws/index.cfm. Accessed November 12, 2019.

From all these charges filed by employees, the EEOC filed 199 discrimination lawsuits against employers in 2018 (1). According to the EEOC, it was 95.7 percent successful in all these lawsuits (1). Whether the various federal employment discrimination laws apply to a fitness facility depends on its size as an employer. For example, the Equal Pay Act applies to employers with one or more employees, Title VII of the Civil Rights Act and the ADA apply to employers with 15 or more employees, and the Age Discrimination in Employment Act applies to employers with 20 or more employees.

Fitness managers and exercise professionals must not only be aware of employment discrimination risks, but also discrimination against individuals who participate in fitness facilities or exercise programs/services. Title II of the Civil Rights Act of 1964 prohibits discrimination because of race, color, religion, or national origin in certain **places of public accommodation** such as health clubs, hotels, restaurants, and places of entertainment. The Department of Justice can bring a lawsuit under Title II when there is reason to believe that a person has engaged in a pattern or practice of discrimination in violation of Title II. The Department can obtain injunctive, but not monetary, relief in such cases. Individuals can also file suit to enforce their rights under Title II and other federal and state statutes may also provide remedies for discrimination in places of public accommodation. The case described below, *Jalal v. Lucille Roberts Health Clubs, Inc.*, dealt with a Title II discrimination claim.

In addition to federal anti-discrimination laws, most states have both employment and public accommodation anti-discrimination laws. Many times, these state anti-discrimination laws are more protective of employee or consumer rights than the federal law. For example, Wisconsin's employment discrimination law protects employees not only from discrimination based on sex, national origin, race and religion, like Title VII, but also prohibits employment discrimination based on marital status, sexual orientation, conviction record, and use of lawful products off the employer's premises during non-working hours (2). Although a full analysis of each state's anti-discrimination law is beyond the scope of this chapter, a summary by the National Conference of State Legislatures (NCSL) of each state's anti-discrimination laws in employment and public accommodation can be found on the NCSL website as follows:

▶ **Discrimination—Employment Laws:**
Available at: www.ncsl.org/research/labor-and-employment/discrimination-employment.aspx. (Accessed November 12, 2019).

▶ **State Public Accommodation Laws:**
Available at: http://www.ncsl.org/research/
civil-and-criminal-justice/state-public-
accommodation-laws.aspx. (Accessed
November 12, 2019).

Fitness managers and exercise professionals should be aware of the state laws in which they operate to ensure that they are complying with those laws, in addition to the various federal laws.

Discrimination: Application to Fitness Facility Employees and Participants

The following five subsections highlight various types of discrimination (religious, sexual, disability, race, and age) that fitness managers and exercise professionals may encounter and the laws that prohibit such discrimination.

Religious Discrimination

People practice many different types of religions. Some religions require observers to behave or dress in certain ways. Because the United States Constitution and the Civil Rights Act give individuals the right to exercise their religious beliefs without discrimination, fitness managers and exercise professionals must be aware of potential religious discrimination claims that may occur. The following case involves a religious discrimination claim made against a health club based on Title II of the Civil Rights Act.

In *Jalal v. Lucille Roberts Health Clubs, Inc.* (3), Yosef Jalal was a Jewish member of Lucille Roberts Health Clubs in New York, which limits membership to women only. Lucille Roberts had a dress code policy that required members to "dress appropriately" while working out. For religious reasons, Ms. Jalal wore a "knee-length, fitted but comfortable skirt" while working out. Health club staff told Ms. Jalal on multiple occasions that she could not wear a skirt while working out at the facility. Management suggested to Ms. Jalal that instead of skirt she wear a long t-shirt. Ms. Jalal noted to health club staff that the dress code did not specifically prohibit wearing skirts. During a kickboxing class, where Ms. Jalal once again was wearing a skirt, the class instructor stopped the music and class

and asked Ms. Jalal to take off her skirt. Ms. Jalal refused, and the health club terminated her membership.

Ms. Jalal sued Lucille Roberts Health Clubs for religious discrimination under Title II of the Civil Rights Act as well as under New York state and city laws. Ms. Jalal argued that the health club treated her differently from other members because of her religion. But, the court disagreed, stating that the health club treated her differently because she insisted on wearing an article of clothing that, according to the health club, was inappropriate gym attire (3). There was no evidence that the health club allowed other non-Jewish women to wear skirts while exercising, or allowed non-Jewish women to violate any other rule of the club. This was significant in the court's decision to dismiss the case. According to the court: "Absent more, the fact that a proprietor has decided to offer his or her services to the public in a way which could impact a religious practice or belief, whether it be by conducting business only on Sundays, failing to keep a Kosher kitchen, by failing to include fish on the menu during Lent, or by prohibiting smoking, raises no inference of discrimination or other conduct which Congress sought to censure through the enactment of Title II" (3, p. 608).

Takeaway lesson from *Jalal*: Even though the court dismissed Ms. Jalal's case for religious discrimination, fitness managers and exercise professionals must be aware that some policies may impact the religious beliefs of fitness clientele. As a result, fitness managers and exercise professionals must be vigilant to ensure that they do not adopt policies that intentionally discriminate against individuals who hold those religious beliefs.

Sexual Discrimination

Each of the following forms of sexual discrimination are described: Employment Discrimination, Sexual Harassment, and Discrimination of Fitness Participants.

Employment Discrimination

Title VII prohibits discrimination based on sex in the employment setting (4). Many state laws prohibit sex discrimination in places of public accommodation, such as fitness facilities. Sex discrimination may take different forms, such as sexual harassment, pregnancy discrimination, sexual orientation discrimination and transgender discrimination. Title VII protects employees from discrimination regardless of their gender and regardless of the gender of the person who is doing the discriminating act. Same-sex discrimination, like opposite-sex discrimination, is actionable under Title VII (5). Thus, a female fitness facility manager can discriminate against a female employee in violation of Title VII, and a male manager can discriminate against a male employee in violation of Title VII.

Sex discrimination under Title VII involves denying equal employment opportunities to any person because of that person's sex, or because a woman is pregnant or based on a gender stereotype. Sex discrimination may include:

- Refusing to hire
- Discharge/firing
- Failing to promote
- Cut in pay or benefits
- Demotion
- Reassignment of duties
- Reassignment to an undesirable position or location
- Denial of opportunities for training and advancement
- Harassment
- Otherwise discriminating against a person with respect to any other term, condition or privilege of employment (6).

In *Bostock v. Clayton County*, the U.S. Supreme Court found that Title VII protects homosexual and transgender employees from discrimination (7). This conclusion aligns with previous EEOC rulings and contradicts the U.S. Department of Justice position, at least under the Trump Administration (8). Fitness managers and exercise professionals should note that given the June 2020 Supreme Court decision on homosexual and transgender employees, it is now illegal to discriminate against these employees under Title VII. In addition, many states have much broader anti-discrimination laws for employees than Title VII. Before the U.S. Supreme Court case found that Title VII protects employees from discrimination based on sexual orientation and gender identity, twenty-one states had those protections already in place through state law (9). For an interesting legal case involving gender identity and fitness centers, see the spotlight case, *Cormier v. Planet Fitness.*

Sexual Harassment

Sexual harassment is a type of employment discrimination based on sex. The U.S. Department of Justice describes sexual harassment as "verbal or physical conduct of a sexual nature" (10, p. 3). The Department of Justice reasons that when an employee is harassed because of their sex, the employer is treating that employee less favorably than employees of another gender (10). "Sexual harassment, if committed or tolerated by the employer, becomes a new and onerous term of employment" (10, p. 3). As an example, a fitness manager who frequently pressures an employee to have sex, and the employee does so for fear of losing his or her job, can constitute "hostile environment" sexual harassment (10). Whether sexual harassment constitutes a violation of Title VII depends on whether a reasonable person would find the work environment hostile and abusive (10). All fitness facilities should have a sexual harassment policy as well as employee training regarding the policy. See the chapter's appendix for a sample of an anti-harassment policy. A case involving hostile environment sexual harassment is featured in the following spotlight case, *Waller v. Blast Fitness Group, LLC.*

KEY POINT

Sexual Harassment

To help avoid claims of sexual harassment and assault, fitness facilities should have policies and procedures that prohibit such behavior and discipline employees who exhibit such behavior. See this chapter's appendix for a sample anti-harassment policy. As with all policies and procedures, fitness facilities should train all employees on the policies and procedures and have employees sign an acknowledgement confirming such training. As demonstrated in the *Waller* case, sexual harassment can occur without physically touching someone. This is in contrast to sexual assault, which involves unwanted touching. See Chapter 5 for further discussion on sexual assault.

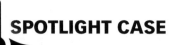

SPOTLIGHT CASE

Waller v. Blast Fitness Group, LLC
No. 4:15CV00586 AGF, 2017 WL 6731721 (E.D. Mo., 2017)

FACTS

Historical Facts:

The regional manager for Blast Fitness, Edgar Thompson, interviewed Terry Waller and offered him a job. Soon after the job offer, Thompson began sending Waller text messages, emphasizing his authority as regional manager, inviting him to spend time with him outside of work. In an in-person interview, Thompson told Waller that "he would get the job only in return for sexual favors" (p. 1). Waller refused and was not hired.

Procedural Facts:

Waller, the plaintiff, filed a charge of sexual harassment and retaliation with the Missouri Human Rights Act (MHRA) and the Equal Employment Opportunity Commission (EEOC). He filed an action against several defendants (collectively "Blast Fitness") including Thompson. He brought two claims under the MHRA—hostile work environment and quid pro quo harassment. The court ruled that Blast Fitness and Thompson were liable on the plaintiff's quid pro quo claim but not on the hostile work environment claim because the plaintiff never began working for Blast Fitness.

Waller testified about his lifelong struggles with asthma and how regular exercise allowed him to live without medication and inhalers. Waller testified that he had dreamed to be a personal trainer and hoped to fulfill this dream with a job at Blast Fitness. However, after being harassed by Thompson, he stopped exercising and his symptoms of asthma returned resulting in a hospital stay—his first since being a teenager. He also testified that he had to seek professional treatment for emotional suffering including depression and anxiety. In addition, Waller testified that he had financial troubles after the incident including a period of homelessness and an inability to maintain employment. Although he had applied for many jobs, he struggled with nervousness during interviews, especially interviews with men because of the harassment by Thompson.

Waller presented a spreadsheet into evidence including loss wages (e.g., the difference between what he would have earned had he been employed by Blast Fitness and his actual wages earned) as well as documents providing evidence of psychotherapy treatments and spreadsheets for the hours billed and costs incurred by his attorneys. Waller requested a judgment totaling more than $2.5 million including (a) economic damages of $28,435.72, (b) compensatory damages for pain and suffering of approximately $1 million, (c) punitive damages of $1.5 million, (d) $94,728.40 in attorney's fees and (d) $2,338.63 in court costs.

ISSUE

Did the court award Waller, the plaintiff, the economic, compensatory, and punitive damages he requested as well as the amounts for attorney fees and court costs?

COURT'S RULING

Yes, the court granted Waller's request for the economic damages he requested and the compensatory and punitive damages but at significantly reduced amounts with all damages totaling $148,435.72. The court reduced the attorney fees to 50% of the requested amount and maintained the court costs.

Waller continued...

COURT'S REASONING

Regarding the economic damages of $28,435.72, the court indicated that the plaintiff provided sufficient evidence to support this request. Regarding compensatory damages for pain and suffering, the court stated, "that he is entitled to compensatory damages for pain and suffering, but the Court cannot sustain Plaintiff's request for approximately $1 million in such damages. Upon review of the record and analogous MHRA cases, the court will award Plaintiff an additional $45,000 in compensatory damages for emotional distress" (p. 2). The court indicated that punitive damages are available under MHRA if the plaintiff provides clear and convincing proof of culpable mental state from actions that are wanton, willful, outrageous or reflect reckless disregard. The court concluded "that Thompson's conduct was quite egregious and that he acted with reckless disregard for the negative consequences his conduct would have upon Plaintiff. Upon review of punitive damages in comparative cases, the Court will award Plaintiff an additional $75,000 in punitive damages" (p. 2).

Regarding the employer's liability, the court stated that "Blast Fitness, as Thompson's employer, is vicariously liable for the above damages...When an employer's liability is vicarious, the employer may raise a 'good faith' defense to punitive damages by proving that the discriminatory employment decisions of managerial agents are contrary to the employer's good-faith efforts to comply with [the MHRA]" (p. 3). A good faith defense requires two necessary elements: "(a) that the employer exercised reasonable care to prevent and correct promptly any sexually harassing behavior, and (b) that the plaintiff employee unreasonably failed to take advantage of any preventative or corrective opportunities provided by the employer to avoid harm otherwise" (p. 3). The court concluded that Blast Fitness did not establish a good faith defense with respect to punitive damages and therefore, "damages will be assessed jointly and severally against Blast Fitness and Thompson" (p. 3).

Lessons Learned from *Waller*:

Legal

- Inappropriate behavior such as sexual harassment by an employee can result in a variety of claims against the employee and the employer through vicarious liability.

- Compensatory damages awarded for such behavior can be economic (e.g., medical costs, lost wages) and non-economic (e.g., pain and suffering). Punitive damages can also be awarded when the behavior is egregious (willful, wanton, reckless) as in this case.

- Regarding vicarious liability, an employer may have a 'good faith' defense to punitive damages if certain elements are met (e.g., the employer acted reasonably to prevent and promptly correct any sexually harassing behavior).

- Joint and several liability allows the plaintiff to demand payment for damages awarded from one or more of the defendants separately or all of them together.

- In addition to compensatory and punitive damages, defendants may also need to pay for the plaintiff's attorney fees and court costs.

Risk Management/Injury Prevention

- Establish a written sexual harassment policy consistent with federal and state laws.

- Train all employees on the policy to help ensure they fully understand it and the importance of following it.

- Provide regular supervision of employees to monitor their conduct/performance while on the job.

- Once informed of sexually harassing behavior by an employee or participant, managers and/or employers need to take prompt, corrective action.

Discrimination of Fitness Participants

To protect the gender-based rights of fitness participants, fitness managers and exercise professionals need to review state anti-discrimination laws. Title VII of the Civil Rights Act only addresses employment discrimination and Title II of the Civil Rights Act does not include gender as a protected class. According to the National Conference of State Legislatures, all but five states (Alabama, Georgia, Mississippi, North Carolina, and Texas) have a public accommodation law that prohibits discrimination on the grounds of gender (11). For example, California's public accommodation law is quite broad and states the following:

> *All persons within the jurisdiction of this state are free and equal, and no matter what their sex, race, color, religion, ancestry, national origin, disability, medical condition, marital status, or sexual orientation are entitled to the full and equal accommodations, advantages, facilities, privileges, or services in all business establishments of every kind whatsoever (12).*

A case from California highlights the problems that can arise for fitness managers and exercise professionals that are accused of sexual harassing participants. A client of Equinox health clubs in San Francisco claimed he was sexually harassed by a yoga instructor (13). The client claimed he reported the harassment and was subsequently banned for life from being a member at the clubs. The client sued outlining nine complaints against the club including discrimination, gender- and/or sex-motivated violence, sexual battery, emotional distress, assault and battery, and retaliation. The club denied the allegations. Regardless of whether the allegations are true, the club's response to the former member has resulted in negative news stories and blog posts about the fitness facility (13).

Fitness managers and exercise professionals who work in states like California must be vigilant in ensuring that their actions and policies for delivering fitness programs/services do not treat individuals, who may be in one of the state's "protected classes," differently. Regarding sexual discrimination

specifically, fitness managers and exercise professionals must avoid sexually harassing participants. They should try to make accommodations to individuals in protected classes so that they can have equal enjoyment of the fitness services they offer. It is important to remember, however, that even when fitness managers and exercise professionals try to accommodate an individual who is part of a protected class, that does not mean they will not face a legal challenge. A good example of a lawsuit that occurred, despite a fitness facility's attempt to accommodate a transgender participant, is described in the following spotlight case, *Cormier v. PF Fitness-Midland, LLC.*

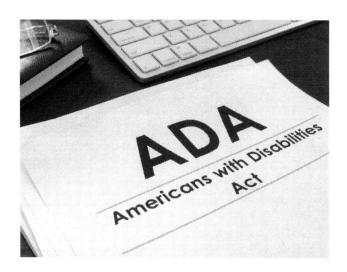

Disability Discrimination

The Americans with Disabilities Act (ADA) was enacted in 1990 by Congress. It contains five titles (14). Titles I and III apply to fitness facilities and programs/services. Title I focuses on employment discrimination and Title III focuses on prohibiting discrimination in places of public accommodation and commercial facilities. Congress revised Title III in 2014 which included increases in the maximum civil penalties. The first violation increased from $55,000 to $75,000 and for subsequent violations, the maximum is $150,000 (15).

Title II of the ADA prohibits discrimination by state and local governments. Fitness facilities and programs/services provided by these government entities need to be familiar with Title II requirements. In addition, Titles II and III require accessibility standards

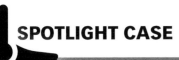

SPOTLIGHT CASE

Cormier v. PF Fitness-Midland, LLC
No. 331286, 2018 LEXIS 2938 (Mich. Ct. App., 2018)

FACTS

Historical Facts:

Plaintiff Yvette Cormier entered into a membership agreement with Defendant PF Fitness-Midland, LLC (Planet Fitness) to use defendant's gym facility in Midland, Michigan on January 28, 2015. On February 28, 2015, she entered the women's locker room and encountered a transgender individual (a man who identified as a woman). Plaintiff left the locker room and told the front desk that there was a man in the women's locker room. Plaintiff was advised that it was defendant's policy that people have access to the facility that corresponds with whatever sex an individual self-identifies. Defendant's corporate office later advised plaintiff that this was consistent with their policy of not judging whether an individual is a man or a woman. Plaintiff returned to the gym several times in the ensuing days and warned other women about the policy and to be careful when using the women's facilities. On March 4, 2015, defendants terminated plaintiff's membership.

Procedural Facts:

Plaintiff sued Planet Fitness in Michigan state court for invasion of privacy, sexual harassment, and retaliation in violation of Michigan law, breach of contract, intentional infliction of emotional distress and violation of the Michigan Consumer Protection Act (MCPA). Defendant moved for summary judgment asserting that plaintiff failed to plead any valid claim. The trial court agreed and granted Defendant's motion. Plaintiff appealed. During the first round of appeal, the Court of Appeals for Michigan upheld the trial court's decision in full. The Michigan Supreme Court (909 N.W.2d. 266, April 2018) then asked the Court of Appeals to reconsider its decision relating to the MCPA claim, which requires businesses, among other things, to reveal facts that are material to a transaction in light of representations of fact made in a positive manner as specified in Michigan Compiled Laws, MCL 445.903(1)(cc).

ISSUE

Did Planet Fitness violate the plaintiff's rights under the MCPA when it failed to disclose to her its policy that assigned men who self-identify as women can use the women's locker room and restrooms?

COURT'S RULING

Yes, plaintiff stated a claim that her MCPA rights may have been violated when Planet Fitness failed to inform her of its policy that assigned men who self-identify as women can use the women's locker room and restrooms. According to the appellate court, a jury could view this as a material fact that would affect the plaintiff's decision to join as a member of the gym.

COURT'S REASONING

Plaintiff's actions indicate that she strongly preferred a locker room and a restroom in which individuals who are assigned biologically male are not present, and it is thus reasonable to infer that defendant's failure to inform plaintiff of the unwritten policy affected her decision to join the gym. "The fact that plaintiff continued to use the gym after learning of the unwritten self-identification policy does not preclude an inference that defendant's failure to inform her of the unwritten policy affected her decision to join the gym. That is because plaintiff was already a member of the gym when she learned of the unwritten policy and was thus subject to a financial penalty if she canceled her membership earlier than provided in the membership agreement" (pp. 13-14). Thus, plaintiff could continue her case at the trial court level on her MCPA claim.

Cormier continued...

Lessons Learned from *Cormier*

Legal

▶ Failing to disclose material facts about gym membership agreements may violate a state's consumer protection laws.

▶ Allowing individuals into locker rooms and restrooms based on gender identity did not violate Michigan's invasion of privacy, breach of contract, sexual harassment, and intentional infliction of emotional distress laws.

▶ Terminating a client's membership because she complained about the fitness center's policy on gender identity did not violate Michigan's invasion of privacy, breach of contract, sexual harassment, and intentional infliction of emotional distress laws.

Risk Management/Injury Prevention

▶ Sometimes fitness managers and exercise professionals may believe they are doing the legally right thing for their participants but may not realize that it can still create a legal case for a certain participant.

▶ To avoid being accused of material misrepresentation, fitness managers and exercise professionals need to evaluate all their written and unwritten policies that a reasonable person would want to know and disclose those policies to participants before they join the fitness facility or receive programs/services.

▶ Fitness facilities may want to consider providing universal changing rooms that can meet the needs of a variety of participants.

under 2010 revisions (16). These standards, the *2010 ADA Standards for Accessible Design*, address requirements for new construction and alterations and are briefly described below and in more detail in Chapter 10. ADA issues involving inclusive exercise equipment are covered in Chapter 9.

It is essential that fitness managers and exercise professionals adhere to the ADA, not only to avoid huge monetary civil penalties, but perhaps, more importantly, to properly serve individuals with disabilities. This population represents many Americans with about one in five reporting they have a disability (17). In addition, according to *Healthy People 2020,* only 36.5% of persons with disabilities are meeting physical activity objectives whereas 58.5% of persons without disabilities are meeting physical activity objectives (18). Therefore, there is a real need to reach these individuals and provide safe and effective exercise programs/services for them.

The following discussion focuses on Titles III and I as they apply to fitness facility programs/services and employment, respectively. However, first, it is important to understand the ADA definition of disability. See Exhibit 3-1. Fitness managers and exercise professionals also need to be familiar with the ADA Amendments

Act (ADAAA) of 2008 (19). With this Act, Congress made it easier for individuals seeking protection under the ADA to establish that they had a disability within the meaning of the statute. For more information on this Act, see "Fact Sheet on the EEOC's Final Regulations Implementing the ADAAA" (19).

Title III—Discrimination of Fitness Participants

As noted above, one of the places that is subject to ADA requirements are places of public accommodation. Places of public accommodation are businesses that are generally open to the public and that fall into one of 12 categories listed in the ADA. Some of these categories include hotels, restaurants, schools, doctors' offices, movie theaters, and fitness facilities (20). Thus, fitness facilities, as places of public accommodation, must comply with the ADA. Often, people believe that Title III only addresses accessibility by providing ramps, etc. but it also requires providing programs/services to meet the needs of individuals with disabilities (e.g., providing reasonable accommodations so that these individuals can fully participate in fitness activities).

Title III requires newly constructed or altered places of public accommodation—as well as commercial facilities

---

Exhibit 3-1: ADA Definition of Disability, In Part*

Disability means, with respect to an individual:

- **A physical or mental impairment that substantially limits one or more of the major life activities of such individual**
- **A record of such an impairment**
- **Being regarded as having such an impairment**

Physical or mental impairment means:

(i) Any physiological disorder or condition, cosmetic disfigurement, or anatomical loss affecting one or more body systems, such as: neurological, musculoskeletal, special sense organs, respiratory (including speech organs), cardiovascular, reproductive, digestive, genitourinary, immune, circulatory, hemic, lymphatic, skin, and endocrine; or (ii) Any mental or psychological disorder such as intellectual disability, organic brain syndrome, emotional or mental illness, and specific learning disability.

Major life activities include, but are not limited to:

(i) Caring for oneself, performing manual tasks, seeing, hearing, eating, sleeping, walking, standing, sitting, reaching, lifting, bending, speaking, breathing, learning, reading, concentrating, thinking, writing, communicating, interacting with others, and working; and (ii) The operation of a major bodily function...

Record of such an impairment:

An individual has a record of such an impairment if the individual has a history of, or has been misclassified as having, a mental or physical impairment that substantially limits one or more major life activities.

Being regarded as having such an impairment:

An individual is "regarded as having such an impairment" if the individual is subjected to a prohibited action because of an actual or perceived physical or mental impairment, whether or not that impairment substantially limits, or is perceived to substantially limit, a major life activity, even if the public accommodation asserts, or may or does ultimately establish, a defense to the action prohibited by the ADA.

---

*Americans with Disabilities Act Title III Regulations. Part 36 Nondiscrimination on the Basis of Disability in Public Accommodations and Commercial Facilities (current as of January 17, 2017). 36.105 Definitions of Disability. Available at: https://www.ada.gov/regs2010/titleIII_2010/titleIII_2010_regulations.htm#a105. (Accessed November 13, 2019).

(privately owned, nonresidential facilities such as factories, warehouses, or office buildings)—to comply with the ADA Standards for Accessible Design (21). The U.S. Department of Justice, Civil Rights Division, has enforcement authority over Title III of the ADA (22). Despite the ADA's requirement that fitness facilities provide equal opportunity to individuals with disabilities to enjoy the facilities, many fitness facilities fall short. Recent studies found that fitness facilities, in general, had a high degree of inaccessibility in several different areas. Areas of greatest inaccessibility concern include customer-service desks, restrooms/locker rooms, drinking fountains, and areas around the exercise equipment (23).

One study focused on sixteen fitness facilities in rural western Wisconsin and found that none of the facilities were 100% ADA compliant (24). Areas in which the facilities received low ratings included training in wheelchair transfer techniques (offered by 0% of facilities), annual continuing education opportunities to prepare employees for adapted programming (7%), and training employees in providing services to individuals with disabilities (8%) (24). These statistics regarding employee education and training are concerning. For more on this topic, see Chapters 5 and 7. The following case, *Neal v. PFTN Murfreesboro South, LLC*, illustrates how fitness facilities may face legal challenges from participants who believe the facility is not accommodating their disability. Another ADA case, described after the *Neal* case, *Class v. Towson University*, involves a student-athlete.

In *Neal v. PFTN Murfreesboro South, LLC* (25), the plaintiff, Deanna Neal suffers from reflexive sympathetic dystrophy (RSD), also known as complex regional pain syndrome (CRPS), which causes chronic pain in her right foot. As a result of the chronic pain, she cannot wear a closed-toe shoe on her right foot but instead wears a flip-flop type shoe at all times when in public. Deanna applied for a membership with Planet Fitness, the defendant, in December 2018. A manager at Planet Fitness contacted her about her application stating it was denied because, if she did not wear closed-toe shoes, it would be a "liability" for the facility. The manager specifically mentioned that Planet Fitness would have to admit other people with disabilities if it allowed her to join and that it did not wish to admit others with disabilities.

The plaintiff filed her complaint on May 14, 2019 alleging that the defendant had discriminated against her in violation of Title III of the ADA. She primarily asked the court to order the defendant to make all "readily achievable alterations to the facility, or to make such facility readily accessible to and usable by individuals with disabilities to the extent required by the ADA" (25, p. 5). The defendant answered the complaint on June 27, 2019 denying that the plaintiff was not allowed to join the facility or that it violated Title III of the ADA. The defendant did not deny, however, that the plaintiff visited its facility and that she presented the facility's manager with a clinical note indicating that she suffers chronic pain from RSD.

Although this case is in the early stages of a lawsuit and the court had not yet ruled at the time of this writing, there are some legal lessons to learn. The primary lesson is that individuals who have disabilities may want to join a fitness facility and participate in the programs/services. The ADA does not require fitness facilities to meet every need of individuals with disabilities. However, if these individuals feel like they are denied access to the facility and its programs/services, they may try filing a lawsuit under Title III of the ADA. Even if the fitness facility succeeds in defending the lawsuit, it is still an expensive venture. It is essential that fitness managers develop/implement policies and procedures that reflect the requirements of the ADA. See Exhibit 3-2 for resources to enhance compliance with ADA Title III.

In *Class v. Towson University* (26), Gavin Class, a Towson University football player, suffered serious heat stroke injuries, including liver failure, in August 2013. After receiving a liver transplant, he experienced several medical complications including a defect in his abominable wall. However, after a long and arduous rehabilitation process, he made a remarkable recovery according to one of his treating physicians, Dr. William Hutson, an expert in liver disease and liver transplant. In fall of 2015, Dr. Hutson indicated that Gavin was able to return to playing football but recommended that he wear protective padding to protect his abdominal wall. In addition, Dr. Douglas Casa, the Chief Operating Officer of The Korey Stringer Institute, indicated that Gavin was able to return to playing football in the fall of 2015 and recommended various safety precautions including the use of a Core Temp Monitoring system. Between August 2014 and June of 2015, the Korey Stringer Institute had Gavin complete several tests including heat tolerance tests to determine his readiness to play football again. "Dr. Casa testified that Class would not have a reoccurrence of heat stroke or heat illness if the Core Temp Monitoring System was used (in conjunction with the other recommendations)" (p. 841).

However, the Towson University's Medical Director of Athletics and Head Team Physician, Dr. Kari Kindschi, blocked Gavin's return to play. The University's Return to Play policy stated that the team physician (or designee) has final authority in deciding if and when an injured student-athlete may return to practice or competition. Despite other medical expert testimony, Dr. Kindschi believed that it was unsafe for Gavin to return to play and that the University would be faced with undue financial or administrative burdens to meet the safety recommendations. Gavin contended that the university discriminatorily refused to provide his reasonable accommodation in violation of Title II of the ADA (Towson University is a public entity so Title II applies) and the Rehabilitation Act. To prove these violations, Gavin had to show he had a disability, he was qualified to receive the benefits of a public service, program, or activity, and he was excluded from participation or denied the benefits.

Citing previous case law regarding the ADA, the court stated that a public entity is not required "to undertake measures that would impose an undue financial or administrative burden ... or effect a fundamental alteration in the nature of a service" (26, p. 850). However, the court concluded that "the accommodations Plaintiff seeks are procedures already in place by Towson University and will therefore not create any undue burden on Towson staff" (p. 850). Therefore, the court ruled in favor of Gavin. This case demonstrates that a University's compliance with its own procedures cannot supersede federal dictates of the ADA and Rehabilitation Act.

Title I—Employee Discrimination

Title I of the ADA requires employers with fifteen or more employees to provide **reasonable accommodations** to qualified individuals with a disability unless the employer can demonstrate undue hardship. "Qualified individuals" are those individuals who can perform the essential functions of their jobs with or without reasonable accommodation. "Qualified" means that the individual satisfies the requisite skill, experience, education, and other job-related requirements of the position. Thus, unless an employer can show undue hardship, an employer must provide reasonable accommodations to those employees who can otherwise perform the fundamental job duties of the position. Reasonable accommodations include modifications or adjustments to the work environment. They also include modifications or adjustments that allow an employee with a disability to enjoy equal benefits and privileges of employment as are enjoyed by similarly situated employees without a disability.

Title I of the ADA is enforced by the Equal Employment Opportunity Commission (EEOC) and prohibits discrimination by employers on the basis of disability in regard to terms, conditions, and privileges of employment. Terms, conditions, and privileges of employment can include participating in wellness programs, receiving benefits like paid time off or free memberships, as well as schedules, hours and pay. Thus, employers such as fitness facilities must ensure

---

Exhibit 3-2: Resources to Enhance Compliance with the ADA

ADA Title III

1. ADA Regulations compiled by the U.S. Department of Justice
   Available at: https://www.ada.gov/regs2010/titleIII_2010/titleIII_2010_regulations.pdf. (Accessed January 12, 2020).

2. Removing Barriers to Health Clubs and Fitness Facilities A Guide for Accommodating All Members, Including People with Disabilities and Older Adults
   Available at: https://fpg.unc.edu/sites/fpg.unc.edu/files/resources/other-resources/NCODH_RemovingBarriersToHealthClubs.pdf (Accessed January 12, 2020).

3. The National Center on Health, Physical Activity and Disability (NCHPAD) is an on-line resource for research and practice information in the area of health promotion and physical activity for persons with disabilities.
   Available at: https://www.nchpad.org, (Accessed January 12, 2020).

4. United States Access Board Guide for Sports Facilities
   Available at: https://www.access-board.gov/guidelines-and-standards/recreation-facilities/guides/sports-facilities. (Accessed January 12, 2020).

5. International Health, Racquet and Sportsclub Association (IHRSA): (a) Does the Americans With Disabilities Act Apply to Your Website (March 2019), and (b) What If a Member at My Club Has an Eating Disorder (August 2018)
   Available at: https://www.ihrsa.org/ (under Improve Your Club-Legal)

ADA Title I

1. Information and Technical Assistance for ADA Title I
   Available at: https://www.ada.gov/ada_title_I.htm. (Accessed January 12, 2020).

2. Job Accommodation Network (JAN)
   Available at: https://askjan.org/publications/ada-specific/Technical-Assistance-Manual-for-Title-I-of-the-ADA.cfm. (Accessed January 12, 2020).

that all employees, regardless of disability, have an equal opportunity in hiring, scheduling, wage and promotion opportunities, as well as in the participation of workplace activities. Fitness facilities must offer reasonable accommodations to employees with disabilities if needed. See Exhibit 3-2 for resources to enhance compliance with ADA Title I.

Is Obesity a Disability Under the ADA?

Since the enactment of the ADA in 1991, there have been a number of court cases determining whether obesity qualifies as a disability under the ADA. The decisions have been mixed according to researchers who have examined these court cases. Nevertheless, most courts require individuals who are obese to also have an underlying physiological condition, such as diabetes or heart disease, in order for the individual to fall within ADA protections (27). The EEOC takes the position that (1) weight is not an impairment when it is in the "normal" range and lacks a physiological cause but (2) may be an impairment when it is outside the "normal" range or occurs as a result of a physiological disorder (28).

Some state laws include obesity as a protected category in and of itself (27). For example, Michigan and the District of Columbia prohibit discrimination based on weight or appearance (27). In other states, state courts are interpreting state anti-discrimination laws more broadly than the ADA. In one recent case from Washington State, *Taylor v. Burlington N. R.R. Holdings, Inc.* (28), the Washington Supreme Court stated that obesity qualifies as an impairment under the plain language of the Washington law that protects people with disabilities (29). Thus, in Washington State, it is illegal for employers to refuse to hire qualified potential employees because the employer perceives them to be obese.

Race Discrimination

Both Title VII and II of the Civil Rights Act of 1964 protect individuals in the United States from discrimination because of their race, color, religion, or national origin. The difference between the two laws is that Title VII protects individuals from such discrimination in employment and Title II involves places of public accommodation. Title VII also adds "sex" to the list of protected classes. Thus, under Title VII, but not Title II, discrimination based on sex is prohibited. Sex discrimination is discussed above. This part of Chapter 3 focuses on race discrimination. An earlier section addressed Title II in regard to religious discrimination.

Race Discrimination Against Fitness Participants

Race discrimination against participants in fitness facilities or programs is protected by Title II of the Civil Rights Act of 1964. As noted earlier, Title II prohibits discrimination in places of public accommodation (30). The U.S. Department of Justice enforces Title II and it can bring a lawsuit against a place of public accommodation when there is reason to believe a person working at the facility has engaged in a **pattern or practice** of discrimination based on race, color, religion or national origin (31). So, just like with Title III of the ADA or the *Jalal* case that was based on religious discrimination, Title II of the Civil Rights Act prohibits race discrimination in places of public accommodation, which includes fitness facilities.

An accusation of a pattern or practice of race discrimination can occur if a fitness facility has rules or practices that target, whether intentionally or unintentionally, members of a certain race or national origin. For example, one outdoor recreation pool in North Carolina faced criticism for being racist when someone posted its "Pool Rule" on social media. One of the rules stated that "baggy pants" and "dreadlocks/weaves/extensions" were banned at the pool. Even though the pool operators explained, at least with regard to the hair limitations, that hair extensions can get into the pool pumping equipment, a number of people were not satisfied with the explanation and vowed to ban use of the pool (32).

In another incident involving a fitness facility, three employees were fired for racial profiling of male customers of the facility. The fitness facility manager and two other employees accused the men of not paying to use the gym. The men denied the accusations saying that they had a membership. Rather than working through the situation, the facility employees called the police and demanded that the men leave the facility. The company fired all three employees (33).

The lesson to be learned from these situations is that even though the situation may not result in a lawsuit, exclusion from a fitness facility based on race or national origin, whether perceived or real, can hurt business. Facility rules and practices must be mindful of racial stereotypes and implicit bias. For example, if the North Carolina pool was truly concerned about harm to the pool pumping equipment from hair extensions, its rules could have asked all swimmers with long hair to wear swim caps because long hair can clog the pool pumping equipment. Applying the rule to everyone who has long hair and offering an explanation as to why the rule is needed may have mitigated a risk of racial discrimination. Employee training on racial discrimination may also mitigate risk. Indeed, a great example of employee training about race discrimination is Starbucks' recent training on the issue. The company closed all of its stores for one day in May 2018 to train all of its employees on racial anxiety and implicit bias after a viral video created outrage over the inappropriate arrest of two black men at a Philadelphia Starbucks. The training video is titled: I'm Not Aware of That: Starbucks Employees Receive Racial Bias Training (34). See Exhibit 3-3 for resources to enhance compliance with Title II of the Civil Rights Act.

Race Discrimination Against Employees

Race discrimination against employees is prohibited under Title VII of the Civil Rights Act of 1964 (4). Race discrimination can occur on the basis of a characteristic associated with race, such as skin color, hair texture, or certain facial features, even though not all members of the race share the same characteristic. It can also occur on the basis of a condition which predominantly affects one race unless the practice is job related and consistent with business necessity. For example, sickle cell anemia predominantly occurs in African-Americans. Thus, a policy which excludes individuals with sickle cell anemia is discriminatory unless the policy is job related and consistent with business necessity. Similarly, a "no-beard" employment policy may discriminate against African-American men who have a predisposition to pseudofolliculitis barbae (severe shaving bumps) unless the policy is job-related and consistent with business necessity (35).

Title VII also prohibits employers from having neutral policies that disproportionately affect minorities and those policies are not job-related (35). To avoid race discrimination against employees, fitness managers and exercise professionals must treat all employees equally, regardless of their race, in all terms, privileges, and conditions of employment. This means equal treatment in terms of: (a) recruitment, (b) hiring, (c) advancement opportunities, (d) benefits, (e) work assignments, (f) performance evaluations, (g) training, (h) discipline, (i) discharge, and (j) any other area of employment (35).

Exhibit 3-3: Resources to Enhance Compliance with Titles II and VII of the Civil Rights Act

Title II of the Civil Rights Act

1. U.S. Department of Justice Fact Sheet, Title II
   Available at: https://www.justice.gov/crt-22. (Accessed January 12, 2020).

2. Library of Congress, The Civil Rights Act of 1964—Titles II and III: Right to Go Where You Want (February 13, 2014)
   Available at: https://blogs.loc.gov/teachers/2014/02/the-civil-rights-act-of-1964-titles-ii-and-iii-the-right-to-go-where-you-want/. (Accessed August 1, 2019).

3. 42 USC § 2000a, et seq.

Title VII of the Civil Rights Act

1. EEOC Enforcement Guidances and Related Documents (for various civil rights laws)
   Available at: https://www.eeoc.gov/laws/guidance/enforcement_guidance.cfm. (Accessed August 1, 2019).

2. EEOC, Title VII of the Civil Rights Act
   Available at: https://www.eeoc.gov/laws/statutes/titlevii.cfm. (Accessed August 1, 2019).

3. Sample Anti-Harassment Policy (Sexual Harassment and Other Types of Harassment)—See Appendix.

Table 3-2	EEOC Facts about Race/Color Discrimination*
DISCRIMINATORY ACTION	**DESCRIPTION/EXAMPLES**
Harassment	Ethnic slurs, racial "jokes," offensive or derogatory comments, or other verbal or physical conduct based on an individual's race/color
Retaliation	Adverse employment action (demotion, termination, relocation, etc.) for opposing discrimination or participating in an EEOC proceeding by filing a charge, testifying, assisting, or otherwise participating in an agency proceeding.
Segregation/ Classification of Employees	Physically isolating employees from other employees or customer contact; assigning primarily minorities to predominantly minority establishments or geographic areas; excluding minorities from certain positions or group or categorize employees or jobs so that certain jobs are generally held by minorities; engaging in racially motivated decisions driven by business concerns—like concerns about the effect on employee relations or negative reaction of clients or customers; coding applications or resumes to designate applicant's race (including facially benign coding that implicates race, such as by area codes where many racial minorities may or are presumed to live).
Pre-employment Inquiries and Requirements	Asking for an applicant's race without a legitimate need, such as for affirmative action purposes or to track applicant flow; using an applicant's race in the selection process for the job; using criminal records in the application process as a substitute for asking about an applicant's race and basing a discriminatory hiring decision on the person's race.

*Facts About Race/Color Discrimination. U.S. EEOC. Available at: https://www.eeoc.gov//eeoc/publications/fs-race.cfm (Accessed November 19, 2019).

Race discrimination can also occur in the ways described in Table 3-2. According to the EEOC, if an employer needs racial information for legitimate purposes such as for affirmative action or to track applicant flow, one way to obtain such information and simultaneously guard against discriminatory selection is to use "tear-off sheets." Tear-off sheets can identify the applicant's race, but after the applicant completes the tear-off portion of the application, the employer separates the tear-off sheet from the rest of the application and does not use the tear-off sheet in the selection process (35). See Exhibit 3-3 for resources to enhance compliance with Title VII of the Civil Rights Act.

Age Discrimination

The Age Discrimination in Employment Act of 1967 (ADEA) prohibits employers with 20 or more employees from discriminating against individuals who are age 40 or older (36). Just like other federal anti-discrimination laws in employment, the ADEA prohibits all forms of discrimination, which can occur in hiring, firing, promotion, wages, job assignments, layoffs, training, benefits, and any other term, condition or privilege of employment (36). Also, like other federal anti-discrimination laws in employment, the ADEA is enforced by the EEOC (36).

Age discrimination can also occur in the form of harassment. Harassment may include derogatory remarks or jokes regarding a person's age. Although simple teasing, offhand comments or minor isolated incidents may not violate the ADEA, if the harassing behavior is so severe that it creates a hostile or offensive work environment, that type of behavior could violate the ADEA. The harassment does not have to come from the employee's supervisor. Illegal harassment can also come from a co-worker, a supervisor in another area of the workplace, an independent contractor, client, or customer (36). As stated earlier, an anti-harassment policy should be in place. See this chapter's appendix for a sample policy.

If an employer has a policy or practice that has a negative impact on applicants or employees age 40 or older, and the policy or practice is not based on a reasonable factor other than a person's age, such policy or practice may be in violation of the ADEA (36). An example of age discrimination in an athletic workplace occurred in *Moore v. University of Notre Dame* (37). The plaintiff was a football coach at the University of Notre Dame. At 64 years old, he was fired. Mr. Moore claimed that the head football coach told him that he was being fired because he was "too old" and would not be an effective coach for another 5-year contract. Notre Dame claimed it had its own reasons for firing Coach Moore, namely that he mistreated the football players. Nevertheless, the jury found that the University fired Coach Moore because of his age (38).

A plaintiff who is successful in an ADEA lawsuit like Coach Moore can ask for reinstatement, back pay, injunctive relief, declaratory judgment, and attorney fees (38). In Coach Moore's case, the court declined to reinstate him to his old job, but he was able to get front pay. Front pay equals the difference between the pay the employee would have earned in his old job and the earnings he may possibly earn in his current and future employment. "Front pay is especially appropriate when the plaintiff has no reasonable prospect of obtaining comparable employment or when the time period for which front pay is to be awarded is relatively short" (38, para. 7). Because of the award of front pay, back pay (what his pay would have been had he not been fired) and attorney fees to Coach Moore, Notre Dame ended up paying more than $500,000. It also suffered negative press from the lawsuit (38).

Employees do not need to be full-time in order to be protected by the ADEA for age discrimination. The ADEA can also protect seasonal or part-time employees (38). That was the case in *Austin v. Cornell University* (39). In that case, Cornell did not rehire two seasonal employees at its golf course and so the seasonal employees sued Cornell for age discrimination. The court found both the head golf professional and the associate director of athletics personally liable for damages because of their discriminatory conduct (39).

Resources for ADEA Compliance

1. **U.S. Department of Labor Fact Sheet on Age Discrimination** Available at: https://www.dol.gov/general/topic/discrimination/agedisc. (Accessed August 3, 2019).
2. **EEOC Fact Sheet, ADEA Regulations and Guidance** Available at: https://www.eeoc.gov/eeoc/history/adea50th/regs.cfm. (Accessed August 3, 2019).

PRIVACY AND COMMUNICATIONS

In the United States there is a legal right to privacy. Which law may apply in a privacy violation (there are state and federal privacy laws) depends on who is infringing the privacy right. A government intrusion into a person's right to privacy may be in violation of the United States Constitution. A privacy violation by a health care provider may implicate the federal Health Insurance Portability and Accountability Act (HIPAA), the Federal Trade Commission Act (FTCA) or a similar state law. An intrusion into one's private affairs by a fellow citizen may be in violation of a state's privacy laws. Table 3-3 (40) illustrates typical state "tort" laws relating to invasions of privacy by private parties:

Table 3-3	Complex of Four Potential Torts for Invasion of Privacy Civil Action*
TORT	
1. Intrusion upon a person's seclusion or solitude, or into his private affairs.	
2. Public disclosure of embarrassing private facts about an individual.	
3. Publicity placing one in a false light in the public eye.	
4. Appropriation of one's likeness for the advantage of another.	

*Rule the Rules of Workplace Wellness Programs (40). ©2020 by the American Bar Association. Reprinted with permission. All rights reserved. This information or any portion thereof may not be copied or disseminated in any form or by any means or stored in an electronic database or retrieval system without the express written consent of the American Bar Association.

The actions of fitness facility managers and exercise professionals may implicate privacy laws when they collect health information about employees, clients or customers; when there is an expectation of privacy by clients or customers (such as in locker rooms); or when fitness facility employees or exercise professionals post photos or statements on websites or social media. Because fitness facility managers and exercise professionals are most likely to encounter possible violations of federal statutory or state privacy laws, this section will focus on those laws and how to mitigate risk with regard to those laws.

Employer-Sponsored Fitness and Wellness Programs

Fitness managers and exercise professionals as well as vendors that provide programs/services in employer-sponsored fitness/wellness programs must be aware and comply with many laws. The laws that apply will depend on whether the program is a **group health plan wellness program** or a non-group health plan wellness program. A group health plan is defined as "welfare benefit plan to the extent that the plan provides medical care to employees or their dependents directly or through insurance or otherwise" (41).

Group health plan wellness programs need to comply with laws such as the Affordable Care Act (ACA), Health Insurance Portability and Accountability Act (HIPAA), Genetic Information Nondiscrimination Act (GINA), and ADA. Employer-sponsored wellness programs often involve collecting **protected health information (PHI)** from employees such as health histories and biometric screenings as well as offering financial incentives and/or disincentives. These types of programs/services are subject to various privacy and other laws. It is beyond the scope of this textbook to cover all these laws and their application to employer-sponsored fitness/wellness programs. However, another textbook covers these laws in detail—*Rule the Rules of Workplace Wellness Programs* (40). Noncompliance to these laws can result in hefty fines. Those involved directly or indirectly with workplace fitness/wellness programs need to become well-educated on these laws and comply with them. They include the following:

- Fitness/wellness managers hired/contracted to oversee the company's employee fitness/wellness program
- Management companies that contract with companies to manage an in-house employee fitness facility and related programs/services
- Fitness facilities that want to offer their fitness/wellness programs and services to employees of local businesses
- Wellness vendors who contract with employers to provide fitness/wellness programs for the company's employees
- Fitness facilities that want to provide an employer-sponsored fitness/wellness program for their own employees

Privacy and communication laws that are (or can be) applicable to all fitness facilities and programs/services—the HIPAA and Federal Trade Commission Act (FTCA)—are described next.

Health Insurance Portability and Accountability Act (HIPAA)

HIPAA protects the use and disclosure of "health information" by "covered entities" and "business associates." HIPAA defines health information quite broadly. Specifically, it can be oral or written information that: a) is created or received by a covered entity; and b) relates to the physical or mental health of an individual, the provision of health care to an individual, or the payment of health care provided to an individual (42). That definition is broad enough to include a lot of information that a fitness facility or exercise professional might collect and use. The following regulations regarding covered entities, business associates, and the HIPAA Privacy and Security Rules come from the Code of Federal Regulations (CFR), Parts 160 and 164 and various subparts.

Covered entities include health plans, health care clearinghouses, and health care providers that transmit any health information in electronic form in connection with a covered transaction (42). For example, covered entities might be hospitals or medical clinics that submit insurance claims electronically. A fitness facility would not be a covered entity unless it provided health care to its participants and submitted information about the care to a health insurer or some other third party, for example.

Business associates are not employees of a covered entity but provide services to a covered entity that requires use or disclosure of PHI (42). Common examples of business associates are vendors of health care providers or health plans that provide services to the providers or plans that involve the use of individual health information. In the fitness world, a fitness facility or exercise professional might be a business associate if they work with employee health plans to help those employees achieve better health. In that situation, the fitness facility or exercise professional may have access to insurance claims data from the health plan to help develop an optimal wellness program for the employees. Because the fitness facility or exercise professional would have access to health information, HIPAA requires such "business associates" to protect the privacy and security of that information.

Generally speaking, the **HIPAA Privacy Rule** requires covered entities to have safeguards in place to ensure the privacy of protected health information. The rule also describes when covered entities may use or disclose an individual's protected health information. Finally, the privacy rule gives individuals rights with respect to their protected health information, including rights to examine and obtain a copy of their health records and to request corrections. Covered entities that engage business associates to work on their behalf must have contracts or other arrangements in place with their business associates to ensure that the business associates safeguard protected health information, and use and disclose the information only as permitted or required by the Privacy Rule (43).

According to Health and Human Services (HHS), the **HIPAA Security Rule** establishes national standards designed to protect individuals' electronic personal health information that is created, received, used, or maintained by a covered entity (44). It is also important to note that Health Information Technology for Economic and Clinical Act (HITECH) expanded compliance with the Security Rule to business associates (45). The Security Rule requires covered entities and business associates to implement appropriate administrative, physical, and technical safeguards to ensure the confidentiality, integrity, and security of electronic protected health information (46). Unlike the Privacy Rule, which applies to PHI in any format (i.e., oral or written), the Security Rule does not apply to PHI that is transmitted orally or in paper form; it applies only to electronic PHI or "e-PHI" (46). The administrative, physical, and technical safeguards that covered entities and business associates must implement under the Security Rule aim to do the following:

1. Ensure the confidentiality, integrity and availability of all e-PHI the covered entity or business associate creates, receives, maintains or transmits.
2. Protect against any reasonably anticipated threats or hazards to the security or integrity of such information.

3. Protect against any reasonably anticipated uses or disclosures of such information that are not permitted or required under the Privacy Rule.
4. Ensure compliance with the Security Rule by the covered entity or business associate's workforce (47).

The **HIPAA Breach Notification Rule** requires covered entities and business associates to notify individuals whose **"Unsecured" PHI** is breached, as well as the Secretary of Health and Human Services and the media under certain methods and circumstances (48). Business associates have a duty to notify the covered entity of a breach (49). Breach means the acquisition, access, use or disclosure of PHI in a manner not permitted by the HIPAA Privacy Rule which compromises the security or privacy of the PHI. Unsecured PHI essentially means PHI that was not encrypted (for electronic PHI) or destroyed (for hard copies of PHI). If the PHI was encrypted or destroyed, even if an electronic device housing the PHI is lost, there is no breach and therefore no duty to report (50, 51).

Not all inadvertent disclosures constitute a breach. For example, unintentional access or use of PHI by a workforce member acting under the authority of a covered entity or a business associate, if such access or use was made in good faith and within that person's scope of authority, does not constitute a breach so long as the PHI is not further used or disclosed in violation of HIPAA (50). A disclosure of PHI by a person who is otherwise authorized to access the PHI at a covered entity or business associate to another person authorized to access the PHI is not a breach (50). Disclosures to unauthorized persons who are not reasonably likely to retain the information disclosed also do not constitute breaches under the HIPAA Breach Notification rule (50).

Compliance with the HIPAA Privacy and Security Rules require covered entities and business associates to expend a lot of resources. A sample, but not exhaustive, list of the various requirements imposed by the Privacy and Security Rules are (43):

Covered Entities Need To:

- Create and implement HIPAA Privacy, Security and Breach Notification Policies & Procedures

⬧ Appoint HIPAA Privacy and Security Officials
⬧ Create and distribute a Notice of Privacy Practices
⬧ Create and distribute Patient Authorizations
⬧ Create and enter into Business Associate Agreements
⬧ Adhere to Minimum Necessary Standards
⬧ Adhere to Breach Standards
⬧ Adhere to Plan Sponsor Disclosure Standards

Business Associates Need To:

⬧ Comply with the Business Associate Agreement (BAA) requirements, such as, for example, using PHI only for purposes needed to conduct the services under the agreement with the covered entity and to report any breaches of PHI to the covered entity
⬧ Implement applicable HIPAA Privacy, Security and Breach Notification Policies and Procedures
⬧ Enter into a BAA with their subcontractors.
⬧ Cooperate with government investigations into HIPAA compliance
⬧ Designate a Security Official and for best practice, a Privacy Official
⬧ Notify Covered Entities of breaches

One other important point to note about HIPAA and its relationship to various state privacy laws is that HIPAA sets a floor of protection for PHI. If a state law is "more stringent" compared to HIPAA, the state law governs (52). A "more stringent" state law is one that is more protective of a person's privacy by being more restrictive in allowing PHI uses or disclosures or, one that permits greater rights of access to or amendment of a person's own PHI (53).

When Does HIPAA Apply to Fitness Facilities and Exercise Professionals?

The HIPAA privacy, security and breach notification rules may apply to fitness facilities and exercise professionals as "covered entities" if either conduct HIPAA standard transactions, such as billing a client's health insurer for covered services. For example, if a fitness facility employed a physical therapist or dietitian that could bill a client's health insurance for services

rendered, that fitness facility may be a HIPAA covered entity. Other "standard transactions" that might result in a fitness facility or exercise professional becoming a HIPAA covered entity is electronically sending health information for any of the following purposes:

⬧ Claims and encounter information
⬧ Payment and remittance advice
⬧ Claims status
⬧ Eligibility
⬧ Enrollment and disenrollment
⬧ Referrals and authorizations
⬧ Coordination of benefits
⬧ Premium payment (54)

If a fitness facility or exercise professional does not electronically send a client's health information for any of the above purposes, it is likely not a HIPAA covered entity subject to the privacy, security, or breach notification rules discussed above.

However, if the fitness facility or exercise professional contracts with a health plan or health care provider to provide services to the plan's enrollees or the provider's patients, then the facility or professional would likely be subject to HIPAA as a business associate. If these situations do not apply to the facility or professional, then it is likely that neither the facility nor professional is subject to HIPAA privacy, security, or breach notification rules. However, the fitness facility or exercise professional could be subject to other federal or state privacy laws with regard to their clients or customers, such as state privacy laws or the Federal Trade Commission Act (FTCA), discussed below.

The Integration of Exercise Programs and Medical Care

With national initiatives such as Exercise is Medicine® (described in Chapter 7) increasing, fitness managers and exercise professionals involved with these efforts need to be fully aware of and comply with HIPAA and other privacy laws. For example, as stated above, if fitness facilities and/or exercise professionals partner with a medical clinic, health care provider, or health care plan, they will likely be considered a business associate. Medical clinics, health care providers, and/or health care plans may require that fitness managers and exercise professionals provide evidence (i.e., have written policies and procedures in place that reflect their compliance with HIPAA Privacy, Security, and Breach Notification rules as well as any relevant state laws). Therefore, before marketing fitness program/services to medical or health care entities, it would be wise for fitness managers/exercise professionals to demonstrate their knowledge of and compliance with these laws. In addition, providing evidence that only credentialed and competent exercise professionals, such as clinical exercise physiologists as described in Chapter 7, will be providing the fitness program/services for individuals with medical conditions will be important from a marketing and risk management perspective.

As described in more detail in Chapter 6, fitness facilities and exercise professionals need to have their participants complete pre-activity screening or a medical history as well as obtain medical clearance when indicated before having their participants begin an exercise program. Obtaining these data is essential in order to design/deliver a safe and effective exercise program. This process may involve acquiring medical records from the various health care providers of the participant such as his/her physician, physical therapist, occupational therapist. These health care providers will not disclose any medical records (e.g., Graded Exercise Test results, physical therapy prescriptions) to a third party until their patient has signed a HIPPA compliant authorization form. See this chapter's appendix for a sample authorization form. This authorization may also be needed before a health care provider can return a medical clearance form to the fitness facility or exercise professional because it too, may contain PHI. As described in Chapter 7, it is essential when working with individuals with medical conditions to maintain two-way communications with the participant's health care provider. Therefore, exercise professionals may need to have their participants sign a similar authorization form before sending any records, such as progress reports, to the participant's health care provider. Even if HIPPA privacy and security regulations may not apply to fitness facilities, there may be other laws that do (e.g., the Federal Trade Commission Act (described next) and state privacy laws). In addition, there are published, professional codes of conduct that all exercise professionals need to follow that include keeping all individual health/fitness data private and secure.

KEY POINT

Medical Exercise Programs

Fitness facilities and exercise professionals who want to be actively involved with initiatives such as Exercise is Medicine® and partner with medical clinics, health care providers, or health care plans may be classified as "business associates" under HIPPA. Therefore, they need to be able to demonstrate their knowledge of and compliance with HIPAA Privacy, Security and Breach Notification rules as well as any state privacy laws. Prior to marketing to medical/health care entities, fitness managers and exercise professionals should have written policies and procedures in place that reflect these laws and their commitment to following them. It is likely that medical/health care entities will require such evidence.

Federal Trade Commission Act (FTCA)

While there may be some question whether HIPAA applies to fitness facilities and exercise professionals, if the fitness facility or exercise professional collects personal information through its website, advertises or posts on social media, it is almost certain that the Federal Trade Commission Act (FTCA) applies to them. The Federal Trade Commission (FTC) is an independent U.S. law enforcement agency charged with protecting consumers and enhancing competition across broad sectors of the economy (55). The FTC's primary legal authority comes from Section 5 of the FTC Act (FTCA), which prohibits unfair or deceptive practices in the marketplace (55). The legal standards for unfairness and deception are independent of each other (56). Depending on the facts, an act or practice may be unfair, deceptive or both (56). An act or practice is unfair where it:

- Causes or is likely to cause substantial injury to consumers,
- Cannot be reasonably avoided by consumers, and
- Is not outweighed by countervailing benefits to consumers or to competition (56).

Public policy, as established by statute, regulation, or judicial decisions, may be considered with all other evidence in determining whether an act or practice is unfair (56). An act or practice is deceptive where:

- A representation, omission, or practice misleads or is likely to mislead the consumer;
- A consumer's interpretation of the representation, omission, or practice is considered reasonable under the circumstances; and
- The misleading representation, omission, or practice is material (56).

The FTC's enforcement authority extends over most companies doing business in the United States (57). Although there are some exceptions, the FTCA would cover most fitness facilities and exercise professionals.

The FTCA and Data Privacy/Security

The FTC uses Section 5 of the FTCA to protect consumer data privacy and security. Indeed, the FTC has brought enforcement actions addressing a wide range of privacy issues, including spam, social networking, behavioral advertising, pretexting, spyware, peer-to-peer file sharing and mobile technology uses (55). Some recent enforcement examples include:

- **FTCA Case #1:** PaymentsMD, LLC, an online billing portal, and its Chief Executive Officer, failed to adequately inform consumers that the company would seek highly detailed medical information from pharmacies, medical labs, and insurance companies (55). According to the Complaint, the authorization language included a statement that "health records related to your treatment may be used or disclosed pursuant to this Authorization" (58, p. 7). However, the FTC found that the website design made the statement hard to read and easy to skip over by having the consumer click on a single check box that preceded all of the authorizations (58). The FTC found the acts and practices by PaymentsMD, LLC to be deceptive and in violation of federal law.
- **FTCA Case #2:** The FTC alleged that Genelink, Inc. and Foru International violated the FTCA in two ways. (59) First, the companies deceived consumers by advertising that a cheek swab DNA test would provide them with customized dietary supplements and skincare products that mitigate or compensate for an individual's genetic disadvantages. The FTC found those claims to be untrue and lacking in scientific proof. The FTC also accused the companies of failing to employ reasonable and appropriate measures to prevent unauthorized access to consumers' personal information. The companies used third parties to receive, process or maintain customers' personal information and the companies stored the personal information on their corporate network. The companies had a privacy policy that stated that they send personal customer information to third-party subcontractors and agents. The privacy policy further stated that the third parties did not have the right to use the personal customer information beyond what was necessary to assist the companies and fulfill customer orders. The companies entered into contracts with these third-parties requiring them to maintain the confidentiality and security of the personal customer information and restricted them from using such information in any way not expressly authorized by the companies. Yet, despite having this privacy policy, the FTC found that the companies failed to protect the security of consumers' personal information. They failed to require by contract that the third-parties implement and maintain appropriate safeguards for consumers' personal information. The companies did not provide reasonable oversight of the third-parties by requiring them to implement simple, low-cost, and readily available defenses to protect the personal information.

Some of the specific security failures include:
- Maintaining consumers' personal information, including names, addresses, email addresses, telephone numbers, dates of birth, social security numbers and bank account numbers in clear text
- Providing company employees, regardless of business need, with access to consumers' complete personal information
- Providing third-party service providers with access to consumers' complete personal

information, rather than, for example, to fictitious data sets, to develop new applications

- ⦚ Failing to perform assessments to identify reasonably foreseeable risks to the security, integrity, and confidentiality of consumers' personal information on respondents' network
- ⦚ Providing a service provider that needed only certain categories of information for its business purposes with access to consumers' complete personal information
- ⦚ Not using readily available security measures to limit wireless access to their network (40, p. 302).

Because of the discrepancy between what the companies claimed both in terms of the success of their products as well as in their data security, the FTC alleged that the companies acts and practices were unfair, deceptive and in violation of the FTCA (59).

Lessons to be Learned from FTCA Cases

Although many fitness facilities or exercise professionals may not be subject to HIPAA privacy and security protections, the FTC has prosecuted cases against companies for failing to implement HIPAA-like privacy and security policies and procedures. To the extent that a fitness facility or exercise professional collects personal information from clients or customers, the facility or professional should create and implement robust privacy and security policies and procedures and ensure its downstream subcontractors do the same. As seen from the above FTCA cases, having a privacy policy is not enough. In fact, having a privacy policy that states personal information is handled with care and is protected but in practice, little is done to follow through on that promise, could be deemed unfair and deceptive under the FTCA.

Advertising and Social Media Posts

The FTCA also governs advertising and social media posts either directly from the fitness facility or exercise professional, or endorsers of the fitness facility or exercise professional. As noted earlier, FTCA § 5 requires that all claims be truthful and non-misleading. With this one requirement, the FTCA sweeps everything into FTC's jurisdiction, everything a company says publicly

(including online) in its marketing materials about its services or products. FTC can require that a company disgorge its unlawful profits; penalties can be in the millions. One of the core requirements behind FTC's enforcement authority is that all claims be substantiated. As FTC explains in the FTC Policy Statement Regarding Advertising Substantiation, the underlying requirement is that advertisers have a reasonable basis for advertising claims before they are disseminated (60). Failure to have a reasonable basis for the claims is an unfair and deceptive act or practice in violation of the FTCA. This requirement severely limits the claims that can be made, independent of the Food and Drug Administration (FDA) concerns. However, for claims involving healthcare services or products, those claims must be substantiated by **competent and reliable evidence**. FTC defines "competent and reliable scientific evidence" as:

> *tests, analyses, research, studies, or other evidence based on the expertise of professionals in the relevant area, that have been conducted and evaluated in an objective manner by persons qualified to do so, using procedures generally accepted in the profession to yield accurate and reliable results (61, pp. 2-3).*

According to FTC, well-controlled clinical studies are the most reliable form of evidence, and that "replication of research results in an independently-conducted study adds to the weight of the evidence." (62, p. 10). Among other things, advertisements must ensure that necessary qualifying information is presented clearly and prominently (for example, disclosing if subjects in a trial engaged in regular exercise and followed a restricted-calorie diet as part of the study regimen, and clarifying that users should follow the same to expect similar results). FTC does not guarantee that following its guidance will *not* result in enforcement action; rather, it encourages industry to avoid puffery and over-stating results of studies that are not supported by the data, methods, and results. In addition to the above guidelines, FTC also addresses claims based on consumer experiences or expert endorsements (63). FTC has different rules for *consumer* endorsements and *expert* endorsements.

For consumer endorsements, among other things (64):

- The advertiser must possess and rely upon adequate substantiation, including, when appropriate, competent, and reliable scientific evidence, to support such claims made through endorsements in the same manner the advertiser would be required to do if it had made the representation directly.
- The endorser's experience should be representative of what consumers will generally achieve with the advertised product or service in actual, albeit variable, conditions of use.

For expert endorsements, among other things (65):

- The endorser's qualifications must in fact give him/her the expertise that he/she is represented as possessing with respect to the endorsement.
- The "endorsement must be supported by an actual exercise of his/her expertise in evaluating product features or characteristics with respect to which he/she is expert and which are both relevant to an ordinary consumer's use of or experience with the product and also are available to the ordinary consumer. This evaluation must have included an examination or testing of the product at least as extensive as someone with the same degree of expertise would normally need to conduct in order to support the conclusions presented in the endorsement." (65, § 255.3(b)).

Thus, according to FTC, the advertiser must possess and rely upon adequate substantiation, including, when appropriate, competent and reliable scientific evidence, to support such claims made through endorsements in the same manner the advertiser would be required to do if it had made the representation directly (i.e., without using endorsements). Consumer endorsements themselves are not competent and reliable scientific evidence. FTC guidance gives detailed examples of consumer endorsements that could be considered misleading. See Exhibit 3-4 for an example relevant to the exercise profession.

Because so many health-related companies rely heavily on consumer testimonials and expert endorsements, it is important to have legal counsel review these for potential

---

Exhibit 3-4: FTC Guidance Example of Consumer Endorsement*

An advertisement for a weight-loss product features a formerly obese woman. She says in the ad, "Every day, I drank 2 WeightAway shakes, ate only raw vegetables, and exercised vigorously for six hours at the gym. By the end of six months, I had gone from 250 pounds to 140 pounds." The advertisement accurately describes the woman's experience, and such a result is within the range that would be generally experienced by an extremely overweight individual who consumed WeightAway shakes, only ate raw vegetables, and exercised as the endorser did. Because the endorser clearly describes the limited and truly exceptional circumstances under which she achieved her results, the ad is not likely to convey that consumers who weigh substantially less or use WeightAway under less extreme circumstances will lose 110 pounds in six months. (If the advertisement simply says that the endorser lost 110 pounds in six months using WeightAway together with diet and exercise, however, this description would not adequately alert consumers to the truly remarkable circumstances leading to her weight loss.)

The advertiser must have substantiation, however, for any performance claims conveyed by the endorsement (e.g., that WeightAway is an effective weight loss product). If, in the alternative, the advertisement simply features "before" and "after" pictures of a woman who says "I lost 50 pounds in 6 months with WeightAway," the ad is likely to convey that her experience is representative of what consumers will generally achieve. Therefore, if consumers cannot generally expect to achieve such results, the ad should clearly and conspicuously disclose what they can expect to lose in the depicted circumstances (e.g., "most women who use WeightAway for six months lose at least 15 pounds"). If the ad features the same pictures but the testimonialist simply says, "I lost 50 pounds with WeightAway," and WeightAway users generally do not lose 50 pounds, the ad should disclose what results they do generally achieve (e.g., "most women who use WeightAway lose 15 pounds") (64).

* Guides Concerning the Use of Endorsements and Testimonials in Advertising, 16 CFR § 255.2(c) (2009).

FTC exposure. Where the endorser has a financial interest in the advertised product, that could materially affect the weight or credibility of the endorsement, it should be disclosed (66, at "When Does the FTC Act Apply to Endorsements?"). The disclosure of the financial relationship does not need to be complicated and does not necessarily need to specify the amount paid (66, at "How Should I Disclose That I was Given Something for my Endorsement?"). A sentence such as "Company X gave me [name of product], and I think it's great" is sufficient. Or, on Twitter, the FTC suggests that the paid endorsement use words like "Sponsored," "Promotion," "Paid ad" or starting a tweet with "Ad:" or "#ad" (66, at "What about a platform like Twitter? How can I make a disclosure when my message is limited to 140 characters?"). On Instagram, you can superimpose words over images that indicate a paid endorsement. According to the FTC, the important point is that the disclosure about the paid endorsement should be easy to notice and read in the time that your Company's followers have to look at the image or read the post (66, at "How can I make a disclosure on Snapchat or in Instagram Stories?"). In general, the requirement is that disclosures be clear and conspicuous. The FTC coordinates enforcement with other federal agencies, including FDA and the state Attorney General (AG), particularly where the product or the claims represent a high risk to the consumer.

FTC Statements Regarding the Limitation of Disclaimers

FTC notes that "vague" disclaimers such as "results may vary" do not cure a deceptive claim. Similarly, overstating the qualifications of an expert can be considered deceptive and misleading. For example, referring to someone as a "leading clinician in joint health" is deceptive if the expert has not conducted sufficient trials to support this endorsement. In addition, the expert's connection to the company affects the "weight and credibility" of the endorsement. Even if the expert is adequately qualified, his or her position with the company must be clearly disclosed.

FTC also cautions against misleading consumer endorsements: FTC states that an advertisement employing endorsements by one or more consumers about the performance of an advertised product or service will be interpreted as representing that the product or service is effective for the purpose depicted in the advertisement. FTC focuses enforcement efforts, in particular, on weight loss claims and considers these "red flag" kinds of claims (67).

KEY POINT

Overstating Credentials of Exercise Professionals

Example #1: Because there are varying levels of credentials and expertise among exercise professionals as described in Chapter 5, fitness facilities need to be sure their marketing and advertising materials accurately reflect the credentials of their fitness instructors and trainers. See spotlight case, *D'Amico v. LA Fitness* in Chapter 5. This court ruled that the fitness facility violated the Connecticut Unfair Trade Practices Act because the facility claimed, in their advertising, they hired only persons who were experienced and qualified in personal fitness training. The plaintiff proved otherwise.

Example #2: Exercise professionals promoting themselves as a "clinical exercise physiologist" need to be sure they have the credentials commensurate with this title (e.g., degree and/or certification in clinical exercise physiology). If not, they may face criminal charges for violating the FTCA or similar state laws as well as civil lawsuits (e.g., negligence) if their actions/inactions led to harming someone. See Chapter 7 for more on this topic regarding the standard of care for exercise professionals working with individuals with medical conditions.

State Privacy and Communications Laws

The FTC is not the only agency paying attention to misleading online endorsements. Among other enforcement agencies, state attorneys general may also bring enforcement actions for deceptive online testimonials and reviews. For example, the New York attorney general recently settled several cases for alleged deceptive online advertising. In one case, Machinima Inc., an online YouTube channel for gamers, paid "influencers" to post videos endorsing Microsoft's Xbox One console and a small handful of games. One of the endorsers was paid $30,000 for their videos, but the compensation was not disclosed in the reviews.

The New York attorney general alleged that such conduct violated New York's Executive Law and General Business Law, which prohibit misrepresentation and deceptive acts or practices in the conduct of any business (68).

State laws also offer consumers privacy protections. This is especially important in light of the fitness trend that **wearable technology,** which collects all kinds of different personal information, is steadily gaining in popularity. According to the American College of Sports Medicine (ACSM) survey of worldwide fitness trends, wearable technology was the number one trend in 2020. An article describing this survey is available at: https://journals.lww.com/acsmhealthfitness/Fulltext/2019/11000/WORLDWIDE_SURVEY_OF_FITNESS_TRENDS_FOR_2020.6.aspx?WT.mc_id=H-PxADx20100319xMP (Accessed January 31, 2020).

Wearable technology includes fitness trackers, smart watches, heart rate monitors and GPS tracking devices. This means that fitness providers are collecting volumes of personal data from wearable technology products as well as the vendors of those products. Through geolocation technology, these devices can reveal locations of individuals. To reduce this operational security risk, the military banned Fitbits, and fitness-tracking devices for deployed troops in 2018 (69). The more data that one collects the greater risk that a data breach may occur. Even if the HIPAA Breach Notification Rule does not apply to fitness facilities or exercise professionals, it is likely a state data breach notification law will apply. All 50 states have data breach notification laws which, generally, require entities to report a data breach to persons whose personal information is affected, as well as to government authorities (70).

In addition to the breach notification laws discussed above and general state tort laws relating to invasion of privacy listed in Table 3-3, many states have other privacy laws that impact fitness facilities or exercise professionals specifically. These laws may address data destruction and disposal, safeguarding personal data, or requiring businesses to conduct due diligence before sharing or disclosing certain categories of personal information to a third party service provider (70). For example, Wisconsin has the following law involving privacy in locker rooms:

175.22 Policy on privacy in locker rooms. (1) In this section:

   a) "Person" includes the state.

   b) "Recording device" means a camera, a video recorder, or any other device that may be used to record or transfer images.

   c) Any person that owns or operates a locker room in this state shall adopt a written policy that does all of the following:

   d) Specifies who may enter and remain in the locker room to interview or seek information from any individual in the locker room.

   e) Specifies the recording devices that may be used in the locker room and the circumstances under which they may be used.

   f) Reflects the privacy interests of individuals who use the locker room.

   g) Specifies that no person may use a cell phone to capture, record, or transfer a representation of a nude or partially nude person in the locker room. (71, p. 3)

Hence, fitness managers and exercise professionals must make an effort to research and understand their own state's laws regarding privacy and communication, as well as the federal laws discussed in this chapter. It is always a good idea for the fitness manager to hire competent legal counsel to help them navigate the various laws that apply to their business. See Exhibit 3-5 for risk management strategies and resources related to privacy and communication.

KEY POINT

Privacy and Communications

As with any legal area, but especially with privacy and communications, fitness managers and exercise professionals should adopt policies and procedures that govern the collection, use, storage, and disclosure of sensitive information. This includes health information as well as personal information such as credit cards, identification information, and other sensitive information. If subject to HIPAA, such policies and procedures are required. However, even if not subject to HIPAA, having such policies and procedures and training staff on those policies and procedures will help reduce the risk of violating various federal and state laws that protect the privacy and security of personal data collected.

Exhibit 3-5: Risk Management Strategies and Resources: Privacy and Communications

Risk Management Strategies for Achieving Privacy and Security of Information

1. Determine when, where and how you collect personal information from employees and fitness participants; document your inventory of personal information.

2. Implement policies and procedures about safeguarding all personal information that is collected from employees and fitness participants.

3. Determine whether you are subject to HIPAA, if so, consult with legal counsel about implementing HIPAA-compliant policies and procedures in accordance with the privacy and security rule.

4. Review advertisements and social media posts and policies to ensure that those ads and posts do not violate FTCA.

Resources for Privacy and Communications Compliance

1. FTC Policy Statement Regarding Advertising Substantiation, Fact Sheet.
   Available at: https://www.ftc.gov/public-statements/1983/03/ftc-policy-statement-regarding-advertising-substantiation. (Accessed August 4, 2019).

2. FTC Enforcement Policy Statement on Marketing Claims for OTC Homeopathic Drugs.
   Available at: https://www.ftc.gov/system/files/documents/public_statements/996984/p114505_otc_homeopathic_drug_enforcement_policy_statement.pdf. (Accessed June 9, 2019).

3. HIPAA for Professionals. U.S. Department of Health and Human Services.
   Available at: https://www.hhs.gov/hipaa/for-professionals/index.html. (Accessed November 21, 2019).

4. IHRSA: See (a) 7 Ways to Protect Your Club From a Data Breach (August 2019), (b) Protecting Your Health Club Members' Health & Data Privacy (July 2019), and (c) Why Sending a Text Has Big Implications for Your Health Club (July 2018)
   Available at: https://www.ihrsa.org/ (under Improve Your Club-Legal)

EMPLOYEE WAGE AND HOUR LAWS

Fitness managers and exercise professionals should be aware of federal laws that govern wages and hours of employees. Two of those laws are the Fair Labor Standards Act (FLSA) and the Equal Pay Act (EPA). See Exhibit 3-7 at the end of this section for risk management strategies and resources that can help increase compliance to wage and hour laws.

Fair Labor Standards Act (FLSA)

The major provisions of the Fair Labor Standards Act of 1938 (FLSA) (72) guarantee minimum wage and overtime pay. The FLSA was intended to establish a minimum standard of living for American workers (73). It also sets recordkeeping and child labor standards (73). The FLSA, along with other labor laws strengthening workers' rights such as the National Labor Relations Act of 1935, was one piece of President Franklin Roosevelt's New Deal during the Great Depression (73).

Employees are covered under the FLSA if they work for covered "enterprises" with at least two employees engaged in commerce or in the production of goods for commerce and have annual revenues of at least $500,000 (74). Private and public hospitals, medical care facilities, schools, and public agencies are also covered "enterprises" under the FLSA (74). Even if an employer is not considered a covered "enterprise," the FLSA covers domestic service workers (i.e., housekeepers) and individuals "engaged in interstate commerce or in the production of goods for commerce" (74, p. 38545). For instance, workers in small businesses that ship goods out-of-state would be covered under FLSA even if the employer is not considered an "enterprise" (75). Thus, if a personal fitness trainer or wellness coach ships goods such as wellness products out of state, those individuals would be engaged in interstate commerce and, therefore, subject to FLSA requirements.

The minimum wage under the FLSA is currently $7.25 per hour (76). The FLSA also requires that covered employees who work more than 40 hours per week receive compensation "at a rate not less than one and one-half times the regular rate at which he is employed" (77). Alternatively, covered employees may receive "compensatory time off at a rate not less than one and one-half hours for each hour of employment for which overtime compensation is required" (77). Under FLSA's so-called "white collar" exemption," executive, administrative, professional, computer, and outside sales employees are exempt from minimum wage and overtime pay (78). In general, white collar workers are exempted if their salaries exceed a certain amount, set at $35,568 per year or $684 per week (79). The U.S. Department of Labor (DOL) increased the salary threshold to these amounts to be effective in January 2020 (80). That means a much larger number of U.S. workers will be required to receive overtime pay (or compensatory time off) if they work more than 40 hours per week. There are other commonly-used exemptions for FLSA requirements. The following may be applicable to certain fitness facilities:

⯈ Commissioned sales employees of retail or service establishments are exempt from overtime if more than half of the employee's earnings come from commissions *and* the employee averages at least one and one-half times the minimum wage for each hour worked.

⯈ Seasonal and recreational employees employed by certain seasonal and recreational establishments are exempt from both the minimum wage and overtime pay provisions of the FLSA (81).

Fitness facilities can be subject to FLSA requirements. For example, in response to an inquiry from an association of over 4,300 health and athletic clubs in the United States (82), the Department of Labor (DOL) concluded that the clubs were not likely exempt from FLSA requirements under the commissioned employees of retail or service establishments exemption. To meet that exemption, an employee: (a) must be employed by a retail or service establishment, (b) the employee's regular rate of pay must exceed 1.5 times the applicable minimum wage under Section 6 of the FLSA, and (c) more than half of the employee's total earnings in a representative period must consist of commissions on goods or services.

The DOL agreed that it is possible the clubs were retail or service establishments. But, the DOL disagreed with the association's argument that the employees met the commission requirement. The association indicated that many of the personal trainers or instructors were paid a flat dollar amount per lesson or session. According to the DOL, flat fees paid without regard to the value of the service performed do not represent commissions on goods or services. Because those employees do not meet the third criterion for the commissioned sales employees exemption, those fitness facility employees would not be exempt from FLSA minimum wage and overtime requirements (82).

Indeed, in 2016, the DOL required Life Time Fitness to pay 15,909 employees across the United States a total of $976,765 in back wages and liquidated damages for violating the FLSA. The DOL found that Life Time Fitness, Inc. took deductions for uniform costs, which resulted in workers making less than the required federal minimum wage per hour (83).

Application to Student Interns

Students majoring in exercise science (or a related area) often complete a required internship (or other student work experiences) at various fitness and athletic facilities. Most often, these are unpaid internships. However, in some cases, certain fitness facilities (e.g., for-profit employers) may need to pay interns in accordance with the FLSA. The law requires "for profit" employers to pay employees for their work. Unpaid internships are generally permissible in the public sector (e.g., government agency such as a city/county parks and recreation department, state-funded university) and non-profit charitable organizations. However, if an internship is completed in a for-profit setting (e.g., health clubs, corporate fitness/wellness programs, some hospitals, professional athletics), the intern may need to be paid for his/her work if classified as an employee under the FLSA. However, if the internship meets a "primary beneficiary test" (see the seven factors listed in Exhibit 3-6), the for-profit business may not be required to pay interns because they would not be considered employees. A key factor is that the work of the intern is not displacing the work of an employee.

Exhibit 3-6: Primary Beneficiary Test for Unpaid Interns and Students*

Courts have used this seven-factor test to determine if the intern or student is an employee under the FLSA when working in a for-profit setting:

1. The extent to which the intern and the employer clearly understand that there is no expectation of compensation. Any promise of compensation, express or implied, suggests that the intern is an employee—and vice versa.

2. The extent to which the internship provides training that would be similar to that which would be given in an educational environment, including the clinical and other hands-on training provided by educational institutions.

3. The extent to which the internship is tied to the intern's formal education program by integrated coursework or the receipt of academic credit.

4. The extent to which the internship accommodates the intern's academic commitments by corresponding to the academic calendar.

5. The extent to which the internship's duration is limited to the period in which the internship provides the intern with beneficial learning.

6. The extent to which the intern's work complements, rather than displaces, the work of paid employees while providing significant educational benefits to the intern.

7. The extent to which the intern and the employer understand that the internship is conducted without entitlement to a paid job at the conclusion of the internship.

*Fact Sheet #71: Internship Programs Under the FLSA. U.S Department of Labor Wage and Hour Division. Available at: https://www.dol.gov/whd/regs/compliance/whdfs71.pdf. (Accessed December 14, 2018).

Application to Volunteers

The FLSA defines, in part, a volunteer as follows:

a) An individual who performs hours of service for a public agency for civic, charitable, or humanitarian reasons, without promise, expectation or receipt of compensation for services rendered…

b) Congress…expressed its wish to prevent any manipulation or abuse of minimum wage or overtime requirements through coercion or undue pressure upon individuals to "volunteer" their services.

c) Individuals shall be considered volunteers only where their services are offered freely and without pressure or coercion, direct or implied, from an employer.

d) An individual shall not be considered a volunteer if the individual is otherwise employed by the same public agency to perform the same type of services as those for which the individual proposes to volunteer (84).

Public Agencies

Individuals may volunteer at fitness facilities that are a public agency (e.g., local, state government) if offered freely. However, employers who are offering unpaid volunteer work to their employees must ensure the offer is not coerced directly or indirectly by anyone in the agency. In addition, the volunteer work cannot be the same type of work that an employee performs while employed. For example, a city recreational department should not expect an employee who leads a nature hiking group to volunteer to do the same "introductory" activity on a weekend. However, if the employee chooses to volunteer at a fundraiser for the agency by staffing a booth, that may be acceptable under the FLSA.

Nonprofit Organizations

Nonprofit employers (e.g., YMCAs, JCCs) need to follow similar procedures. A volunteer will not, generally, be considered an employee for FLSA purposes if the individual volunteers freely for public service, religious or humanitarian objectives, and without contemplation or receipt of compensation. Typically, such volunteers serve on a part-time basis and do not displace regular employed workers or perform work that would otherwise be performed by regular employees. In addition, paid employees of a nonprofit organization cannot volunteer to provide the same type of services to their nonprofit organization that they are employed to provide (85).

For-Profit Businesses

The FLSA provides guidelines for volunteers in public and nonprofit sectors in which payment of minimum wage and overtime would not be required. However, under the FLSA, employees may not volunteer services in for-profit businesses (i.e., any individual that performs work that benefits the employer must be paid the required wages). However, employees who want to volunteer (not coerced) at a community charity run on the weekend, in which the employer is a sponsor is likely permissible (86).

Summary: Volunteers in Public, Nonprofit, and For-Profit Fitness Facilities

It will be important for fitness facilities and programs that utilize volunteers to follow the FLSA based on their type of facility/program—public, nonprofit, or for-profit. Fitness managers and exercise professionals should consult with their legal counsel to help ensure compliance with the FLSA. See Figure 3-1 for a Decision Algorithm regarding volunteers.

FLSA and Compensation for Meetings/Trainings

Another interesting provision of the FLSA concerns payment for attendance at lectures, meetings, training programs and similar activities. The FLSA considers such attendance "working time," and, therefore, subject

Figure 3-1: Decision Algorithm: Volunteers in Public and Non-Profit Settings

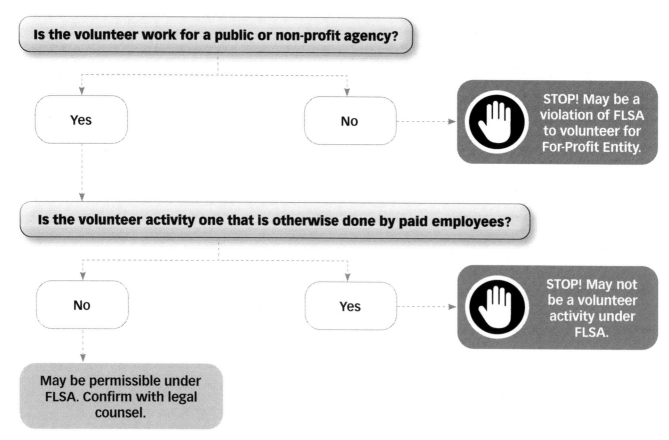

to FLSA minimum wage and overtime provisions, unless the following four criteria are met:

a) Attendance is outside of the employee's regular working hours;

b) Attendance is in fact voluntary;

c) The course, lecture, or meeting is not directly related to the employee's job; and

d) The employee does not perform any productive work during such attendance (87).

All four of these criteria must be met (87). Thus, if an activity takes place during the employee's regular working hours or attendance is mandatory, the employer should consider such participation compensable work time.

A court evaluates whether an activity is mandatory from the employee's reasonable perspective (88, 89). "Attendance is not voluntary, of course, if it is required by the employer. It is not voluntary in fact if the employee is given to understand or led to believe that his present working conditions or the continuance of his employment would be adversely affected by nonattendance" (88, p. 5).

Employees have sued their employers for FLSA violations for failing to pay them for time spent in "mandatory" trainings (88). In one case, the employees viewed the trainings as mandatory because their attendance was tied to wage increases and the company president would call employees who missed the training (88). Similar arguments could be made in the workplace wellness context if employee participation in wellness programs affected an employee's working conditions or employment at a company. For example, if an employer tied wellness program participation to a large incentive or had supervisors "encourage" employee participation, an employee may view participation as mandatory. In such a case, if an employer did not pay an employee for his or her time spent participating in the wellness activity, an employee could raise a FLSA claim.

Employers can reduce their FLSA risk by paying employees for the time spent participating in various activities encouraged by the employer. For example, one recent news article highlighted how one gym was not paying its personal trainers for duties like attending meetings, cleaning weights, or organizing the gym. The personal trainers alleged that they were not being paid for 15-21 hours per week for performing those duties and sued under the state wage laws (90). An example of how a fitness facility may be sued under the FLSA is featured in the spotlight case, *Mogilevsky v. Wellbridge Club*.

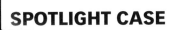

SPOTLIGHT CASE

Mogilevsky v. Wellbridge Club Mgmt., Inc.
905 F. Supp. 2d 405 (D. Mass., 2012)

FACTS

Historical Facts:

Boris Mogilevsky was a personal trainer for Wellbridge Club Management, a health club in Cambridge, Massachusetts. He worked there from July 2002 until June 2010 when Wellbridge fired him. In 2007, Mogilevsky brought a class action lawsuit against Wellbridge under the FLSA and the Massachusetts Wage Act alleging that he and other personal trainers were not being paid overtime wages for work in excess of forty hours per week. Wellbridge paid trainers a commission when providing personal training services and hourly wages only when performing "noncommissionable" work. After Mogilevsky sued Wellbridge, he claimed that Wellbridge sought revenge against him by shunting away potential clients (thereby reducing his income), taking unwarranted disciplinary actions, and using those disciplinary actions to fire him.

Procedural Facts:

Wellbridge sought a court ruling to close the case because it believed Mogilevsky failed to bring any evidence that links his Wage Act lawsuit to any adverse employment action. Wellbridge submitted evidence that Mogilevsky's discipline

Mogilevsky continued...

and firing were warranted. Specifically, Wellbridge brought evidence that Mogilevsky mistreated clients and co-workers. Mogilevsky characterizes Wellbridge's evidence of misconduct as false.

ISSUE

Could a jury believe that Wellbridge disciplined and fired Mogilevsky because he brought a lawsuit for overtime wages under the FLSA and Massachusetts Wage Act?

COURT'S RULING

Yes, a jury could believe that, so the case must go to trial.

COURT'S REASONING

Although the court said Mogilevsky's evidence countering Wellbridge's argument that it disciplined and fired him for good reason was scant, it was enough to present to the jury. The court said Mogilevsky's evidence that Wellbridge took disciplinary actions against him despite having positive annual evaluations could be seen by a jury as resentment at him for filing the FLSA and Wage Act lawsuit.

Lessons Learned from *Mogilevsky*

Legal

▶ Unless they are exempt under the FLSA, employees such as personal trainers are owed overtime if they work more than 40 hours per week.

▶ What constitutes "work" that is compensable may be a subject of dispute.

▶ Once an employee complains about wages and hours and invokes the FLSA or state law equivalent, disciplining that employee may result in a retaliation claim (i.e., retaliating against the employee for exercising his or her rights under the law).

Risk Management

▶ Pay all employees for all time worked, including overtime.

▶ Set clear expectations of job duties and behavior towards clients and co-workers and apply any discipline consistently across all employees (no favorable or unfavorable treatment).

▶ Keep lines of communication open between employees and management about working conditions.

Equal Pay Act (EPA)

The Equal Pay Act (EPA) is part of the FLSA (91). The EEOC enforces the EPA as it does with other workplace discrimination laws. According to the EEOC, the EPA requires employers to pay men and women who work for the same establishment the same pay for the same work. Thus, equal pay must be given for substantially equal jobs. To determine if two jobs are substantially equal, an employer must compare the job's content, not title.

Job content comprises of skill, effort, responsibility, and working conditions in the same establishment. Each of these factors in job content are described by the EEOC as shown in Table 3-4. Pay differentials are permitted when they are based on seniority, merit, quantity or quality of production, or a factor other than sex. These are known as "affirmative defenses" and it is the employer's burden to prove that they apply. In correcting a pay differential, no employee's pay may be reduced. Instead, the pay of the lower paid employee(s) must be increased (92).

Table 3-4	Job Content Factors to Determine Substantially Equal Jobs and Pay (92)
JOB FACTOR	**DESCRIPTION**
Skill	Measured by factors such as the experience, ability, education, and training required to perform the job. The issue is what skills are required for the job, not what skills the individual employees may have. For example, two bookkeeping jobs could be considered equal under the EPA even if one of the job holders has a master's degree in physics, since that degree would not be required for the job.
Effort	The amount of physical or mental exertion needed to perform the job. For example, suppose that men and women work side by side on a line assembling machine parts. The person at the end of the line must also lift the assembled product as he or she completes the work and place it on a board. That job requires more effort than the other assembly line jobs if the extra effort of lifting the assembled product off the line is substantial and is a regular part of the job. As a result, it would not be a violation to pay that person more, regardless of whether the job is held by a man or a woman.
Responsibility	The degree of accountability required in performing the job. For example, a salesperson who is delegated the duty of determining whether to accept customers' personal checks has more responsibility than other salespeople. On the other hand, a minor difference in responsibility, such as turning out the lights at the end of the day, would not justify a pay differential.
Working Conditions	This encompasses two factors: (1) physical surroundings like temperature, fumes, and ventilation; and (2) hazards.
Establishment	The prohibition against compensation discrimination under the EPA applies only to jobs within an establishment. An establishment is a distinct physical place of business rather than an entire business or enterprise consisting of several places of business. In some circumstances, physically separate places of business may be treated as one establishment. For example, if a central administrative unit hires employees, sets their compensation, and assigns them to separate work locations, the separate work sites can be considered part of one establishment.

Exhibit 3-7: Risk Management Strategies and Resources: Wage and Hour Laws

Risk Management Strategies:

- If employers expect their employees to attend a meeting or event, they need to pay them their regular wage.
- Employers who use interns or volunteers should not assume that those individuals can work without pay, especially if they do the same or similar work of paid employees.
- If an individual complains about their wages or hours, avoid discipline that could be interpreted as retaliation for lodging a wages/hours complaint.

Resources:

- U.S. Department of Labor Wage and Hour Division.
  Available at: https://www.dol.gov/whd/. (Accessed November 21, 2019).
- Compliance Assistance—Wages and the Fair Labor Standards Act (FLSA).
  Available at: https://www.dol.gov/whd/flsa/. (Accessed November 21, 2019).

EMPLOYEE SAFETY

Two federal laws, the Occupational Safety and Health Act of 1970 (OSHA), and the Clinical Laboratory Improvement Amendments (CLIA) and related state laws can impact fitness facilities and exercise professionals. Each of these laws and their implications for the fitness industry are discussed, below. See Exhibit 3-8 at the end of this section for risk management strategies and resources that can help increase compliance to employee safety laws.

Occupational Safety and Health Act (OSHA)

The Occupational Safety and Health Act (OSHA) of 1970 (93) requires most private sector employers (e.g., any business with one or more employees) and federal agency employers to ensure a safe work environment for employees (state and local government workers may be protected by a state program) (94). Self-employed workers are not covered by OSHA. Congress enacted the law because it found that personal injuries and illnesses arising out of work situations impose a substantial burden upon, and are a hindrance to, interstate commerce in terms of lost production, wage loss, medical expenses, and disability compensation payments (95). The regulations provide specific standards employers must meet to ensure a safe work environment and are found at 29 CFR § 1910 (96).

It is the employer's duty to find and correct safety and health problems. OSHA further requires that employers first try to eliminate or reduce hazards by making feasible changes in working conditions rather than relying on personal protective equipment such as masks, gloves, or earplugs, switching to safer chemicals, enclosing processes to trap harmful fumes, or using ventilation systems to clean the air are examples of effective ways to eliminate or reduce risks. Employers must also:

- Prominently display the official OSHA Job Safety and Health—It's the Law poster that describes rights and responsibilities under the OSH Act. This poster is free and can be downloaded from www.osha.gov.
- Inform workers about chemical hazards through training, labels, alarms, color-coded systems, chemical information sheets and other methods.
- Provide safety training to workers in a language and vocabulary they can understand.
- Keep accurate records of work-related injuries and illnesses.
- Perform tests in the workplace, such as air sampling, required by some OSHA standards.
- Provide required personal protective equipment at no cost to workers.
- Provide hearing exams or other medical tests required by OSHA standards.

- Post OSHA citations and injury and illness data where workers can see them.
- Notify OSHA within 8 hours of a workplace fatality or within 24 hours of any work-related inpatient hospitalization, amputation or loss of an eye (1-800-321-OSHA [6742]).
- Not retaliate against workers for using their rights under the law, including their right to report a work-related injury or illness.
- Pay for most types of required personal protective equipment. (94, pp. 9-10)

Under OSHA, workers are entitled to working conditions that do not pose a risk of serious harm. Workers have the right to:

- File a confidential complaint with OSHA to have their workplace inspected.
- Receive information and training about hazards, methods to prevent harm, and the OSHA standards that apply to their workplace. The training must be done in a language and vocabulary workers can understand.
- Receive copies of records of work-related injuries and illnesses that occur in their workplace.
- Receive copies of the results from tests and monitoring done to find and measure hazards in their workplace.
- Receive copies of their workplace medical records.
- Participate in an OSHA inspection and speak in private with the inspector.
- File a complaint with OSHA if they have been retaliated against by their employer as the result of requesting an inspection or using any of their other rights under the OSH Act.
- File a complaint if punished or retaliated against for acting as a "whistleblower" under the 21 additional federal laws for which OSHA has jurisdiction. (94, p. 10)

OSHA is administered and enforced by the Occupational Safety and Health Administration, a division of the U.S. Department of Labor, and applies to most private sector employers and workers in all 50 states, the District of Columbia, and other US jurisdictions either directly through OSHA or through an OSHA-approved state plan (94). State plans are safety and health programs operated by a state instead of the federal government. To be approved by OSHA, state plans must be at least as effective at protecting worker safety as the federal OSHA program (94).

OSHA requires employers to meet certain safety standards or face financial penalties for noncompliance. Financial penalties can be up to $7,000 per violation for less serious violations, and up to $70,000 per violation for willful or repeat violations (97). Three important standards for fitness facilities are OHSA's General Duty Clause, Hazard Communication Standard, and Bloodborne Pathogens Standard (BBP). The BBP is covered in Chapter 11.

General Duty Clause

OSHA's General Duty Clause at Section 5(a)(1) of OSHA, requires employers to provide their employees with a place of employment that is free from recognizable hazards that are causing or likely to cause death or serious harm to employees (98). The courts have interpreted the General Duty Clause to mean that an employer has a legal obligation to provide a workplace free of conditions or activities that either the employer or industry recognizes as hazardous and that cause, or are likely to cause, death.

Hazard Communication Standard

If employees work excessively with chemicals, such as cleaning products (that is, more than the average consumer of the chemical product), it may be required under OSHA (or at least a good idea) for the fitness facility to provide employees a list of the hazardous chemicals present in the workplace, properly label those chemicals, train employees on how to properly use those chemicals and the hazards they may present, and provide employees with protective equipment to minimize any adverse effect from use of those chemicals. For more information, see: Fact Sheet on OSHA Hazard Communication, available at: https://www.osha.gov/dsg/hazcom/HCSFinalRegTxt.htmlhttps://www.osha.gov/dsg/hazcom/HCSFinalRegTxt.html (Accessed January 12, 2020).

Case Examples: Fitness Facility OSHA Hazard Communication Violations

Case #1: The failure to provide personal protective equipment as well as the failure to develop and implement a hazard communication program resulted in penalties totaling $60,000 for repeat violations (99). The fitness facility did not provide eye, face, and hand protection for employees using liquid and other hazardous chemicals and did not meet the requirements of a hazard communication program such as having a written plan.

Case #2: The fitness facility failed to install proper emergency washout stations for its employees that handled a range of chemicals that were potentially dangerous (100). The facility was initially fined $195,300, but because they failed to address the problem despite having years to do so, the fines continued to accrue at a rate of $300/day and reached over $500,000.

Clinical Laboratory Improvement Amendments (CLIA)

In addition to the BBP, another law involving human blood or other specimens is the Clinical Laboratory Improvement Amendments (CLIA) of 1988 and state laws that govern drawing of blood and laboratory testing. Fitness facilities or exercise professionals may sponsor blood tests or conduct finger prick tests to measure certain health markers, such as cholesterol or glucose levels, as part of a pre-activity health screening procedure or as a periodic service to participants. For more information regarding pre-activity health screening procedures, see Chapter 6. This section focuses on CLIA compliance that governs the testing of human blood or other specimens.

CLIA Compliance

The federal Centers for Medicare and Medicaid Services (CMS) regulates all laboratory testing (except research) performed on humans in the United States through CLIA (101). CLIA was established to strengthen federal oversight of clinical laboratories to ensure the accuracy and reliability of patient test results (102). Federal law defines a **laboratory** to be a facility that performs certain testing on human specimens in order to obtain information that can be used for the diagnosis, prevention, or treatment of any disease or impairment of a human being; or the assessment of the health of a human being; or procedures to determine, measure or otherwise describe the presence or absence of various substances or organisms in a human body (102). Given this broad definition, many workplace wellness **biometric screening** activities involve a CLIA "laboratory" at some point during the testing process as well as fitness facilities that conduct biometric screening.

All facilities that meet the definition of "laboratory" under CLIA must obtain an appropriate CLIA certificate prior to conducting patient testing (102). However, facilities that only collect or prepare specimens (or both) or only serve as a mailing service and do not perform testing are not considered laboratories under CLIA. CLIA's regulatory requirements vary according to the kind of tests each laboratory conducts (102). Tests are categorized as:

- Waived
- Moderate Complexity
- High Complexity (102).

Most on-site, point-of-care biometric screens fall within the CLIA waived test category (101). Laboratories that perform waived tests must obtain a certificate of waiver under CLIA (103). Waived tests must meet the following criteria:

- Are cleared by the FDA for home use;

- Employ methodologies that are so simple and accurate as to render the likelihood of erroneous results negligible; or
- Pose no reasonable risk of harm to the patient if the test is performed incorrectly (103)

A full list of the tests that are waived under CLIA, and those tests' manufacturers can be found in a document titled: Waived Tests and CPT Codes, available at: https://www.doh.wa.gov/portals/1/Documents/Pubs/681018.pdf (Accessed November 24, 2019).

The significance of being categorized as a waived test is that there are fewer regulatory requirements for the laboratory conducting those tests. Laboratories eligible for a certificate of waiver must: (a) follow the manufacturers' instructions for performing the test, and (b) meet the certificate of waiver requirements found at 42 CFR § 493.35-39 (103). The certificate of waiver requirements includes:

- Filing an application with the Department of Health and Human Services (HHS)
- Making records available and submitting reports to HHS to ensure compliance with 42 CFR § 493.15(e)
- Agreeing to permit announced and unannounced inspections by HHS
- Remitting a certificate of waiver fee (104).

The certification is good for two years (105). After that, the laboratory must renew the certificate (105). It is

---

Exhibit 3-8: Risk Management Strategies and Resources: Employee Safety Laws

Risk Management Strategies:

1. Determine whether your fitness facility exposes your employees or participants to any hazards, such as tripping hazards, chemical hazards, bloodborne pathogen hazards, etc.

2. Remove the risk of those hazards by investing in protective equipment, rearrangement of equipment, etc.

3. Train your employees on OSHA and CLIA standards.

Resources:

1. OSHA Training Tools
   Available at: https://www.osha.gov/dte/library/. (Accessed November 24, 2019).

2. Free OSHA On-site Consultation Program (available to small and medium-sized businesses)
   Available at: https://www.osha.gov/consultation. (Accessed November 24, 2019).

3. CLIA Resources:
   Available at: https://www.fda.gov/medical-devices/ivd-regulatory-assistance/clinical-laboratory-improvement-amendments-clia. (Accessed November 24, 2019).

important that fitness/wellness managers and professionals and organizations that include screening activities involving laboratory testing assess whether the appropriate CLIA certificates have been issued.

State laws can sometimes override or go beyond CLIA requirements, including for waived tests (101). State regulations may limit the tests that can be run, dictate who can run certain tests, require certain practitioner oversight, or regulate the way results can be provided or reported to employees (101). There are also state laws that address transport, storage, and disposal of biometric specimens (106). Some states also prohibit Direct Access Testing (DAT), which are laboratory tests that are allowed without a physician's order (101). In those states that prohibit DAT, physicians must order the test and the results must be reported to the ordering physician (101). The examination of each state's laws that govern biometric screening is beyond the scope of this textbook. Nevertheless, fitness managers and exercise professionals should be aware that such state laws exist and should consult with legal counsel when assessing a screening program's compliance with those laws.

WELLNESS PRODUCTS AND DEVICES

A threshold question is whether a given product is a regulated medical device (107). To decide whether a device is subject to FDA medical device regulation is to determine the device's "intended use." To determine the intended use, the FDA looks at a product's labeling claims, advertising matter, or oral or written statements by manufacturers or their representatives (108). Generally, products, including software, are considered medical devices if they are intended for a medical purpose (108). If a product is considered a medical device, the manufacturer must comply with certain FDA regulatory requirements (108). See Exhibit 3-9 at the end of this section for risk management strategies and resources that can help increase compliance to laws involving wellness products and devices.

Mobile Apps

A "**mobile medical app**" is "a software application that can be run on a smart phone, tablet or other portable computer, or a web-based software platform tailored to a mobile platform but executed on a server, that meets the definition of device in § 201(h) of the FDCA [Food, Drug, and Cosmetic Act] and is intended either: (a) to be used as an accessory to a regulated medical device; or (b) to transform a mobile platform into a regulated medical device. Generally, if a mobile app is intended for use in performing a medical device function (i.e., for diagnosis of disease or other conditions, or the cure, mitigation, treatment, or prevention of disease) it is a medical device, regardless of the platform on which it is run... the FDA looks at a product's labeling claims, advertising materials or oral or written statements by manufacturers or their representatives to determine a device's intended use" (40, p. 341).

"The key for wellness professionals and organizations is to determine whether a mobile app constitutes a mobile *medical* app or just a **mobile app**. If the latter, the FDA will exercise enforcement discretion, which means the FDA is choosing not to enforce compliance of those apps under the FDCA. If the app is a mobile "medical" app, then the FDA will apply its regulatory oversight over those apps" (40, p. 341).

Low-Risk Wellness Devices

Because low-risk wellness devices are, generally, not considered medical devices, the FDA does not regulate them. The FDA released draft guidance regarding low risk wellness devices on January 20, 2015 (109). According to the FDA, low-risk products generally promote a healthy lifestyle and meet the following two factors: (a) are intended for only general wellness use, and (b) present a very low risk to users' safety (109). In evaluating the second factor, FDA considers a product to present an inherent risk to a user's safety if the product:
- Is invasive;
- Involves an intervention or technology that may pose a risk to a user's safety if device controls are not applied, such as risks from lasers, radiation exposure, or implants;
- Raises novel questions of usability; or
- Raises questions of biocompatibility (109, p. 5).

Examples of such products include:
- Sunlamp products promoted for tanning purposes (exposure to ultraviolet radiation creates an increased risk of skin cancer);

- Implants promoted for improved self-image or enhanced sexual function (creates in increased risk of rupture or adverse reaction to implant materials, as well as from the implantation procedure);
- A laser product that claims to improve confidence in user's appearance by rejuvenating the skin (laser technology presents risk of skin and eye burns and presents usability considerations that may be addressed with labeling and other device controls) (109, p. 6).

Another way to determine whether a wellness device qualifies as low risk is to investigate whether the FDA already regulates products of the same type as the product in question (109). Fitness managers and exercise professionals may visit the FDA website at: http://www.accessdata.fda.gov/scripts/cdrh/cfdocs/cfpcd/classification.cfm (accessed November 24, 2019) to search for similar products that the FDA might already regulate.

INTELLECTUAL PROPERTY

In an effort to help people become fit and healthy, fitness companies, organizations, facilities, or exercise professionals may create programs, names, tools, equipment, technology, or other works that would benefit from intellectual property protection. Fitness managers and exercise professionals may also use creative works, such as music, within their facilities or programs. This section first describes the types of protection available for various creations. Next, a brief description of U.S. intellectual property law (e.g., trademarks, patents, and copyright law) is provided and its application to the exercise profession.

Seeking the Correct Type of Protection

It is important to know which intellectual property concept protects which unique creation so that companies, organizations, facilities, or exercise professionals can seek the correct type of protection. See Table 3-5.

Exhibit 3-9: Risk Management Strategies and Resources: Wellness Products and Devices

Risk Management Strategies:

1. To lower FDA enforcement risk, use only low-risk wellness devices.

2. To determine whether a device qualifies as a low-risk wellness device, evaluate its intended use.

    a. Ask: Is the device intended for only general wellness use?

    b. Does the device present a very low risk to users' safety?

3. To determine whether the device presents a very low risk to users' safety, look at whether the device:

    a. Is invasive;

    b. Involves an intervention or technology that may pose a risk to a user's safety if device controls are not applied, such as risks from lasers, radiation exposure, or implants;

    c. Raises novel questions of usability; or

    d. Raises questions of biocompatibility.

4. It would not be within the scope of practice of exercise professionals to use a medical device that is used within the legal scope of practice of licensed professionals such as physicians or physical therapists.

Resources:

1. FDA Guidance Document for Low Risk Wellness Devices
   Available at: https://www.fda.gov/regulatory-information/search-fda-guidance-documents/general-wellness-policy-low-risk-devices.(Accessed November 25, 2019).

2. FDA Medical Devices
   Available at: https://www.fda.gov/medical-devices. (Accessed November 25, 2019).

Table 3-5	Types of Protection for Various Creations					
CREATION TYPE	**COPYRIGHT**	**TRADEMARK**	**SERVICE MARK**	**PATENT**	**STATE BUSINESS REGISTRATION DEPARTMENT**	**WEBSITE DOMAIN NAME**
Business Name					✔	✔
Invention (new technology, tool or exercise equipment)				✔		
Slogan for a workout			✔			
Slogan for a product		✔				
Logo for a workout			✔			
Logo for a product		✔				
Book about fitness	✔					
Music for fitness	✔					

It is a good idea to hire an intellectual property lawyer to assist in seeking such protection. See Exhibit 3-10 at the end of this section for risk management strategies and resources regarding intellectual property laws.

Trademarks

If a fitness company, professional organization or individual, or facility creates a unique name, program, logo, or product, for example, it may be wise to obtain protection for that unique creation by seeking help from the U.S. Patent and Trademark Office (USPTO) (for trademarks and patents) or the U.S. Copyright Office for copyrights. It is important to know which intellectual property concept protects which unique creation so that organizations, facilities, or exercise professionals can seek the correct protection.

To put it simply, **trademarks** protect words or symbols that identify goods and **service marks** protect words or symbols that identify services. However, people often use the term "trademark" in reference to both goods and services (110). Fitness organizations, facilities and exercise professionals may use trademarks to protect the name, slogan and/or logo of their facility or specific fitness or wellness programs they created.

As long as the trademark is used in commerce (i.e., for business purposes), it has common law protection. This means that if someone else tries to use your trademark for a similar product or service within your geographic area, you might be able to stop them by using state unfair competition laws and the common law. Unregistered trademarks use TM for goods or SM for services, to indicate "common law" protection for the trademark or service mark (110).

To obtain further protection for trademarks, fitness organizations, facilities, or exercise professionals can register the trademark or service mark with the USPTO. Federal registration of a trademark with the USPTO provides notice to the public of the registrant's claim of ownership of the mark, a legal presumption of ownership nationwide, and the exclusive right to use the mark on or in connection with the goods or services set forth in the registration. Registered trademarks use the ® symbol for the mark (110) such as in Exercise is Medicine®.

Patents

A **patent** is a limited duration property right relating to an invention, granted by the USPTO in exchange for public disclosure of the invention. Patentable materials include machines, manufactured articles, industrial processes, and chemical compositions. In the exercise profession, a patentable invention might be a new piece of exercise equipment, wearable technology, or weight loss product. Patents protect the product or process between, approximately, 15 to 20 years depending on whether it is a design, utility, or plant patent (110).

Copyright

A **copyright** protects original works of authorship including literary, dramatic, musical, and artistic works, such as poetry, novels, movies, songs, computer software, and architecture. (110). Copyrights can protect the original work of art for many, many years. For individual works of art (whether music or books, for example), copyright protects the work for the life of the author plus 70 years (110). Individuals can register their copyrighted material with the U.S. Copyright Office at: https://www.copyright.gov/registration/. Examples of items one can register for copyright include literary works, performing arts (music, sound recordings, scripts, stage plays), visual arts (artwork, illustrations, jewelry, fabric, architecture), computer programs, databases, blogs, websites, motion pictures and photographs (111).

Copyright infringement occurs when someone uses copyrighted material without permission of the author/creator. For example, to reprint information from textbooks such as this textbook, it will be necessary to obtain permission from the publisher prior to reprinting a portion of it in another publication. Also, regarding using music in a fitness facility, it will be necessary to purchase licensing agreements from Performing Rights Organizations (PROs) such as:

- Broadcast Music, Inc. (BMI): www.bmi.com
- American Society of Composers, Authors, and Publishers (ASCAP): www.ascap.com
- Society of European Stage Authors and Composers (SECAC): www.sesac.com

Some fitness facilities may be exempt from paying these fees based on the Fairness in Music Licensing Act (FMLA). Before using music, videos, software, or other forms of creations that are copyrighted, fitness managers and exercise professionals need to consult with a competent intellectual property lawyer to be sure they are not violating any copyright laws, otherwise they may face costly penalties. Fitness companies, facilities, and programs have been involved in copyright infringement cases as demonstrated in the following cases.

Case #1—Peloton

Peloton, an on-demand fitness streaming company was founded in 2012. In 2019, a number of music publishing companies, led by Downtown Music Publishing, LLC (hereinafter "plaintiffs"), sued Peloton Interactive, Inc. for copyright infringement (112). The plaintiffs argued that Peloton failed to obtain authorization from owners of over 1,000 copyrighted works in the form of a synchronization license. Obtaining a synchronization license is different than purchasing a music licensing agreement as described above. "A synchronization license allows the licensee lawfully to reproduce a protected work in connection with or in timed relation with a visual image, such as videos that Peloton records, archives and makes available to its customers" (112, p. 4). For example, Peloton's streaming fitness classes combine visual fitness instruction with copyrighted music which requires Peloton to secure the synchronization rights for each copyrighted song (112, 113). Because Peloton's brand relies on music, and because Peloton sought synchronization licenses from certain other copyright owners, the plaintiffs alleged that Peloton was willfully infringing federal copyright law and should pay the plaintiffs over $150,000,000 in damages. Fitness managers and exercise professionals may want to review an article titled: Why All Gyms Need to Follow the Peloton Music Copyright Case (113). In this article, the plaintiffs were referred to as the National Music Publishers' Association (NMPA)—a group of music publishers. In February 2020, this case was settled out-of-court and terms of the settlement were not disclosed (114).

Case #2—Workout America Facilities

Another copyright infringement case involved Workout America facilities located in Georgia. Workout America played copyrighted music through at least thirteen ceiling mounted stereo speakers and floor box speakers throughout its facilities. Participants had to pay a $5.00 admission charge to use Workout

America facilities. It is illegal under the Copyright Act of 1976 to play musical compositions without a license over a stereo system in a business establishment for the entertainment of customers. Because Workout America failed to obtain a license to use the copyrighted songs to use in its fitness facilities, the court found Workout America to have violated federal copyright law and ordered Workout America to pay damages to the music publisher companies who sued (115).

Case #3—University of Iowa Football Program

The University of Iowa's football team's Twitter account was suspended due to music copyright infringement (116). The University's women's gymnastics team account was also suspended for similar infractions. The athletic director stated that efforts were underway to help ensure that future posts are complying with copyright law. The Iowa State University football team's account was also suspended.

Exhibit 3-10 Risk management Strategies and Resources: Intellectual Property Laws

Risk Management Strategies:

1. Conduct a thorough search for use of any proposed symbols or phrases to determine whether there is a registered or common law trademark use of the symbol or phrase.

2. Register a created work (symbol, word, phrase) with the USPTO to strengthen protection of your trademark or service mark.

3. Obtain formal permission and/or required licenses to use copyrighted materials in fitness facilities or fitness programs.

Resources:

1. United States Patent and Trademark Office
   Available at: https://www.uspto.gov/. (Accessed November 26, 2019).

2. United States Copyright Office
   Available at: https://www.copyright.gov/. (Accessed November 26, 2019).

3. US Copyright Office Fact Sheet on How to Obtain Permission to Use Copyrighted Material
   Available at: https://www.copyright.gov/circs/m10.pdf. (Accessed November 2019).

 KEY TERMS

- Biometric Screening
- Business Associates
- Competent and Reliable Evidence
- Copyright
- Covered Entities
- Group Health Plan Wellness Program
- HIPAA Breach Notification Rule
- HIPAA Privacy Rule
- HIPAA Security Rule
- Laboratory
- Mobile App

- Mobile Medical App
- Patent
- Pattern or Practice
- Places of Public Accommodation
- Protected Health Information (PHI)
- Reasonable Accommodation
- Service Marks
- Trademarks
- Unsecured PHI
- Wearable Technology

STUDY QUESTIONS

The Study Questions for Chapter 3 can be found on the Fitness Law Academy website (www.fitnesslawacademy.com) under Textbook. They are provided in a fillable format for convenience.

APPENDIX

This chapter's appendix follows the References.

REFERENCES

1. EEOC Releases Fiscal Year 2018 Enforcement and Litigation Data. U.S. Equal Employment Opportunity Commission. April 10, 2019. Available at: https://www.eeoc.gov/eeoc/newsroom/release/4-10-19.cfm. Accessed June 27, 2019.

2. Wisconsin Fair Employment Act, Wis. Stat. §§ 111.31-111.395.

3. *Jalal v. Lucille Roberts Health Clubs Inc.*, 254 F. Supp. 3d 602 (S.D.N.Y. 2017).

4. The Civil Rights Act of 1964, 42 U.S. Code § 2000e–2(a).

5. *Oncale v. Sundowner Offshore Services, Inc.*, 118 S. Ct. 998 (U.S., 1998).

6. Esmaili T. Employment Discrimination. Legal Information Institute. Last Updated June 2017. Available at: https://www.law.cornell.edu/wex/employment_discrimination. Accessed January 6, 2020.

7. *Bostock v. Clayton County, Georgia,* 140 S. Ct. 1731 (U.S., 2020). Available at: https://www.supremecourt.gov/opinions/19pdf/17-1618_hfci.pdf. Accessed June 23, 2020.

8. Lipak A. Supreme Court to Decide whether Landmark Civil Rights Law Applies to Gay and Transgender Workers. *The New York Times.* April 22, 2019. Available at: https://www.nytimes.com/2019/04/22/us/politics/supreme-court-gay-transgender-employees.html. Accessed July 23, 2019.

9. Equality Maps: State Non-Discrimination Laws. Movement Advancement Project. January 5, 2020. Available at: http://www.lgbtmap.org/equality-maps/non_discrimination_laws. Accessed July 23, 2019.

10. Ford C. Employment Discrimination: Gender Discrimination and Hostile Work Environment. United States Department of Justice, Executive Office for United States Attorneys. May 2009. Available at: https://www.justice.gov/sites/default/files/usao/legacy/2009/05/07/usab5702.pdf. Accessed July 23, 2019.

11. Teigan A. State Public Accommodation Laws. National Conference of State Legislatures. April 08, 2019. Available at http://www.ncsl.org/research/civil-and-criminal-justice/state-public-accommodation-laws.aspx. Accessed July 22, 2019.

12. Unruh Civil Rights Act, Cal. Civ. Code § 51(b).

13. Uffalussy JG. Equinox Gym Bans Man 'For Life' After He Reported Sexual Misconduct by Yoga Teacher: Lawsuit Filed. *Yahoo Beauty.* October 24, 2017. Available at: https://www.yahoo.com/lifestyle/equinox-gym-bans-man-life-reported-sexual-misconduct-yoga-teacher-lawsuit-filed-185730889.html. Accessed November 12, 2019.

14. Americans with Disabilities Act of 1990, as Amended. Available at: https://www.ada.gov/pubs/adastatute08.htm. Accessed November 13, 2019.

15. Civil Monetary Penalties Inflation Adjustment under Title III. Information and Technical Assistance on the Americans with Disabilities Act. Available at: https://www.ada.gov/civil_penalties_2014.htm. Accessed November 13, 2019.

16. ADA Standards for Accessible Design. Information and Technical Assistance on the Americans with Disabilities Act. Available at: https://www.ada.gov/2010ADAstandards_index.htm. Accessed November 13, 2019.

17. Nearly 1 in 5 People have a Disability in the U.S. Census Bureau Reports. July 25, 2012. Available at: https://www.census.gov/newsroom/releases/archives/miscellaneous/cb12-134.html. Accessed November 13, 2019.

18. *Healthy People 2020.* Physical Activity Objectives. Available at: https://www.healthypeople.gov/2020/data-search/Search-the-Data#objid=5069. Accessed May 14, 2019.

19. Fact Sheet on the EEOC's Final Regulations Implementing the ADAAA. Available at: https://www.eeoc.gov/laws/regulations/adaaa_fact_sheet.cfm. Accessed November 13, 2019.

20. The Americans With Disabilities Act, 42 U.S.C. § 12181(7).

21. Public Accommodations and Commercial Facilities (Title III). Information and Technical Assistance on the Americans with Disabilities Act. Available at: https://www.ada.gov/ada_title_III.htm. Accessed November 13, 2019.

22. Americans with Disabilities Act Title III Regulations. Nondiscrimination on the Basis of Disability by Public Accommodations and in Commercial Facilities. Department of Justice. September 15, 2010. Available at: https://www.ada.gov/regs2010/titleIII_2010/titleIII_2010_regulations.pdf. Accessed July 29, 2019.

23. Rimmer JH, Padalabalanarayanan S, Malone, LA, et al. Fitness Facilities Still Lack Accessibility for People With Disabilities, *Disability and Health Journal,* 10(2), 214-221, 2017.

24. Johnson MJ, Stoelzle HY, Finco KL, et al. ADA Compliance and Accessibility of Fitness Facilities in Western Wisconsin. *Topics in Spinal Cord Injury Rehabilitation,* 18(4), 340-353, 2012.

25. *Neal v. PFTN Murfreesboro South, LLC,* Civ. Complaint. Action No. 3:19-cv-00398 (M.D. Tenn. 2019). Available at: https://www.

References continued...

courtlistener.com/recap/gov.uscourts.tnmd.79042/gov.uscourts.
tnmd.79042.1.0.pdf. Accessed July 29, 2019.

26. *Class v. Towson University*, 118 F. Supp. 3d 833 (D. Md., 2015).

27. Moorman AM, Eickhoff-Shemek JM. The Legal Aspects: Is Obesity
a Disability Under the ADA? *ACSM's Health & Fitness Journal*, 9(1),
29-31, 2005.

28. *Taylor v. Burlington N. R.R. Holdings, Inc.*, 193 Wn.2d 611 (Wash.,
2019).

29. Corte RL. Washington Court: Obesity Covered by Anti-discrimination
Law. *The Seattle Times*. July 12, 2019. Available at: https://www.
seattletimes.com/seattle-news/washington-court-obesity-covered-
by-antidiscrimination-law/. Accessed July 31, 2019.

30. The Civil Rights Act of 1964, 42 U.S.C. § 2000a(a).

31. Title II of the Civil Rights Act (Public Accommodations). The United
States Department of Justice. August 6, 2015. Available at: https://www.
justice.gov/crt-22. Accessed August 1, 2019.

32. Keister K. Social Media Stir Surrounds Swimming Pool Rules in Wendell,
NC. *The News & Observer*. June 17, 2019. Available at: https://www.
newsobserver.com/news/local/article231653263.html. Accessed
August 1, 2019.

33. Berg A. Three Fired at LA Fitness on Race Profiling Accusations.
Athletic Business E-Newsletter. April 2018. Available at: https://www.
athleticbusiness.com/facilities/three-fired-at-la-fitness-over-racial-
profiling.html. Accessed August 1, 2019.

34. Rose J. I'm Not Aware of That: Starbucks Employees Receive Racial
Bias Training. May 28, 2018. Available at: https://www.npr.
org/2018/05/29/615263473/thousands-of-starbucks-stores-close-
for-racial-bias-training?jwsource=cl. Accessed November 19, 2019.

35. Facts about Race/Color Discrimination. U.S. Equal Employment
Opportunity Commission. Available at: https://www.eeoc.gov/eeoc/
publications/fs-race.cfm. Accessed August 1, 2019.

36. Age Discrimination. U.S. Equal Employment Opportunity Commission.
Available at: https://www.eeoc.gov/laws/types/age.cfm. Accessed
August 1, 2019.

37. *Moore v. University of Notre Dame*, 22 F. Supp. 2d 896 (N.D. Ind., 1998).

38. Wolohan JT. Age Discrimination Illegal, Potentially Expensive for
Athletic Departments. *Athletic Business E-Newsletter*. March 2000.
Available at: https://www.athleticbusiness.com/civil-actions/
age-discrimination-illegal-potentially-expensive-for-athletic-
departments.html. Accessed August 1, 2019.

39. *Austin v. Cornell University*, 891 F. Supp. 740 (N.D.N.Y., 1995).

40. Zabawa BJ, Eickhoff-Shemek, JM. *Rule the Rules of Workplace Wellness
Programs*. Chicago, IL: American Bar Association, 2017.

41. Employee Retirement and Income Security Act of 1974 (ERISA), 29
U.S.C. §§ 1167 and 1183.

42. The Social Security Act, 45 C.F.R. § 160.103.

43. The HIPAA Privacy Rule, 45 C.F.R §§ 160.101 - 160.552 (2013); 45 C.F.R.
§§ 164.102 - 164.106 (2013); 45 C.F.R. §§ 164.500 - 164.534 (2013).

44. The Security Rule. Office for Civil Rights. May 12, 2017. Available at:
https://www.hhs.gov/hipaa/for-professionals/security/index.html.
Accessed April 16, 2016.

45. Health Information Technology for Economic and Clinical Health
(HITECH) Act, Pub. L. No. 111-5, §§ 13400 – 13411 (2009).

46. Summary of the HIPAA Security Law. Office for Civil Rights. July 26,
2013. Available at: https://www.hhs.gov/hipaa/for-professionals/security/
laws-regulations/index.html. Accessed April 16, 2016.

47. The HIPAA Privacy Rule, 45 C.F.R. § 164.306 (2013).

48. The HIPAA Privacy Rule, 45 C.F.R. § 164.400 (2009).

49. The HIPAA Privacy Rule, 45 C.F.R. § 164.410 (2013).

50. The HIPAA Privacy Rule, 45 C.F.R. § 164.402 (2013).

51. Guidance to Render Unsecured Protected Health Information
Unusable, Unreadable, or Indecipherable to Unauthorized Individuals,
Office for Civil Rights. July 26, 2013. Available at: http://www.hhs.
gov/hipaa/for-professionals/breach-notification/guidance/index.html.
Accessed October 2, 2016.

52. The HIPAA Privacy Rule, 45 C.F.R. § 160.203(b) (2002).

53. The HIPAA Privacy Rule, 45 C.F.R. § 160.201 (2013).

54. Transactions Overview. Centers for Medicare & Medicaid Services. July
26, 2017. Available at https://www.cms.gov/Regulations-and-Guidance/
Administrative-Simplification/Transactions/TransactionsOverview.html.
Accessed August 4, 2019.

55. 2014 Privacy and Data Security Update. Federal Trade
Commission. Available at: https://www.ftc.gov/system/files/
documents/reports/privacy-data-security-update-2014/
privacydatasecurityupdate_2014.pdf. Accessed April 16, 2016.

56. Federal Trade Commission Act Section 5: Unfair or Deceptive Acts or
Practices. Federal Trade Commission. December 2016. Available at:
https://www.federalreserve.gov/boarddocs/supmanual/cch/ftca.
pdf. Accessed April 16, 2016.

57. The Federal Trade Commission Act, 15 U.S.C. § 45(a) (2012).

58. Complaint. *In re PaymentsMD, LLC*, Dkt. No. C-4505, ¶ 9 (Fed. Trade
Comm. January 27, 2015) Available at: https://www.ftc.gov/system/
files/documents/cases/150206paymentsmdcmpt.pdf. Accessed April
16, 2016.

59. Complaint. *In re Genelink, Inc. and Foru International Corp.*, Dkt. No.
C-4456 (Fed. Trade Comm. May 8, 2014). Available at: https://www.
ftc.gov/system/files/documents/cases/140512genelinkcmpt.pdf.
Accessed April 17, 2016.

60. FTC Policy Statement Regarding Advertising Substantiation. Federal
Trade Commission. March 11, 1983. Available at https://www.ftc.
gov/public-statements/1983/03/ftc-policy-statement-regarding-
advertising-substantiation. Accessed August 4, 2019.

61. Enforcement Policy Statement on Marketing Claims for OTC
Homeopathic Drugs. Federal Trade Commission. Available at: https://
www.ftc.gov/system/files/documents/public_statements/996984/
p114505_otc_homeopathic_drug_enforcement_policy_statement.
pdf. Accessed June 9, 2019.

62. Dietary Supplements: An Advertising Guide for Industry. Federal Trade
Commission. April 2001. Available at: https://www.ftc.gov/tips-advice/
business-center/guidance/dietary-supplements-advertising-guide-
industry. Accessed June 9, 2019.

63. Guides Concerning the Use of Endorsements and Testimonials in
Advertising, 16 CFR §§ 255.0 – 255.5 (2009).

64. Guides Concerning the Use of Endorsements and Testimonials in
Advertising, 16 CFR § 255.2 (2009).

65. Guides Concerning the Use of Endorsements and Testimonials in
Advertising, 16 CFR § 255.3 (2009).

66. The FTC's Endorsement Guides: What People are Asking, available at
https://www.ftc.gov/tips-advice/business-center/guidance/ftcs-
endorsement-guides-what-people-are-asking (Accessed January 12,
2020).

67. Gut Check: A Reference Guide for Media on Spotting False Weight Loss
Claims. Federal Trade Commission. January 2014. Available at: https://www.
ftc.gov/tips-advice/business-center/guidance/gut-check-reference-
guide-media-spotting-false-weight-loss. Accessed January 11, 2020.

68. A.G. Schneiderman Announces Settlement with Machinima and Three
Other Companies for False Endorsement. New York State Officer of the
Attorney General. February 11, 2016. Available at: https://ag.ny.gov/press-

References continued...

release/2016/ag-schneiderman-announces-settlement-machinima-and-three-other-companies-false. Accessed January 11, 2020.

69. Copp T. Fitbits and Fitness Tracking Devices Banned for Deployed Troops. August 6, 2018. Your Military. Available at: https://www.militarytimes.com/news/your-military/2018/08/06/devices-and-apps-that-rely-on-geolocation-restricted-for-deployed-troops. Accessed November 20, 2019.

70. Joseph JM. Data Breach Notifications Laws: A Fifty State Survey. 1st Ed., pp. vi-vii. Washington D.C.: American Health Lawyers Association, 2011.

71. Miscellaneous Police Provisions, Wis. Stat. § 175.22 (2018).

72. The Fair Labor Standards Act of 1938, 29 U.S.C. § 201, et seq (2018).

73. Williams P. Historical Overview of the Fair Labor Standards Act, *Florida Coastal Law Review,* 10, 657-69, 2009.

74. Defining and Delimiting the Exemptions for Executive, Administrative, Professional, Outside Sales and Computer Employee, 80 Fed. Reg. 38516 (proposed July 6, 2015; to be codified at 29 C.F.R. pt. 541).

75. Fact Sheet #14: Coverage Under the Fair Labor Standards Act (FLSA). U.S. Department of Labor Wage and Hour Division. July 2009. Available at: https://www.dol.gov/sites/dolgov/files/WHD/legacy/files/whdfs14.pdf. (Accessed January 11, 2020).

76. Fair Labor Standards Act of 1938, 29 U.S.C. § 206 (2016).

77. Fair Labor Standards Act of 1938, 29 U.S.C. § 207 (2010).

78. 29 C.F.R. §§ 541.100 to 541.504 (2004).

79. 29 C.F.R. § 541.600 (2019).

80. Defining and Delimiting the Exemptions for Executive, Administrative, Professional, Outside Sales and Computer Employee, 81 Fed. Reg. 32391 (proposed May 23, 2016; to be codified at 29 C.F.R. pt. 541).

81. Fair Labor Standards Act Advisor, Exemptions. U.S. Department of Labor. Available at: https://webapps.dol.gov/elaws/whd/flsa/screen75.asp. Accessed September 17, 2019.

82. Opinion Letter. U.S. Department of Labor Wage and Hour Division. November 14, 2005. Available at: https://www.dol.gov/whd/opinion/FLSA/2005/2005_11_14_53_FLSA.htm. Accessed September 17, 2019.

83. Life Time Fitness to Pay More than $976K in Back Minimum Wages, Damages to 15K Employees at Locations in 26 States. *U.S. Department of Labor.* November 29, 2016. Available at: https://www.dol.gov/newsroom/releases/whd/whd20161129. Accessed September 17, 2019.

84. 29 C.F.R. § 553.101 (1987).

85. Fact Sheet #14A: Non-Profit Organizations and the FLSA. U.S. Department of Labor Wage and Hour Division. August 2015. Available at: https://www.dol.gov/whd/regs/compliance/whdfs14a.pdf (Accessed September 24, 2019).

86. Fair Labor Standards Act Advisor, Volunteers. U.S. Department of Labor. Available at: https://webapps.dol.gov/elaws/whd/flsa/docs/volunteers.asp. Accessed September 24, 2019).

87. 29 C.F.R. § 785.27 (1961).

88. *Wicke v. L&C Insulation, Inc.,* No. 12-cv-638-wmc, 2014 LEXIS 89193 (W.D. Wis. 2014).

89. 29 CFR § 785.28 (1961).

90. Marsh J. Personal Trainers Sue Crunch Gym for up to $200K in Unpaid Wages. *New York Post.* April 20, 2016. Available at: https://nypost.com/2016/04/20/personal-trainers-sue-crunch-gym-for-up-to-200k-in-unpaid-wages/. Accessed August 5, 2019.

91. The Equal Pay Act of 1963, 29 U.S.C. § 206(d) (2016).

92. Facts about Equal Pay and Compensation Discrimination. U.S. Equal Employment Opportunity Commission. Available at: https://www.eeoc.gov/eeoc/publications/fs-epa.cfm. Accessed August 4, 2019.

93. The Occupational Safety and Health Act of 1970, 29 U.S.C. § 651, et seq. (1970).

94. All About OSHA. U.S. Department of Labor Occupational Safety and Health Administration. Available at: https://www.osha.gov/Publications/all_about_OSHA.pdf. Accessed August 5, 2019.

95. The Occupational Safety and Health Act of 1970, 29 U.S.C. § 651 (1970).

96. Occupational Safety And Health Standards, 29 C.F.R. § 1910 (1974).

97. The Occupational Safety and Health Act of 1970, 29 U.S.C. § 666 (1990).

98. The Occupational Safety and Health Act of 1970, 29 U.S.C. § 654 (1970).

99. OSHA Cites Xsport Fitness Facility in Libertyville Illinois for Failing to Provide Workers with Personal Protective Equipment. Available at: http://advancedsafetyhealth.com/newsletter-blog/2013/01/01/fitness-center-receives-repeat-osha-citations. Accessed November 22, 2019.

100. Club Fails to Update Safety Feature, Faces Heavy $200,000 Fines. Schoenfeld & Schoenfeld, P.C. Available at: https://www.schoenfeldlawyers.com/blog/2017/08/club-fails-to-update-safety-features-faces-heavy-200000-fines/. Accessed June 25, 2020.

101. Biometric Health Screening for Employers: Consensus Statement of the Health Enhancement Research Organization, American College of Occupational and Environmental Medicine, and Care Continuum Alliance. *Journal of Occupational and Environmental Medicine,* 55(10), 1244-1251, 2013.

102. Direct Access Testing (DAT) and the Clinical Laboratory Improvement Amendments (CLIA) Regulations. Centers for Medicare & Medicaid Services. Available at: https://www.cms.gov/Regulations-and-Guidance/Legislation/CLIA/Downloads/directaccesstesting.pdf. Accessed June 5, 2016.

103. 42 C.F.R. § 493.15 (2017).

104. 42 C.F.R. § 493.35 (1995).

105. 42 C.F.R. § 493.37 (1995).

106. Wis. Admin. Code § NR 526.07 (2006); Wis. Admin. Code § NR 526.08 (1996); Wis. Admin. Code § NR 526.10 (2013).

107. The Food, Drug and Cosmetic Act, 21 U.S.C. § 321 (2016).

108. How to Determine if Your Product is a Medical Device. U.S. Food and Drug Administration. December 16, 2019. Available at: https://www.fda.gov/medical-devices/classify-your-medical-device/how-determine-if-your-product-medical-device. Accessed January 12, 2020.

109. Guidance Document. General Wellness: Policy for Low Risk Devices. U.S. Food and Drug Administration Center for Devices and Radiological Health. January 20, 2015. Available at: https://www.fda.gov/media/90652/download. Accessed May 20, 2016.

110. Trademark, Patent, or Copyright? U.S. Patent and Trademark Office. Available at: https://www.uspto.gov/trademarks-getting-started/trademark-basics/trademark-patent-or-copyright. Accessed October 19, 2019.

111. Registration Portal. U.S. Copyright Office. Available at: https://www.copyright.gov/registration/. Accessed January 12, 2020.

112. Amended Complaint. *Downtown Music Publishing, LLC, et al. v. Peloton Interactive,* Inc., No. 19-02426 (S.D. N.Y. 2019).

113. Durkin H. Why All Gyms Need to Follow the Peloton Music Copyright Case. July 30, 2019. IHRSA. Available at: https://www.ihrsa.org/improve-your-club/why-all-gyms-need-to-follow-the-peloton-music-copyright-case/. Accessed November 25, 2019.

114. Berg A. Peloton Settles with the NMPA Over Music Rights Lawsuit. *Athletic Business E-Newsletter.* February 2020. Available at: https://www.athleticbusiness.com/contract-law/peloton-settles-with-nmpa-over-music-rights-lawsuit.html. Accessed March 13, 2020.

115. *Blue Seas Music, Inc. v. Fitness Surveys, Inc.,* 831 F. Supp. 863 (N.D. Ga. 1993).

116. Berg A. University of Iowa Football's Twitter Account Suspended. *Athletic Business E-Newsletter.* May 2019. Available at: https://www.athleticbusiness.com/web-social/university-of-iowa-football-s-twitter-account-suspended.html. Accessed November 25, 2019.

*From: Center for Health and Wellness Law, LLC (https://www.wellnesslaw.com). Reprinted with permission.

EDITORIAL NOTE: CAUTION!!!

Regarding the Forms in this Appendix: *No form should be adopted by any program until it has first been reviewed by legal counsel in the state where a form is to be used as well as by the medical director/advisor/risk manager for the program. To be acceptable, each form must be written in accordance with prevailing state and federal laws by knowledgeable legal counsel.*

FORM A: ANTI-HARASSMENT POLICY

All Unlawful Harassment Prohibited

[EMPLOYER NAME] strictly prohibits and does not tolerate unlawful harassment against employees or any other covered persons [including interns] because of race, religion, creed, national origin, ancestry, sex (including pregnancy), gender (including gender nonconformity and status as a transgender or transsexual individual), age, physical or mental disability, citizenship, genetic information, past, current or prospective service in the uniformed services, [OTHER PROTECTED CLASSES RECOGNIZED BY APPLICABLE STATE OR LOCAL LAW] or any other characteristic protected under applicable federal, state, or local law.

Sexual Harassment

All [EMPLOYER NAME] employees, other workers and representatives (including [vendors/patients/customers/subscribers/clients] and visitors) are prohibited from harassing employees and other covered persons based on that individual's sex or gender (including pregnancy and status as a transgender or transsexual individual) and regardless of the harasser's sex or gender.

Sexual harassment means any harassment based on someone's sex or gender. It includes harassment that is not sexual in nature (for example, offensive remarks about an individual's sex or gender), as well as any unwelcome sexual advances or requests for sexual favors or any other conduct of a sexual nature, when any of the following is true:
- Submission to the advance, request or conduct is made either explicitly or implicitly a term or condition of employment.
- Submission to or rejection of the advance, request or conduct is used as a basis for employment decisions.
- Such advances, requests or conduct have the purpose or effect of substantially or unreasonably interfering with an employee's work performance by creating an intimidating, hostile or offensive work environment.

[EMPLOYER NAME] will not tolerate any form of sexual harassment, regardless of whether it is:
- Verbal (for example, epithets, derogatory statements, slurs, sexually-related comments or jokes, unwelcome sexual advances or requests for sexual favors).
- Physical (for example, assault or inappropriate physical contact).
- Visual (for example, displaying sexually suggestive posters cartoons or drawings, sending inappropriate adult-themed gifts, leering or making sexual gestures).
- Online (for example, derogatory statements or sexually suggestive postings in any social media platform including Facebook, Twitter, Instagram, Snapchat, etc.).

This list is illustrative only, and not exhaustive. No form of sexual harassment will be tolerated.

Harassment is prohibited both at the workplace and at employer-sponsored events.

Other Types of Harassment

[EMPLOYER NAME]'s anti-harassment policy applies equally to harassment based on an employee's race, religion, creed, national origin, ancestry, age, physical or mental disability, citizenship, genetic information, past, present or prospective service in the uniformed services, [OTHER PROTECTED CLASSES RECOGNIZED BY APPLICABLE STATE OR LOCAL LAW] or any other characteristic protected under applicable federal, state, or local law.

Such harassment often takes a similar form to sexual harassment and includes harassment that is:
- Verbal (for example, epithets, derogatory statements, slurs, derogatory comments or jokes).
- Physical (for example, assault or inappropriate physical contact).
- Visual (for example, displaying derogatory posters, cartoons, drawings or making derogatory gestures).
- Online (for example, derogatory statements or sexually suggestive postings in any social media platform including Facebook, Twitter, Instagram, Snapchat, etc.).

This list is illustrative only, and not exhaustive. No form of harassment will be tolerated.

Harassment is prohibited both at the workplace and at employer-sponsored events.

FORM A continued...

Complaint Procedure

If you are subjected to any conduct that you believe violates this policy or witness any such conduct, you must promptly speak to, write or otherwise contact your direct supervisor or, if the conduct involves your direct supervisor, the [next level above your direct supervisor/[DEPARTMENT NAME] Department], ideally within [ten (10)/[NUMBER]] days of the offending conduct. If you have not received a satisfactory response within [five (5)/[NUMBER]] days after reporting any incident of what you perceive to be harassment, please immediately contact [[POSITION]/[DEPARTMENT NAME] Department]. [This individual/These individuals] will ensure that a prompt investigation is conducted. [Although not mandatory, a Complaint Form is available at [LOCATION] to make your complaint if you wish to use it.]

Your complaint should be as detailed as possible, including the names of all individuals involved and any witnesses. [EMPLOYER NAME] will directly and thoroughly investigate the facts and circumstances of all claims of perceived harassment and will take prompt corrective action, if appropriate.

Additionally, any manager or supervisor who observes harassing conduct must report the conduct to [[POSITION]/[DEPARTMENT NAME] Department] so that an investigation can be made and corrective action taken, if appropriate.

No Retaliation

No one will be subject to, and [EMPLOYER NAME] prohibits, any form of discipline, reprisal, intimidation or retaliation for good faith reporting of incidents of harassment of any kind, pursuing any harassment claim or cooperating in related investigations. [For more information on [EMPLOYER NAME]'s policy prohibiting retaliation, please refer to [EMPLOYER NAME]'s Anti-Retaliation Policy or contact the [DEPARTMENT NAME] Department.]

[EMPLOYER NAME] is committed to enforcing this policy against all forms of harassment. However, the effectiveness of our efforts depends largely on employees telling us about inappropriate workplace conduct. If employees feel that they or someone else may have been subjected to conduct that violates this policy, they should report it immediately. If employees do not report harassing conduct, [EMPLOYER NAME] may not become aware of a possible violation of this policy and may not be able to take appropriate corrective action.

Violations of This Policy

Any employee, regardless of position or title, whom [[POSITION]/[DEPARTMENT NAME] Department] determines has subjected an individual to harassment or retaliation in violation of this policy, will be subject to discipline, up to and including termination of employment.

Administration of This Policy

The [DEPARTMENT NAME] Department is responsible for the administration of this policy. If you have any questions regarding this policy or questions about harassment that are not addressed in this policy, please contact the [DEPARTMENT NAME] Department.

Employees Covered Under a Collective Bargaining Agreement

The employment terms set out in this policy work in conjunction with, and do not replace, amend or supplement any terms or conditions of employment stated in any collective bargaining agreement that a union has with [EMPLOYER NAME]. [Employees should consult the terms of their collective bargaining agreement. Wherever employment terms in this policy differ from the terms expressed in the applicable collective bargaining agreement with [EMPLOYER NAME], employees should refer to the specific terms of the collective bargaining agreement, which will control.]

FORM A continued...

Conduct Not Prohibited by this Policy

This policy is not intended to preclude or dissuade employees from engaging in [legally protected activities/activities protected by state or federal law, including the National Labor Relations Act,] such as discussing wages, benefits or terms and conditions of employment[, forming, joining or supporting labor unions] [, bargaining collectively through representatives of their choosing] [, raising complaints about working conditions for their and their fellow employees' mutual aid or protection], or legally required activities.

OR

This policy is not intended to restrict communications or actions protected or required by state or federal law.

Acknowledgment of Receipt and Review

I, _____ (employee name), acknowledge that on _____ (date), I received a copy of [EMPLOYER NAME]'s [NAME OF POLICY] and that I read it, understood it and agree to comply with it. I understand that [EMPLOYER NAME] has the maximum discretion permitted by law to interpret, administer, change, modify or delete this policy at any time [with or without notice]. No statement or representation by a supervisor or manager or any other employee, whether oral or written, can supplement or modify this policy. Changes can only be made if approved in writing by the [POSITION] of [EMPLOYER NAME]. I also understand that any delay or failure by [EMPLOYER NAME] to enforce any work policy or rule will not constitute a waiver of [EMPLOYER NAME]'s right to do so in the future. I understand that neither this policy nor any other communication by a management representative or any other employee, whether oral or written, is intended in any way to create a contract of employment. I understand that, unless I have a written employment agreement signed by an authorized [EMPLOYER NAME] representative, **I am employed at will and this policy does not modify my at-will employment status.** If I have a written employment agreement signed by an authorized [EMPLOYER NAME] representative and this policy conflicts with the terms of my employment agreement, I understand that the terms of my employment agreement will control.

OR

I, _____ (employee name), acknowledge that on _____ (date), I received and read a copy of the [EMPLOYER NAME]'s [NAME OF POLICY][, dated [EDITION DATE]] and understand that it is my responsibility to be familiar with and abide by its terms. [I understand that the information in this Policy is intended to help [EMPLOYER NAME]'s employees to work together effectively on assigned job responsibilities.] This Policy is not promissory and does not set terms or conditions of employment or create an employment contract.]

[SIGNATURE PAGE FOLLOWS]

_____

Signature

_____

Printed Name

_____

Date]

FORM B: AUTHORIZATION FOR RELEASE OF PROTECTED HEALTH INFORMATION

1. _____   _____
(Name of Patient)   (Date of Birth)

_____   _____
(Street Address)   (City, State, Zip Code)

I authorize the use and/or release of my protected health information (PHI) as described below. I understand that this authorization is voluntary and is made to confirm my instructions. I also understand that the information used and/or released as a result of this authorization may no longer be protected by federal privacy laws and may be further used and/or released by persons or organizations receiving it without obtaining my authorization.

2. I AUTHORIZE: **3. TO RELEASE PHI TO:**

_____   _____
(Name of Physician/Health Care Facility) (Name of Physician/Health Care Facility/Other)

_____   _____
(Street Address)   (Street Address, City, State, Zip Code)

_____   _____
(City, State, Zip Code)   (Phone Number and/or Email Address)

4. PHI TO BE RELEASED:

Please describe the health information you would like released: _____

_____

For the following dates: _____

Unless checked below, it is assumed I want the following records included in the release:

❑ Mental Health *(excluding   ❑ HIV (AIDS)   ❑ Developmental Disabilities
psychotherapy notes)   ❑ Drug Abuse   ❑ Alcoholism

* Please note that the "Authorization for Release of Psychotherapy Notes" must be completed for the release of psychotherapy notes.

5. PURPOSE OR NEED FOR DISCLOSURE: (Check applicable categories)

❑ Transfer of Medical Care   ❑ Application for Insurance   ❑ Disability Determination
❑ Specialty Consultation   ❑ Vocational Rehab Evaluation   ❑ Visual Inspection of Records
❑ Legal Investigation   ❑ Personal   ❑ Other:_____

6. EXPIRATION DATE: This authorization will expire on _____/_____/_____(MM/DD/YYYY). If I do not specify a date, this authorization will remain in effect until this request is processed.

7. SIGNATURE: I understand that by signing this form, I am confirming my authorization for the health care provider named in Section 2 to use and/or disclose the protected health information described above, to the persons and/or organizations named in Section 3. I understand written notification is necessary to cancel this request.

_____   _____
(Signature of Patient)*   (Date)

* If this authorization is signed by a representative of the patient, please complete the following:

Representative's Name: _____

Patient is:
❑ Minor   ❑ Incompetent   ❑ Disabled   ❑ Deceased

Legal Authority:
❑ Parent of Minor   ❑ Legal Guardian   ❑ Power of Attorney   ❑ Next of Kin

** SEE REVERSE SIDE OF FORM FOR IMPORTANT INFORMATION ABOUT YOUR RIGHTS **

FORM B continued...

ADDITIONAL INFORMATION REGARDING THE RELEASE OF PROTECTED HEALTH INFORMATION (PHI)

[PROVIDER] recognizes the patient's right to confidentiality of protected health information in accordance with the federal privacy rule and Wisconsin law. Patients should be aware of the following information when requesting the release of protected health information:

Right to Refuse to Sign this Authorization

A patient has the right to refuse to sign this authorization form and [PROVIDER] will not condition treatment or payment of claims upon the provision that the patient sign this authorization form.

Right to Inspect or Copy the Information to be Used or Disclosed

A patient has the right to inspect or obtain a copy of the protected health information to be used or disclosed by signing this authorization form and may arrange a time to do so by contacting the medical records department.

Right to Receive a Copy of this Authorization

A patient has the right to request a copy of the signed authorization.

Right to Revoke Authorization

A patient has the right to revoke an authorization at any time by giving a written notice of revocation to the Privacy Officer listed below. Revocation of this authorization will not apply to information that has been released in compliance with this authorization prior to the receipt of the written notice of revocation. The revocation will not apply to the patient's insurance company when the law provides the insurer with the right to contest a claim under the patient's policy.

Redisclosure of Information by Recipient

Any disclosure of protected health information carries with it the potential for an unauthorized redisclosure. If the person(s) and/or organization listed in Section 3 are not health care providers, health plans or health care clearinghouses subject to the federal privacy rule, the protected health information disclosed as a result of this authorization may no longer be protected by the federal privacy standards and may be redisclosed without obtaining my authorization.

Multiple Releases of Information

A patient may request multiple releases of information described on the authorization form (Section 6). However, all releases based on this form are limited to records dated up to and including the date of the patient's signature unless otherwise specified. A new authorization is necessary for release of information related to care provided after the date of the patient's signature, unless the authorization specifies release of future records of a specific test or a specific clinic appointment.

Marketing

If [PROVIDER] uses this authorization for marketing activities, the patient will be informed if [PROVIDER] receives any direct or indirect payment in connection with the use or disclosure of the patient's information.

HIV Test Results

A patient's HIV test results may be released without authorization to persons/organizations that have access under State law and a list of those persons/organizations is available upon request.

Who May Sign Authorization

Wisconsin Statutes recognize the need for informed consent. Generally, all patients 18 years of age and over must sign for release of their own medical records unless the following conditions apply:

- The patient is incompetent.
- The patient is disabled and cannot sign the form.
- The patient is deceased. (A surviving spouse or personal representative of the estate may sign. If no such person exists, then an adult member of the immediate family may sign).

Patients *less than 18 years of age* must sign for release of their medical records when:

- The patient is 14 years of age or older and the records involve mental health treatment or developmental disabilities (parents retain the right to access this information)
- The patient is 14 years of age or older and the records involve HIV test results
- The patient is 12 years of age or older and the records involve alcoholism or drug dependence
- The patient is an emancipated minor who is married or in the military
- The patient's records for release include abortion procedure.

All persons signing for release of protected health information on behalf of a patient must state their relationship to the patient and provide proof of their legal authority to act on behalf of the patient.

Privacy Officer: [NAME]_____ , who can be reached at [PHONE] _____ , [EMAIL] _____ .

NOTE TO RECIPIENT OF INFORMATION: This protected health information has been disclosed according to federal and state privacy rules. Unless you have further authorization, these rules may prohibit you from redisclosing this information without the specific written consent of the patient or the patient's legal representative.

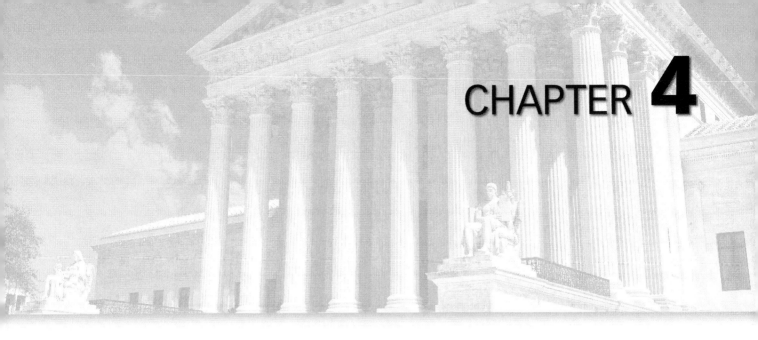

CHAPTER 4

Negligence and Common Defenses to Negligence

LEARNING OBJECTIVES

After reading this chapter, fitness managers and exercise professionals will be able to:

1. Obtain a sufficient understanding of negligence.

2. Explain how courts determine duty in negligence cases and the role of expert witnesses (1).

3. Realize that duties can arise based on relationships that are formed (1).

4. Describe the reasonable person standard of care and the standard of care of a professional.

5. Distinguish standards of care and standards of practice.

6. Explain the potential legal impact published standards of practice can have in negligence lawsuits (1).

7. Explain the connection between "competence" of an exercise professional and breach of duty.

8. Describe the duties owed to invitees.

9. Describe the standard of care related to children and its application to fitness facilities that serve children (1).

10. Obtain an appreciation of two common defenses to negligence—the primary assumption of risk defense and the waiver (release of liability) defense (1).

11. Describe the similarities and differences between express assumption of risk and primary assumption of risk.

12. Using the facts, the court's ruling, and the court's reasoning from negligence lawsuits, explain the differences between the primary

assumption of risk defense and the waiver (release of liability) defense (1).

13. Describe risk management strategies that will help strengthen the primary assumption of risk defense.

14. Explain the sections and certain language that should be considered in the development of a waiver (release of liability) to help increase its enforceability.

15. Realize the importance of having competent legal counsel prepare assumption of risk and waiver (release of liability) documents.

16. Describe recommendations for the administration of waivers (releases of liability) to participants by facility staff members (1).

INTRODUCTION

This chapter provides a comprehensive overview of negligence and common defenses to negligence. This chapter focuses on duties that can arise out of relationships formed between fitness managers and exercise professionals and the participants they serve. The potential legal impact of standards of practice published by professional and independent organizations in negligence cases is also described. This chapter explains two common defenses to negligence —primary assumption of risk and waiver (release of liability). Several spotlight cases and other cases are described to help understand how these two common defenses are applied in negligence lawsuits involving fitness facilities. Risk management strategies that can strengthen the primary assumption of risk defense are provided and recommendations regarding preparation and administration of an enforceable waiver are also presented. It is especially important for fitness managers and exercise professionals to understand the many concepts covered in this chapter because it provides the foundation for the information that follows in chapters 5-11.

Editorial Note: *Some of the content in the following sections titled "understanding negligence" and "standards of care" and their subsections reflect content from Chapter 3 in Risk Management for Health/Fitness Professionals: Legal Issues and Strategies (1). The publisher transferred the rights to this textbook to the authors in 2017. Permission to reprint and revise/update this content was granted by the author of Chapter 3.*

UNDERSTANDING NEGLIGENCE

Almost all lawsuits occurring in the fitness field and described throughout this textbook involve negligence cases. Therefore, it is essential that fitness managers and exercise professionals obtain a good understanding of negligence. As presented in Chapter 1, negligence is one of three categories under tort liability. The other two are intentional and strict liability. Negligence can be defined as failing to do something that a reasonable prudent person would have done (omission) or doing something that a reasonable prudent person would not have done

(commission) given the same or similar circumstances (2). See Figure 4-1. As discussed in Chapter 1, in a negligence lawsuit the plaintiff must first prove that the defendant owed him/her a certain duty determined by reference to a "standard of care." But how is duty determined? First, it is important to understand the court (or judge) determines duty—not juries, or lawyers. However, whether a defendant breached a duty will be determined by the jury (or by the judge if there is no jury).

Figure 4-1: Negligent Conduct: Omission and Commission*

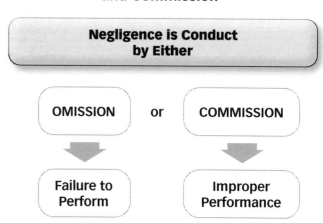

Rule the Rules of Workplace Wellness Programs (60). ©2020 by the American Bar Association. Adapted and reprinted with permission. All rights reserved. This information or any portion thereof may not be copied or disseminated in any form or by any means or stored in an electronic database or retrieval system without the express written consent of the American Bar Association.

Courts determine duty in a variety of ways. This chapter will describe those that are most relevant for fitness managers and exercise professionals (1). Betty van der Smissen (3) states that duty is formed from three primary origins: (a) inherent in the situation, (b) voluntary assumption, and (c) mandated by statute.

Inherent in the Situation

According to van der Smissen, "the existence of duty is inherent in nearly every situation in which a teacher, coach, recreation leader, fitness specialist, administrator, manager... et al. might be actively engaged" (3, p. 40). In the fitness field, these individuals would include fitness managers, supervisors, and exercise professionals such as personal fitness trainers, group exercise leaders, and strength and conditioning coaches. For example, a fitness manager has a duty to provide a *reasonably safe* environment for members and a personal fitness trainer has a duty to provide a reasonably safe exercise program for a client. Reasonably safe means taking steps to protect another from harm. There are many examples of negligence cases in this textbook involving fitness managers and exercise professionals who failed to take steps to protect their participants from harm. To properly carry out this duty to provide reasonably safe facilities and programs, fitness managers and exercise professionals need to develop and implement risk management strategies to prevent "foreseeable" risks of injuries. Many of the plaintiffs' injuries in the cases described in this textbook resulted from foreseeable risks associated with participation exercise programs such as fractures, herniated discs, exertional rhabdomyolysis, stroke, and cardiac arrest. See Table 2-3 Chapter 2. Many of these injuries could have been prevented if fitness managers and exercise professionals had properly carried out their duty to provide reasonably safe facilities and programs.

KEY POINT

Fitness managers and exercise professionals have a duty to provide *reasonably safe* facilities and programs. "Reasonably safe" means taking steps (i.e., developing and implementing risk management strategies) to help prevent "foreseeable" risks of injuries. In many of the negligence cases described in this textbook, the courts determined that fitness managers and exercise professionals had a duty to provide reasonably safe facilities and programs.

Voluntary Assumption

A legal duty can be created through a voluntary assumption of duty, based on the action or conduct of an individual, even when no relationship initially existed. For example, in *Parks v. Gilligan* (4), the defendant volunteered to spot for the plaintiff while he performed a bench press exercise using dumbbells. As the plaintiff placed the dumbbells on the floor, his left index finger was crushed when his left hand came in contact with a weight on the floor. The plaintiff claimed that the volunteer spotter had assumed a duty owed him and he failed to carry out that duty (i.e., failed to ensure that floor area where the exercise was taking place was free of weights or other objects that could cause an injury) and thus, proximately caused the plaintiff's injury. The case resulted in a settlement and the defendants, the facility and the volunteer spotter paid $15,000 and $5,000, respectively, to the plaintiff. This case demonstrates how those who voluntarily assume a duty can be potentially liable for an injury. It is important to realize that even though no legal duty may exist (e.g., to assist another individual), once that duty is voluntarily assumed, a relationship is formed which results in an obligation (or duty) to provide reasonable care.

Mandated by Statute

A legal duty can be established by requirements specified in certain statutes such as employment, supervisory requirements, or rendering first aid in certain situations (3). For example, in the state of Wisconsin, there is a statute that requires fitness centers to have "at least one employee who has satisfactorily completed a course or courses in basic first aid and basic cardiopulmonary resuscitation… and at least one employee who has current proficiency in the use of an automated external defibrillator" present on the premises during all hours the fitness center is open (5). Several states have also enacted statutes that require fitness facilities to have an automated external defibrillator (AED) as discussed in Chapter 11. Violation of statutes in these situations can result in **negligence per se**—a legal doctrine in which the plaintiff does not have to prove negligence as he/she would in an ordinary negligence case, but does have to show that the violation of the statute did *cause* the harm that the statute was intended to prevent, and that the victim was in the class of persons that statute was designed to protect (6).

STANDARDS OF CARE

The following section describes standards of care (or duties) of various individuals. Each of the following are presented: reasonable person, professional, land owner/occupier, children, and licensed health care provider.

Standard of Care: Reasonable Person

Keeton et al. (7) state that the reasonable person standard, when used in reference to demonstrating negligence, requires one to act as a reasonable person, or a person of ordinary/reasonable prudence. But how do the courts determine what is reasonable conduct? A reasonable person is one who has taken steps to avoid foreseeable, unreasonable risks of harm (7). The *Turner* case described below explains how the concept of foreseeability is used in determining negligence. But what are unreasonable risks? Two factors are weighed: (a) the defendant's burden of taking precautions and (b) the gravity (seriousness) and probability (frequency) of the risk which the conduct creates. See Figure 4-2.

The defendant's burden of providing safeguards is weighed against the seriousness and likelihood of potential injury, resulting in a risk-benefit analysis to determine negligence using the ordinary standard of care (7). To illustrate, imagine your car breaks down in the middle of a busy street, what would a reasonable person do? A reasonable person might put on their emergency flashers, put the car's hood up, and then call for a tow truck. None of these steps create an undue burden for the driver (e.g., cost a lot of money), in light of the

Figure 4-2: Balance Between Two Factors to Determine Unreasonable Risks

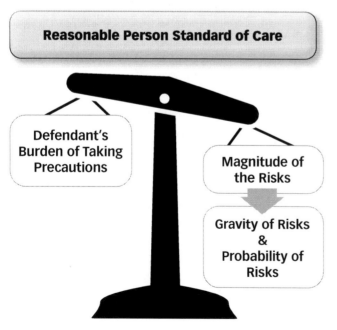

magnitude of the risks (gravity and probability) that a stalled car on a busy street can create. It is likely that a stalled car on a busy street could be struck by another vehicle. Further, the severity of harm caused by a car accident can be substantial. Therefore, in this situation, the burden of the defendant to take precautions is low, whereas the magnitude of risk is high. In a situation where a driver did not take these steps and harm resulted because of the driver's omissions, the driver could be found negligent under the reasonable person standard of care.

The *Turner v. Rush Medical College* (8) case is described to help understand foreseeable, unreasonable risks and application of the reasonable person standard of care. The plaintiff, a 23-year-old medical student at Rush Medical College, was required to run one mile in eight minutes as part of an experiment in his pathology class. The plaintiff suffered many serious and debilitating injuries including "extreme exertional rhabdomyolysis" requiring over two months of hospitalization at a cost of approximately $250,000. (Exertional rhabdomyolysis is described in Chapter 8). The plaintiff contended that the defendant, Rush Medical College, breached its duty to exercise reasonable care by requiring the plaintiff to run a timed mile without:

a) learning what forms of physical exercise the plaintiff did and, specifically, whether the plaintiff had ever performed a timed-mile run (a pre-activity health screening issue);

b) conducting a physical examination of the plaintiff to check on his respiration and blood pressure (a pre-activity health screening issue);

c) having medical personnel present to assist the plaintiff during and after the timed mile run (an emergency response issue);

d) making oxygen available to the plaintiff if he needed the same during and after the timed mile run (an emergency response issue);

e) providing for water to be available to the plaintiff, if needed, during and after the timed mile run (a safety issue involving program delivery).

The trial court granted the defendant's motion to dismiss stating that "the complaint did not allege facts which established that the defendants owed plaintiff a duty" (8, p. 894). The trial court ruled that "lack of foreseeability of harm and public policy considerations required dismissal of plaintiff's complaint as a matter of law" (8, p. 894). On appeal, the court stated, "that at the time of the defendant's conduct a reasonably prudent person would not have foreseen plaintiff's injury" (8, p. 892). The defendant viewed the plaintiff as a healthy 23-year-old man. Regarding the public policy concerns, the court held that to impose a duty in similar cases would impose an expensive financial burden on schools (i.e., a duty to provide medical precautions). The appellate court upheld the trial court's decision to grant the motion to dismiss.

In this case, the court decided the burden of taking precautions (such as those suggested by the plaintiff) was too great of a financial burden for Rush Medical College when weighed against the magnitude of risk (e.g., low probability of the plaintiff being harmed and severity of any harm that might occur). In other words, the defendant's burden to take precautions outweighed the magnitude of the risk. Therefore, pursuant to the ruling in this case, the defendant had no duty to take additional precautions and, therefore, did not breach any duty and was not liable for the plaintiff's injury.

The *Turner* case is interesting because most exercise professionals would likely disagree with the court's decision, instead, favoring Justice Pincham's dissenting view. Justice Pincham opined, "it is practically a matter of common knowledge that running an eight-minute mile may cause injury…An injury from such an undertaking is certainly reasonably foreseeable" (8, p. 895). Regarding the public policy concerns, Justice Pincham stated, "schools and facilities have a duty to exercise reasonable care in supervising track and field events…and a duty to provide medical care when needed" (8, p. 897).

Justice Pincham's opinion in *Turner*, regarding a school's duty to provide reasonable care, reflects a more common opinion of courts in similar cases. For example, in *Kleinknecht v. Gettysburg College* (9), the trial court held that it was not "reasonably foreseeable" that Drew Kleinknecht, a 20-year old lacrosse player for Gettysburg College, would suffer a cardiac arrest and, therefore, determined that the defendant College owed him no duty to provide emergency medical care. However, the appellate court disagreed, ruling that the College had a duty toward Drew to provide emergency medical care while engaged in a school-sponsored activity. The College was held liable for Drew's death. See also *Limones v.*

School District of Lee County, spotlight case in Chapter 11, in which the Florida Supreme Court ruled that the school district had a duty to act with reasonable care (i.e., a duty to take appropriate action to avoid or mitigate further aggravation of the student's injury).

Note: *It is likely that courts will apply the reasonable person standard of care in fitness facilities that have no staff supervision such as apartment complexes, hotels, and outdoor fitness areas in city parks. However, in fitness facilities that offer structured programs and services provided by professional staff members, courts are more likely to apply the standard of care of a professional.*

Standard of Care: Professional

The previous discussion addressed the reasonable person standard of care, which is a standard that requires all of us to act as a person of ordinary prudence. However, if a person holds himself out as having special skills or knowledge superior to that of an ordinary person, the law will demand of that person conduct consistent with their skillset (7). The *Restatement of Law Third, Torts* states: "If an actor has skills or knowledge that exceed those possessed by most others, these skills or knowledge are circumstances to be taken into account in determining whether the actor has behaved as a reasonably careful person" (6, pp. 82-83). Keeton et al. state that "experienced milk haulers, hockey coaches, expert skiers, construction inspectors, and doctors must all use care which is reasonable in light of their superior learning and experience and any special skills, knowledge or training they may personally have over and above what is normally possessed by persons in the field" (7, p. 185). Professional persons or those whose work require special skills, are required not only to exercise reasonable care, but to also possess special knowledge and ability (7). Because the jobs of fitness managers and exercise professionals require specialized knowledge and skills, they will likely be held to a **standard of care of a professional**. **Note:** For purposes of this textbook, "standard of care of a professional" will be also referred to as the **professional standard of care**.

Medical malpractice (negligence of a licensed health care provider) is a common type of negligence. In medical malpractice cases, expert medical testimony is used to determine if a health care provider breached a duty (standard of care). State statutes specify requirements for expert medical testimony. The purpose of **expert testimony** is to educate the court as to the duty the defendant owed to the plaintiff and if the defendant breached that duty. Keeton et al. (7) state that juries composed of laymen are normally incompetent to pass judgment on matters of medical science and, therefore, there can be no finding of negligence in the absence of expert testimony. Keeton et al. (7) also state that the ultimate result of all expert testimony is "that the standard of conduct becomes one of good medical practice which is to say what is customary and usual in the profession" (7, p. 189). However, courts have indicated that *customary practice* should be just one factor in determining what good medical practice is and it is not conclusive. See *Darling v. Charleston Community Memorial Hospital* (10) where the court stated that just because the evidence showed that the physician followed the customary practice, it is not the sole test of malpractice.

Another factor, *locality*, in medical malpractice cases was used by courts to establish the standard of care, which involved comparing the physician to other physicians in the same location. For example, a country doctor should not be held to the same standard as an urban doctor. However, see *McGuire v. DeFrancesco* (11) where the court ruled that the physician should have followed a nationwide standard versus a statewide standard.

As in medical malpractice cases, fitness managers and exercise professionals should understand that customary practice and locality will, likely, not be factors courts will consider when determining the standard of care. Courts in many of the negligence cases described throughout this textbook have relied on expert testimony to help educate the court as to the standard of care (duty) the defendant owed to the plaintiff and whether or not the defendant met the standard of care. Often in their testimony, experts will provide their opinions regarding situational factors (see Exhibit 4-1) and reference published standards of practice as evidence of the standard of care. See section later in this chapter—Published Standards of Practice.

As described in Chapter 5, the credentials of exercise professionals working in the field vary tremendously. It is important for exercise professionals to realize they will be held to a standard of care regarding the special knowledge and skills expected of exercise professionals. However, if an exercise professional holds himself/herself out as having a higher level of knowledge and skill than he/she possesses or takes on responsibilities beyond his/her level of education and training (e.g., a professional who markets himself/herself as a clinical exercise physiologist but does not possess credentials/competence in clinical exercise), the professional will likely be held to that higher standard. Therefore, it is important for exercise professionals to accurately represent their credentials and always stay within their **scope of practice** (i.e., practice within the limitations of their education, training, experience, and certification). More information on scope of practice is covered in Chapter 7. False marketing of the credentials of fitness staff members can lead to violations of state statutes such as unfair or deceptive acts. See *D'Amico v. LA Fitness* (12), spotlight case described in Chapter 5.

KEY POINT

Because the jobs of fitness managers and exercise professionals require specialized knowledge and skills, they will likely be held to a standard of care of a professional (or the professional standard of care), which is a different standard of care than the reasonable person standard of care. Expert witnesses educate the court regarding the standard care (or duty owed to the plaintiff) given the circumstances. They often include in the testimony situational factors such as the (a) nature of the activity, (b) type of participants, and (c) environmental conditions.

Situational Factors: Standard of Care of Exercise Professionals

According to Betty van der Smissen, "If one accepts responsibility for giving leadership to an activity or providing a service, one's performance is measured against the standard of care of a qualified professional *for that situation*" (13, p. 40). In this context, a qualified professional means a competent professional with credentials. In negligence lawsuits, courts will consider the credentials of an exercise professional such as degrees, certifications, and experience but, more importantly, courts will consider the competence, or the *behavior* of the professional given the situation. Remember, a breach of duty is some type of behavior—a failure to act or improper action. The phrase that van der Smissen emphasizes—*for that situation*—involves considering three situational factors: (a) nature of the activity, (b) type of participants, and (c) environmental conditions (13). See Exhibit 4-1 for a description of these three factors. Expert witnesses, who provided testimony in many of the negligence cases included in this textbook, described how the exercise professional did not address one or more of these three situational factors when designing and delivering an exercise program. To further demonstrate how these situational factors are included in expert testimony, see two articles written by well-known expert witness, Dr. Anthony Abbott, describing cardiac arrest litigations (14) and injury litigations (15) in which he served as an expert witness.

Standard of Care: Special Relationships

In addition to the legal duties reflected in both the reasonable person standard of care and the professional standard of care, duties can also arise out of special relationships. According to the *Restatement of Law Third, Torts* (6), the following are examples of special relationships that give rise to a duty of reasonable care: (a) a common carrier with its passengers, (b) an innkeeper and its guests, (c) employer and its employees, (d) a school and its students, and (e) a landlord and its tenants (6). An additional special relationship, land owner/occupier and person(s) on land (18) will be the focus of this next section because of its relevance to fitness facilities.

Land Owner/Occupier and Person(s) on Land

A special relationship is formed between a land owner/occupier, such as the owner/manager of a fitness

---

Exhibit 4-1: Situational Factors* Courts Consider When Determining the Standard of Care of Exercise Professionals

Nature of the activity—the professional must be aware of the skills and abilities the participant needs to participate "safely" in the activity, e.g., the exercise professional must possess adequate knowledge and skills to lead "reasonably safe" exercise programs.

> *Example:* Exercise professionals that lead "advanced" exercise programs that can increase the risk of injury, such as Olympic lifting and extreme conditioning, need to have advanced knowledge and skills necessary to safely teach these types of programs. They need to be fully informed of precautions that must be taken.

Type of participants—the professional must be aware of individual factors of the participant, e.g., medical conditions that impose increased risks and know how to minimize those risks.

> *Example:* Exercise professionals that design/deliver exercise programs for individuals with medical conditions, such as diabetes and back problems, need to possess credentials and competence in clinical exercise through clinical academic coursework, clinical certifications, and clinical experience (16). It is essential that the professional fully understands any additional or unique risks imposed by such medical conditions and how to minimize those risks. Advanced credentials are needed for exercise professionals who work with clinical population programs because courts may rule that these types of programs impose different duties (e.g., a different standard of care) than other, general population programs. See *Bartlett v. Push to Walk* (17), spotlight case in Chapter 7.

Environmental conditions—the professional must be aware of any conditions that may increase risks, e.g., weather conditions such as heat/humidity, floor surfaces, exercise equipment, and know how to minimize those risks.

> *Example:* Exercise professionals need to have the necessary knowledge and skills to properly implement important safety precautions to help prevent heat injuries. Knowing and implementing precautions to minimize risks associated with slippery floor surfaces and improper maintenance of equipment is also important.

*van der Smissen (13)

facility, and person(s) on land (e.g., a participant(s) who use a fitness facility). The law classifies persons that enter a fitness facility (or any business) as trespassers, licensees, or invitees. The court in *Duncan v. World Wide Health Studios* (19) describes the differences in the legal duties that the fitness managers and exercise professionals have toward persons in each classification. In *Duncan*, the plaintiff was seriously injured while using a leg press. On the day of the injury, the plaintiff was visiting the health club accompanied by a friend who was a regular member of the club. To determine whether the defendant health club was negligent, the court first examined the relationship between the plaintiff and the health club. The court stated that the standard of care owed to a person entering the land of an owner/occupier is determined by the circumstances surrounding his/her entry. The court in *Duncan* described the relationship between a land owner/occupier and a trespasser, licensee, and invitee as follows:

1. A trespasser is one who enters the premises without the permission of the occupier or without a legal right to do so; and towards the trespasser no duty exists in most instances except to refrain from willfully or wantonly injuring him.

2. A licensee is one who enters the premises with the occupier's express or implied permission, but only for his own purposes which are unconnected with the occupant's interests; and to him in addition to the duty owed to a trespasser, is owed the duty of warning the licensee of latent dangers of the premises if actually known by the occupier.

3. An invitee is a person who goes on the premises with the express or implied invitation of the occupant…for their mutual advantage; and to him, the duty owed is that of reasonable and ordinary care, which includes the prior discovery of reasonably discoverable conditions of the premises that may be unreasonably dangerous, and correction thereof or a warning to the invitee of the danger (19, p. 837).

An example of a **trespasser** would be a golfer entering the land of a homeowner to retrieve his/her ball without the permission of the homeowner. Although no duty exists other than to not intentionally or willfully injure the trespasser, land owners/occupiers do have duty to warn if they know of trespassers or if

trespassing is frequent and it would be likely for trespassers to confront a dangerous activity/condition on their land. A special legal doctrine in reference to this concept called *attractive nuisance* applies to the child trespasser—see section below: Child Trespasser and Attractive Nuisance.

Examples of a **licensee** is sales representative entering a business to sell a product or a social guest in one's own home. Generally, there is no duty to warn of any dangerous condition unless the land owner/occupier knows that a dangerous condition exists, knows that it is likely that the licensee will confront the dangerous condition, and knows it is unlikely that the licensee will recognize the dangerous condition.

An example of an **invitee** would be a member, participant, or guest who participates in the programs/services offered by a fitness facility. Invitees are owed a different standard of care than a trespasser or a licensee because a mutual benefit exists between an invitee and the land owner/occupier. For example, an owner of a fitness facility receives a monetary benefit from the fees that a member pays, and the member receives all the benefits that the membership provides. The land owner/occupier owes a duty to act reasonably toward invitees regarding the activities/conditions on their land. This involves reasonable inspection of the property for dangers and to reasonably repair and/or warn of dangers.

After examining whether the plaintiff in *Duncan* was a trespasser, licensee, or an invitee, the court determined that the plaintiff was an invitee because he was "in the position of one who may confer a future benefit upon the defendant" (19, p. 838). In other words, the plaintiff was a prospective purchaser of the health club's services. The court stated that the defendant health club had a duty of ordinary and reasonable care toward invitees that includes an obligation to inspect the premises making them safe to visit. There was no evidence that the health club had breached its duty to inspect the leg press machine that the plaintiff was hurt on, or that the leg press was dangerous in any way. The manager of the defendant health club testified that the leg press machine was functioning properly and that the plaintiff's injury was due to his own misuse of it. Though the defendant health club clearly had a duty toward its members and guests (invitees) to inspect the leg press machine to ensure its safe use, the court found no breach of this duty and, therefore, concluded that the plaintiff's injury was not due to negligence on part of the health club. Additional cases are described in Chapter 10 regarding duties toward invitees, including spotlight case, *Crossing-Lyons v. Towns Sports International, Inc.* (20).

The Child Trespasser and Attractive Nuisance

The general rule for **attractive nuisance** is that if land owners/occupiers keep something on their property which they have reason to believe could attract and injure a child, the land owner/occupier must take reasonable steps to protect the child's safety such as remove the hazard or prevent accessibility to the hazard (21).

Smith v. AMLI Realty Co. (22) is an excellent case that demonstrates the attractive nuisance doctrine. Nine-year-old Lucas Smith was visiting an apartment complex where his father lived. He was approached by another child, Dana Faulkenberg who lived in the area, who asked him to go to the apartment complex weight room, so she could show him a trick she had learned. A Universal weight machine was in the room which had a "lat" exercise device which a user could pull down by using the lat bar. By doing so, the weights would be raised. Dana took the pin to the lat exercise and set the weights at 70 pounds. Both children pulled the lat bar down and so that Dana could straddle it. As Lucas released the bar, it rose up in the air and Dana was hanging by her knees. After hanging in this position for a while, Dana asked Lucas to help her down. Lucas placed his hands under the suspended weight stack and lifted it up causing the bar to go down. While he was doing this, Dana jumped off the bar causing the 70 pounds to exert downward with force pinning Lucas' left hand between the descending weights and the weights in the bottom stack. Lucas' fingers were seriously injured.

Smith's (Lucas' mother) lawsuit against AMLI Realty Co., owner of the apartment complex, was based on the attractive nuisance theory. In this type of negligence action, Smith had to show that the condition on AMLI's property (i.e., the weight machine in the apartment complex weight room) was *dangerous*. Whether a condition is considered dangerous will depend upon the plaintiff's knowledge, understanding, and appreciation of the risk the condition creates. The defendant claimed the weight machine was not dangerous because Lucas had actual knowledge of the specific risk, understood, and appreciated the risk. The trial court agreed with AMLI and dismissed the case. However, upon appeal, the appellate court reversed the trial court's decision stating that the weight machine was dangerous because "a child (of plaintiff's age, knowledge, judgment, and experience would not have recognized the danger presented by attempting to hold the suspended weights while his friend endeavored to extricate herself from the bar" (22, p. 62). The court stated that Lucas had knowledge and appreciation that 70 pounds could injure his hand, but it was not apparent to him that he could not hold up the weights once Dana jumped off the bar. Therefore, Lucas appreciated some, but not all, of the risks and the weight machine was dangerous to him.

Another factor courts will evaluate under an attractive nuisance theory claim is whether the land owner/occupier took *reasonable* steps to protect the child. To determine what the court would consider *reasonable*, the courts will examine the defendant's burden to eliminate the danger compared to the risk to children the danger can create—the same elements described above regarding the reasonable person standard of care. If the burden is light in comparison to the risk, the defendant could be found negligent under the attractive nuisance theory. In *Smith*, the court stated that the burden of defendant AMLI to eliminate the danger entailed installing a lock and providing tenants with keys, which is, arguably, a very minor burden in comparison to the possibility of weights injuring children.

Standard of Care: Children

In *Smith*, Lucas, a nine-year old boy did not understand and appreciate all the risks involved when playing with the exercise equipment at the apartment complex. At what age do children fully understand and appreciate risks associated with any type of physical activity? This is especially important for fitness facilities offering programs and services to children and highlights the need for adult supervision. The *Restatement of Law Third, Torts* states that a "child's conduct is negligent if it does not conform to that of a reasonably careful person of the same age, intelligence, and experience" except when "a child less than five years of age is incapable of negligence" or "when the child is engaging in a dangerous activity that is characteristically undertaken by adults" (6, p. 77). Most American jurisdictions follow this approach, but some jurisdictions follow a different approach as follows:

- **Under seven years of age:** Incapable of committing negligence.
- **Seven to 14 years of age:** A rebuttable presumption against a child's capacity to commit negligence may exist.
- **Above 14 years of age:** A rebuttable presumption in favor of the child's capacity to commit negligence exists (6).

In *Campbell v. Morine* (23), a 15-year-old boy was struck and killed by a motorist on a rural road in the evening. He was jogging with a friend (also 15 years old) in the same direction as traffic. The decedent's mother brought a negligence lawsuit against the defendant motorist. The trial court found the defendant 65% negligent and the decedent 35% negligent, mainly because he failed to jog against oncoming traffic. On appeal, the defendant claimed that the decedent's conduct should have been based on an adult standard of care and not a child's standard of care. The defendant claimed that if the trial court would have used an adult standard of care in determining the amount of negligence, a larger proportion of negligence would have been attributed to the decedent. However, the court held that "even though a minor could be held to the same standard of care as an adult, he is not held to that standard, unless the trier of fact determines that his age, abilities, and experience require application of the adult standard of care" (23, p. 1202). A dissenting opinion agreed with the defendant, arguing that the decedent should have been treated as an adult.

Standard of Care: Licensed Health Care Provider

The federal government defines a health care provider in 29 C.F.R § 825.125 (24). This Act, in part, states the following:

a) The Act defines *health care provider* as:
    (1) A doctor of medicine or osteopathy who is authorized to practice medicine or surgery (as appropriate) by the State in which the doctor practices; or

    (2) Any other person determined by the Secretary to be capable of providing health care services.
b) Others capable of providing health care services include only…

Note: *A list of these "others" are provided in the Act (24).*

---

c) The phrase authorized to practice in the State as used in this section means that the provider must be authorized to diagnose and treat physical or mental health conditions.

As described above, expert medical testimony is used in medical malpractice cases to determine if a health care provider breached a duty.

In *Mikkelsen v. Haslam* (25), five orthopedic surgeons testified that failure to advise a total hip replacement patient that the prosthesis was a walking hip only, and that the patient should not ski or jog, is a departure from orthopedic medical profession standards. This case also demonstrates how patients rely upon and trust the advice they receive from their physician. In *Mikkelsen*, the plaintiff was born with a congenitally dislocated right hip. After a total hip replacement surgery in 1974, the plaintiff contended that her physician told her she had no physical limitations and that she could ski and play tennis. The physician testified that he told the plaintiff to not run, twist, or lift. Five years after the surgery, the plaintiff felt she was ready to begin skiing and contacted her physician for clearance to do so. She, along with two of her co-workers who heard her conversations with the physician, testified that the physician endorsed the skiing. In 1979, the plaintiff went skiing 10 times with no problems. In 1980, she severely fractured her femur while skiing and the hip replacement was adversely affected and could not be repaired. She would need to use a wheelchair or crutches for the rest of her life.

The trial court provided an instruction to the jury that the plaintiff could have assumed the risks (contributory negligence) which would bar any recovery. The jury found the defendant negligent (medical experts testified that downhill skiing was contraindicated for patients with hip replacement), but the plaintiff was also negligent and, therefore, the plaintiff was precluded from any recovery.

Note: This case was decided before the state of Utah adopted a comparative negligence rule. On appeal, the plaintiff contended that "she could not, as a matter of law be contributorily negligent or have assumed the risk when she skied, if... [the defendant physician] advised her she could ski" (25, p. 1387). The appellate court held that "a physician has a duty to warn his patient of how to avoid injury following treatment..." and that "the physician-patient relationship permits a patient to rely on a doctor's professional skill and advice" (25, p. 1388). The appellate court found that "it is not contributory negligence to follow the advice of a physician" (25, p. 1388). Therefore, the defenses of contributory negligence and assumption of risk did not apply, and the court returned the case to the trial court for a new trial.

Implications for exercise professionals arise from *Mikkelsen*. As discussed above, the relationship between an exercise professional and his/her client requires a standard of care of a professional—a duty to provide a reasonably safe exercise program. Clients believe that their degreed and/or certified exercise professional is an exercise expert and, thus, will trust the instruction and advice the professional provides. The instruction and advice provided to a client must be appropriate given the client's health and fitness status in order to meet the standard of care. Failure to do so could result in negligence if the client is harmed when following the instruction/advice, as demonstrated in many of the cases described in this textbook. In addition, exercise professionals need to follow any instructions (e.g., limitations, contraindications) a client's physician (or other health care provider) may have indicated on the medical clearance form. See Chapter 6 for more on medical clearance.

Editorial Note: The content in the first three paragraphs in the following section titled "published standards of practice" and the first subsection (description of the Elledge case) reflect content from Chapter 3 in Risk Management for Health/Fitness Professionals: Legal Issues and Strategies (1). The publisher transferred the rights to this textbook to the authors in 2017. Permission to reprint and revise/update this content was granted by the author of Chapter 3.

PUBLISHED STANDARDS OF PRACTICE

Published standards of practice are generally classified into two categories: (a) **desirable operating practices**, and (b) **technical physical specifications** (26). Desirable operating practices are published by professional organizations such as the American College of Sports Medicine (ACSM) and National Strength and Conditioning Association (NSCA). Examples include standards, guidelines, position papers, or other similar publications. Technical physical specifications are, primarily, published by independent organizations such as the Consumer Product Safety Commission (CPSC), American Society for Testing and Materials (ASTM) and manufacturers of exercise equipment. Examples include ASTM International standard statements that reflect exercise equipment and fitness facility specifications and owner's manuals published by exercise equipment manufacturers that include specifications for proper installation, maintenance, etc. for each piece of equipment. However, professional organizations that publish desirable operating practices also include some technical specifications in their publications.

Desirable operating practices, primarily, include job functions of fitness managers and exercise professionals such as conducting pre-activity health screening, hiring qualified staff members, and providing emergency care when an injury occurs. These are described in Chapters 5-8 and 11. Job functions regarding technical physical specifications such as conducting proper maintenance of exercise equipment and providing proper facility safety signage are described

KEY POINT

The major purpose of published standards of practice is to enhance the safety of participants. They reflect "best practices" that should be followed. Fitness managers and exercise professionals should interpret them as the minimal level of service owed to participants. It cannot be assumed that they cover the major legal liability exposures facing fitness facilities and programs. Following laws (statutory, administrative, and case law) is also necessary.

in Chapters 9 and 10. The major purpose of published standards of practice is to enhance the safety of participants. They reflect "best practices" that fitness managers and exercise professionals should follow. They should be interpreted as the minimal level of service owed to participants. It cannot be assumed they cover all major legal liability exposures facing fitness facilities and programs. Following laws (statutory, administrative, and case law) is also necessary.

Fitness managers and exercise professionals need to understand the distinction between "standards of care" and "standards of practice" as shown in Figure 4-3. As previously described regarding standards of care, if the plaintiff proves there was a duty, then the issue is whether or not the defendant breached the duty (standard of care) owed to the plaintiff. Regarding published standards of practice, it is important to understand their potential legal impact. Because most courts allow published standards of practice to be introduced as admissible evidence (usually via expert testimony), courts will consider them when determining duty. If the judge or jury accepts the expert testimony, then the standards of practice become the standard of care. As stated by the courts in the *Elledge v. Richland/Lexington School District Five* (27), industry safety standards

Figure 4-3: Distinguishing Standards of Care and Standards of Practice

are not substantive law but can be admitted as evidence to establish the standard of care in negligence cases.

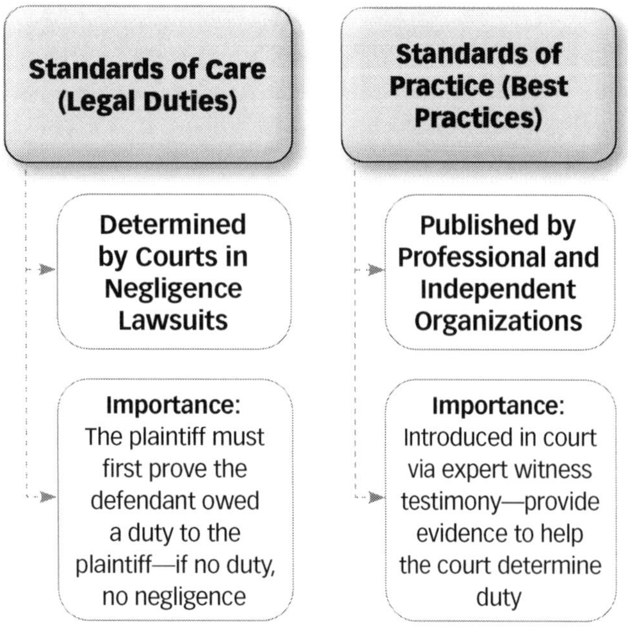

Elledge v. Richland/Lexington School District Five

In 1994, Ginger Sierra, a nine-year-old fourth grader, was injured while playing on modified monkey bars on the school's playground. Three years earlier the school principal noticed children climbing on top of the bars rather than lying on the bench running underneath. Feeling that the original monkey bars were unsafe, the principal contracted with a playground equipment sales representative, who was not trained or licensed as an engineer, to modify the monkey bars. This modification resulted in removing the bench and lowering the bars forming an inclined ladder ranging from 20 to 30 inches above the ground. Neither handrails nor a non-slip surface were added to the newly modified monkey bars.

While walking across the bars after a light rain, Ginger's foot slipped on a narrow bar resulting in a fall that trapped her right leg between the bars. She suffered a severe "spiral-type" fracture in her femur that resulted in damage to her femur's growth plate. Ginger's mother, Christine Elledge, sued the school district for injuries sustained by her daughter. Elledge claimed that the school district was negligent because it deviated from the accepted standard of care (i.e., the modification of the monkey bars did not meet standards published by ASTM and guidelines published by CPSC for playground equipment). However, the trial court excluded Elledge's evidence that included video deposition testimony from an expert in playground equipment. This expert testimony would have clearly shown that the district did not adhere to industry standards as outlined by ASTM and CPSC. The trial court found for the defendant school district and Elledge appealed.

On appeal, Elledge asserted that the trial court erred in excluding evidence of ASTM standards and CPSC guidelines, arguing that such evidence was relevant to establish the appropriate standard of care. The appellate court agreed and reversed the trial court's ruling. Citing a variety of other cases to support its decision, the appellate court stated:

Safety standards promulgated by government or industry organizations in particular are relevant to the standard of care for negligence... Courts have become increasingly appreciative of the value of national safety codes and other guidelines issued by governmental and voluntary associations to assist in applying the standard of care in negligence cases...A safety code ordinarily represents a consensus of opinion carrying the approval of a significant segment of an industry, and it is not introduced as substantive law but most often as illustrative evidence of safety practices or rules generally prevailing in the industry that provides support for expert testimony concerning the proper standard of care (27, pp. 477-478).

This case was further appealed to the South Carolina Supreme Court. This court upheld the appellate court's decision stating:

The general rule is that evidence of industry safety standards is admissible to establish the standard of care in a negligence case. The evidence of CPSC guidelines and ASTM standards which respondents sought to have admitted in the instant case is exactly the type of evidence contemplated by this general rule. The Court of Appeals correctly held the trial court committed reversible error in excluding the evidence (28, p. 189).

To support the ruling in *Elledge,* the court also referenced an article published in the American Law Reports (ALR)—*Admissibility of Evidence, on Issue of Negligence, of Codes or Standards of Safety Issued or Sponsored by Governmental Body of by Voluntary Association* (58 A.L.R 3d. 148, 1974). For examples of negligence lawsuits (spotlight cases in this textbook) in which published standards of practice were introduced as evidence of the duty, see Table 4-1.

Published Standards of Practice: Perspectives of Expert Witnesses

Experienced expert witnesses who testify in cases involving fitness facilities and programs have articulated their views on published standards of practice. Referring to *ACSM's Health/Fitness Facility Standards and Guidelines,* Harvey C. Voris and Dr. Marc Rabinoff, who each have over 30 years of experience serving as expert witnesses, state that they have referenced this ACSM publication as well as other prominent standards published by the NSCA and ASTM to inform the courts and juries as to what is appropriate (29). When describing the *Jimenez v. 24 Hour Fitness* (30) case (spotlight case described in Chapter 9), Voris stated, "The published standards by ASTM, ACSM and NSCA do establish a standard of care for the fitness industry that manufacturers and operators can be held accountable to if they elect to ignore them" (31, p. 97). Even though it has been over 20 years that these documents

Table 4-1	Spotlight Cases: Published Standards of Practice Introduced as Evidence of Duty
SPOTLIGHT CASE (CHAPTER)	**PUBLISHED STANDARDS OF PRACTICE**
	DESIRABLE OPERATING PRACTICES
Covenant Health System v. Barnett **(7)**	ACSM's Guidelines for Exercise Testing and Prescription
Miller v. YMCA of Central Massachusetts **(10)**	Medical Advisory Committee Recommendations: A Resource for YMCAs
Miglino v. Bally Total Fitness **(11)**	AHA and ACSM Joint Position Statement: Automated External Defibrillators in Health/Fitness Facilities
	TECHNICAL PHYSICAL SPECIFICATIONS
Stelluti v. Casapenn Enterprises, LLC **(4)**	Manufacturer's Owner's Manual—Indoor Cycle
Scheck v. Soul Cycle **(8)**	Manufacturer's Owner's Manual—Indoor Cycle
Chavez v. 24 Hour Fitness **(9)**	Manufacturer's Owner's Manual—Cross Trainer
Jimenez v. 24 Hour Fitness **(9)**	Manufacturer's Owner's Manual—Treadmill

have evolved with the goal to improve safety, some defendants still plead ignorance when it comes to being aware of these published standards (31). For example, the defendants in *Jimenez* claimed they did not know about the spacing specifications for treadmills in the manufacturer's manual (30, 31). Of course, ignorance is not a legal defense.

Regarding the *ACSM's Health/Fitness Facility Standards and Guidelines,* another experienced expert witness, Doug Baumgarten, stated, "There have been occasions in which the court…says, 'Well, those are just recommendations. There's no legal requirement,'…"But when I get hired by a plaintiff…I always use the ACSM manual as a published standard, and very often it carries a lot of weight" (32). In addition to expert witnesses referring to published standards of practice in their testimony, plaintiffs may cite negligent claims such as "failed to follow industry standards" against the defendants in their complaint. For example, see *Baldi-Perry v. Kaifas and 360 Fitness Center* (33) described in Chapter 2.

Examples of Published Standards of Practice

To help minimize legal liability and maximize safety, fitness managers and exercise professionals need to adhere to both desirable operating practices and technical physical specifications. Below is a list and short description of "selected" publications that focus on desirable operating practices but also contain technical specifications. It is not an inclusive list. In addition, it is important to realize that professional organizations have published numerous position stands, white papers, or other similar documents that also contain operating practices and technical specifications. It is the responsibility of fitness managers and exercise professionals to be familiar with all these types of publications. Please note the "special notice" that follows regarding published standards of practice.

1. *ACSM's Health/Fitness Facility Standards and Guidelines,* 5th edition, 2019 (34)

    This publication contains 34 standards and 37 guidelines that cover a variety of topics such as screening, facility orientation, emergency procedures, staff qualifications, facility operations, equipment maintenance, and signage as well as many supplemental appendices. Standards are defined, in part, as "minimum requirements that…each health/fitness facility must meet to provide a relatively safe environment … standards are not intended…to supersede…laws and regulations" (p. xiii). Guidelines are defined in part as "recommendations that…health/fitness operators should consider using to improve the quality of the experience they provide to users" (p. xiii).

2. *ACSM's Guidelines for Exercise Testing and Prescription,* 10th edition, 2018 (35)

    This publication has numerous guidelines regarding screening, testing, prescription, exercise prescription for healthy and clinical populations, behavior change theories as well as several appendices. It states that the "views and information… are provided as guidelines—as opposed to standards of practice. This distinction is an important one because specific legal connotations may be attached to standards of practice that are not attached to guidelines" (p. ix).

3. *NSCA Strength & Conditioning Professional Standards & Guidelines,* 2017 (36)

    This publication contains 11 standards and 14 guidelines that cover a variety of topics such as screening, personnel qualifications, supervision/instruction, emergency procedures, programs for children, equipment set-up/maintenance, and signage as well as several appendices. It defines a standard as "a required procedure that probably reflects a legal duty or obligation for the standard of care" and a guideline as "a recommended operating procedure formulated and developed to further enhance the quality of services provided" (p. 2). This publication is unique when compared to the others listed here regarding its definition of standard and other related information provided on scope of practice, legal concepts, liability exposures, and risk management.

4. IHRSA (International Health, Racquet & Sportsclub Association) Club Membership Standards in *IHRSA's Guide to Club Membership & Conduct,* 3rd edition, 2005 (37)

    This publication contains 12 standards that address a variety of issues such as equal access, membership contracts, screening, emergency procedures, supervisor competence, supervision of youth programs, signage, and maintenance of exercise equipment. No definition of standard is provided.

5. *Medical Fitness Association's Standards and Guidelines for Medical Fitness Center Facilities,* 2nd edition, 2013 (38)

This publication contains 31 standards and over 100 guidelines that cover a variety of topics such as medical oversite, quality management, screening, emergency procedures, staff qualifications, youth programs, aquatics facilities, and facility operations as well as many appendices. It states that "standards and guidelines are not intended to be a 'legal' requirement..." (p. 5).

6. *Exercise Standards & Guidelines Reference Manual,* 5th edition, 2010, published by Aerobics and Fitness Association of America (AFAA) (39)

The standards and guidelines in this publication focus on principles of safe and effective exercise for instructors who teach group exercise programs. Practices such as screening, testing, emergency response are covered for both general and special populations (e.g., prenatal, youth, and seniors). Standards and guidelines are also provided for various types of group exercise programs such as aqua fitness, kickboxing, and step aerobics. No definitions are provided for standards and guidelines and these terms appear to be used interchangeably.

7. *Safeguarding Health and Well-Being, Medical Advisory Committee Recommendations: A Resource Guide for YMCAs,* 2011 (40)

These YMCA recommendations cover many areas such as aquatics, exercise and fitness, facility and member safety, general health and safety, infectious diseases, nutrition, sports, and youth health and safety. These recommendations often cite standards and guidelines published by other organizations such as ACSM, NSCA, American Heart Association, and American Academy of Pediatrics. It states that

"YMCA executive directors are encouraged to review these recommendations with their staff and local medical advisory committees, determine if they need to be adapted for their community, and then implement the recommendations as approved by their own board of directors" (p. x).

8. American Association for Cardiovascular and Pulmonary Rehabilitation (AACVPR), *Guidelines for Cardiac Rehabilitation and Secondary Prevention Programs,* 5th edition, 2013 (41)

This publication provides numerous guidelines for professionals who lead cardiac rehabilitation (CR) programs and secondary prevention (SC) programs. Regarding operating practices and technical specifications, topics include medical evaluation

KEY POINT

Special Notice Regarding Published Standards of Practice

Although there are similarities among the many professional organizations that have published standards of practices, inconsistencies exist. Inconsistencies are concerning from a legal perspective because expert witnesses will decide which standards of practices they will include in their testimony and it is unlikely that defendants will know which standards of practice these might be when faced with a negligence lawsuit.

It is impossible to list and describe all these published standards of practice in this textbook, although some are briefly summarized. Therefore, it is recommended that fitness managers and exercise professionals, along with their risk management advisory committee, select those that are "the most authoritative or safety oriented in their approach regardless of how they are defined and/or stated..." (1, p. 53), e.g., required (mandatory) versus recommended (voluntary) as well as those that are most applicable to their type of facility and programs.

The first step is to become aware of these many published standards of practice. In addition to reviewing those listed above, another helpful resource is: *Physical Activity and Health Guidelines: Recommendations for Various Ages, Fitness Levels and Conditions from 57 Authoritative Sources* (43).

As described in Chapter 2, published standards of practice are continually being updated and, thus, it is important to stay abreast of these updates, as well as changes in any laws, and then revise the facility's Risk Management Policies and Procedures Manual accordingly.

and testing, program administration (facilities/ equipment, organizational policies/procedures, documentation, personnel), and management of medical problems and emergencies. Regarding the guidelines, it states "that all programs may not have the resources to provide specific expertise in each area, but the core competencies should be some part of every program" (p. xii). See also *Guidelines for Pulmonary Rehabilitation Programs* (42).

Fitness managers and exercise professionals may ask questions such as, "why are there so many published standards of practice in the exercise profession" and "why can't there be just one set of standards as there is in the athletic training profession." The exercise profession is not a unified profession like athletic training which has established (a) standards for academic programs such as required accreditation, (b) one major national professional organization—the National Athletic Trainers' Association (NATA), (c) one national, independent board of certification that oversees the national certification exam (44), and (d) state licensure. The exercise profession is a young, evolving profession and someday it may become unified. But that is doubtful given the numerous organizations, certification programs, academic programs, etc., that all seem to do their own thing. No true collaborative effort has been made or been successful in developing one set of uniform standards of practice for fitness facilities and programs (45).

Future Direction for Published Standards of Practice

It is recommended that professional organizations, as they continue to revise and update their published standards and guidelines, refer to the Appraisal of Guidelines for Research & Evaluation (AGREE) II Instrument (46). The original AGREE Instrument was developed by a group of international guideline developers and researchers in 2003. Although it focuses on clinical practice guidelines, it states that the clinical guidelines "have evolved to cover topics across the health care continuum, e.g., health promotion, screening, diagnosis" (p. 0). It also states that the "potential benefits of guidelines are only as good as the quality of the guidelines themselves" (p. 0). The major purposes in developing this instrument were to "address the issue of variability in guideline quality" and to assess "the methodological rigor and transparency in which a guideline is developed" (p. 0).

Because the exercise profession continues to develop a positive, working relationship with the healthcare industry through initiatives such as Exercise is Medicine® (EIM) and because it may become a licensed profession in the future, it may be wise for leaders in the exercise profession to follow the same criteria in the development of published standards of practice that are used in the healthcare industry. The AGREE II Instrument contains six domains and several guidelines within each domain (46). For example, one guideline under Domain 2 (Stakeholder Involvement) involves pilot testing the guideline among end users. An example of a guideline under Domain 3 (Rigor of Development) addresses the use of systematic methods and evidence (46). It is recommended that professional organizations that published standards of practice review the 23 AGREE II guidelines to assess their level of compliance with each.

Although the published standards of practice, listed above, reference some statutory and administrative laws such as the OSHA's Bloodborne Pathogens Standard and AED state statutes, they typically do not cite case law. Legal research involving the issues and types of claims that often arise in negligence and other lawsuits against fitness facilities is essential for identifying and developing safety standards and guidelines. Although many standards of practice reflect certain negligence claims, such as the failure to conduct screening and carry out emergency procedures, common negligence claims are often not reflected in the standards of practice.

For example, published standards of practice often specify credentials that fitness managers and exercise professionals should possess. However, they do not address competence such as practical skills needed to perform the job safely and effectively. It is important to realize that (a) possessing credentials (degrees, certifications, experience) does not necessarily mean the individual is competent and, (b) competence is essential from a safety and legal perspective. There are several examples of negligence lawsuits in this textbook in which a personal fitness trainer possessed a certification but was incompetent or an exercise professional with a degree in exercise science (or related area) was incompetent. Unfortunately, the defendants in these cases faced negligence claims such as the failure to provide proper instruction. Competence is described in more detail in Chapter 5.

The failure to provide proper instruction is considered by legal experts as one of the most common claims of negligence (29, 47). A standard of practice that could address "improper instruction" would be to require fitness facilities to have their fitness staff members complete a practical training program that focuses on safe teaching and training before they begin their jobs. Academic exercise science programs may or may not have required coursework in which students develop skills regarding proper instruction and certification programs (written-only examinations) do not assess practical skills such as teaching. It is unlikely that academic and certification programs will be held liable (e.g., educational malpractice) for their failure to adequately address these important skills, but employers can be. More information regarding liability of employers is addressed in Chapter 5.

COMMON DEFENSES TO NEGLIGENCE

When faced with a negligence lawsuit, defendants have several legal defenses they can utilize. Of course, the best defense is not to breach a duty. If the defendant has acted in accordance with the applicable standard of care (no breach of a duty owed to the plaintiff), there can be no negligence. Legal defenses include comparative negligence, statutes of limitations, and immunity statutes as described in Chapter 1. However, the two most common defenses are the primary assumption of risk and waiver (release of liability), as used by defendants in many of the negligence cases described in this textbook. Fitness managers and exercise professionals should understand how these defenses work and the circumstances in which they are effective protecting the defendants and ineffective not protecting the defendants.

KEY POINT

For purposes of this textbook, a waiver (release of liability) will be referred to as a defense. However, as referenced in the Headnotes in the *Jimenez* case (30), a waiver is more appropriately characterized as an express assumption of risk. The defendant is relieved of legal duty owed to the plaintiff; and being under no duty, cannot be charged with negligence.

As described in Chapter 2, a waiver is a contractual transfer of risk; meaning the fitness participant, who signed the waiver, bears all financial and legal responsibility for any loss (harm/damages) for which the transferring organization (fitness facility) might have otherwise been liable.

Assumption of Risk Defense

The assumption of risk doctrine "involves a participant's voluntarily knowing, understanding, and agreeing to assume those ordinary and reasonable risks associated with certain activities" (1, p. 64). The assumption of risk defense is available to defendants when facing negligence claims/lawsuits involving injuries from sport, risky activities (e.g., skydiving), and fitness activities. **Express assumption of risk** and **primary assumption of risk** will be the focus of this discussion.

Express assumption of risk "arises when a plaintiff explicitly consents to relieve the defendant of a duty owed by the defendant regarding specific known risks" (48, p. 1212). Explicit consent requires an individual to sign a written document (contract) prior to participation. Examples are provided in Exhibit 4-2 (Express Assumption of Risk for Participation in a Specified Activity), Exhibit 4-3 (Assumption of Risk and Waiver of Liability, included in the membership agreement, signed by the plaintiff in *Locke v. Life Time Fitness, Inc.*, spotlight case in Chapter 11), and Exhibit 4-4 (Waiver & Release Form, signed by the plaintiff in *Stelluti v. Casapenn Enterprises*, spotlight case presented later in this chapter). These documents describe the risks of the activity (e.g., minor, major, life-threatening, and death) and include a statement such as: "I understand and voluntarily accept this risk. I agree to specifically assume all risk of injury", as provided in *Locke*. When signing such a document, the individual affirms his/her knowledge and understanding of the risks and voluntarily assumes the risks.

EDITORIAL NOTE: CAUTION!!!

Regarding Form in Exhibit 4-2: No form should be adopted by any program until it has first been reviewed by legal counsel in the state where a form is to be used as well as by the medical director/advisor/risk manager for the program. To be acceptable, each form must be written in accordance with prevailing state laws by knowledgeable legal counsel and should state to the participant the reasons for the procedure, the risks and benefits, etc., in a manner specific to the program activities for which consent, or other form of contractual document, is being obtained. The form (Exhibit 4-2) hereinafter reproduced is protected by copyright and may not be reproduced in any form, by any means. It is reproduced here with permission of the copyright holder, PRC Publishing, Inc., 3976 Fulton Drive NW, Canton, Ohio 44718, 1-800-336-0083, www.prcpublishingcorp.com.

Primary assumption of risk "follows from the plaintiff engaging in risky conduct from which the law implies consent" (48, p. 1213). For example, it is implied that one who engages in sport activities assumes the reasonably foreseeable **risks inherent in the activity**. "To the extent a risk inherent in the sport injures a plaintiff, the defendant has no duty and there is no negligence" (48, p. 1214). Risks inherent in the sport are those that are inseparable from the activity and happen because of participation (i.e., they cannot be eliminated). For example, in *Main v. Gym X-Treme* (49), the court stated that "the doctrine of primary assumption of risk requires an examination of the activity itself. If the activity involves risks that cannot be eliminated, then a finding of primary assumption of risk is appropriate" (p. 6). The spotlight cases (*Corrigan* and *Santana*) and other cases presented in this section, demonstrate how the courts examine the activity when analyzing the primary of assumption of risk defense.

Note: *Some of the courts in the negligence cases described in this textbook use the term* **inherent risks** *when referring to risks inherent in an activity or sport. Therefore, the term inherent risks is also used in this textbook to mean the same as risks inherent in the activity.*

The primary assumption of risk defense is always available to defendants in a negligence claim. However, for this defense to be effective, the evidence must show three elements "(1) the plaintiff possessed full subjective understanding, (2) of the presence and nature of the specific risk, and (3) voluntarily chose to encounter the risks (48, p. 1214). The knowledge and understanding of the risks that the plaintiff possessed is a question for the court. For example in *Corrigan*, the appellate court, citing previous case law, stated:

> It is true that relieving an owner or operator of a sporting venue from liability for inherent risks of engaging in a sport is justified when a consenting participant is aware of the risks; has an appreciation of the nature of the risks; and voluntarily assumes the risks...If the risks of the activity are fully comprehended or perfectly obvious, the plaintiff has consented to them and the defendant has performed its duty. In our view...defendant did not establish as a matter of law that the risks associated with the use of the treadmill to plaintiff, a novice, were fully appreciated or perfectly obvious (*Corrigan, pp. 862-863*).

The *Corrigan* court also stated it did not find "under the doctrine of primary assumption of risk, that plaintiff assumed the risks inherent in using this piece of equipment. Primary assumption of the risk may be applied in cases where there is an elevated risk of danger, typically in sporting and recreational events... We are unpersuaded that plaintiff's first time on the treadmill falls within the reach of this principle...the risk of being ejected from this machine was not readily apparent. Under these circumstances, a jury should assess whether plaintiff's injuries are the result of any breach of duty by defendant" (*Corrigan*, p. 863).

Exhibit 4-2: Express Assumption of Risk for Participation in Specified Activity*

I, the undersigned, hereby expressly and affirmatively state that I wish to participate in _____.
I realize that my participation in this activity involves risks of injury, including but not to limited to *(list)* _____
_____ and even the possibility of death. I also recognize that there are many other risks of injury, including serious disabling injuries, which may arise due to my participation in this activity and that it is not possible to specifically list each and every individual injury risk. However, knowing the material risks and appreciating, knowing and reasonably anticipating that other injuries and even death are a possibility, I hereby expressly assume all of the delineated risks of injury, all other possible risk of injury and even death which could occur by reason of my participation.

I have had an opportunity to ask questions. Any questions which I have asked have been answered to my complete satisfaction. I subjectively understand the risks of my participation in this activity and knowing and appreciating these risks I voluntarily choose to participate, assuming all risks of injury or even death due to my participation.

_____   _____   Dated: _____

Witness   Participant

NOTES OF QUESTIONS AND ANSWERS

_____

_____

This is, as stated, a true and accurate record of what was asked and answered.

_____

Participant

TO BE CHECKED BY PROGRAM STAFF

		CHECKED	INITIALS
I.	RISKS WERE ORALLY DISCUSSED	_____	_____
II.	QUESTIONS WERE ASKED AND THE PARTICIPANT INDICATED COMPLETE UNDERSTANDING OF THE RISKS	_____	_____
III.	QUESTIONS WERE NOT ASKED, BUT AN OPPORTUNITY TO QUESTION WAS PROVIDED AND THE PARTICIPANT INDICATED COMPLETE UNDERSTANDING OF THE RISKS	_____	_____

_____   _____

Staff Member   Date

*Reproduced and adapted with permission from Herbert & Herbert, LEGAL ASPECTS OF PREVENTIVE, REHABILITATIVE AND RECREATIONAL EXERCISE PROGRAMS, FOURTH EDITION (PRC Publishing, Inc., Canton, Ohio 2002). All other rights reserved.

Exhibit 4-3: Assumption of Risk and Waiver of Liability*

ASSUMPTION OF RISK AND WAIVER OF LIABILITY

I understand that there is an inherent risk of injury, whether caused by me or someone else, in the use of or presence at a Life Time Fitness center, the use of equipment and services at a Life Time Fitness center, and participation in Life Time Fitness' programs. This risk includes, but is not limited to:

1. Injuries arising from the use of any Life Time Fitness' centers or equipment, including any accidental or 'slip and fall' injuries;

2. *Injuries arising from participation in supervised or unsupervised activities and programs within a Life Time Fitness center or outside a Life Time Fitness center, to the extent sponsored or endorsed by Life Time Fitness;*

3. *Injuries or medical disorders resulting from exercise at a Life Time Fitness center, including,* but not limited to, heart attacks, strokes, heart stress, sprains, broken bones and torn muscles or ligaments; and

4. *Injuries resulting from the actions taken or decisions made regarding medical or survival procedures.*

I understand and voluntarily accept this risk. I agree to specifically assume all risk of injury, whether physical or mental, as well as all risk of loss, theft or damage of personal property for me, any person that is a part of this membership and any guest under this membership while such persons are using or present at any Life Time Fitness center, using any lockers, equipment, or services at any Life Time Fitness center or participating in Life Time Fitness' programs, whether such programs take place inside or outside of a Life Time Fitness center. I waive any and all claims or actions that may arise against Life Time Fitness, Inc., its affiliates, subsidiaries, successors or assigns (collectively, 'Life Time Fitness') as well as each party's owners, directors, employees or volunteers as a result of any such injury, loss, theft, or damage to any such person, including and without limitation, personal bodily or mental injury, economic loss or any damage to me, my spouse, my children, or guests resulting from the negligence of Life Time Fitness or anyone else using a Life Time Fitness center. If there is any claim by anyone based on any injury, loss, theft or damage that involves me, any person that is a part of my membership, or any guest under this membership, I agree to defend Life Time Fitness against such claims and pay Life Time Fitness for all expenses relating to the claim, and indemnify Life Time Fitness for all obligations resulting from such claims (Locke, p. 672).

I agree to and accept the terms and conditions above and I have received a complete copy of my Member Usage Agreement.

*Locke v. Life Time Fitness, Inc., 20 F. Supp. 3d 669 (D. Ill., N.D., 2014)

In *Santana*, the appellate court examined the risks inherent in step aerobics, stating

> *…in an activity like step aerobics, defendant owes no duty to protect against the risks inherent in the exercise of stepping on and off a platform, such as a sprained ankle. However, defendants generally do have a duty to use due care not to increase the risks to a participant over and above those inherent in the sport… In this case, defendants…provided the instructor who decided what would be done and for how long. They provided the instructor who also gave direction on techniques. An instructor/student relationship is to be considered in determining the scope of the defendant's duty… Under these circumstances, defendants owed a duty to plaintiff and the other participants not to increase the risks inherent in step aerobics… (Santana, pp. 26-27).*

The *Santana* court further stated, "step aerobics does not inherently require exercises which are designed in such a way as to create an extreme risk of injury, such as, by combining movements that affect the balance and draw the participant's focus away from the platform while stepping on and off it or requiring the use of a mirror for orientation instead of looking where one's feet are going…" (*Santana*, pp. 26-27).

Spotlight Cases: Primary Assumption of Risk an Ineffective Defense

In the following spotlight cases, *Corrigan* and *Santana*, the primary assumption of risk defense was ineffective in protecting the defendants. In *Corrigan*, the personal trainer failed to properly instruct the plaintiff on how to use the treadmill because the plaintiff was a novice—she did not know, understand, and appreciate the risks of using a treadmill. In *Santana*, the group exercise instructor exacerbated the risks inherent in step aerobics.

In addition to *Corrigan* and *Santana*, see the following spotlight cases in other chapters in which the primary assumption of risk was ineffective in protecting the defendants:

1. *Levy v. Town Sports International, Inc.* (Chapter 7): Trainer created unreasonable increased risks.

2. *Layden v. Plante* (Chapter 7): Trainer created unreasonable increased risks.
3. *Scheck v. Soul Cycle* (Chapter 8): Instructor was negligent— failed to properly instruct a novice.
4. *Lotz v. The Claremont Club* (Chapter 8): Instructor of youth activity created unreasonable increased risks.
5. *Butler v. Seville et al.* (Chapter 9): Trainer was negligent—improper instruction and supervision.
6. *Locke v. Life Time Fitness, Inc.* (Chapter 11): Decedent did not assume a risk that facility's employees would not be properly trained to carryout emergency procedures.

Following the *Corrigan* and *Santana* spotlight cases, are descriptions of cases in which the primary assumption of risk defense was *effective* in protecting the defendants. See "Cases: Primary Assumption of Risk an Effective Defense." In reviewing all of the cases involving the primary assumption of risk defense, note the factors courts consider when determining if the plaintiff assumed the risks (e.g., did the plaintiff know/understand the risks inherent in the activity, was the plaintiff a novice or experienced exerciser, and was the plaintiff participating in a sport or in a physical activity program to improve health/fitness).

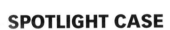

SPOTLIGHT CASE

Corrigan v. MuscleMakers Inc.
258 A.D.2d 861 (N.Y. App. Div., 1999)

FACTS

Historical Facts:

The plaintiff in *Corrigan* was a 49-year-old woman who was participating in her first personal training session. Toward the end of her session, her personal trainer in-structed her to get on a treadmill. He set it at 3.5 miles per hour for 20 minutes. He provided her with little or no instruction on how to use the treadmill and then left her unattended. After a short while she began to drift back on the belt and though she attempted to walk faster she was thrown from the treadmill resulting in a fractured ankle. The plaintiff was a novice—she had never participated in a fitness facility of this type nor had she ever been on a treadmill.

Procedural Facts:

The plaintiff filed a negligence claim against the defendants (the personal trainer and the health club) seeking recovery for her injuries. The defendants filed a motion for summary judgment claiming that the plaintiff voluntarily participated in

Corrigan continued...

an athletic activity, and therefore, assumed the risks. The defendants appealed the court's decision to deny their motion for summary judgment.

ISSUE

Was the primary assumption of risk doctrine an effective defense to dismiss the plaintiff's negligence claim and grant the defendant's motion for summary judgment?

COURT'S RULING

No, the appellate court ruled that the primary assumption of risk was not an effective defense to dismiss the plaintiff's negligence claim; the decision to deny the defendant's motion for summary judgment was affirmed.

COURT'S REASONING

Relying on previous case law decisions, the appellate court ruled that the "doctrine of primary assumption of risk... maybe applied in cases where there is an elevated risk of danger, typically in sporting and recreational events" (p. 863). The court stated that this doctrine does not apply in this case because the fitness activity (exercising on a treadmill) was not an athletic or sporting event in which a lesser standard of care should be applied.

In addition, the plaintiff was a novice who did not fully know, understand, and appreciate the risks associated with using the treadmill—a requirement for the primary assumption of risk to apply. The court concluded that the personal trainer failed to ensure that plaintiff knew how to use the treadmill, referring to a guideline in the machine's manual that stated knowledge on how to use the treadmill was necessary for safe operation. The court indicated that a jury would need to determine if the plaintiff's injuries were due to the defendant's negligence (breach of duty).

Lessons Learned from *Corrigan*:

Legal

▸ Primary assumption of risk was not an effective defense for negligent instruction which occurred in this case. (A waiver was not addressed in this case).

▸ Primary assumption of risk is an effective defense for injuries due to risks inherent in the activity but only if:

• The plaintiff is a *not* a novice. A novice will not be able to fully know, understand, and appreciate the risks of the activity until he/she acquires more experience.

• The injury results from participation in sporting and recreational activities, not fitness activities. For example, individuals who participate in sports assume an elevated risk of danger inherent in the sport whereas fitness activities taught by a trainer should not have an elevated risk of danger.

▸ Instructional guidelines in the equipment owner's manual may provide evidence of duty or the standard of care.

Risk Management/Injury Prevention

▸ Personal fitness trainers need to be well-trained on the importance of providing proper instruction to their clients on how to use exercise equipment and direct supervision of their clients, especially clients that are novices.

▸ Facility fitness staff members who teach and train participants on how to use exercise equipment should be aware of (and follow) the instructional guidelines set forth in the equipment owner's manual and inform their participants of any warnings also specified in the manual.

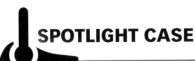

SPOTLIGHT CASE

Santana v. Women's Workout and Weight Loss Centers, Inc.
No. H021377, 2001 LEXIS 1186 (Cal. Ct. App., 2001).

FACTS

Historical Facts:

Marleen Santana was injured while participating in a modified step aerobics class at the *Women's Workout and Weight Loss Centers, Inc.* that combined step aerobics and overhead arm strength training exercises using a Dyna-Band. Santana was experienced in "normal" step aerobics; however, this was her first step experience that also involved the use of the Dyna-Band. The participants were instructed to "keep their heads facing forward and not to look at their feet while doing the exercise but to look straight ahead at their reflections in a mirror for orientation" (p. 2). While participating in the activity, Santana fell and fractured her ankle. The injury required surgical intervention involving inserting pins in her leg.

When the plaintiff joined the defendant's facility, she signed a membership application (signature was placed on the front page) which contained a release of liability on the back. She claimed that she was not informed of the release on the back (it was not indicated on the form and she was not told by an employee) and was not offered time to read it. The back of the application contained two columns of 8-point type with paragraphs labeled in 12-point type. The last paragraph on the bottom right was headed: ASSUMPTION OF RISK RELEASE & INDEMNITY.

Procedural Facts:

The plaintiff, Santana, filed a negligence lawsuit and alleged that the "peculiar design of the exercise was 'unnecessarily hazardous' in that the simultaneous performance of multi angled upward/downward steps and vigorous overhead arm exercises, combined with the forced inability to see one's feet in relation to the step platform made normal balance unduly difficult and dangerous" (p. 6). The defendant, *Women's Workout and Weight Loss Centers, Inc.*, moved for summary judgment contending that the membership agreement that contained a release of liability barred her negligent action and asserted that she assumed the risks. The trial court ruled that the plaintiff's fall was a risk inherent in the "sport of step aerobics" and thus found that the defendants had no duty to the plaintiff. The trial court granted the motion for summary judgment, and the plaintiff appealed.

ISSUE

Did the defenses, release of liability and primary assumption of risk, bar the plaintiff's negligence claims made against the defendant?

COURT'S RULING:

No, the appellate court ruled the release to be unenforceable and the primary assumption of risk defense did not apply in this case. The trial court's ruling to grant summary judgment to the defendant was reversed.

COURT'S REASONING:

Regarding the waiver defense and citing previous case law, the court stated:

> An exculpatory clause is unenforceable if not distinguished from other sections, if printed in the same typeface as the remainder of the document, and if not likely to attract attention because it is placed in the middle of a document...In other words, a release must not be buried in a lengthy document, hidden among other verbiage, or so encumbered with other provisions as to be difficult to find...Here, the release clause is a separate paragraph on the back of the document. It is printed in 8-point type and is differentiated from other paragraphs by a

Santana continued...

heading in 12-point type, all capital letters. However, the ink is very light and the heading is actually lighter than the regular text on the front of the document. In addition, the waiver is the last paragraph on the back of the document and the signature line is on the front. No advisement that there is a release of liability clause on the back of defendant's form appears on the front of the form (pp. 18-19).

Regarding the primary assumption of risk defense, the court relied on previous case law to distinguish participation in sports and a step aerobics exercise class as follows:

...an activity falls within the meaning of 'sport' if the activity is done for enjoyment or thrill, requires physical exertion as well as elements of skill, and involves a challenge containing a potential risk of injury" and involves 'elements like physical contact between participants...competition aimed at scoring points, racing against time, or accomplishing feats of speed...' (p. 25). Duty is constricted in the sports setting because the activity involves inherent risks which cannot be eliminated without destroying the sport itself (p. 24).

...in an activity like step aerobics, defendant owes no duty to protect against the risks inherent in the exercise of stepping on and off a platform, such as a sprained ankle. However, defendants generally do have a duty to use due care not to increase the risks to a participant over and above those inherent in the sport . . . In this case, defendants ...provided the instructor who decided what would be done and for how long. They provided the instructor who also gave direction on techniques. An instructor/student relationship is to be considered in determining the scope of the defendant's duty...Under these circumstances, defendants owed a duty to plaintiff and the other participants not to increase the risks inherent in step aerobics...However, step aerobics does not inherently require exercises which are designed in such a way as to create an extreme risk of injury, such as, by combining movements that affect the balance and draw the participant's focus away from the platform while stepping on and off it or requiring the use of a mirror for orientation instead of looking where one's feet are going (pp. 26-27).

In forming its ruling/reasoning, the court referred to the expert testimony provided by Dr. Peter Francis as admissible evidence. The court also clarified that the duty owed to the plaintiff is determined by courts/judges, not experts. Dr. Francis stated that athletes are well informed of the risks involved in sports by their own experiences. In other words, they assume the risks inherent in the sport because they fully understand and appreciate these risks and voluntarily accept them. But this does not apply to individuals who participate in group exercise programs. "These individuals do not expect to be at significant risk for injury...participants rely upon the exercise instructor to provide safe forms of exercise" (pp. 9-10). Dr. Francis also stated that "the unorthodox combination of the two forms of exercise [aerobic and an overhead strength exercise], together with the use of a mirror for visual orientation, created a situation that was inherently dangerous. This combination of factors did not meet the standard of care in the industry" (p. 8). However, he also stated that although combining two or more forms of exercise is inefficient, they are not always inherently dangerous as they were in this case.

Lessons Learned from *Santana:*

Legal

- Primary assumption of risk is an effective defense for 'sport' activities because:
  - The risks inherent in the sport cannot be altered without destroying the sport itself (i.e., sports involve physical contact, competition, racing against time which elevate the risk of danger/injury).
  - Participants in sport activities voluntarily participate knowing these risks.
- Primary assumption of risk may not be an effective defense when a group exercise leader instructs participants to perform exercises that increase the risks over and above those inherent in the activity.

Santana continued...

> ◆ The exculpatory clause within a release of liability must be distinguished (e.g., highlighted using caps, large and bold font) from other sections in the document to be enforceable.
>
> ◆ Courts often rely on the testimony of an expert witness to help determine the duty owed to the plaintiff.
>
> **Risk Management/Injury Prevention**
> ◆ Group exercise instructors need to be well-trained on the importance of providing safe instruction to their participants.
>
> > • For each exercise taught, instructors need to consider factors such as what is the purpose of the exercise, does it create any safety concerns.
>
> ◆ Direct supervision/evaluation of group exercise leaders is needed to be sure they are properly teaching their classes. If not, corrective measures may be needed. For example, providing re-training on how to teach safely and having the instructor submit lesson plans that can reviewed by an exercise professional/supervisor to determine if they are appropriate.

Cases: Primary Assumption of Risk Defense an Effective Defense

In a spotlight case described in Chapter 6, *Rostai v. Neste Enterprises* (50), the defendants successfully invoked the primary assumption of risk defense. The *Rostai* court made no distinction between participation in sports and a structured exercise program as the courts had in *Corrigan* and *Santana*. Although the actions of the trainer in *Rostai* may be considered negligent by most exercise professionals (the trainer instructed his sedentary client to perform high intensity exercise in the first session), the court ruled the plaintiff had assumed the risks created by the trainer's conduct. According to the court, only intentional or reckless conduct by the trainer would have constituted a breach of the duty owed to the plaintiff.

In *Main v. Gym X-Treme* (49), a 10-year-old girl, Brenna Main, attended a birthday party at defendant's facility. An employee of the facility opened the door to the gymnasium so that the girls attending the party could jump on the spring floor. While jumping on the spring floor, Brenna fell and broke her arm. Brenna Main and Danielle Main filed a complaint against the defendant alleging negligent supervision. The defendant filed a motion for summary judgment which the trial court granted. The appellate court agreed and upheld the trial court's ruling. The court stated, "primary assumption of risk completely negates a negligence claim because the defendant owes no duty to protect the plaintiff against the inherent risks of the recreational activity in which the plaintiff engages" (p. 5).

The court also stated, "a plaintiff who voluntarily engages in a recreational activity or sporting event assumes the inherent risks of that activity and cannot recover for injuries sustained in engaging in the activity unless the defendant acted recklessly or intentionally in causing injuries" (49, p. 4). According to the court, application of the primary assumption of risk doctrine applies regardless of "whether the activity was engaged by children or adults, or was unorganized, supervised or unsupervised" (p. 4). The court determined that jumping on a spring board in a gymnasium at a birthday party was a "recreational" activity and, thus, the plaintiff assumed the risks.

In *Tadmor v. New York Jiu Jitsu, Inc.* (51), the plaintiff was injured while participating in an advanced martial arts class for the first time. The plaintiff was encouraged to take the advanced class by his instructor after participating in the beginner classes for over a month and half. The injury occurred while sparring with a stocky guy after he had first sparred with a tall thin guy and lost that match. When the plaintiff was instructed to spar with the stocky guy, he told his instructor "It doesn't look like a match" but his instructor assured him by saying "Don't worry about it" and "I got your back" (p. 442). The plaintiff claimed that the stocky guy used an unfamiliar, advanced, maneuver that forced him to the floor causing injuries and subsequent knee surgeries.

The plaintiff filed a complaint against the defendant and the defendant filed a motion of summary judgment which the trial court dismissed. However, the appellate court reversed the trial court's decision and granted the defendant's motion for summary judgment. The court stated, "it is well established that the doctrine of assumption of risk generally applies where the plaintiff is injured while voluntarily participating in a sport or recreational activity, and the injury-causing event is a known, apparent or reasonably foreseeable consequence of the participation" (51, p. 440). The court indicated that the plaintiff knew and appreciated the risk of sparring and that matching him with a heavier wrestler did not unreasonably increase the risk of injury. The plaintiff argued he was not aware of the potential risks at the time and only accepted the risk of sparring with the stocky guy once the instructor reassured him. A dissenting opinion agreed with the plaintiff and stated that there is a question as to "whether defendant's assurances concealed or unreasonably heightened the risk of injury in a martial arts match with a more advanced opponent, such that the risk was not assumed by the plaintiff" (p. 445).

In *Blume v. Equinox* (52), the plaintiff injured his back while performing a squat exercise with 300 pounds during a personal training session. He had a long history of performing weighted exercises (including squats) under the supervision of a different personal trainer who had informed him of the potential risk of injury while squatting. The plaintiff typically performed squats with 200 pounds but had never attempted more than 220 pounds prior to the day of his injury. In his complaint, the plaintiff claimed that his trainer failed to design a safe program by asking him to squat with 300 pounds. The court granted the defendants' motion of summary judgment based on the primary assumption of risk defense.

The defendants cited many cases that found no duty is owed to an injured party who engages in athletic or recreational activity. However, the plaintiff argued that the primary assumption of risk doctrine does not apply to him because he was not involved in playing a game on a field as were the plaintiffs in almost all the cases the defendants cited. The court stated that even though the plaintiff was engaged in an exercise under the supervision of a paid expert in a controlled setting, the activity "is still simply exercise and the primary assumption of risk defense generally applies" and because "a squat carries commonly known risks including back injury" (52, p. 4).

In another case, *Rutnik v. Colonie Center Court Club, Inc.* (53), the primary assumption of risk defense was,

again, effectively raised by the defendant. In *Rutnik*, A wrongful death action was filed against the defendant Club after an experienced racquetball player collapsed during a Club-sponsored racquetball tournament and died from cardiac arrest (1). The defendant claimed the player assumed the risks when he volunteered to participate in the tournament (1) The appellate court agreed stating "relieving an owner or operator of a sporting facility from liability for the inherent risk of engaging in sports is justified when the consenting participant is aware of the risk, has an appreciation of the nature of the risks and voluntarily assumes the risk" (p. 452). The court indicated that because the decedent was an experienced racquetball player, he must have known and appreciated the risk of cardiac arrest while playing racquetball (1). The court also stated that the staff members at the Club carried out emergency procedures properly, so defendants performed their respective duties in a reasonable manner.

Summary: Assumption of Risk

Whether or not the assumption of risk will be an effective defense, insulating defendants from liability for negligence, will likely depend upon the court's examination of the activity, the conduct of the defendants, and rulings from prior cases in that jurisdiction. Generally, the assumption of risk doctrine serves as an effective defense for injuries caused by risks inherent in the activity if the injured party knew and understood those risks and voluntarily participated regardless. Fitness managers and exercise professionals can strengthen the assumption of risk defense by adopting the following risk management strategies:

1. Prior to participation, have all participants sign an express assumption of risk document such as those presented in Exhibits 4-2, 4-3, and 4-4. It is essential that this document is prepared by a competent lawyer.
   a) The language in the document includes informing participants of the risks inherent in the activity—minor, major, life-threatening, and even death.
   b) This language can also help refute negligent claims such as the failure to warn of risks.
   c) The document needs to be properly administered—see "administration of waiver/release of liability" later in this chapter.

2. Train all exercise professionals (e.g., personal fitness trainers, group exercise instructors) on how to provide sufficient information (especially to new participants) regarding the risks related to the exercises they will be performing.
   a) See Chapter 8 that describes the importance of offering "beginner" classes
   b) See Chapter 10 that describes the facility/equipment orientation for new participants
3. Train all exercise professionals so they fully understand situations when they are training/teaching that create increased risks over and above those inherent in the activity and the potential consequences.
   a) Consider providing a training session discussing the case law examples such as those above.
   b) Supervise exercise professionals and evaluate their job performance.
4. Do not have exercise professionals teach advanced exercises to participants until they are well-experienced and skilled with beginning and intermediate level exercise activities. Be sure exercise professionals who teach individuals with medical conditions know how to design/deliver a proper exercise program such as knowing the precautions that need to be taken to minimize risks.
5. When a participant is ready for an advanced exercise, be sure the exercise professional informs the participant of any risks that may exist and employs a safe, gradual progression when introducing the advanced exercise. For example, certain risks are "increased" with heavy resistance training compared to moderate intensity weight lifting, as described in Chapter 9.

Note: *All documents and records of the above risk management strategies should be stored in a secure location—they may provide important evidence if ever faced with a negligence lawsuit.*

Waiver (Release of Liability) Defense

For purposes of this textbook, the terms *waiver, release,* and *release of liability* will be used interchangeably. The courts, in the negligence cases described in this textbook, referred to these documents as titled by the fitness facility. For example, in the spotlight cases described later in this section, the documents signed by the plaintiffs were titled Personal Training Agreement and Release of Liability (*Evans* spotlight case) and Waiver & Release Form (*Stelluti* spotlight case).

Waivers are commonly used in fitness facilities. A waiver is often referred to as a prospective release, meaning it is signed *prior* to participation. A waiver is a contract and like all contracts, it must meet the four elements of a valid contract as described in Chapter 1—Agreement, Consideration, Contractual Capacity and Legality. See Table 1-4 in Chapter 1 for an example of how these four elements are applied in a waiver contract.

Waiver law is quite complex and varies from state to state. Therefore, it is necessary that fitness managers and exercise professionals consult with a competent lawyer to prepare a waiver that will be enforceable in their jurisdiction. A waiver or release includes an **exculpatory clause.** Exculpatory means "clearing or tending to clear from alleged fault or guilt" and an exculpatory clause is defined as "a contract clause which releases one of the parties from liability for his or her wrong doing" (54, p. 392).

Most of the cases described throughout this textbook are negligence lawsuits involving personal injury and wrongful death actions against exercise professionals and fitness facilities. As described in Chapter 1, in a negligence lawsuit the plaintiff must prove that the defendant had a duty, breached that duty, and that the breach of duty caused the harm/damages. "Waivers and releases, where effective, circumvent or nullify the duty element necessary to establish a cause of action for negligence...the party so released is waived of his/her obligations imposed by the duty element otherwise required by law for negligence actions… (1, p. 72). Courts will analyze a variety of factors to determine if a waiver is an effective defense. Many of these factors are addressed in the *Evans* and *Stelluti* spotlight cases and other cases described below.

One factor that courts will often examine is if the waiver was contrary to or against **public policy.** Public policy is defined as "community common sense and common conscience, extended and applied throughout the state to matters of public morals, health, safety, welfare, and the like" (54, p. 857). To gain an understanding and appreciation of the concept of public policy as it relates to waivers, see Exhibit 4-5, a dissenting opinion written by two justices in the *Stelluti* case. When analyzing public policy issues in waiver cases, courts often rely on

Tunkl v. Regents of the University of California (55). In this case, the California Supreme Court developed a test to determine the factors in which a waiver would violate public policy and thus be unenforceable. These factors are:

1. Is the business in question of a type generally thought suitable for public regulation;

2. Is the party seeking exculpation engaged in performing a service of great importance to the public, which is often a matter of practical necessity for some members of the public;

3. Does the party performing the service hold himself out as willing to perform this service for any member of the public who seeks it, or at least for any member coming within certain established standards;

4. As a result of the essential nature of the service and in the economic setting of the transaction, does the party invoking exculpation possess a decisive advantage of bargaining strength against any member of the public who seeks his services;

5. In exercising a superior bargaining power does the party seeking an adhesion contract of exculpation make no provision whereby a purchaser may pay additional reasonable fees and obtain protection against negligence;

6. As a result of the transaction, is the person or property of the purchaser placed under the control of the seller, thereby subject to the risk of carelessness by seller or his agents (55, pp. 98-101).

Factors #4 and #5 from *Tunkl* are often addressed in waiver cases involving fitness facilities such as in the *Stelluti* and *Butler* cases described below.

The enforceability of waivers is based on state law. Some states have statutes that have prohibited waivers and in other states, courts have ruled waivers as against public policy for personal injury. In *Waivers & Releases of Liability* (56), using a general rating scale of excellent, good, fair, and poor, the following states were rated "poor" regarding the likelihood of enforcement of waivers: Connecticut, Hawaii, Louisiana, Virginia, and Wisconsin. Two states, Massachusetts and New York were rated good. However, both of these states have statutes that prohibit health club waivers. For example, the New York statute is titled: Agreements Exempting Pools, Gymnasiums…and Similar Establishments from Liability for Negligence Void and Unenforceable" (N.Y. Gen. Oblig. Law § 5-326). Therefore, specific to fitness

facilities, a "poor" rating would be assigned to these states. Hawaii and Louisiana also have similar state statutes and in the other states listed, waivers were rated poor based on Supreme Court rulings (56). For example, the Supreme Court of Virginia ruled, in *Hiett v. Lake Barcroft Community Association,* 418 S.E.2d 894 (Va., 1992), that waivers to protect against negligence for personal injuries were against public policy and unenforceable.

Waivers & Releases of Liability (56) may be a helpful resource for fitness managers and exercise professionals as well as lawyers. It provides an analysis of waiver law in each state such as the (a) exculpatory clause requirements such as does this clause need to explicitly include the word negligence, and (b) enforceability of parental waivers. The specific language that is needed to help ensure the exculpatory clause will be enforceable varies from state to state. Children do not have contractual capacity and, therefore, they cannot enter into a contract like a waiver. However, in some states, parents (or legal guardians) can waive the rights of the child and a parental waiver will be enforced. This book covers many other important topics regarding waivers and releases (e.g., limitations to waivers and why they sometimes fail, eleven steps for writing stand-alone waivers, administration of waivers including electronic/online waivers, group waivers, waiver considerations for unsupervised facilities, waivers and rights of non-signing spouse/child with regard to a **loss of consortium** (interference with a relationship) claim, other protective documents, and indemnification clauses). It is impossible to address all these aspects of waivers and releases in this textbook, but some of the key issues related to the enforceability of waivers in fitness facilities are described in the spotlight and other cases below. The authors of *Waivers & Releases of Liability* have a website (see www.sportwaiver.com) covering current waiver cases and much more.

Spotlight Cases: Waiver Defense

Before describing the spotlight cases, it is important to realize that many courts generally disfavor waivers for personal injury. However, they do not want to interfere with the freedom of two parties to contract. Therefore, waivers are often enforced if they are not against public policy (e.g., if any of the six factors specified in *Tunkl* are present, the waiver may violate public policy and, thus, is unenforceable) and meet other requirements as well. In the *Santana* spotlight case described earlier, the waiver was ineffective primarily because the exculpatory clause was not conspicuous within the document—it was not distinguishable from other sections in the document. The waivers in the following spotlight cases *Evans v. Fitness & Sports Clubs, LLC* (57) and *Stelluti v. Casapenn Enterprises, LLC* (58) absolved (protected) the defendants from any liability due to their own ordinary negligent conduct. In *Evans*, the court ruled that the waiver did not violate public policy (met all three prongs of a valid exculpatory clause) and that the exculpatory clause was sufficiently conspicuous and unambiguous.

In *Stelluti v. Casapenn Enterprises LLC, dba Powerhouse Gym* (58), the court ruled that even though the wavier was an adhesion contract, Stelluti did not have a 'position of unequal bargaining power' such that the contract violated public policy. She could have taken her business to another fitness club. See Exhibit 4-4: Waiver in *Stelluti* and take note of the various sections within the waiver. Also see Exhibit 4-5: Dissenting Opinion in *Stelluti*. Two judges prepared a dissent to the majority's opinion. This will help explain why courts disfavor waivers. What do you think? Do you agree or disagree with the dissent?

Expert testimony was an interesting factor in *Stelluti* (58). Although testimony of expert witnesses was reviewed by the New Jersey Supreme Court, it did not appear to have much influence in the decision to uphold the waiver. The defendants and the plaintiff provided expert testimony in this case. The expert for the defendants noted that, regarding the handlebar on the bike, there is "no noticeable difference between the appearance of the post when it is locked in place or when the post merely is resting on top of an elevation locking pin," (p. 295) and, therefore, concluded the plaintiff's accident occurred unexpectedly and without warning. The plaintiff's expert stated, "Powerhouse was 'negligent in providing a safe environment' and, specifically, that the spinning instructor 'failed to provide effective specific supervision, instruction and assistance' to Stelluti..." (p. 296). Stelluti's expert also referenced a protocol stating that "every certified spinning instructor should follow, including, 'proper handlebar height adjustment' before each class 'to help ensure a comfortable position on the bike and avoid undue strain on the back'...The protocol noted that students should be reminded to 'check that the 'pop pin' is fully engaged in to make sure that the handlebars are secure.' The expert also referred to the Star Trac Group Cycles Owners Guide, which emphasized that 'proper instruction from a certified Spinning instructor should be used to properly fit the group cycle for use' and that 'users should be aware of the features, functions and proper operation of the cycle *before* using the cycle for the first time'" (pp. 296-297).

SPOTLIGHT CASE

Evans v. Fitness & Sports Clubs, LLC
No. 15-4095, 2016 WL 5404464 (E.D. Pa., 2016)

FACTS

Historical Facts:

Patricia Evans, a 61-year-old female, was participating in a personal training session at the defendant's club (Fitness & Sports Clubs, LLC d/b/a LA Fitness) when she was instructed to perform "suicide runs". Her trainer had her run forward to a weight and run backwards to the start line. Evans claimed her trainer instructed her to go "faster, faster", and as she was backpedaling she fell, which resulted in the plaintiff fracturing both of her wrists.

When Evans became a member of the club, she signed a three-page Membership Agreement. The exculpatory clause in the Membership Agreement included, in part, the following:

Evans continued...

> Member hereby releases and holds LA Fitness...harmless from all liability to Member...for any loss or damage and forever gives up any claim or demands therefore, on account of injury to Member's person..., whether caused by the active or passive negligence of LA Fitness or otherwise, to the fullest extent permitted by law (p. 5).

Evans also was required to sign a three-page Personal Training Agreement and Release of Liability. The following statement was included on the first page:

> By signing this Agreement Client acknowledges that Client has read, understood and agreed with all terms and conditions of this Agreement, after having the opportunity to have it reviewed by an attorney at the discretion of Client. Client further acknowledges Client has received a filled-in and completed copy of this entire Agreement, which includes the **ACKNOWLEDGMENT & ASSUMPTION OF RISK** and the **LIMITATION OF LIABILITY & FULL RELEASE OF LAF** on page 2... (p. 2).

The following exculpatory language appeared on the second page printed in larger font than the rest of the information on page two:

> **LIMITATION OF LIABILITY & FULL RELEASE OF LAF:** Client agrees to fully release LAF [LA Fitness], its owners, employees, affiliates, authorized agents and independent contractors from any and all liability, claims, demands or other actions that Client may have for injuries, disability or death or other damages of any kind, including but not limited to, direct, special, incidental, indirect, punitive or consequential damages, whether arising in tort, contract, or breach of warranty, arising out of participation in the Services, including, but not limited to, the Physical Activities, even if caused by the negligence or fault of LAF, its owners, employees, affiliates, authorized agents, or independent contractors. Client is urged to have this Agreement reviewed by an attorney before signing (p. 2)

The third page contained a New Client Checklist that included the following statement: "I have received and read a copy of my entire Personal Training Agreement…" (p. 3).

Procedural Facts:

The plaintiff, Patricia Evans, filed a negligence lawsuit against the defendant club LA Fitness. Evans claimed that the exculpatory language in the Agreements was not sufficiently conspicuous and therefore the agreements were invalid and unenforceable. She claimed the employee perused through the Agreement but did not go over all the pages of the document and therefore, she did not have any understanding of the waiver of liability. The defendant club filed a motion for summary judgment, claiming the agreements signed by Evans were valid and barred her negligence lawsuit.

ISSUE

Did the membership and personal training agreements, signed by the plaintiff Patricia Evans, absolve the defendant LA Fitness of liability for its own negligence?

COURT'S RULING

Yes, the exculpatory clauses in the membership and personal training agreements barred Evans' negligence lawsuit against LA Fitness. Therefore, the court granted the defendant's motion for summary judgment.

COURT'S REASONING

Regarding the validity of exculpatory clauses, the court stated:

> An exculpatory clause is valid if the following conditions are met 1) the clause does not contravene public policy, 2) the contract is between parties relating entirely to their own private affairs; and 3) the contract is not one of adhesion … A valid exculpatory clause is only enforceable if 'the language of the parties is clear that a person is being relieved of liability for his own acts of negligence' (p. 3).

Evans continued...

Relying on court rulings in previous cases, the court stated that the exculpatory language in the agreements that Evans signed met all three prongs of a valid exculpatory clause. Public policy is violated only if it is a matter of interest to the public or state such as public services, public utilities, common carriers, and hospitals and LA Fitness does not provide services related to a matter of interest to the public or state. Regarding the second prong, the court ruled that the agreements signed by Evans were "contracts between private parties and pertained only to the parties' private rights" (p. 4). The court also ruled that the agreements signed by Evans were not contracts "of adhesion because exercising at a gym is a voluntary recreational activity and the plaintiff was under no compulsion to join the gym" (p. 4).

The court continued with its reasoning by stating that although an exculpatory clause is facially valid, there are standards to guide a court's determination for it to be enforceable as follows:

1) the contract language must be construed strictly, since exculpatory language is not favored by the law; 2) the contract must state the intention of the parties with the greatest particularity, beyond doubt by express stipulation, and no inference from words of general import can establish the intent of the parties; 3) the language of the contract must be construed, in cases of ambiguity, against the party seeking immunity from liability; and 4) the burden of establishing the immunity is upon the party invoking protection under the clause (p. 5).

The court determined that the exculpatory clauses in both Agreements, unambiguously, established the defendant's intent to relieve itself of liability for negligence.

Regarding Evan's claim that the exculpatory language in the Agreements was not sufficiently conspicuous, the court referred to the following three factors established in *Beck-Hummel v. Ski Shawnee, Inc.*, 902 A.2d 1266 (Pa. Super. Ct. 2006) to determine conspicuity: "1) the waiver's placement in the document; 2) the size of the waiver's font; and 3) whether the waiver was highlighted by being printed in all capital letters or a different font or color from the remainder of the text" (p. 5). The exculpatory language on the second page of the Personal Trainer Agreement that Evans signed was in large font and the title of this section was bolded and in caps.

Lessons Learned from *Evans:*

Legal

▸ Exculpatory clauses in agreements are not favored by law but they can be valid if certain conditions are met such as:

- The exculpatory clause does not violate public policy. The defendant in this case did not provide services of public interest such as common carriers and hospitals.
- The agreement/contract is between private parties as demonstrated in this case.
- The agreement/contract is not one of adhesion. The plaintiff in this case had a choice to join the facility.

▸ Factors to determine if the exculpatory clause is sufficiently conspicuous (e.g., highlighted in caps, size of font) within the agreement may also be considered by a court to confirm its validity.

Risk Management/Injury Prevention

▸ Personal fitness trainers need to be sure that all exercises taught to their clients are appropriate for "each" client. For example, why did the trainer in this case have a 61-year-old female perform suicide runs and run backwards?

- For each exercise taught, trainers need to consider factors such as what is the purpose of the exercise, does it create any safety concerns?

▸ Direct supervision/evaluation of personal fitness trainers is needed to be sure they are properly designing and delivering exercise programs based on the client's fitness level, age, and medical conditions. If not, corrective measures may be necessary. For example, require that the trainer participate in additional training and/or have the trainer submit prepared lesson plans that can be reviewed by an exercise professional/supervisor to determine if they are appropriate.

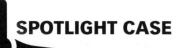

SPOTLIGHT CASE

Stelluti v. Casapenn Enterprises, LLC, dba Powerhouse Gym
203 N.J. 286 (N.J., 2010).

FACTS

Historical Facts:

After signing the paperwork including a "Waiver & Release Form" to join Powerhouse gym, Gina Stelluti participated in her first spinning class. She advised the instructor of her inexperience and the instructor helped her to adjust the seat bike and feet pedals and told Stelluti to watch and imitate her during the class. Shortly after the class began, Stelluti rose to a standing position, the handlebars dislodged from the bike, and as a result she fell forward while her feet remained strapped to the pedals. After some assistance to detach herself from the bike and resting for 15 minutes, she tried to resume her participation but had too much pain and had to quit. Stelluti visited the hospital to receive medical attention after the incident occurred. She was diagnosed with several injuries including back and neck injuries. Her medical expert stated, "that three years after her accident Stelluti suffers from chronic pain associated with myofascial pain syndrome" (p. 294). The waiver that Stelluti signed (required of all members) can be found in Exhibit 4.4.

Procedural Facts:

The plaintiff, Stelluti, filed the following negligence claims against Powerhouse Gym: "1) failing to properly maintain and set up the stationary bike, 2) failing to properly instruct the plaintiff as to how to use the bike or exercise proper care, 3) causing a dangerous and hazardous condition to exist, 4) allowing a nuisance to exist, 5) failing to provide proper safeguards or warnings on the bike, 6) failing to provide proper and safe equipment, 7) maintaining the bike in an unsafe, hazardous and/or defective manner..." (p. 295).

Given the waiver that Stelluti signed, the defendants, Powerhouse Gym and others, filed a motion for summary judgment, which was granted, by the trial court. Upon appeal, the intermediate New Jersey appellate court upheld the trial court's ruling. Stelluti then appealed to the New Jersey Supreme Court.

ISSUE

Did the New Jersey Supreme Court uphold the trial and intermediate appellate court rulings to grant summary judgment to the defendants on the basis that the waiver & release form was enforceable?

COURT'S RULING

Yes, the New Jersey Supreme Court ruled that the waiver & release form signed by Stelluti was enforceable citing factors regarding the enforceability of waivers from *Gershon v. Regency Diving Center,* 386 N.J Super. 237 (2004) and *Tunkl v. Regents of the University of California,* 60 Cal. 2d 92 (1963).

COURT'S REASONING

Although the court analyzed several factors from *Gershon* and *Tunkl,* two of them will be discussed (a) was the waiver an adhesion contract, and (b) did the waiver/release violate public interest? Regarding a contract of adhesion, the New Jersey Supreme Court ruled:

> A contract of adhesion is defined as one 'presented on a take-it-or-leave-it basis, commonly in a standardized printed form, without opportunity for the 'adhering' party to negotiate'... Although a contract of adhesion may require one party to choose either to accept or reject the contract as is, the agreement nevertheless may be enforced... Here, Powerhouse's agreement was a standard pre-printed form presented

Stelluti continued...

to Stelluti and other prospective members on a typical 'take-it-or-leave-it basis.' No doubt, this agreement was one of adhesion... (p. 301).

Giving her the benefit of all inferences from the record, including that Powerhouse may not have explained to Stelluti the legal effect of the contract that released Powerhouse from liability, we nevertheless do not regard her in a classic 'position of unequal bargaining power' such that the contract must be voided...Stelluti could have taken her business to another fitness club, could have found another means of exercise aside from joining a private gym, or could have thought about it and even sought advice before signing up and using the facility's equipment...we hold that the agreement was not void based on any notion of procedural unconscionability (p. 302).

Regarding a violation of public interest, the New Jersey Supreme Court stated:

To properly balance the public-policy interests implicated in the instant matter one must consider the nature of the activity and the inherent risks involved... By its nature, exercising entails vigorous physical exertion. Injuries from exercise are common; indeed minor injuries can be expected—for example, sore muscles following completion of a tough exercise or workout may be indicative of building or toning muscles. Those injuries and others may result from faulty equipment, improper use of equipment, inadequate instruction, inexperience or poor physical condition of the user, or excessive exertion... (p. 310).

Although there is public interest in holding a health club to its general common law duty to business invitees—to maintain its premises in a condition safe from defects that the business is charged with knowing or discovering—it need not ensure the safety of its patrons who voluntarily assume some risk by engaging in strenuous physical activities that have a potential to result in injuries. Any requirement to so guarantee a patron's safety from all risk in using equipment, which understandably is passed from patron to patron, could chill the establishment of health clubs... (p. 311).

Although it would be unreasonable to demand that a fitness center inspect each individual piece of equipment after every patron's use, it would be unreasonable, and contrary to the public interest, to condone willful blindness to problems that arise with the equipment provided for patrons' use. Thus, had Powerhouse's management or employees been aware of a piece of defective exercise equipment and failed to remedy the condition or to warn adequately of the dangerous condition, or if it had dangerously or improperly maintained equipment, Powerhouse could not exculpate itself from such reckless or gross negligence. That showing was not made on this record... (pp. 311-312).

With respect to its agreement and its limitation of liability to the persons who use its facility and exercise equipment for the unique purpose of the business, we hold that it is not contrary to the public interest, or to a legal duty owed, to enforce Powerhouse's agreement limiting its liability for injuries sustained as a matter of negligence that result from a patron's voluntary use of equipment and participation in instructed activity. As a result, we find the exculpatory agreement between Powerhouse and Stelluti enforceable as to the injury Stelluti sustained when riding the spin bike (p. 313).

Lessons Learned from *Stelluti:*

Legal

▸ A waiver/release, if properly written and administered, can be effective in protecting defendants from their own negligence such as the negligent instruction of a group exercise leader. However, in some jurisdictions, waivers are not valid for personal injuries caused by negligent conduct because they violate public policy, based on a state's Supreme Court ruling or statute.

Stelluti continued...

> ◗ Courts will often rely on factors (e.g., was the waiver an adhesion contract) identified from previous case law such as *Tunkl* to determine if a waiver is enforceable or not.
>
> ◗ Fitness facilities have a "common law" duty (e.g., maintain premises free from dangers) owed to invitees. Given this duty, a defendant cannot exculpate itself (via a waiver) from gross/reckless conduct such as being aware of a defective/dangerous piece of equipment and failing to correct it or adequately warn of it.
>
> ◗ Waiver law is always evolving, and court rulings/state statutes can change at any time.
>
> **Risk Management/Injury Prevention**
>
> ◗ Spinning instructors (and all group exercise instructors) need to be well-educated and trained before they teach any classes.
>
> ◗ Spinning instructors (and all group exercise instructors) may need a checklist of all safety instructions that need to be reviewed with all new participants before they begin the class, such as proper instruction on the use/set up of equipment as described in the owner's manual, principles of safe exercise such as beginning with light-moderate intensity, and signs/symptoms of overexertion.
>
> ◗ Spinning instructors (and all group exercise instructors) need to closely observe and provide additional instruction, if needed, for all new participants until they know and understand the risks inherent in the activity.

Additional Cases: Waiver Defense

As demonstrated in *Evans* and *Stelluti*, courts will consider various factors to decide if the waiver defense will protect defendants in negligence lawsuits. The following is a brief description of the court decisions regarding the enforceability of waivers in additional spotlight cases presented throughout the textbook and why the waiver was either enforceable or unenforceable.

- *Bartlett v. Push to Walk* (Chapter 7): Waiver was enforceable on two counts of ordinary negligence but not a third count of gross negligence (instruction provided by the trainer was gross negligence).
- *Layden v. Plante* (Chapter 7): Waiver was unenforceable—the exculpatory clause did not clearly state "negligence" or "fault" and even it had, it would not have been enforceable in New York, due to a state statute that prohibits waivers in fitness facilities.
- *Scheck v. Soul Cycle* (Chapter 8): It was unknown if the plaintiff signed a waiver—online/onsite waiver procedures were questionable but even if there was evidence that the plaintiff signed a waiver, it would have been unenforceable in New York for the same reason as in *Layden*.
- *Jimenez v. 24 Hour Fitness* (Chapter 9): Waiver was unenforceable for two reasons

(a) gross negligence—the defendant facility knew it did not follow the owner's manual specifications regarding treadmill clearance, and (b) waiver was administered with fraud and misrepresentation (i.e., it was not provided in Spanish and no Spanish-speaking employee went over the terms of the waiver with a participant who only spoke Spanish).

- *Chavez v. 24 Hour Fitness* (Chapter 9): Waiver was unenforceable due to the defendant's gross negligence—there was evidence (documentation) of the facility improperly maintaining a cross-trainer machine as set forth in the owner's manual specifications.
- *Grebing v. 24 Hour Fitness* (Chapter 9): Waiver was enforceable because the defendant properly assembled, inspected, and maintained a low row machine and had records of such—there was no gross negligence on part of the defendant as the plaintiff claimed.
- *Butler v. Seville et al.* (Chapter 9): The Connecticut court ruled that waiver was unenforceable—it violated public policy because it was an adhesion contract (Note: As listed above, Connecticut is one of the states that was rated "poor" regarding the enforceability of waivers).

Exhibit 4-4: Waiver in *Stelluti v. Casapenn Enterprises, dba Powerhouse Gym, LLC* (57)

WAIVER & RELEASE FORM

Because physical exercise can be strenuous and subject to risk of serious injury, the club urges you to obtain a physical examination from a doctor before using any exercise equipment or participating in any exercise activity. **You (each member, guest, and all participating family members) agree that if you engage in any physical exercise or activity or use any club amenity on the premises or off premises including any sponsored club event, you do so entirely at your own risk.** Any recommendation for changes in diet including the use of food supplements, weight reduction and or body building enhancement products are entirely your responsibility and you should consult a physician prior to undergoing any dietary or food supplement changes. **You agree that you are voluntarily participating in these activities and use of these facilities and premises and assume all risks of injury, illness, or death.** We are also not responsible for any loss of your personal property.

These bolded sections reflect an Express Assumption of Risk that addresses injuries, illness, and even death and "voluntary" participation.

This waiver and release of liability includes, without limitation, all injuries which may occur as a result of, (a) your use of all amenities and equipment in the facility and your participation in any activity, class, program, personal training or instruction, (b) the sudden and unforeseen malfunctioning of any equipment, (c) our instruction, training, supervision, or dietary recommendations, and (d) your slipping and/or falling while in the club, or on the club premises, including adjacent sidewalks and parking areas.

In this section, a comprehensive list of activities that the waiver and release covers.

You acknowledge that you have carefully read this "waiver and release" and fully understand that it is a release of liability. **You expressly agree to release and discharge the health club, and all affiliates, employees, agents, representatives, successors, or assigns, from any and all claims or causes of action and you agree to voluntarily give up or waive any right that you may otherwise have to bring a legal action against the club for personal injury or property damage.**

To the extent that statute or case law does not prohibit releases for negligence, this release is also for negligence on the part of the Club, its agents, and employees.

These bolded sections reflect the exculpatory clause (absolves defendants of liability for their own negligence)

If any portion of this release from liability shall be deemed by a Court of competent jurisdiction to be invalid, then the remainder of this release from liability shall remain in full force and effect and the offending provision or provisions severed here from.

This section is the severability clause

By signing this release, I acknowledge that I understand its content and that this release cannot be modified orally (p. 293).

Acknowledgement statement (signature and date below)

Exhibit 4-5: Dissenting Opinion, in part, *Stelluti v. Casapenn Enterprises, LLC, dba Powerhouse Gym* (57)

Justices ALBIN and LONG, dissenting.

Today the Court has abandoned its traditional role as the steward of the common law. For the first time in its modern history, the Court upholds a contract of adhesion with an exculpatory clause that will allow a commercial, profit-making company to operate negligently—injuring, maiming, and perhaps killing one of its consumer-patrons—without consequence. Under the Court's ruling, a health club will have no obligation to maintain its equipment in a reasonably safe manner or to require its employees to act with due care toward its patrons. That is because, the Court says, a health club patron has the right to contract not only for unsafe conditions at a health club, but also for careless conduct by its employees. The Court's decision will ensure that these contracts of adhesion will become an industry-wide practice and that membership in health clubs will be conditioned on powerless consumers signing a waiver immunizing clubs from their own negligence. The Court's ruling undermines the common-law duty of care that every commercial operator owes to a person invited on to its premises.

Without the incentive to place safety over profits, the cost to the public will be an increase in the number of avoidable accidents in health clubs. And like the plaintiff in this case, the victims of the clubs' negligence will suffer the ultimate injustice—they will have no legal remedy.

Tens of thousands of New Jersey citizens join health clubs to stay healthy—to reduce the prospect of suffering from heart disease or a stroke, to battle obesity, and to improve the likelihood of living a longer life. The irony is that those who seek to live a better lifestyle through membership at a health club, now, will have a greater likelihood of having their well-being impaired through the careless acts of a club employee.

The ruling today is not in the public interest, not consistent with this Court's long-standing, progressive common-law jurisprudence protecting vulnerable consumers, and not in step with the enlightened approaches taken by courts of other jurisdictions that have barred the very type of exculpatory clause to which this Court gives its imprimatur…

In the past, this Court has struck down exculpatory clauses that violated public policy, expressed either in the common law or a statute, particularly when there was inequality in bargaining power between the parties to the contract…

Never before in the modern era has this Court upheld an exculpatory clause in which a commercial enterprise protects itself against its own negligence at the expense of a consumer, who had no bargaining power to alter the terms of the contract. The high courts of other states have struck down exculpatory clauses similar to the type that our Court now validates…

It is hard to imagine how the public interest could be served by permitting health clubs to exempt themselves from the common law governing premises liability. Tens of thousands of people in this State go to health clubs to maintain healthy lifestyles and to improve their health…

The benefits of exercise are beyond dispute. The Surgeon General has declared 'that Americans can substantially improve their health and quality of life by including moderate amounts of physical activity in their daily lives'…The health benefits of exercise include lower risks of early death, coronary heart disease, stroke, high blood pressure, obesity, adverse blood lipid profile, type 2 diabetes, metabolic syndrome, colon cancer, and breast cancer, to name a few…Some health clubs even have rehabilitation/physical therapy programs for accident or stroke victims.

Whatever the Court says in its opinion, people will continue to go to health clubs, even if they are compelled to sign away their rights in a contract of adhesion. Most people do not have at their individual disposal the sophisticated exercise machinery and equipment, indoor tracks, pools, and trainers offered at health clubs. Gina Stelluti is a perfect example—a waitress without health insurance, who could not possibly afford to purchase the equipment available at a health club.

Ms. Stelluti does not claim that Powerhouse should be the general guarantor for every injury suffered in its facility. This case is not about a health club patron asserting that the facility is legally responsible for an injury caused by over-exertion, misuse of equipment, or from the act of another patron over whom the club has no control. Rather, Ms. Stelluti merely argues that a health club should be held responsible if it does not maintain its equipment in a reasonably safe manner and if its instructors do not exercise due care—matters over which a club does have control. It is one thing to assume a risk of which one is

Exhibit 4-5 continued...

aware. It is another thing to say, as the Court does, that one should assume the risk for a dangerous condition of which one is unaware and over which one has no control...

Tort law is not just about compensating victims, but also about preventing accidents. By allowing a health club to eliminate its duty to exercise a reasonable degree of care, the majority has decreased the incentives for health clubs to provide a reasonably safe environment for their patrons. This will inevitably lead to more preventable accidents. Because health clubs will not have a legal incentive to maintain their equipment in a reasonably safe manner, how many cases will there be of handlebars flying off of spin bikes, of cables to weight machines breaking, of pools mistakenly treated with the wrong amounts or kinds of chemicals? Increasing profits is the dominant force motivating most commercial establishments; increasing public safety had been one of the objectives of tort law...

The exculpatory clause to which the Court gives its blessing should be void as against public policy. That is so because the exculpatory clause in this case unfairly allocates the risk from the commercial operator, who is in the best position to remove and prevent the dangers on the premises, to the unwary patron, and because it encourages lack of due care. Exalting the right to contract—a contract of adhesion, no less—over the public interest is not in keeping with this Court's development of a progressive and enlightened common law... (pp. 314-325).

⬥ *Crossing-Lyons v. Towns Sport International, Inc.* (Chapter 10): Waiver was unenforceable because the facility failed to carry out its common law duties to invitees (i.e., to guard against any dangerous conditions that the owner knows about or should have known).

⬥ *Miller v. YMCA of Central Massachusetts et al.* (Chapter 10): Waiver unenforceable—it was signed by a participant in the Silver Sneaker's program held at the YMCA. The Silver Sneaker's waiver did not include the YMCA, so the YMCA was not protected. Even if the waiver had included the YMCA, it likely would have been unenforceable due to the gross negligence of the YMCA.

⬥ *Locke v. Life Time Fitness, Inc.* (Chapter 11): Waiver (see Exhibit 4-3) was enforceable for several of the negligence claims made by the plaintiff (wife of the decedent) but it was unenforceable because the exculpatory clause did not specifically include inadequate training of employees on how to deal with health emergencies.

Summary: Waivers and Releases of Liability

In most of the above cases, the waiver was unenforceable and, thus, did not protect the fitness facility and its employees because of one of the following: (a) gross negligence of the defendants, (b) violations of public policy (e.g., *Tunkl* factors, state statutes, court rulings), (c) the exculpatory clause was inconspicuous or the language within the waiver was not written properly to cover all activities/negligent acts, and (d) improper administration. Before providing a list of recommendations, it is essential that fitness managers and exercise professionals always have a knowledgeable lawyer prepare waiver/release of liability contracts—never just use one from a book or the Internet. As stated above, waiver law is quite complex and many factors need to be considered so the waiver will be enforceable in any given jurisdiction. The authors of *Waivers and Releases of Liability* (56) recommend using a stand-alone "participant agreement" and they provide eleven steps to consider when preparing the written agreement.

Waivers do nothing to help ensure participant safety. They are only an effective risk management strategy after an injury occurs and subsequent litigation. Fitness managers and exercise professionals that use a waiver as their only risk management strategy need to realize the importance of developing many

KEY POINT

It is essential that fitness managers and exercise professionals always have a competent lawyer prepare waiver/release of liability contracts—never just use one from a book or the Internet. Waiver law is quite complex and many factors need to be considered so the waiver/release of liability will be enforceable in any given jurisdiction.

other risk management strategies that do focus on safety, which is their #1 responsibility. The many other risk management strategies presented throughout this textbook focus on injury prevention and need to be seriously considered and implemented in order to create a true safety culture. The following are general recommendations and are based on some of the court rulings in the cases previously described involving waivers. By no means is it an inclusive list of everything that needs to be considered.

Note: *As described in Chapters 8 and 10, non-traditional exercise programs (e.g., Internet training, home training, outdoor training) and facilities (e.g., unsupervised, partially supervised, outdoor) should have a lawyer prepare a protective legal document (with assumption of risk/release of liability provisions) that specifically addresses the risks and limitations associated with these types of programs and facilities.*

Recommendations

1. Use a "stand-alone" waiver (release of liability) versus including exculpatory language in a membership contract or some other document. Sections to include:

    a) A section that informs the participant of the risks of participation in the facility's activities and programs/services (i.e., list injuries that include minor, major, life-threatening, and even death). This section will help strengthen the assumption of risk defense.

    b) A section that describes all the activities/situations that the waiver intends to cover. As demonstrated from the above cases, if an activity is missing, the waiver may not be enforceable for that activity. Broad language such as "any and all" activities may be effective, but language that is overly broad such as "harm from any cause" may not be effective.

    c) A section that includes the exculpatory clause. This section should be (1) conspicuous (e.g., labeled "waiver and release of liability" in large, bold font), (2) include the phrase "ordinary negligence" (even though some states might not require this explicitly, it helps to make the

clause clear and unambiguous), and (3) clearly communicates the exchange of consideration (i.e., the legal rights the participant is waiving in exchange for participation in the facility's programs/services).

    d) A section that includes a severability clause. If one section within the agreement is determined to be unenforceable, the other sections of the agreement remain in effect. For example, if a court rules that the exculpatory clause is unenforceable, the assumption of risk section remains effective.

    e) Acknowledgement and signature section. This section helps affirm that the participant read and understood the terms within the agreement and is of age to enter into a legally binding contract. Include a space for the participant's signature and date.

2. Additional factors to be considered in the preparation of the waiver (release of liability):

    a) Consider language such as the following from *Stelluti* (58), to cover all parties:

    i. "release and discharge the health club, and all affiliates, employees, agents, representatives, successors, or assigns, from any and all claims or causes of action and you agree to voluntarily give up or waive any right that you may otherwise have to bring a legal action against the club for personal injury or property damage" (p. 293).

    ii. Note the above includes "property damage" but also consider adding property loss and theft.

    b) Consider language that relinquishes claims made by parties other than the signer such as spouse, heirs, estate, etc. Depending on state law, this type of language may bar claims such as a loss of consortium claim (interference with a relationship) and a **loss of parental consortium** (interference with the parent-child relationship). For example, in the *Locke* case, briefly described above, the wife of the decedent was not barred from pursuing a wrongful death action against the defendant in Illinois. Having a signer's spouse also sign a waiver/agreement should be discussed with legal counsel.

c) Consider including an **indemnification** clause. With this clause, the "participant or another party agrees to reimburse the service provider for any monetary loss resulting from an injury to the participant or an injury or loss caused by the participant" (56, p. 107). Generally, indemnification clauses/agreements are between two businesses. In some jurisdictions, these types of clauses are unenforceable when a participant indemnifies a provider for the negligence of the provider (56).

d) Consider indicating the timeframe of the waiver, incorporating phrases such as "any and all present and future claims." For example, in *Nimis v. St. Paul Turners, et al.* (59), the participant signed a waiver as part of her membership contract. Her membership (and the waiver) expired, and she did not renew until over a year later. She was not asked to sign a waiver when she renewed her membership. Therefore, the original waiver was not in effect at the time of her injury.

e) Discuss with legal counsel whether parents/legal guardians should sign a waiver relinquishing the rights of their child. Some states may enforce these waivers, but most will not (56). In lieu of a waiver, seek legal counsel to use an "agreement to participate" which is not considered a contract (56). It does not contain exculpatory language. Its purpose is to inform participants (and parents/guardians) of the nature of the activity, the risks of participation in the activity, and the behaviors expected of the participant (56).

f) Fitness facilities that offer in-house child care need to consider protections for children participating in the facility's child care services.

g) If an employee is injured while participating in employer-sponsored fitness and/or recreation programs, will workers' compensation apply? Employees injured while on-the-job generally receive workers' compensation benefits (a form of strict liability) and the employee cannot sue the employer for negligence even if the injury was caused by the employer's negligence. Application of workers' compensation depends upon several factors that vary from state to state. If workers' compensation does not apply, a waiver may be considered. Case law examples were described in Chapter 1. For more on this topic, see *Rule the Rules of Workplace Wellness Programs* (60).

3. Administration of the waiver (release of liability):
   a) Give the participant ample time to read the waiver.
   b) After it has been read by the participant, have a well-trained staff member review the purpose of each section in the agreement with the participant to help ensure he/she understands the terms and can ask questions.
   c) Ensure the participant is of legal age. Ask for an ID if age is questionable.
   d) If a couple joins the facility, be sure each reads and signs their own waiver.
   e) If an outside group, such as Silver Sneakers in the *Miller* case, is renting or leasing space in the facility to provide a program, be sure participants sign the facility's waiver as well as the outside group's waiver.
   f) Read the agreement to non-readers and/or provide the agreement in other languages for members who do not speak English. For example, for participants who only speak/read Spanish, have the waiver translated into Spanish and/or have a Spanish-speaking employee administer the waiver.
   g) Once completed, offer to make a copy of the waiver to give to the participant.
   h) If a facility wishes to obtain a waiver electronically, discuss these procedures with a knowledgeable lawyer.
   i) Retain and store the waiver in a safe, secure location and consider making a duplicate copy (e.g., scan the document and store it on a secure computer). Retain the documents at least until the state's statute of limitations has expired and in consultation with legal counsel.

Note: *If the facility's personnel can use the facility and/or participate in the facility's programs while they are not on the job, ensure they sign the facility's assumption of risk/waiver and complete the same procedures as new participants such as pre-activity health screening.*

KEY TERMS

- Attractive Nuisance
- Desirable Operating Practices
- Exculpatory Clause
- Expert Testimony
- Express Assumption of Risk
- Indemnification
- Inherent Risks
- Invitee
- Licensee
- Loss of Consortium
- Loss of Parental Consortium

- Medical Malpractice
- Negligence per se
- Primary Assumption of Risk
- Professional Standard of Care
- Public Policy
- Risks Inherent in the Activity
- Scope of Practice
- Standard of Care of a Professional
- Technical Physical Specifications
- Trespasser

STUDY QUESTIONS

The Study Questions for Chapter 4 can be found on the Fitness Law Academy website (www.fitnesslawacademy.com) under Textbook. They are provided in a fillable format for convenience.

REFERENCES

1. Eickhoff-Shemek JM, Herbert DL, Connaughton, DP. *Risk Management for Health/Fitness Professionals: Legal Issues and Strategies.* Baltimore, MD: Lippincott Williams & Wilkins, 2009.

2. Dougherty NJ, Goldberger AS, Carpenter LJ. *Sport, Physical Activity, and the Law.* 3rd Ed. Champaign, IL: Sagamore Publishing, 2007.

3. van der Smissen B. *Legal Liability and Risk Management for Public and Private Entities.* Vol. One: § 2.11 Bases or Origins of Duty and § 2.111 Inherent in the Situation. Cincinnati, OH: Anderson Publishing Co., 1990.

4. *Parks v. Gilligan,* Analyzed In: Suit Against Volunteer Spotter Settled. The Exercise Standards and Malpractice Reporter, 12(3), 41, 1998.

5. Fitness Center Staff Requirements. W.S.A. 100.178. West's Wisconsin Statutes Annotated, Thomson/West, 2008.

6. A Concise Restatement of TORTS Third Edition. Compiled by: Bublick EM, Rogers JE. St. Paul, MN: American Law Institute, 2013.

7. Keeton W, Dobbs D, Keeton R, Owen D. Prosser and Keeton on the Law of Torts, 5th Ed., St Paul, MN: West Publishing Company, 1984.

8. *Turner v. Rush Medical College,* 537 N.E.2d 890 (Ill. App. Ct., 1989).

9. *Kleinknecht v. Gettysburg College,* 989 F.2d 1360 (3d Cir., 1993).

10. *Darling v. Charleston Community Hospital,* 211 N.E.2d 253 (Ill., 1965).

11. *McGuire v. DeFrancesco,* 811 P.2d 340 (Ariz. Ct. App., 1990).

12. *D'Amico v. LA Fitness,* 57 Conn. L. Rptr. 242, 2013WL 6912912 (Conn. Super. Ct., 2013).

13. van der Smissen B. Elements of Negligence. In: Cotten DJ, Wolohan JT, eds. *Law for Recreation and Sport Managers,* 4th Ed. Dubuque, IA: Kendall/Hunt Publishing Company, 2007.

14. Abbott AA. Cardiac Arrest Litigations. *ACSM's Health & Fitness Journal,* 17(1), 31-34, 2013.

15. Abbott AA. Injury Litigations. *ACSM's Health & Fitness Journal,* 17(3), 28-32, 2013.

16. Warburton DER, Bredin SSD, Charlesworth SA, et al. Evidence-Based Risk Recommendations for Best Practices in the Training of Qualified Exercise Professionals Working with Clinical Populations. *Applied Physiology Nutrition and Metabolism* 36, S232-S265, 2011.

17. *Bartlett v. Push to Walk,* No. 2:15-cv-7167-KM-JBC, 2018 WL 1726262 (D. N.J., 2018).

18. Restatement of the Law Third, Torts: Liability for Physical and Emotional Harm. Philadelphia, PA: American Law Institute, Vol. 1, 2009, Vol. 2, 2012.

19. *Duncan v. World Wide Health Studios,* 232 S.2d 835 (La. Ct. App., 1970).

20. *Crossing-Lyons v. Towns Sport International, Inc., d/b/a New York Sports Club,* No. L-2024-14, 2017 WL 2953388 (N.J. Super. Ct. App. Div., 2017).

21. Attractive Nuisance Doctrine. USLegal. Available at: https://premisesliability.uslegal.com/attractive-nuisance-doctrine. Accessed December 26, 2018.

22. *Smith v. AMLI Realty Co.,* 614 N.E.2d 618 (Ind. App., 1993).

23. *Campbell v. Morine,* 585 N.E.2d 1198 (Ill. App. Ct., 1992).

24. Electronic Code of Federal Regulations. 29 C.F.R § 825.125. Definition of Health Care Provider. Available at: https://www.ecfr.gov/cgi-bin/text-idx?SID=b9511cd59a65dfbfd8d9e638035bb44c&mc=true&node=se29.3.825_1125&rgn=div8. Accessed June 9, 2020.

25. *Mikkelsen v. Haslam,* 764 P.2d 1384 (Utah, 1988).

26. van der Smissen B. Standards and How They Relate to Duty and Liability. Paper presented at the 13th annual conference for The Society for the Study of the Legal Aspects of Sport and Physical Activity, Albuquerque, NM, 2000.

27. *Elledge v. Richland/Lexington School District Five,* 341 S.C. 473 (S.C. Ct. App., 2000).

28. *Elledge v. Richland/Lexington School District Five,* 352 S.C. 179 (S.C., 2002).

29. Voris HC, Rabinoff M. When is a Standard of Care Not a Standard of Care? *The Exercise Standards and Malpractice Reporter,* 25(2), 20-21, 2011.

30. *Jimenez v. 24 Hour Fitness,* 188 Cal. Rptr. 3d. 228 (Cal. Ct. App., 2015).

31. Voris HC, Ignorance has Never Been a Good Defense. The Exercise, Sports and Sports Medicine Standards & Malpractice Reporter, 4(6), 97, 2015.

32. Brown N. Opportunities for Injury Abound in Rec Centers, Health Clubs. *Athletic Business E-newsletter.* June 2018. Available at: https://www.athleticbusiness.com/athlete-safety/opportunities-for-injury-abound-in-rec-centers-health-clubs.html#lightbox/0/. Accessed November 5, 2018.

33. *Baldi-Perry v. Kaifas and 360 Fitness Center, Inc.* Compliant. Index No. 2010-1927, Supreme Court, Erie County, New York. February 19, 2010.

34. ACSM's Health/Fitness Facility Standards and Guidelines. Sanders ME. (ed). 5th Ed. Champaign, IL: Human Kinetics, 2019.

35. ACSM's Guidelines for Exercise Testing and Prescription. Riebe D. (ed). 10th Ed. Philadelphia, PA: Lippincott Williams & Wilkins, 2018.

36. NSCA Strength and Conditioning Professional Standards and Guidelines. *Strength and Conditioning Journal,* 39(6), 1-24, 2017. Available at: https://www.nsca.com/education/articles/nsca-strength-and-conditioning-professional-standards-and-guidelines/. Accessed November 5, 2018.

37. IHRSA Club Membership Standards. In: *IHRSA's Guide to Club Membership & Conduct.* 3rd Ed. Boston, MA: International Health, Racquet & Sportsclub Association, 2005. Available at: http://download.ihrsa.org/pubs/club_membership_conduct.pdf. Accessed November 5, 2018.

38. *Medical Fitness Association's Standards & Guidelines for Medical Fitness Center Facilities,* Roy B. (ed.). 2nd Ed. Monterey, CA: Healthy Learning, 2013.

39. *Exercise Standards & Guidelines Reference Manual.* 5th Ed. Sherman Oaks, CA: Aerobics and Fitness Association of America, 2010.

40. *Safeguarding Health and Well-Being, Medical Advisory Committee Recommendations: A Resource Guide for YMCAs.* Chicago, IL: YMCA of the USA, February 2011. Available at: http://safe-wise.com/downloads/MAC_2010a_Collection.pdf. Accessed November 5, 2018.

41. American Association for Cardiovascular and Pulmonary Rehabilitation (AACVPR). *Guidelines for Cardiac Rehabilitation and Secondary Prevention Programs.* Williams MA, Roitman JL (eds). 5th Ed. Champaign, IL: Human Kinetics, 2013.

42. American Association for Cardiovascular and Pulmonary Rehabilitation (AACVPR). *Guidelines for Pulmonary Rehabilitation Programs.* 4th Ed. Champaign, IL: Human Kinetics, 2011.

References continued...

43. Rahl RL. *Physical Activity and Health Guidelines: Recommendations for Various Ages, Fitness Levels, and Conditions from 57 Authoritative Sources.* Champaign, IL: Human Kinetics, 2010.

44. *BOC Standards of Professional Practice.* Version 3.2. Board of Certification for the Athletic Trainer, October 2018. Available at: http://www.bocatc.org/system/document_versions/versions/171/original/boc-standards-of-professional-practice-2019-20181207.pdf?1544218543. Accessed July 22, 2020.

45. Herbert DL. ANSI Directs the Withdrawal of NSF Standard as an American National Standard for Health/Fitness Facilities. *The Exercise, Sports and Sports Medicine Standards & Malpractice Reporter,* 3(6), 93, 2014.

46. Appraisal of Guidelines for Research & Evaluation (AGREE) II. *The AGREE II Instrument.* AGREE Next Steps Consortium, December 2017. Available at: https://www.agreetrust.org. Accessed November 5, 2018.

47. van der Smissen B. *Legal Liability and Risk Management for Public and Private Entities,* Vol. 2. Cincinnati, OH: Anderson Publishing Company, 1990.

48. *Pellham v. Let's Go Tubing, Inc.* 398 P.3d 1205 (Wash. Ct. App. 2017).

49. *Main v. Gym X-Treme,* No. 11AP-643, 2012 LEXIS 1139 (Ohio Ct. App., 2012).

50. *Rostai v. Neste Enterprises, d/b/a Gold'sGym,* 41 Cal. Rptr. 3d 411 (Cal. Ct. App., 2006).

51. *Tadmor v. New York Jiu Jitsu,* 109 A.D.3d 440, 2013 LEXIS 5636 (N.Y. App., 2013).

52. *Blume v. Equinox,* 975 N.Y.S.2d 707, 2013 LEXIS 3161 (N.Y. Misc., 2013).

53. *Rutnik v. Colonie Center Court Club, Inc.,* 672 N.Y.S.2d 451, 1998 LEXIS 4845 (N.Y. App. Div.,1998).

54. Black DC, Nolan JR, Nolan-Haley JM., et al. *Black's Law Dictionary,* 6th Ed. St. Paul, MN: West Publishing Company, 1991.

55. *Tunkl v. Regents of the University of California,* 60 Cal.2d 92 (Cal., 1963).

56. Cotten DJ, Cotten MB. *Waivers & Releases of Liability,* 10th Ed. Sport Risk Consulting: Statesboro, GA, 2019.

57. *Evans v. Fitness & Sports Clubs, LLC.,* No. 15-4095, 2016 WL 5404464 (E.D. Pa., 2016).

58. *Stelluti v. Casapenn Enterprises, LLC, dba Powerhouse Gym,* 203 N.J. 286 (N.J., 2010).

59. *Nimis v. St. Paul Turners,* 521 N.W.2d 54 (Minn. Ct. App., 1994).

60. Zabawa BJ, Eickhoff-Shemek JM. *Rule the Rules of Workplace Wellness Programs.* Chicago, Illinois: American Bar Association, 2017.

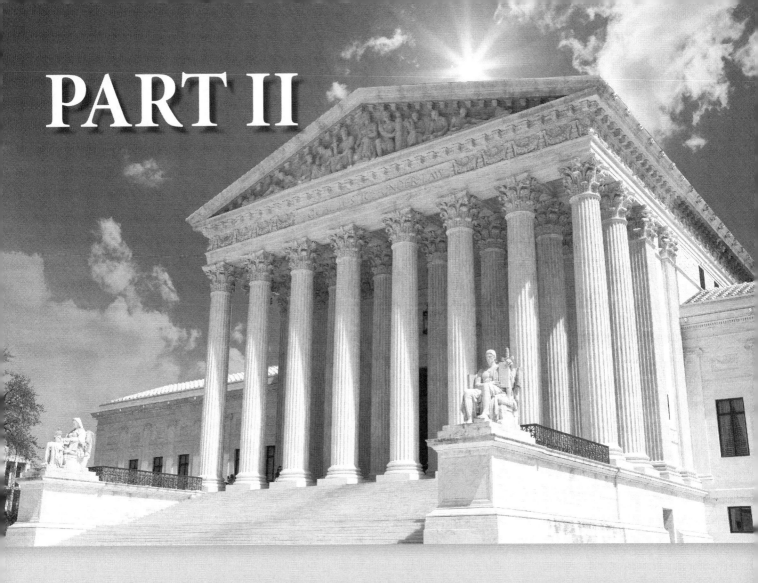

PART II

Legal Liability Exposures and Risk Management Strategies

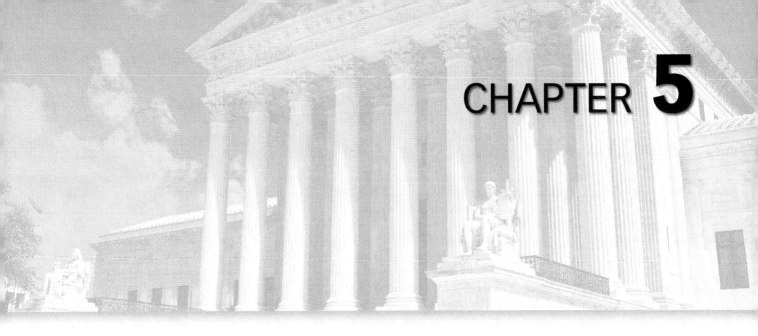

CHAPTER 5

Hiring Credentialed and Competent Personnel

LEARNING OBJECTIVES

After reading this chapter, fitness managers and exercise professionals will be able to:

1. Recognize that many federal and state laws exist that are applicable to employment issues such as those covered in this chapter and in Chapter 3 and the importance of complying with them (1).

2. Describe self-regulated and government-regulated types of credentialing in reference to accreditation, certification, licensure, and statutory certification (1).

3. Explain why it is essential, from a legal liability perspective, to hire only credentialed and competent personnel to design and deliver exercise programs and services.

4. Discuss why existing educational preparation programs may not be preparing competent exercise professionals and practitioners.

5. Explain how educational preparation programs will, likely, not be liable for educational malpractice (inadequate education) but how employers can face liability if they fail to properly hire, train, and supervise their personnel.

6. Recognize that the assessment of practical skills in educational programs is often missing and explain the connection between the lack of practical skills and legal liability.

7. Distinguish between vicarious liability and direct liability of employers and how they each apply to employees and independent contractors.

8. Describe the importance of conducting criminal background checks on certain personnel and why there is a need to have policies and procedures in place to address criminal conduct, such as sexual misconduct, and why.

9. Explain the potential legal liability consequences of untruthful marketing or advertising of the credentials of a fitness facility's personnel.

10. Discuss legal liability issues associated with independent contractors, vendors, interns, and volunteers.

11. Describe the differences between general and professional liability insurance and why both are needed (1).

12. Explain why fitness managers and other exercise professionals in supervisory roles need to possess excellent pedagogy skills.

13. Describe the components of classroom training and practical training and why both types of training are essential for all newly-hired exercise professionals and practitioners.

14. Develop and implement 10 risk management strategies that will help minimize legal liability exposures associated with personnel credentialing and competence issues.

INTRODUCTION

This textbook describes many negligence lawsuits, yet, these cases are just a small sample of the many negligence claims and lawsuits made against exercise professionals and their employers. It is important to realize that "about 95% of pending lawsuits end in a pre-trial settlement. This means that just one in 20 personal injury cases is resolved in a court of law by a judge or jury" (2, p. 1). These statistics are supported by noted expert witness, Thomas Bowler. He has served as an expert witness in about 400 cases over 25 years with only 11 going to trial. This equates to about 97% of the cases being settled or disposed by way of summary judgment (T. Bowler, personal communication, January 14, 2020). Settled cases are usually not made public.

Given these statistics, it is difficult to know how many negligence claims/lawsuits are filed against exercise professionals and their employers each year. However, it appears that the number of negligence lawsuits (personal injury lawsuits) against exercise professionals and fitness facilities continues to increase as well as the costs of liability insurance (3). One thing is certain regarding these negligence lawsuits—most are based on allegations of improper conduct or incompetence of exercise professionals and their employers. Therefore, educational preparation of fitness managers and exercise professionals as well as hiring credentialed and competent personnel is the focus of this chapter. This chapter describes the various types of credentialing in the exercise profession with a focus on credentialing challenges that employers face. This chapter also describes legal liability exposures of hiring personnel and risk management strategies that will help minimize those liability exposures.

TYPES OF CREDENTIALING

Over the last several decades, the exercise science profession has experienced several challenges with how to best prepare professionals to enter the field. Because the exercise profession is self-regulated and not government-regulated, almost anyone can practice in the field. Allied health professions such as athletic training and physical therapy are government-regulated meaning an individual must meet certain requirements before he/she can practice in that profession. For example, in most states where licensure is required to practice athletic training, an athletic trainer must graduate from an academic program that is accredited through the Commission on Accreditation of Athletic Training Education (CAATE), pass the national board of certification (BOC) examination, and then meet the state licensure requirements before he/she can practice. These requirements do not exist in the exercise profession. Self-regulation of the exercise profession has led to voluntary accreditation of academic programs and numerous certifications offered by professional organizations. See Table 5-1 that depicts the various types of credentialing—accreditation, certification,

Table 5-1	Types of Credentialing	
SELF-REGULATED		**GOVERNMENT-REGULATED AT STATE LEVEL**
Accreditation* ▶ Organizations, e.g., hospitals, universities ▶ Academic Programs, e.g., exercise science, athletic training ▶ Certification Examinations, e.g., accredited by NCCA *Obtained through an independent agency		**Licensure** ▶ Individuals—required to practice, e.g., athletic trainers, physical therapists
Certification ▶ Individuals—not required to practice but employers may require it ▶ Individuals—may be required to obtain a license to practice		**Statutory Certification** ▶ Individuals—specific credentials are required to use a certain title, e.g. certified dietitian, certified nutritionist

Figure 5-1: Levels of Exercise Professionals to Demonstrate Varying Credentials

Exercise Professional (or Practitioner) Level I	Exercise Professional (or Practitioner) Level II	Exercise Professional (or Practitioner) Level III	Exercise Professional Level IV	Exercise Professional Level V

• Little or No Formal Education and Practical Training
• Non-Accredited Certification or No Certification
	• Little or No Formal Education and Practical Training
	• Accredited Certification
		• Associate's Degree in Exercise Science or Equivalent Formal Education and Practical Training
		• Accredited Certification
			• Bachelor's Degree
			  ○ Exercise Science
			  ○ Exercise Physiology
			• Accredited Professional Certification that Requires a Degree
				• Master's Degree
				  ○ Clinical Exercise Physiology
				  ○ Fitness/Wellness Management
				• Accredited Professional Certification that Requires a Degree

licensure, and statutory certification. More information regarding each of these types of credentialing is described below.

Licensed professions such as athletic training and physical therapy control "who" can practice in their own fields. However, there is no licensure or government control in the exercise profession (except in Louisiana for clinical exercise physiologists only) and, thus, there are all types of individuals with varying credentials practicing in the field. See Figure 5-1. Note the term "exercise practitioner" is inserted as an alternative for exercise professional in Levels I through III. Many individuals in the profession would argue that an "exercise professional" would only be someone with at least a bachelor's degree in exercise science, exercise physiology, or related area, so the term exercise practitioner might be more appropriate for these three levels. Many challenges and legal implications exist for fitness managers and supervisors when it comes to hiring, training, and supervising personnel given so many varying levels of credentials that exist in the exercise profession. However, one of the purposes of this chapter is to provide strategies that can be implemented to address these many challenges. But first, it will be important to dive a little deeper into academic programs and the coursework often included in the curriculum.

Academic Programs

Undergraduate and graduate degree programs in exercise science, exercise physiology, or related areas have grown tremendously over the last three to four decades. Two professional organizations, the American College of Sports Medicine (ACSM) and the American Society of Exercise Physiologists (ASEP), have established certain academic courses that students must have to be eligible to take their own exercise physiologist certification examination. See Table 5-2. Although these are considered "minimum" requirements, academic

KEY POINT

Because the exercise profession is self-regulated, there are no credentials required to practice in the field. The credentials that exercise professionals possess can vary tremendously as shown in Figure 5-1. Because of this, employers can be faced with various legal liability exposures when hiring and/or contracting with exercise professionals and practitioners. Learning how to minimize these exposures is important for employers who have a general duty to properly hire, train, and supervise their employees and other personnel.

programs offer additional courses that students must take to meet their degree requirements and to help their students acquire **competence** (i.e., the knowledge and skills to properly perform the many job tasks and responsibilities of exercise professionals).

The Gap Between Academic Coursework and Job Responsibilities

Often a gap exists between theory and practice or between knowledge and the application of that knowledge. In addition to courses that focus on obtaining important exercise science knowledge, courses are needed that focus on the attainment of essential practical skills (e.g., teaching/training/coaching) and the knowledge/skills to perform the many administrative responsibilities in professional positions including legal/risk management responsibilities. Exhibit 5-1 provides a list and short descriptions of suggested courses that academic programs can offer that will help their students develop practical skills as well as help prepare them for their many future administrative responsibilities and legal duties. Take note of how these course descriptions reflect the responsibilities listed in the job descriptions for a Fitness Manager, Assistant Fitness Director, Assistant Fitness Manager, Group Exercise Coordinator, and Assistant Strength and Conditioning Coach in Exhibit 5-2. These positions require a degree in an exercise science area and reflect the titles of entry-level positions for exercise professionals.

Note: *A strength and conditioning course is not listed in Exhibit 5-1 because it is listed in Table 5-2 under ACSM. It is not listed under the ASEP required courses. Practical skills such as how to properly teach strength and conditioning exercises, leading groups through conditioning drills, etc. need to be significant components of this course. See Chapters 8 and 9. A nutrition course is not listed in Exhibit 5-1 because it is listed in Table 5-2 under ASEP. It is not listed under the ACSM required courses. In addition to nutrition knowledge, this course also needs to address practical skills on how to properly provide nutrition information within the exercise professional's scope of practice. For more information on scope of practice, see Chapter 7. A Stress Management course should also be considered.*

While a fitness manager position would require advanced administrative knowledge and skills, it is important to realize that many entry-level professional jobs in the field also require administrative knowledge and skills. For example, entry-level professionals such as an assistant fitness director, program coordinator, group exercise coordinator, personal trainer coordinator, assistant clinical exercise physiologist, and assistant strength and conditioning coach will have similar administrative responsibilities as a fitness manager

Table 5-2	Required Academic Courses
ACSM: ELIGIBILITY TO SIT FOR THE EP-C EXAMINATION*	**ASEP: ELIGIBILITY TO SIT FOR EPC EXAMINATION****
Exercise Physiology	Exercise Physiology
Strength and Conditioning	Fitness Assessment and Prescription
Applied Kinesiology or Biomechanics	Exercise Metabolism
Anatomy and Physiology	Kinesiology
Exercise Testing and Prescription	Research Design
Special Populations	Biomechanics
Health Risk Appraisal	Environmental Physiology
	Nutrition
	Exercise and Special Populations
	Documentation of hands-on laboratory experiences in exercise physiology (or related) laboratories

* Degree Requirements for the ACSM Exercise Physiologist Certification: https://www.acsm.org/get-stay-certified/get-certified/health-fitness-certifications/exercise-physiologist/degree-requirements-ep-c, Accessed February 3, 2020.
** ASEP Standards of Practice: https://www.asep.org/organization/practice, Accessed February 3, 2020.

Exhibit 5-1: Suggested Academic Courses to Help Undergraduate Students Gain Knowledge and Practical Skills Reflecting Job Responsibilities and Legal Duties

SUGGESTED COURSES

1. **Theory and Practice of Personal Fitness Training:** In this course, students learn how to apply the many principles of exercise taught in courses such as exercise physiology, applied biomechanics, fitness testing/prescription related to proper design/delivery of an individual exercise program. It is best to have a course where the students have "real-life" experiences to help them obtain these skills. For a description of such a course, see *Educating and Training the Personal Fitness Trainer: A Pedagogical Approach* (4). A course like this is essential for exercise professionals who will work as a personal fitness trainer as well as have oversight of the facility's personal training programs (e.g., personal trainer coordinator).

2. **Theory and Practice of Teaching Group Exercise:** In this course, students learn how to teach a variety of group exercise programs such as step aerobics, strength and conditioning, circuit training, and aquatic exercise. The focus is on developing "teaching" skills, preparing lesson plans, etc. that apply important principles of safe exercise such as how to modify exercises and monitor intensity. The course concludes with a "practical exam" of each student's group exercise teaching skills. A course like this is essential for exercise professionals who will work as a group exercise instructor as well as have oversight of the facility's group exercise program (e.g., group exercise coordinator).

3. **Planning and Evaluation of Fitness/Wellness Programs:** In this course, students obtain the knowledge and skills related to strategic planning and why it is important in the design/delivery of high-quality (safe and effective) programs. The course content addresses: (a) conducting a needs assessment, (b) developing programs based on needs, (c) implementing programs, and (d) evaluating programs at process, impact, and outcome levels. Fitness managers and exercise professionals continually develop new programs and revise current programs and, thus, program planning and evaluation skills are needed.

4. **Fitness and Legal Risk Management:** In this course, students are introduced to the many management responsibilities that they will likely have in most professional positions such as human resource management (e.g., hiring procedures), financial management (e.g., budgeting procedures), marketing/promotion of programs, and of course, legal/risk management. **Note:** It is recommended to offer an entire course in legal/risk management but if that is not doable at the undergraduate level, a unit on legal/risk management should be included in a Fitness Management course. An entire course in Legal/Risk Management should be seriously considered at the graduate level for professionals who are seeking advanced positions in the field, such as middle and upper management positions, where they will have the ultimate responsibility as the legal/risk management manager.

5. **Emergency Response and Planning:** In this course, students earn their certifications such as First-Aid, CPR/AED and also learn how to develop written emergency action plans (EAPs) for a facility. The failure of a fitness facility to have written EAPs and/or the failure to carry them out properly are major liability exposures. Students can develop a hypothetical EAP or develop one for a community fitness facility as a service learning project.

6. **Behavior Change Strategies or Exercise Psychology:** In this course, students develop knowledge and skills regarding various theories related to health behavior change and how to apply them in practice. Although such a course is not listed in the ACSM required courses, it is an important course because 25% of the competencies for ACSM's exercise physiologist examination are under: Exercise Counseling and Behavioral Modification (10).

7. **Professional Development and Ethics:** In this course, students are exposed to many factors related to their professional success and reputation such as preparing an effective resume, strategies for job interviews and informational interviews, codes of conduct published by several organizations, moral/ethical responsibilities, professional communications (email, social media), advocacy, and development of a professional portfolio that showcases their knowledge and skills that can be shared with future employers in job interviews.

8. **Internship:** In this final semester course, students under the direction of an experienced, well-educated site supervisor, work in a facility to obtain real-world experiences to sharpen their knowledge/skills obtained in the academic coursework. The student should come well-prepared for the internship position, e.g., the site supervisor should not have to prepare an intern on the basics of teaching, training, fitness testing, etc.—that is the responsibility of the academic program. The internship exists to provide valuable leadership and learning experiences to further develop the intern's knowledge/skills resulting in increased competence and confidence to perform job tasks.

but, generally, focus on a certain program area versus responsibilities for the entire program. Many of these positions will be supervisory positions involving a general legal duty to properly hire, train, and supervise employees as well as many other management functions. It is likely that most of these positions will require teaching, training, and/or coaching of participants as a part of the job responsibilities. The percentage of time spent on management functions varies, but it can be significant, perhaps 50% or more for an entry-level professional's job. The remaining time is spent on direct service responsibilities (e.g., teaching/training/coaching participants). See this mixture of responsibilities in the job descriptions in Exhibit 5-2. Because entry-level professional positions require competence in carrying out a variety of job responsibilities including administrative and teaching/training/coaching, undergraduate coursework is needed in these areas. As professionals move into advanced positions (middle and upper management positions), more time (e.g., 75-90%, will be spent on management functions).

Accreditation

Accreditation can be awarded to (a) organizations, (b) educational programs, and (c) certification examinations. Organizations such as hospitals earn accreditation through the Joint Commission on Accreditation of Healthcare Organizations (JCAHO) and universities earn accreditation through one of six regional accrediting agencies recognized by the United States Department of Education (USDE) and the Council for Higher Education Accreditation (CHEA) (5). Academic programs in exercise science (undergraduate) and exercise physiology (graduate) can obtain "voluntary" accreditation through the Commission on the Accreditation of Allied Health Education Programs (CAAHEP). Most programs are not accredited but some are as of April 2020: (a) 65 undergraduate exercise science programs, (b) 13 graduate exercise physiology programs (eight clinical exercise physiology and five applied exercise physiology), and (c) five associate degree programs in personal fitness training (6).

Undergraduate programs in exercise physiology can also obtain accreditation through the Board of Accreditation which was created within the administrative infrastructure of the ASEP. Therefore, it is not an "independent" accreditation agency as is CAAHEP. There are four academic programs that have obtained this accreditation (7).

To earn accreditation, organizations and educational programs must meet certain standards established by the accrediting agency. For example, an undergraduate program curriculum in exercise science must cover many competencies (knowledge and skills) listed under each of the following five domains that were revised in 2017 to meet the CAAHEP accreditation standards:

Domain I—Health and Fitness Assessment

Domain II—Exercise Prescription and Implementation

Domain III—Exercise Counseling and Behavior Strategies

Domain IV—Legal/Professional

Domain V—Management (8)

Applying for accreditation is a complex, lengthy, and costly process and includes preparing numerous documents to help demonstrate that the standards have been met in advance of a required site visit by members of the accrediting agency. Once accreditation is obtained, it can be used for marketing and public image purposes to promote the commitment to quality of the organization/program. Maintaining accreditation is also important. An academic program may need to submit an annual report and fee and complete a comprehensive review every 10 years.

Obtaining accreditation for a certification examination requires a different process. Many professional organizations such as the ACSM, National Strength and Conditioning Association (NSCA), and American Council on Exercise (ACE) have opted for accreditation through the National Commission for Certifying Agencies (NCCA), created by the Institute for Credentialing Excellence. The NCCA has 24 standards that the professional organizations must meet for their certification examination(s) to become accredited (9). The NCCA is revising these standards with a public review and comment period set for summer 2020 (9). Many of the standards address various procedures that the certifying organization must follow to help ensure the integrity and quality of the examination. However, one important standard (Standard 14: Job Analysis)

Exhibit 5-2: Job Descriptions, In Part: Fitness Manager, Assistant Fitness Director, Group Exercise Coordinator, and Assistant Strength and Conditioning Coach

Fitness Manager (corporate fitness/wellness) *

- Development of annual strategic plan…
- Budget management…
- Hiring, training and supervision of full and part time staff…
- Successful management of personal training and group exercise programs…
- Development, delivery and evaluation of health promotion, incentive and other specialty programs

Assistant Fitness and Spa Director (private, for profit fitness facility) **

- Develops a comprehensive standard facility operations manual…
- Develops and maintains accurate facility maintenance procedures and checklists through routine preventative maintenance and repair…
- Ensures fiscal responsibility…
- Maintains a fully staffed department and/or facility by recruiting, interviewing, hiring, and training all staff.

Assistant Fitness Manager (community, non-profit fitness facility) ***

- Conducts 16 classes per week…
- Assists in recruiting, supervising, training and evaluating instructors, personal trainers…
- Assist with the maintenance of fitness equipment
- Manager On Duty (MOD) responsibilities
- Assist in planning, development, and implementation of fitness programs

Coordinator, Group Exercise (university, campus recreation center) ****

- Supervision of group fitness personnel
- Personnel management responsibilities include… recruiting, hiring, training, evaluating, mentoring…
- Program delivery responsibilities include the design, implementation, management, evaluation and expansion of group fitness programming…

Assistant Strength and Conditioning Coach (university athletics) *****

Assist the head coach with all aspects of the Strength & Conditioning program including but not limited to practice competition activities…directing and implementing plans for daily practices…, organizing and administering clinics, etc., and overall administrative tasks within the operation of the program.

---

*Startwire. Available at: https://www.startwire.com/express_apply_jobs/MjEyNF9lNjlkZWMwZDVhMTQ1OTIwZjJhN2IwOTI1OWNkNGNkM19sdX-VhX2k=?source=kimble_l2_mediu. (Accessed November 16, 2018).

**Monster. Available at: https://www.monster.com/jobs/search?q=Assistant-fitenss-director&jobid=712caee9-34a7-47c5-a671-04d2eb47de07. (Accessed March 17, 2019).

***Indeed. Available at: https://www.indeed.com/jobs?q=assistant%20fitness%20director&l&vjk=57592e84b3053215. (Accessed December 6, 2018).

****Indeed. Available at: https://www.indeed.com/jobs?q=Health%20Fitness%20Program%20Coordinator&start=30&vjk=c9d9ec43519584dc. (Accessed March 17, 2019).

*****Indeed. Available at: https://www.indeed.com/viewjob?jk=cd4aab8bc6725df6&from=tp-serp&tk=1cu1tb0j319p3003. (Accessed November 16, 2018).

---

requires a **job task analysis** (JTA) that "must lead to clearly delineated domains and tasks that characterize proficient performance" (9, p. 17). The validity of the JTA is critical because the results of the JTA lead to the domains, tasks, and knowledge/skills (competencies) that are then used to develop the content of the certification examination, as shown in Figure 5-2.

Typically, the JTA survey contains a list of certain job tasks (e.g., knowledge and skills) in which individuals who complete the survey provide ratings regarding (a) how important that task is, and (b) how frequently they perform that task. If the individual does not fully understand a certain job task and what it all entails but then rates that task, the validity of the results could

Figure 5-2: Outcomes of a Job Task Analysis: Typical Certification Model for Personal Fitness Trainers and Group Exercise Instructors (5)*

(No formal education and practical skills training are required prior to taking accredited certification examinations)

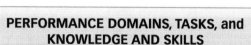

JOB TASK ANALYSIS (JTA)

PERFORMANCE DOMAINS, TASKS, and KNOWLEDGE AND SKILLS

ACCREDITED CERTIFCATION EXAMINATION

be questioned. For example, a job task for an exercise professional might state "exercise professionals apply federal, state, and local laws into the design/delivery of exercise programs" or a job task for a personal fitness trainer might state "personal fitness trainers conduct fitness assessments." If exercise professionals or personal fitness trainers do not have adequate knowledge or skill regarding these tasks, it will be difficult for them to accurately rate their importance and frequency and,

KEY POINT

Almost all entry-level professional positions (e.g., those that require a bachelor's degree such as those described in Exhibit 5-2), will require the professional to have various managerial knowledge and skills. Therefore, managerial competence including legal/risk management competence is essential for fitness managers and exercise professionals serving in supervisory positions.

thus, possibly taint the validity of the JTA. It might be best to first ask the individual their level of knowledge/skill related to each task and if this is rated low, their ratings of importance and frequency should, perhaps, be omitted from the data analysis.

The JTA for the ACSM-EP certification examination resulted in five domains in 2012 (same as those listed above for CAAHEP accreditation) and four domains in 2017 based on an updated JTA (10). Domain IV (legal/professional) and Domain V (management) made up 10% and 15%, respectively, of the EP examination questions in 2012. In 2017, Domain V was eliminated and Domain IV was retitled "risk management and professional responsibilities" (10). The competencies in Domain IV (legal/professional) in 2012 reflect many of the same competencies in Domain IV (risk management and professional responsibilities) in 2017 (8, 11). However, the percentage of questions on the EP examination in these two similar domains decreased from 10% to 5% (10). Given that most entry-level professional positions (e.g., Assistant Director, Personal Trainer Coordinator) involve many legal and management responsibilities, it is interesting that the updated JTA resulted in these major changes. The deletion of the management domain is concerning in that employers will expect entry level professionals to have knowledge and skills in this area as demonstrated in the job descriptions in Exhibit 5-2. Management competence including legal/risk management competence is essential for fitness managers and exercise professionals.

State Licensure

As shown in Table 5-1, **licensure** is decided by state governments, not the federal government. Most allied health professionals need to possess a license to practice in their field, but not all. For example, individuals must possess the registered dietitian (RD) credential to qualify for licensure in most states, but in some states (e.g., Arizona, Michigan), licensure is not required to practice (12). In these States, anyone can practice dietetics—credentials are not needed. In other states, through **statutory certification**, individuals need to possess certain credentials before they can use a title such as certified dietitian or certified nutritionist (12), as described in Table 5-1. Eligibility requirements for the RD examination are described in Table 5-3.

Table 5-3	Eligibility Requirements for Registered Dietitian (RD) Examination*

1. Complete the minimum of a Baccalaureate degree from a U.S. regionally accredited college or university or foreign equivalent.

2. Complete an accredited Didactic Program in Dietetics (accredited by the Accreditation Council for Education in Nutrition and Dietetics (ACEND).

3. Complete an ACEND-accredited Dietetic Internship (DI) program that includes at least 1200 hours of supervised practice experience.

*Commission on Dietetic Registration, Academy of Nutrition and Dietetics, Option 1- Dietetic Internship. Available at: https://www.cdrnet.org/rd-eligibility. Accessed February 3, 2020.

The purpose of state licensure is to prevent unqualified individuals from practicing in a certain profession. It helps ensure the public is receiving quality (safe and effective) services from individuals who meet minimum educational requirements. Because certain educational requirements are needed to qualify for licensure, it raises the bar from certifications which may not require any formal education, which is the case for most certifications in the fitness field as described below.

The preparation of a state licensure bill involves addressing several factors such as (a) qualifications for licensure and renewal, (b) definition of the scope of practice distinguishing it from other licensed professions, (c) qualifications of the members of the licensing board and their powers/duties, and (d) criminal penalties for violations of the licensing statutes (5). Other issues such as determining the need for government regulation also need to be considered. In July 2015, the White House published a document entitled: *Occupational Licensing: A Framework for Policy Makers*. See Table 5-4 for Licensing Best Practices, provided in this publication, that should be considered when establishing state licensure. Many exercise professionals would agree that item #2 in Table 5-4 under "protecting public health

and safety" would apply to the exercise profession, especially given the continued increase in the number of injuries and subsequent litigations.

As described in many of the negligence lawsuits presented in this textbook, injuries are commonly caused by exercise professionals who have not obtained adequate education and/or important practical skills. Because licensure would likely require formal education and practical training, many believe it is the only remedy to help protect the public. Others believe that government control will create practice limitations and barriers to access for consumers that are not needed and that certifications accredited by NCCA or other accrediting agencies adequately address public health and safety concerns.

Licensure Efforts in the Exercise Profession

Over the past couple of decades, legislative bills to license personal fitness trainers and group exercise leaders have been proposed in several states. Although none of the proposed state licensing bills became law, Washington D.C. did pass a law (13) to regulate personal trainers in 2014. It was repealed before it went into effect (14). Louisiana is the only state that requires licensure for exercise professionals, but only for clinical exercise physiologists who work under

Table 5-4	Licensing Best Practices (In-Part)*

Ensure that Licensing Restrictions are Closely Targeted to Protecting Public Health and Safety, and are Not Overly Broad or Burdensome

1. In cases where public health and safety concerns are mild, consider using alternative systems that are less restrictive than licensing, such as voluntary State certification ("right-to-title") or registration (filing basic information with a State registry).

2. Make sure that substantive requirements of licensing (e.g., education and experience requirements) are closely tied to public health and safety concerns.

3. Minimize procedural burdens of acquiring a license, in terms of fees, complexity of requirements, processing time, and paperwork.

Work to Reduce Licensing's Barriers to Mobility

1. Harmonize licensing requirements to the maximum extent possible across States.

2. Form interstate compacts that make it easier for licensed workers to practice and relocate across State lines, while also enabling State regulators to share practitioners' performance histories.

*Occupational Licensing: A Framework for Policy Makers. 2015. Available at: https://obamawhitehouse.archives.gov/sites/default/files/docs/licensing_report_final_nonembargo.pdf (pp. 42-43). Accessed November 19, 2018.

a physician in a clinical setting. When this law (LSA-R.S. 37:3422) went into effect January 1, 1996, it was believed that other states would implement similar laws to license clinical exercise physiologists, but this has not been the case. For example, Massachusetts proposed a similar bill, but it was met with strong opposition from inside the profession (American Society of Exercise Physiologists) and outside the profession (American Physical Therapy Association of Massachusetts) for different reasons (15).

Proposed licensure bills for personal trainers and group exercise leaders, in their initial drafts, often include formal education and practical training requirements. For example, the proposed licensure bill in New Jersey required an associate degree in the health and fitness field or 200 classroom hours, at least 50 hours of an internship, and passing an examination administered and approved by the state licensing board (16). When the bill was re-introduced later, the requirements were modified which would allow someone to qualify for a license who only needed to possess a NCCA-accredited certification (16). It is important to note that NCCA accredited certifications in personal fitness training and group exercise leadership do not require any educational credentials in these areas to be eligible to sit for a certification examination. Watering down the credentials to obtain a license (e.g., no requirement for formal education, only NCCA-accredited certification) will not raise the bar for entry into the field as licensure does in other professions. When only an NCCA-accredited certification is needed to obtain a license to practice, there virtually is no distinction between self-regulation and government-regulation.

An effective lobbying effort has existed to oppose licensure bills that require formal education and practical experience, generally by those organizations that make a lot of money from certifications or by the health club industry that believes that licensure will increase operating costs and have a negative impact on their bottom line (5). Some people believe that the organizations that oppose licensure are more concerned with their profits than the safety of the public. They also argue that many occupations that require formal education and practical training before obtaining a license to practice (e.g., hair stylists/barbers and massage therapists), pose much less risk of injury to the public than those leading fitness programs.

It is unlikely that states will continue to propose licensure bills for personal fitness trainers and group exercise leaders given the release of the *ACSM Exercise Professional Licensure Statement* (17). It states that it does not support licensure for non-degree personal trainers working in nonclinical/community settings with apparently healthy clients. However, the ACSM does support licensure for "exercise professionals with at least a bachelor's degree in exercise science and related, accredited certification, assuming these professionals are working with patients and clients with medical conditions that require clinical support" (17, p. 2). This approach to licensure is commensurate with other licensed allied health professions. However, realistically, there are many non-degree personal trainers and other fitness instructors who are leading exercise programs for people with medical conditions. Most fitness facilities provide programs/services for people with medical conditions given that 60% of adults in the U.S. have at least one chronic medical condition and 40% have two or more chronic conditions (18).

Because licensure is decided at the state level, it likely will take many years to achieve this goal of licensure for degreed exercise professionals. One major question is: Will these licensure proposals, which will define the scope of practice in the proposed bill, prohibit all others to work with clinical populations (i.e., only those who are licensed can work with individuals with medical conditions?). Another question is: Will the scope of practice for the exercise professional cross over into the scope of practice of other established licensed allied health professions such as nursing, physical therapy, and athletic training? If so, this may create turf battles between the exercise profession and various licensed professions. Moving forward with this goal to obtain licensure for degreed exercise professionals will bring several challenges and will require a collaborative effort among organizations inside and outside the exercise profession.

State Licensure Versus "Licensed" Group Exercise Instructors

Obtaining a state license to practice in an allied health profession is *substantially different* from a group exercise instructor who obtains a license to teach trade-marked exercise programs such as Zumba®, Piloxing®, BollyX® and others. At the time this chapter was written, the credentials to obtain such a license vary with none of them requiring even an accredited group exercise certification.

For example, to obtain a license to teach Zumba® Fitness classes, the company (https://www.zumba.com) requires completion of a ten-hour, one-day training program and Piloxing® (https://www.piloxing.com) requires completion of a nine-hour, one-day training workshop. Neither requires passing a written or practical examination. BollyX® (https://bollyx.com) requires attending a training workshop, replicating given choreography, and passing an online written examination. With these three formats, instructors can elect to pay a monthly fee to maintain their license and to access resources such as music and choreography. Employers cannot assume that a "licensed" group exercise instructor is well-prepared to teach group exercise programs or to substitute for a teacher. They may need to require and/or provide formal education and practical training before having them teach any of the trade-marked exercise programs.

Certification

When certifications began in the exercise profession, it was required for individuals to pass both written and practical examinations. The individual had to first pass the written examination to be eligible to take the practical examination. Employers could be somewhat assured that these certified professionals possessed certain knowledge and practical skills to properly perform the job (5). However, much has changed. Today, obtaining a certification requires passing a written examination only, except in rare cases where a practical examination is also required (e.g., see SCCC below). To help address the lack of a practical skills examination, some certifications require practical experience to be eligible to sit for the written examination.

In 2004, there were as many as 250 fitness certifications offered by 75 organizations (19). "Since then, the number of organizations and certifications has continued to grow, especially in the area of specialty certifications such as senior fitness, mind/body, nutrition/weight management, functional training, health/wellness coaching, and the like" (5, p. 162). Because there is no government regulation, individuals who want to start an organization and offer certifications (or licenses for trade-marked exercise programs) can easily do so. The fees generated from certifications can produce large profits for an organization, not to mention the additional fees obtained when certified

individuals need to submit and pay for continuing education credits or units to the certifying organization.

To help distinguish the "fly-by-night" certifications from those offered by credible professional organizations, a concerted effort was made by professional organizations to have their certifications accredited by NCCA or other accrediting agencies such as the Distance Education Accrediting Commission (DEAC). Employers have been encouraged to hire personal fitness trainers that have an accredited certification from an independent and nationally recognized agency such as NCCA and DEAC. For example, in 2005, the Board of Directors of the International Health, Racquet & Sportsclub Association (IHRSA) recommended that its member clubs hire personal fitness trainers holding at least one current certification that has third-party accreditation (20). IHRSA lists 16 organizations that have acceptable accredited certifications through NCCA and DEAC and are considering a proposal from American National Standards Institute (ANSI) as an additional acceptable accrediting organization (20). Most of the 16 organizations have NCCA accreditation.

The following section provides examples of the eligibility requirements for four levels of individual certifications: (a) personal fitness training/group exercise leadership, (b) exercise professional certifications, (c) exercise professional clinical certifications, and (d) fitness facility director certifications as well as program and facility certifications. This is not a complete list of the certifications offered by these organizations. Many of them offer several other types of health and fitness certifications. Also, there are many other organizations that offer various certifications.

Personal Fitness Training and Group Exercise Leadership Certifications

All the following organizations offer accredited certifications in personal fitness training and/or group exercise leadership. None of them require any formal education (e.g. academic coursework) or practical training prior to taking a written-only examination. They all have minimal eligibility requirements to sit for the examination such as the following: (a) 18 years old, (b) high school diploma or equivalent, and (c) adult CPR/AED. To help prepare for the certification examination, candidates are often encouraged to review resources provided by the organization, attend a workshop, or participate in an online training program. Some of the organizations include preparation materials with their certification fee. The information for the following eight certifying organizations was obtained from their websites. All are NCCA accredited except ISSA which is DEAC accredited.

1. **American Council on Exercise (ACE):** Certified Personal trainer (CPT) and Group Fitness Instructor (GFI)

2. **American College of Sports Medicine (ACSM):** Certified Personal Trainer (CPT) and Group Exercise Instructor (GEI)

3. **Athletics and Fitness Association of America (AFAA):** Certified Group Fitness Instructor (CGFI)

4. **International Sports Sciences Association (ISSA):** Certified Personal Trainer (CPT)

5. **National Academy of Sports Medicine (NASM):** Certified Personal Trainer (CPT)

6. **National Strength and Conditioning Association (NSCA):** Certified Personal Trainer (CPT)

7. **National Council on Strength & Fitness (NCSF):** Certified Personal Trainer (CPT)

8. **National Exercise Trainers Association (NETA):** Certified Personal Trainer (CPT) and Group Exercise Instructor (GEI)

Another organization called the National Board of Fitness Examiners (NBFE) was founded in 2003 (21). It offers a national board certification examination in personal training. Originally, to qualify for this certification, the candidate had to possess a certification from one of the NBFE approved affiliate certification organizations. Now, however, candidates certified through national organizations that have not become NBFE affiliates can qualify to sit for the NBFE written examination. Also, at one time the NBFE had proposed a practical, hands-on examination in addition to the written examination, but due to lack of support, it was not deployed (21). For more information, see the NBFE website: www.nbfe.org.

NCCA Accredited Exercise Professional Certifications that Require a Degree

In addition to the required academic coursework listed in Table 5-2 to be eligible to sit for the ACSM and ASEP Exercise Physiologist examinations, an academic degree is required. ACSM requires a bachelor's degree or higher with a major in exercise science, or equivalent and ASEP requires an academic degree with a major in exercise physiology or related degree programs such as exercise science, kinesiology, sport science, human performance (22). There are no practical examinations nor practical experience requirements for either of these certifications. The following are examples of additional certifications that require a degree:

1. **National Strength and Conditioning Association (NSCA):** Certified Strength and Conditioning Specialist (CSCS) requires a "bachelor's degree or higher granted by an accredited institution, or a degree in physical therapy or chiropractic medicine" (23, p. 13). The examination contains two sections: Scientific Foundations and Practical/Applied. **Note**: NSCA has proposed changes in their eligibility requirements for CSCS to go into effect in 2030 that includes a bachelor's degree in a strength and conditioning related field that is obtained from a program accredited by an NSCA-approved accrediting agency (24).

2. **College Strength & Conditioning Coaches association (CSCCa):** Strength & Conditioning Coach Certified (SCCC) requires a degree in exercise science or related field. A higher level of certification is also available—Master Strength & Conditioning Coach (MSCC). For the SCCC, there is a written examination and an in-person practical examination that is judged by a panel of Master Strength & Conditioning Coaches (25).

NCCA Accredited Exercise Professional Clinical Certifications—Degree and Practical Experience Required

1. **ACSM:** Clinical Exercise Physiologist (CEP) requires a bachelor's degree or equivalent and 1200 hours of clinical experience or a master's degree in clinical exercise physiology or equivalent and 600 hours of clinical experience (26).

2. **American Council on Exercise (ACE):** Certified Medical Exercise Specialist requires a bachelor's degree in exercise science or related area and 500 completed hours of work experience designing/implementing exercise programs for apparently healthy or high-risk individuals (27).

3. **American Association of Cardiovascular and Pulmonary Rehabilitation (AACVPR):** Certified Cardiac Rehabilitation Professional requires 1200 hours in CR/Secondary prevention in Cardiac Rehabilitation (CR) and a minimum of a bachelor's degree in a health-related field or current RN licensure (28). **Note**: This examination is not NCCA accredited.

The NSCA also offers a clinical certification, Certified Special Population Specialist (CSPS), but it does not require a bachelor's degree. Candidates have three options to meet the eligibility requirements: "current NSCA certification...or NCCA-accredited personal trainer certification, OR bachelor's degree or higher granted by an accredited institution in exercise science or related field..., OR current license as a physical therapist, physical therapist assistant, or athletic trainer" (23, p. 13). In addition, 250 hours of practical experience coaching/training individuals from special populations is required. **Note:** As of April 2020, this certification was not listed on the NCCA website (https://www.credentialingexcellence.org/page/get-started-with-accreditation) as being accredited.

Management Certifications

1. **Medical Fitness Association (MFA):** Fitness Facility Director requires three years of management/leadership experience and a bachelor's degree in fitness, business or related field OR five years of management/leadership experience and an associate degree.
2. **Medical Fitness Association (MFA):** Medical Fitness Facility Director requires passing the Fitness Facility Director examination.

Note: *Both require serving (currently or within one year) in a supervisory or management position in a fitness facility or medically integrated fitness facility, respectively (29). NCCA accreditation is pending for both as of April 2020.*

Program and Facility Certifications

The AACVPR offers a program certification for facilities that adhere to standards and guidelines developed and published by AACVPR and other professional organizations (30). The MFA offers a Medical Fitness Facility Certification for facilities that adhere to the MFA's published standards and guidelines (31).

CREDENTIALED: YES, BUT ARE THEY COMPETENT?

The exercise profession has made significant progress in the last three to four decades. There are many academic programs in exercise science (or related areas) and numerous certifications that have helped prepare exercise professionals for their jobs. Excellent resources, based on a wealth of scientific evidence, are available for professionals to help them design and deliver high quality, safe, and effective programs. Professionals can stay abreast of current research by attending conferences and completing continuing education programs. The profession has more well-credentialed professionals working in the field than ever before. So why are exercise injuries continuing to rise significantly and why are there so many negligence claims and lawsuits against exercise professionals and their employers? One answer to these questions is the lack of practical "how to" skills training among exercise professionals.

Academic programs that focus only on "science" courses and do not offer courses that help students obtain important practical skills will not adequately prepare professionals for their many job responsibilities. For example, most academic programs will have a fitness testing/exercise prescription course where students can be formally evaluated on their "fitness testing" practical skills. However, there are many more practical skills that need to be attained and measured such as teaching/training/coaching skills as well as knowledge/skills in administration (e.g., legal/risk management) and strategic program planning. Therefore, academic programs may be preparing a "credentialed" professional, but not a "competent" professional who can properly perform the many tasks that professional jobs in the field require.

Many exercise professionals (or practitioners) lack practical skills because of written-only certification examinations which cannot adequately assess skills like fitness

Figure 5-3: The Connection Between the Lack of Practical Skills and Legal Liability

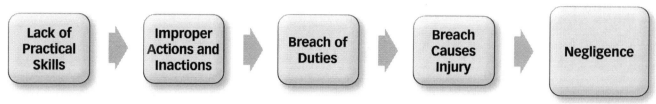

testing and safe/effective teaching and training skills. For example, how can an employer know if a certified personal trainer knows how to (a) properly measure blood pressure during a cardiovascular test, (b) teach a proper warm-up or assist clients who are performing an exercise incorrectly, (c) properly teach a resistance exercise to a client, or (d) apply safe principles of exercise when designing/delivering an exercise program? Knowledge of these skill areas might be covered on a written certification examination, but proof of actual skill attainment cannot. This reality is best expressed by Dr. Anthony Abbott, well-known expert witness, who stated: "…just because one is certified does not necessarily equate with his or her being qualified. To become a truly qualified personal trainer requires in-depth knowledge of anatomy, physiology, kinesiology, biomechanics and principles of exercise science coupled with considerable hands-on practical training" (3, p. 98).

Another valid point Dr. Abbott makes is that certification candidates need to receive comprehensive education and ample practical training taught by exercise physiology academicians or instructors who have had real-world experience themselves (3). Regarding certification examinations, Dr. Abbott has taken over 30 certification examinations including most of the accredited ones. He states that the "concept of accreditation has lost most of its value" (3, p. 100) because the examination questions are poorly written and simplistic and, therefore, do not adequately test the depth of the trainer's knowledge (3).

The Legal Significance of Practical Skills

In the many negligence lawsuits described throughout this textbook, the defendants (e.g., personal fitness trainers, group exercise leaders, strength and conditioning coaches) did not appear to possess important practical skills necessary to design and deliver a safe exercise program resulting in a breach of duty. They failed to provide

a reasonably safe program. Their lack of practical skills led to improper actions and/or inactions (or improper behavior/conduct), which caused the injuries and subsequent negligence claims/lawsuits. See Figure 5-3. It is unknown in these cases if the defendants possessed important knowledge related to safe principles of exercise (progression, signs and symptoms of overexertion, etc.) but it was evident, if they did have the knowledge, they did not know how to properly apply it, often referred to as **theory-practice gap**. In other words, they did not possess the necessary practical skills on how to safely train, teach, or coach the participants in their programs.

It is important to realize that courts may review the credentials of a defendant such as his/her degrees, certifications, experience, but more importantly, courts will judge the "competence" of the defendant by determining if the actions/inactions of the defendant breached any duties owed to the plaintiff. For example, did the personal trainers have their clients perform exercises beyond their limitations given their health/fitness status and did managers fail to meet their general duty to properly hire, train, and supervise their employees? Courts will determine if the defendants were competent when performing their responsibilities.

Preparation of competent professionals requires learning by doing. As Aristotle stated, "For the things

> ### KEY POINT
>
> **Competence and Legal Liability:** In negligence lawsuits, courts will perhaps review the credentials of the defendant (exercise professional), but more importantly, courts will judge the "practical competence" of the defendant—did his/her conduct or actions/inactions breach any legal duties owed to the plaintiff. For fitness managers/supervisors, the courts will review their managerial competence—did they properly hire, train, and supervise employees.

we have to learn before we can do them, we learn by doing them" (32). In an interesting study by Zenko and Ekkekakis (33), an 11-quesiton survey was administered to 1,808 ACSM certified exercise professionals to assess their knowledge of recommended frequency, duration, and intensity ranges regarding heart rate, metabolic equivalents, and ratings of perceived exertion. On average, respondents answered 42.87% of the questions correctly. There were no differences among gender, age, and years of professional experience as well as no differences if the respondents possessed one, two, or three (or more) certifications. Significant differences were found between (a) levels of education ranging from 38.72% for some college to 47.01% for doctorate, and (b) primary job role ranging from 40.59% for personal trainers and 44.18% for clinical exercise physiologists.

Obviously, these guidelines for prescribing exercise are very basic and are, likely, included in academic and certification preparation programs, so why were the findings from the Zenko and Ekkekakis study (33) less than ideal? One possible explanation is that the certified individuals learned these guidelines to help them pass an academic or certification examination, but they were not applying them in practice. If they had been applied in practice, on a regular basis, it would have strengthened and reinforced their knowledge of the guidelines, likely resulting in better scores on the 11-item questionnaire. Another interesting finding from this study was that years of professional experience made no difference. Other studies have also found a similar result to demonstrate a lack of a relationship between years of professional experience and knowledge among exercise professionals (3, 34).

Obtaining a strong knowledge base comes from formal education and related practical "hands-on" supervised training. A key factor related to experience is the "quality" of the professional experience, whether that is in academic coursework, an internship, or the experience requirement for certain certifications. The experience must be under the leadership of a well-credentialed, competent professional who can provide valuable learning experiences across all major job responsibilities including the many legal, risk management, and fitness safety responsibilities. As one author stated, "competence is not about mileage or years; it's about demonstrating abilities in a confident manner. A deep knowledge and

KEY POINT

Obtaining a strong knowledge base comes from "high quality" formal education and related practical "hands-on" training. The practical training needs to be under the supervision of a competent and dedicated exercise professional who can provide valuable learning experiences involving major job tasks and responsibilities including those regarding legal/risk management and fitness safety.

understanding a person has gained within a period of time is what defines them as experienced and ultimately competent for their line of work" (35).

Future Directions: Academics and Licensure

Academics. A survey (36) of more than 32,000 students at 43 randomly-selected four-year institutions revealed that only one-third of students believed they will have the knowledge and skills to be successful in the workplace. In a 2019 report (37), provosts of public colleges reported that their institutions did not prepare students for the real world (e.g., only 41% identified student outcomes and only 25% assessed student outcomes). Most students attend college to obtain the necessary credentials to qualify for professional positions upon graduation. They expect their academic programs to provide the necessary knowledge and skills to adequately prepare them for jobs in the workplace. This should be **the** number one objective of academic programs in exercise science (or related areas). This objective is met if the coursework reflects the many job responsibilities of fitness managers and exercise professionals and if the faculty members truly care about the student's success. There are many published articles addressing the importance of improving college education. For example, an article titled "The Imperative to Improve College Learning" helps explain this issue (37).

As described above and inferred throughout this textbook, there are major challenges facing the exercise profession when preparing professionals for their many job and legal responsibilities. These challenges are evident when academic programs are not offering important coursework and practical experiences needed for most professional jobs and when certification examinations do not require any formal education and practical training as eligibility requirements to take the examination. Until these challenges are addressed, it will be the employer's responsibility to provide the education and training needed for exercise professionals to successfully carry out their many job and legal responsibilities.

There may be little incentive, at least from a legal perspective, to address these challenges in academic and certification programs. It is unlikely that educational programs provided by academic institutions and certifying organizations will be held liable for the failure to provide adequate education and training. There is no real educational malpractice, yet. However, it is evident from court rulings that employers can be liable for the negligent conduct of their employees and for their failure to properly hire credentialed and competent exercise professionals as well as failures to train and supervise their employees. Employers, obviously, have an incentive to encourage academic and certification preparation programs to make improvements in, and standardize, their educational and training programs. It may be in the future that such a "direct call to action" will be made by employers.

Generally, courts have rejected claims of educational malpractice claims, which are most often brought under the theory of negligence (38). In these cases, courts have provided policy reasons against allowing claims/lawsuits for educational malpractice under the theory of negligence such as "the fear of a potential flood of litigation against schools…the fear that an educational malpractice cause of action could entangle the courts into overseeing the day-to-day operations of schools, which might be particularly inappropriate in the university setting due to considerations of academic freedom and autonomy" (38, p. 111). Given these practical and policy reasons, courts have stated that common-law tort remedy (i.e., negligence) is not the best way to address the problem of inadequate education (38).

It is difficult to know why academic programs in exercise science (or related areas) often do not have their students complete courses that will best prepare them for their many job responsibilities including legal, risk management, and fitness safety responsibilities. It may be that the academicians who teach in these programs have never worked as a fitness manager or exercise professional in the "real world" and, thus, do not have a good

KEY POINT

It is unlikely the educational preparation programs (e.g., academic, non-academic, certification) will be liable for their failure to provide adequate education/training (educational malpractice). However, employers can be found liable for the negligent conduct of their employees as well as their failure to properly hire, train, and/or supervise their employees.

understanding or appreciation of what professionals do daily. In addition, it is likely that academicians have never had a Fitness Law/Risk Management course in their own educational preparation programs, so they might not realize the importance of such a course. Another possible reason is best stated by an exercise physiology academician who believes that academic exercise physiologists focus too much on their research. He states:

> They believe there isn't anything else but research…Their academic life is to teach as little as possible…Why, more often than not, they are products of unsound thinking at the administrative level…the problem with such thinking is that the students get left out…Their education is not what it should be (39, p. 3).

This academician also stated that even if exercise physiology professors would consider changing their thinking in this regard, many would not be interested in doing so (39).

It is important to note, though, that these same professors often involve their students in all aspects of their research which provides students with excellent learning experiences to gain an appreciation of the importance of research. However, in addition to developing research skills, acquiring relevant "program evaluation" skills is equally as important if not more important. Exercise professionals who pursue jobs in fitness facilities will have oversight of many fitness/wellness programs. It is unlikely that most professionals working in these settings will be conducting research on a regular basis but will (or should be) continually conducting program evaluation at the process, impact, and outcome levels. Program evaluation skills are essential to design and deliver high quality, safe and effective programs. Therefore, if students are not exposed to coursework in this area, they will likely not have the knowledge and skills on how to properly collect evaluation data and then use the data for decision-making, improvement of program quality, and accountability. Similar program evaluation skills are also needed to evaluate the comprehensive risk management plan (discussed in Chapter 2) for the facility. As listed in Exhibit 5-1, a course that focuses on planning and evaluation of fitness/wellness programs should be seriously considered and incorporate frameworks such as RE-AIM (40).

Licensure. If the exercise profession pursues licensure for degreed exercise physiologists, following the athletic training model may be a wise approach. To apply this model, consistency will be needed among the domains and competencies for CAAHEP accreditation, the domains and competencies for a national board examination, and the required academic coursework that reflects the domains and competencies. In 2017, the following five organizations adopted the CAAHEP accreditation standards and guidelines for undergraduate programs in exercise science (8):

- American College of Sports Medicine
- American Council on Exercise
- American Kinesiotherapy Association
- National Academy of Sports Medicine
- National Council on Strength & Fitness

It would be wise to invite other professional organizations such as ASEP to adopt these accreditation standards. It will be essential to obtain universal support as the profession moves forward with licensure.

In addition to having consistency among the domains and competencies for accreditation, certification, and academic coursework, there will need to be an "independent" national board examination. Neither the ACSM nor the ASEP examinations are independent. To make licensure a reality for exercise physiologists, strong leadership from professional organizations will be needed. Leaders need to step up to make a genuine, concerted effort to work together for the common good and advancement of the profession. A major difference between the athletic training and exercise professions is that athletic training has one major professional organization (National Athletic Trainers' Association), whereas, there are many organizations in the exercise profession. To effectively achieve the goal of licensure, there will need to be buy-in and commitment from all the major professional organizations.

A first logical step, for the leaders within these professional organizations, would be to review the CAAHEP domains/competencies (8)—these competencies would help determine the coursework needed for programs to become accredited as well as serve as the basis for the national board examination. The undergraduate competencies under Domains IV (legal/professional) and V (management) are quite comprehensive and cover many of the major legal liability exposures that exist in fitness programs and facilities as well as risk management strategies to minimize legal liability exposures. They also reflect content provided in this textbook. Examples of competencies under the Legal/Professional and Management domains include:

- Skill in developing…a policy and procedures manual (IV.A.2.a).
- Skill in maintenance of a safe exercise environment… (IV.A.2.c).
- Skill in applying policies, practices and guidelines to efficiently hire, train, supervise… employees (V.A.2.a).
- Knowledge of accepted guidelines, standards, and regulations…for the management of… facilities (V.C.1.a).
- Knowledge of federal, state…laws as they relate to…management (V.C.1.e) (8, pp. 21, 23).

There are 32 competencies under Domain IV and 31 competencies under Domain V. Specific academic courses, such as those listed in Exhibit 5-1, are needed to adequately cover these many competencies, which reflect many of the daily job responsibilities of fitness managers and exercise professionals. None of the above competencies can be adequately covered in a one-hour lecture.

Once the review of the CAAHEP domains and competencies is completed, there will be several other tasks that will need to be completed before a national board certification examination could be offered. This certification could serve as *the* credential needed for state licensure as is the case with athletic training's national Board of Certification (BOC) examination which is the credential that is specified in state licensure statutes. Having one national board certification as the licensing credential would allow exercise professionals to practice in other states without having to obtain individual state credentials which could vary from state to state. However, some states could have additional requirements specified in the statute that are needed for licensure.

Pursuing licensure for clinical exercise physiologists could take a similar approach by first reviewing the CAAHEP competencies for graduate programs (8). There are six domains under the clinical exercise physiology track with Domain VI covering legal and professional responsibilities. The other graduate track, applied exercise physiology, has five domains with Domain V covering legal and professional responsibilities. Neither of these tracks include a "management" domain as they did in prior years. Many exercise professionals who want to obtain a master's degree do so to be eligible or competitive for advanced positions in the field. In addition to courses that cover the competencies in the domains, courses in management including risk management are essential in preparing exercise professionals for these advanced positions. To stay abreast of legislature efforts involving licensure of clinical exercise physiologists, see the website for the Clinical Exercise Physiologist Association (CEPA): https://www.acsm-cepa.org/.

Future Directions: Certification, Accreditation, and Continuing Education

While licensure for personal fitness trainers and group exercise instructors is unlikely and most certifications, including those that are accredited, do not require any practical "hands-on" training, it is predicted that a high number of unnecessary injuries and subsequent litigation will continue. If the profession desires to change these negative outcomes and remain self-regulated regarding personal fitness trainers and group exercise leaders, one option is to consider a model that was successfully implemented by the health and wellness coaching profession. A published article (41) describes the many steps involved in this model as well as the challenges to obtain a consensus among so many diverse individuals and organizations. These steps, that began in 2010 and were completed in 2017, included developing a 3-pronged mission statement based on research and best practices, conducting a JTA to help form the learning domains and competencies, developing education and training standards as well as the national board certification examination. This professional

Figure 5-4: Outcomes of a Job Task Analysis: Professional Model (5)*

(Formal education and practical skills training are required prior to taking a national board certification examination)

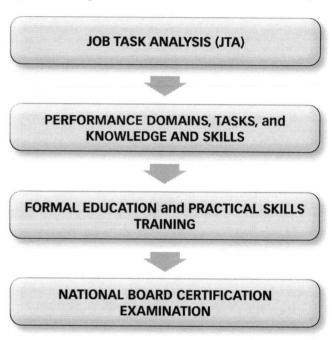

model (see Figure 5-4) is similar to those used to prepare allied health professionals for licensure, which requires formal education and practical training "before" sitting for a national certification examination.

The website of the National Board for Health & Wellness Coaches (42) describes the specific eligibility requirements for the national board examination. Requirements include: (a) an associate degree or higher in any field or 4000 documented hours of health and wellness coaching work experience, (b) completion of an approved education and training program, and (c) a coaching log after passing the Practical Skills Assessment. Once all requirements are met, an individual is eligible to take the national board certification examination and earn the title: National Board Certified Health & Wellness Coach (NBC-HWC). Given the education and training requirements, it is likely that coaches will feel quite confident and well-prepared to be a "competent" coach upon passing the national board examination. There are several standards that approved education and training programs must meet. They are described on the website: https://nbhwc.org/.

This national certification is, obviously, the credential that employers would seek out when hiring health and wellness coaches versus individuals who possess a health and wellness coaching certification that only requires passing a written examination. Given the rigor to earn this certification, employers can be somewhat confident that the prospective employee has the necessary knowledge and skills to provide safe and effective coaching. It also creates less of a burden for employers to provide basic education and training regarding the knowledge and skills needed for coaching. The commitment among all the stakeholders who persevered through this lengthy process are commended. Their commitment to high standards has significantly advanced the health and wellness coaching profession and credibility among health care professionals.

It is interesting to note that personal injury and subsequent litigation resulting from health and wellness coaching is less likely than litigation from leading exercise programs. Health and wellness coaches can be liable for negligence if the advice or instruction they provide to a client results in harm to that client. They may even face criminal charges if their practice crosses over into a licensed profession. However, there does not appear to be much case law in this area. The goal to develop high standards and a national board examination was clearly to advance the reputation and creditability of the profession, more so than to address issues of injuries and litigation. If the exercise profession would consider a similar model, it would not only advance the reputation and credibility of the profession, but it would, likely, lead to a decrease in the number of injuries and subsequent litigation, especially given the practical skills training and formal assessment of practical skills required in this model. Some exercise professional organizations offer one-day or two-day workshops that are provided in an instructor-led, live format or online programs to help individuals prepare for a certification examination. However, it is difficult with these approaches to provide adequate practical training and assessment of practical skills.

It is unlikely that leading exercise professionals and organizations will come together to complete all the lengthy steps that would lead to a national board examination for personal fitness trainers and group exercise leaders requiring formal education and practical training. Too many in the field believe that practical training and assessment of practical skills is not necessary. Some have stated that practical examinations are too costly, create a burden for candidates, and could not be designed to be fair and unbiased (43). Isn't it time to consider the individuals who have experienced a serious injury due to the negligent acts (incompetence) of an exercise professional or practitioner? What about their costs and burdens, not to mention the costs/burdens of the victim's family members? As demonstrated in the many negligent cases described in this textbook, the serious injuries and deaths that occurred could have been prevented by simply having credentialed and "competent" personnel.

Leaders within certifying professional organizations that truly care about this on-going and growing problem could address this problem and set their professional organization apart from the many other organizations that now have accredited certifications. Accredited certification examinations initially distinguished those from the fly-by-night certifications, but it may now be time to distinguish accredited certification examinations. As Dr. Anthony Abbott stated, the "concept of accreditation has lost most of its value" (3, p. 100). Accredited examinations vary in measuring the depth of the individual's knowledge so, obviously, some are better than others, but how do candidates and employers know how to distinguish the many accredited certifications?

Certifying organizations that have NCCA accreditation can require formal education and practical training

KEY POINT

Some commentators in the exercise profession have stated that having practical examinations, in addition to written examinations, to become certified would be too costly, create a burden for candidates, and could not be designed to be fair and unbiased (43). However, what about the individuals who experienced a serious injury due to the incompetence of an exercise professional? What about their costs and burdens not to mention the costs/burdens of the victim's family? Many injuries, as demonstrated in the negligence cases described in this textbook, could have been prevented by having only **competent** personnel design/deliver exercise programs.

as a prerequisite to sit for the examination under NCCA Standard 3: Education, Training, and Certification. It states, "If education/training is a prerequisite for taking the certification examination, a certification program may require graduation from, or completion of, a program accredited or approved by an accrediting or approval body independent from the certification board" (9, p. 9). This is an option for leading professional organizations to consider that would establish standards that almost all other professions and vocations have (i.e., formal education and practical training requirements *before* taking a certification examination). Certifications that have education and practical training requirements would eventually become the certifications that employers would seek out. It also would be *the* certification that true professionals would want to possess because it would set them apart for all the others that have typical accredited certifications.

Continuing Education: Distinguishing Between Certificate and Certification

Most certifications in the exercise profession require continuing education credits (CECs) or continuing education units (CEUs) to keep certifications current. Certified professionals can earn CECs and CEUs in a variety of ways (e.g., completing all types of courses, participation in conferences and workshops, and passing a quiz after reading an approved article). All of the continuing education options first need to be "approved" by the certifying organization. Too often, exercise professionals opt for what is the easiest and quickest way to earn their CECs/CEUs. It might be wise in the future to require a set number of CECs or CEUs that address certain topics such as ethics, updates on safety standards and laws, and reviews/updates on safe methods of teaching, training, and coaching.

Often, there is confusion between a certificate and a certification. It is important to realize that after successfully completing continuing education programs, the professional often receives a "certificate" of completion. This is distinct from a "certification" as described by the NCCA (44). A certification "assesses knowledge, skills, or competencies previously acquired" and is broad in scope, whereas a certificate program "provides instruction and training" to acquire specific knowledge, skills, or competencies and is narrow in scope (44, p. 1). In addition, a certification requires the completion of a proctored examination that is closed-book and a certificate may require completion of some sort of an examination, but, it is not proctored and is open-book. Most certifying organizations make these distinctions clear on their websites. However, some organizations refer to certifications on their websites, but are actually certificate programs. This is confusing for professionals who might not understand the differences and to employers if professionals are not stating these credentials, correctly, on their resumes.

ASSESSMENT OF LEGAL LIABILITY EXPOSURES

Assessment of Legal Liability Exposures Development of Risk Management Strategies Implementation of the Comprehensive Risk Management Plan Evaluation of the Comprehensive Risk Management Plan

Employment law is quite complex and there are many employment laws and regulations that employers must follow. Chapter 3 focuses on these laws, but this chapter and other chapters also address some of these laws. It is recommended that fitness managers as well as exercise professionals working in a supervisory role take a course in employment law, human resource management, and/or familiarize themselves with labor law resources provided by the federal government (45) and books such as *The Employer's Legal Handbook* (46). As employment issues arise, consultation with a competent lawyer is needed.

The discussion above described various issues and challenges facing the exercise profession related to preparing credentialed and competent fitness managers and exercise professionals. The next section will focus on liability exposures facing employers and describe lawsuits involving employers that will help explain these liability exposures. Various other legal issues regarding independent contractors, vendors, and other personnel will also be discussed along with liability insurance issues.

Vicarious and Direct Liability of Employers

Employers have a vested interest to hire credentialed and competent employees because they can be held liable for the negligent acts of their employees while performing their jobs through a legal doctrine called **respondeat superior** that imposes **vicarious liability** on an employer, a form of strict liability. This is evident in almost all the cases described throughout this textbook in which the fitness facility (employer) was named as a defendant based on an employee's negligent conduct. Plaintiffs can also make claims against an employer based on **direct liability** of the employer such as negligent hiring, which is different from vicarious liability of an employer. This was demonstrated in the *Baldi-Perry v. Kaifas and 360 Fitness Center, Inc.* (47) case described in Chapter 2. The plaintiff filed several negligence claims against the facility (employer) for their hiring, training and supervision failures such as:

- Failing to have trainers who were certified and/ or trained to conduct a proper pre-activity screening;
- Negligently hiring trainers who were not qualified to design exercise programs for individuals with injuries;

- Failing to offer appropriate and necessary training to physical trainers;
- Failing to ensure trainers followed internal rules, employee manuals, regulations, and operating and training procedures (pp. 9-10).

The jury returned a large verdict of $1.4 million in favor of the plaintiff in this case. See Table 5-5 for additional examples of these types of direct liability claims made by plaintiffs against fitness facilities.

In negligent hiring lawsuits, as with all negligent lawsuits, the plaintiff will have to prove four elements: (a) the defendant had a legal duty, (b) the duty was breached, (c) the breach of duty caused the injury, and (d) harm/damages. One duty requires an employer to inquire about the competence and credentials of the prospective employee. For example, when "hiring someone for a position that may expose customers or others to danger, you [the employer] must use special care in checking references and other background information" (46, p. 11). Courts will investigate various factors to determine if an employer is liable for negligent hiring.

In *Bartlett v. Push to Walk* (48), spotlight case in Chapter 7, the employer was not liable for negligent hiring. The court stated, "New Jersey courts recognize the tort of negligent hiring where the employer either knew or should have known that the employee was violent or aggressive, or that the employee might engage in injurious conduct toward third persons" (p. 8). The employer had no prior knowledge or evidence of such conduct by the employee (an exercise professional) or any intentional acts committed by the employee.

Table 5-5	Spotlight Cases: Direct Liability Claims Against Fitness Facilities for Failing to Properly Hire, Train, and Supervise Employees
SPOTLIGHT CASE (CHAPTER)	**CLAIMS AGAINST THE FACILITY (EMPLOYER)**
Bartlett v. Push to Walk (7)	Negligent hiring of an exercise professional
Vaid v. Equinox (8)	Negligent retention and supervision of a personal fitness trainer
Lotz v. The Claremont Club (8)	Negligent hiring, training, and supervision of an employee leading a children's activity
Butler v. Saville et al. (9)	Negligent provision of properly trained and qualified fitness trainers
Miller v. YMCA of Central Massachusetts et al. (10)	Negligent training and supervision of employees regarding steam room safety
Locke v. Life Time Fitness, Inc. (11)	Negligent training of employees on how to respond to emergencies

Although the negligent and gross negligent conduct of the exercise professional was the cause of the injury in this case, the injury was not due to negligent hiring. However, the employer was liable for the gross negligent acts of the employee based on vicarious liability.

KEY POINT

Employers have a vested interest to hire only credentialed and competent employees because they can be held *vicariously* liable for the negligent conduct of their employees through a legal doctrine called respondeat superior. They also can be *directly* liable for failing to properly hire, train and supervise their employees.

Criminal Background Checks

Criminal background checks will determine an applicant's criminal convictions (not arrests). They are important because they can help minimize potential civil claims associated with negligent hiring. Employers will be able to show they took reasonable efforts to determine an employee's history. Whether a criminal background check is needed will depend on various factors including the nature of the job. For example, conducting criminal background checks may be needed for employees who will be leading exercise programs for vulnerable populations such as children, older adults, and persons with disabilities (1). In some cases, it may also be necessary to conduct criminal background checks on employees who will have one-on-one relationships with participants such as personal fitness trainers, massage therapists, and coaches working in athletic programs (1). For example, in *Elena Myers Court v. Loews Philadelphia Hotel, Inc.* (49), the court stated that the defendant gym should have taken action to follow-up on the criminal records and employment history of a massage therapist versus solely relying on his massage therapist license which was in good standing based on self-reporting requirements. The massage therapist's past would have put the defendant gym on notice for his propensity for sexual violence. The court ruled that: (a) the defendant gym breached its duty to conduct a reasonable pre-employment investigation, (b) the

breach caused the injuries to the plaintiff, and (c) the plaintiff may include punitive damages.

Government agencies and private employers can perform background checks when hiring an employee. The Federal Bureau of Investigation (FBI) provides contact information for state agencies that conduct background checks (50) and the FBI website has information on how to request a federal background check (51). Certain laws may apply when conducting background checks. For example, the Fair Credit Reporting Act requires providing a copy of the investigative report to the applicant if it is decided not to hire the applicant based on the findings in the report (46).

Employer Liability and Criminal Acts Including Sexual Misconduct

The legal principle of respondeat superior applies when an employee conducts a negligent act while preforming his/her job duties. Committing a criminal act is not within the scope of an employee's employment. Therefore, imposing vicarious liability on an employer will be very difficult. Legal claims/lawsuits regarding employees who commit criminal acts are most often based on negligent hiring (e.g., hiring a known sex offender as a personal trainer or massage therapist) and negligent supervision.

In the following spotlight case, *Jessica H. v. Equinox Holdings, Inc.*, the employer was not found liable through vicarious liability or for negligent hiring, retention, and supervision. This case dealt with sexual assault allegations made by the plaintiff client against her personal fitness trainer. This case clarified that the key issue regarding vicarious liability for an employee's criminal conduct is foreseeability. The key issue regarding negligent hiring, supervision, and retention is whether the employer knew (or should have known) about the employee's tendency for committing such conduct. In this case, the employer did not know of the trainer's conduct until after he was fired for a different reason.

Negative Outcomes: Failing to Address Sexual Misconduct

Sexual misconduct includes sexual assault and rape. States may define these terms differently, but generally,

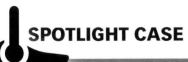

SPOTLIGHT CASE

Jessica H. v. Equinox Holdings, Inc.
No. 103866/08, 2010 LEXIS 1215 (N.Y. Misc., 2010)

FACTS

Historical Facts:

The plaintiff, Jessica H., agreed to a personal training arrangement with Equinox employee, Shalmaine Locaino, in which she would pay him $40 for each training session. This rate was about one-half of what Equinox charged and they both understood that this would circumvent Equinox's personal training contract. After training with Locaino once a week for the first year, she began training with him twice a week and then three-four times per week in both private and group trainings. Plaintiff alleged that Locaino sexually assaulted her 12 times and raped her on the 13th occurrence. The plaintiff testified that in the last 15-20 minutes of a private training session, Locaino would have her go to a spa room on a different floor and it was there where he would pull down her tights and exercise shorts and sexually assault her. The plaintiff never informed anyone what had happened "because she felt ashamed…and also understood that she was paying Locaino 'under the table' and was afraid of having her membership revoked, a fear on which, allegedly, Locaino played" (p. 5). After these occurrences, she continued training with Locaino. It wasn't until Locaino was terminated by Equinox, for an unrelated reason (dishonesty), that the plaintiff informed the manager at Equinox about what had happened. The manager insisted she report the occurrences to the police, which she did.

Procedural Facts:

The plaintiff filed a complaint against the defendants Locaino and Equinox that included allegations of sexual assaults committed by Locaino, vicarious liability based on the doctrine of respondeat superior, negligent supervision, hiring and retention. The defendants filed a motion for summary judgment.

ISSUE

Should the motion for summary judgment be awarded to the defendants?

COURT'S RULING

Yes, summary judgment was granted to the defendants regarding allegations of vicarious liability as well as negligent hiring, retention, and supervision.

COURT'S REASONING

Regarding **vicarious liability** and relying on previous case law, the court stated:

> The doctrine of respondeat superior renders an employer vicariously liable for torts committed by an employee acting within the scope of the employment. Pursuant to this doctrine, the employer may be liable when the employee acts negligently or intentionally, so long as the tortious conduct is generally fore-seeable and a natural incident of the employment. If, however, an employee 'for purposes of his own departs from the line of his duty so that for the time being his acts constitute an abandonment of his service, the master is not lia-ble.' Assuming plaintiff's allegations of sexual abuse are true, it is clear that the employee here departed from his duties for solely personal motives unre-lated to the furtherance of Equinox's business (p. 11).

Jessica H. continued...

Sexual assault is not within the scope of employment and, therefore, an employer cannot be held vicariously liable for criminal acts unless the acts are foreseeable. Because it was after Locaino was terminated that Equinox was informed of his conduct, there was no notice of foreseeability.

Regarding **direct liability**—negligent hiring, retention, and supervision the court stated:

> In those instances where an employer cannot be held vicariously liable for torts committed by its employee, the employer can still be held liable under theories of negligent hiring and negligent retention. The negligence of the employer in such a case is direct, not vicarious, and arises from its having placed the employee in a position to cause foreseeable harm from which the injured party most probably would have been spared had the employer taken reasonable care in making its decision concerning the hiring and retention of the employee. An essential element of a cause of action for negligent hiring and retention is that the employer knew, or should have known, or the employee's propensity for the sort of conduct which caused the injury (pp. 12-13).

When hiring Locaino, Equinox did not conduct a criminal investigation because there was nothing in his application indicating that further investigation was necessary. The court stated there is no common-law duty for further investigation unless the employer knew of facts that would warrant such an investigation. Had Equinox performed such an investigation, it would have found there was nothing in Locaino's background that would have put Equinox on notice of such conduct, as determined after this lawsuit was filed. Regarding negligent retention, the court clarified that it is not viable in sexual abuse cases "unless the employer had notice of prior allegations of an employee's improper conduct and failed to investigate the allegations" (p. 12). Similarly, for negligent supervision, the court stated that the plaintiff's allegations failed based on the issue of notice.

NOTE: The plaintiff filed a motion to have the court reargue this case. See *Jessica H. v. Equinox Holdings, Inc.,* 2010 N.Y. Misc. LEXIS 1864. She argued that further discovery was needed. However, the court indicated that her argument was completely meritless. The defendant Equinox fully responded to all discovery requests and orders prior to making its motion for summary judgment by producing nearly 750 pages of documents. The plaintiff had ample opportunity to raise this issue in her opposition papers to the summary judgment motion and she failed to do so.

Lessons Learned from *Jessica H.*

Legal
- Under the doctrine of respondeat superior, employers can be found liable for the negligent act(s) of an employee if the negligent act(s) occurred within the scope of the employee's job responsibilities.

- Because sexual assault or other criminal acts committed by an employee are not within the employee's scope of employment, employers cannot be held liable for these acts under vicarious liability unless they failed to investigate the acts after becoming aware of them—foreseeability is an important factor.

- Although conducting criminal background checks may not be a common law duty, they might be if facts obtained in the hiring process warranted such an investigation.

- A victim of sexual assault can file criminal charges against the wrong-doer (e.g., file a report with the police) and file a civil lawsuit against the defendants (e.g., intentional tort, negligence)

Risk Management/Injury Prevention
- Managers need to establish and follow proper hiring procedures which may include conducting criminal background investigations, especially with prospective employees who will be working with vulnerable populations (children, elderly, disabled) as well as those working closely with participants such as personal fitness trainers and massage therapists.

Jessica H. continued...

▶ Once an employee/employer becomes aware of sexual misconduct or other criminal acts committed by an employee, independent contractor, vendor, volunteer, or participant, an immediate investigation must take place. It is recommended to consult with legal counsel when establishing the steps in such an investigation.

▶ Upon hiring, managers need to train all employees on the facility's code of conduct as well as policies and procedures that need to be followed while on the job, including locations allowed (and not allowed) for training participants, procedures for payment of services, etc. and inform them of the consequences of not following the facility's code of conduct and policies and procedures.

▶ Managers and program supervisors need to continually supervise their employees and the activities taking place in the facility and take immediate corrective action if they notice any wrong-doing or risks.

▶ Include, perhaps in the membership agreement, that if, as a participant, they observe/experience any criminal conduct, to report it to management immediately.

▶ Document hiring, training, supervision procedures and store documents in a secure location.

sexual assault is unwanted sexual contact that stops short of rape and rape is forced sexual intercourse. Both reflect criminal conduct as well as intentional torts. An individual who commits such conduct can be charged criminally and face civil lawsuits. Once such conduct is brought to the attention of an employee or an employee's supervisor, it is essential, from a legal liability perspective, for the employer to take immediate action to investigate the allegation, and perhaps consult with a competent lawyer. Allegations of sexual harassment (discussed in Chapter 3), another form of sexual misconduct, also need to be addressed immediately. In addition to the traumatic experience suffered by the victim(s), there are many negative outcomes for employers who fail to address sexual misconduct.

A couple of litigations, the Jerry Sandusky cases at Penn State University and the Larry Nassar cases at USA Gymnastics and Michigan State University, received a lot of negative media coverage. If the sexual assaults committed by these individuals had been resolved when they were first reported many years prior, the negative outcomes for these institutions would have been far less. But the alleged sexual assaults and cover-ups continued. In addition to the negative media coverage, the financial losses such as the monies paid out in settlements and fines were significant. Penn State University paid out over $250 million (52) and Michigan State University announced $500 million in payments to victims—the largest payout in history related to a university sexual abuse scandal (53). These settlements are large, but if

these cases had gone to trial, they likely would have resulted in verdicts totaling much more. Of course, the perpetrators, Sandusky and Nassar are serving very long jail sentences for their horrendous crimes against children. Some individuals (e.g., coaches, athletic directors, and administrators) allegedly involved in the cover ups in these institutions lost their jobs and, in some cases, were convicted of child endangerment and sentenced to serve time in jail (54). USA Gymnastics filed bankruptcy due to facing 100 lawsuits from more than 350 sexual-assault victims (55).

To help address these abuses, the U.S. Center for SafeSport was opened in March 2017 and the Protecting Young Victims from Sexual Abuse and Safe Sport Authorization Act was signed into law on February 14, 2018 (56). An article written by Nancy Hogshead-Maker, an Olympic gold medalist swimmer, lawyer, and CEO of Champion Women (legal advocacy organization for girls and women in sport) titled "How to Stop Sexual Abuse in Sports" provides a brief overview/history of this important issue and how she has advocated for change (57). Also see: *Staying in Bounds: An NCAA Model Policy to Prevent Inappropriate Relationships Between Student-Athletes and Athletic Department Personne*l at: https://www.ncaa.org/sites/default/files/Staying%2Bin%2B-Bounds%2BFinal.pdf.

Sexual misconduct prevails throughout all sectors of society. As the "MeToo" movement gained visibility in 2017, so did the firing of many prominent individuals who were accused of sexual misconduct with co-workers or others. Sexual misconduct in athletic/sport settings often receives a great deal of media coverage, as did the Sandusky and Nassar cases. Below are just a few headlines of such stories involving collegiate athletic programs covered in the *Athletic Business E-Newsletter* in September and October 2018 and May and September 2019.

1. New Mexico Settles with Alleged Victim for $200K (September 2018)
   (alleged gang rape by athletes)
2. Report: NCAA Serves Baylor of Notice of Allegations (October 2018)
   (125 sexual assault cases, 2011-2015, many involving football players)
3. a) Title IX Lawsuit: Ohio State Failed to Stop Abuse, and b) School Knew of Ex-Ohio State Team Doctor's Abuse (May 2019)
   (abuse by now-deceased Ohio State University team doctor Richard Strauss was known by coaches, trainers, other team doctors, and school leaders; at least 177 students sexually abused)
4. Michigan State Fined $4.5M Over Nassar Inaction (September 2018)
   (U.S. Dept. of Education fined the university)

Sexual misconduct cases in athletic programs often involve violations of Title IX. Educational programs or activities that receive Federal financial assistance must comply with Title IX of the Education Amendments Act of 1972, prohibiting discrimination based on sex. The Office of Civil Rights (OCR) enforces Title IX regulations which are quite broad and complex. For an overview of the law and the many Title IX issues the OCR addresses, see Sex Discrimination: Overview of the Law (58).

Federal guidelines from the U.S. Department of Education requires Title IX training for all employees at colleges and universities that need to comply with Title IX (58). Since the Nassar case, Michigan State has focused on three initiatives regarding (a) protecting patients, (b) responding to sexual misconduct, and (c) preventing abuse from happening in the first place (59). Universities and colleges, as well as all employers, should have established policies and procedures regarding sexual misconduct and make concerted efforts to inform and train employees (and other personnel such as contractors, interns, volunteers) of these policies and procedures. Exercise professionals working in collegiate athletic programs or in any fitness setting need to report an incident of sexual misconduct following the reporting procedures in the employer's policies and procedures.

There are also procedures for filing a complaint with the OCR for a Title IX violation. A whistleblower who files such a report may be concerned about retaliation that might follow (e.g., being fired or demoted). However, retaliation is prohibited under Title IX for filing an OCR complaint or for advocating for a right protected by Title IX (58). For example, an athletic director and soccer coach for a college in Minnesota received a $100,000 settlement after he claimed he was removed from his job in retaliation for pointing out Title IX violations (60). For fitness managers and exercise professionals who do not work for an employer who is required to follow Title IX regulations, there are other laws that protect whistleblowers. For example, the federal Whistleblower Protection Act (61) that protects federal employees and state whistleblower statutes such as Florida's Fla. Stat. § 448.102 that protects private-sector employees and Fla. Stat. § 112.3187 that protects public-sector employees.

False Marketing/Deceptive Advertising of Employees' Credentials

Fitness managers need to be sure that their marketing and advertising content regarding the credentials of their employees is truthful. As demonstrated in the spotlight case below, *D'Amico v. L.A. Fitness*, the facility violated a state statute that prohibits deceptive advertising. It is important to realize that participants will rely on the marketing and advertising statements that fitness facilities make about the credentials of their employees. The plaintiff in *D'Amico* believed the defendants when they advertised hiring only persons who were experienced and qualified to provide personal training. The plaintiff set forth sufficient facts to show that the personal fitness trainer was not qualified and experienced and that his lack of credentials and competence led to her injury.

Exercise professionals need to be truthful when they promote their credentials on resumes, business cards, Internet sites, social media, etc. For example, if a professional promotes himself/herself as a "clinical exercise physiologist", it will be essential that he/she has the credentials (e.g., degree, certification) to support that title because a prospective client with a medical condition(s) will rely on this expertise when deciding to hire the professional. If the client is injured because the professional did not possess the advanced knowledge and skills necessary to safely design and deliver a program, given the client's medical condition, the exercise professional could face a negligence lawsuit. The exercise professional could also face charges involving violations of state deceptive advertising statutes as well as possible federal laws dealing with unfair or deceptive acts or practices, such as the Federal Trade Commission Act (FTCA). More information regarding the FTCA is provided in Chapter 3.

Academic programs need be sure that the marketing of their programs is not deceptive or misleading. For example, if a program states on its website that their undergraduate exercise science program helps prepare students for national certifications such as ACSM and NSCA, then it will be important that the coursework is designed to do so, and that it covers the competencies associated with the certifications. When deciding which academic program to attend, prospective students will rely on this type of information and assume it is truthful.

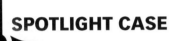

SPOTLIGHT CASE

D'Amico v. LA Fitness
57 Conn. L. Rptr. 242, 2013 WL 6912912 (Conn. Super. Ct., 2013)

FACTS

Historical Facts:

The plaintiff, on the same day she joined defendant LA Fitness, purchased a personal training package from defendant Pro Results. She received five or six personal training sessions all without incident. The plaintiff alleged that on January 25, 2010 she was assigned a new trainer who instructed her to do an intensive exercise, although she advised the trainer that she did not feel safe nor comfortable doing it. Despite her objections, she continued to perform the exercise as directed by her trainer but "was unable to maintain control of herself and her right arm and shoulder twisted violently" (p. 1). The plaintiff claimed the injuries she suffered were a direct result of the employee's actions in instructing her to perform the exercise routine.

Procedural Facts:

The defendants filed a motion for summary judgment in March 2012 on all four counts in the plaintiff's complaint. In her first two counts, the plaintiff claimed the defendants were negligent for failing to (a) properly assess her fitness level and recommending the exercise routine that caused her injury, and (b) properly supervise their employees and/or agents who recommended it. The defendants argued the plaintiff's action against them was not until March 12, 2012, and, therefore, did not commence within the two years of the date of the injury (or discovery of the injury) required by Connecticut General Statutes **§ 52-584** as follows, in part:

> No action to recover damages for injury to the person, or to real or personal property, caused by **negligence,** or by reckless or wanton misconduct...shall be brought but within two years from the date when the injury is first sustained or discovered or in the exercise of reasonable care should have been discovered, and except that no such action may be brought more than three years from the date of the act or omission complained off... (p. 2).

In her third and fourth counts, she stated the defendants held themselves as having "experience and expertise in providing physical fitness and personal training facilities", but "employed and retained inexperienced and and/or unqualified

D'Amico continued...

personnel to supply personal training services" (p. 1). The plaintiff alleged that the defendants violated the Connecticut Unfair Trade Practices Act (CUTPA) because they acted deceptively in the conduct of a trade or business.

ISSUES

1) Were the legal proceedings on the first two counts of negligence initiated within the two-year statute of limitations?

2) Regarding the third and fourth counts: did the defendants violate the CUTPA by deceptively advertising the qualifications and experience of their staff members engaged in personal training?

COURT'S RULING

1) No, legal proceedings were not commenced within two years of the date of injury. Summary judgment was granted for the first two counts.

2) Yes, the defendants were found in violation of the CUTPA. Summary judgment was denied for the third and fourth counts.

COURT'S REASONING

The plaintiff testified that she sought medical attention four days after the incident on January 25, 2010. The court stated that "the plaintiff knew or should have known that the incident which caused the injuries gave rise to this action occurred on January 25, 2010. The statute of limitations therefore began to run on that date and her action was not timely commenced" (p. 4).

Regarding violations of the CUTPA, the court referred to General Statutes § 42-110b, which in part states, "No person shall engage in unfair methods of competition and unfair or deceptive acts or practices in the conduct of any trade or commerce" (p. 4). The court considered three factors based on a rule, established in previous cases, to determine if the defendants' practices were unfair: "(1) whether the practice, without necessarily having been previously considered unlawful, offends public policy as it has been established by statutes, the common law, or otherwise… (2) whether it is immoral, unethical, oppressive or unscrupulous; (3) whether it causes substantial injury to consumers (or competitors or other businessmen)" (p. 4). A practice may be unfair by meeting one criteria to a high degree or meeting two or three criteria to a lesser degree. In this case, the court stated all three prongs were met.

The first prong was satisfied because the defendant's practice met the three requirements of deceptive practice: "(1) there must be a representation, omission or other practice likely to mislead consumers; (2) consumers must interpret the message reasonably under the circumstances; and (3) the misleading representation, omission or practice must be material—that is, likely to affect consumer decisions or conduct" (p. 5). The court stated that the second prong was satisfied because the defendants held themselves out as having the experience and qualifications to operate a safe health club facility and that they hired only persons who were experienced and qualified to provide personal training. The plaintiff set forth sufficient facts to show otherwise. The third prong was satisfied because it met the three requirements of the 'substantial injury' test established by the Federal Trade Commission: "(a) the injury is substantial, (b) the harm exceeds any offsetting benefit, and (c) the harm is one that could not reasonably have been avoided by the consumer" (p. 6).

Lessons Learned from *D'Amico:*

Legal

▶ Plaintiffs need to file their complaints within the statutes of limitations. These statutes vary from state to state. In this Connecticut case, it was two years meaning two years from the date the injury was first sustained or reasonably discovered. These statutes can serve as an effective defense for a defendant as in this case.

▶ Advertising the qualifications and experiences of the facility's fitness staff members needs to be truthful to help prevent violations of state statutes involving unfair or deceptive practices. The Federal Trade Commission (FTC) Act also prohibits unfair or deceptive acts or practices.

D'Amico continued...

> ♦ Courts will use various factors from rules or tests such as the 'substantial injury' test analyzed in this case to determine if the defendant violated any unfair or deceptive practices.
>
> **Risk Management/Injury Prevention**
> ♦ Personal fitness trainers need to be 'qualified' (e.g., possess certain credentials) and 'competent' (e.g., possess important knowledge and skills) to help ensure the safety of their clients.
>
> ♦ Personal fitness trainers need to be well-trained on how to conduct a personal training program, e.g., proper screening, testing, prescription, and listening to their clients.
>
> ♦ Direct supervision/evaluation of personal fitness trainers is needed to help ensure they are performing their job tasks safely and effectively. If not, corrective measures may be needed such as re-training.

Legal Liability Issues: Independent Contractors, Vendors, Interns, and Volunteers

Fitness facilities often contract with independent contractors and vendors to provide programs and services to participants. Many facilities also have interns and volunteers who assist with various programs and services. Each will be discussed regarding legal liability issues that fitness managers and exercise professionals need to know to help comply with relevant laws and regulations.

Independent Contractors

Black's Law Dictionary defines an **independent contractor**, in part, as "one who renders service in course of self-employment or occupation, and who follows employer's desires only as to the results of the work" (62, p. 530). Most often, independent contractors are hired because they have certain skills that an employer may need on occasion and to hedge against liability for negligence. In the exercise profession, employers often hire group exercise leaders and personal fitness trainers (and other workers) as independent contractors who provide services on a continual basis. It is essential that fitness managers and exercise professionals understand the potential legal issues associated with hiring independent contractors.

The Internal Revenue Service (IRS) distinguishes independent contractors and employees based on three categories: (a) behavioral control, (b) financial control, and (c) relationship of the parties. See Exhibit 5-3 that describes each of these. If an employer is unsure regarding the classification of a worker, IRS Form SS-8 (63) can be completed and submitted. After review of the form, the IRS will issue a letter as an advisory that may be helpful in determining the worker status of an individual but only for tax purposes (1). Misclassification of an employee as an independent contractor can lead to significant financial costs for the employer. For example, if such misclassification occurs, the employer may be required to pay for contributions and taxes such as (a) Social Security and Medicare contributions of both the employer and employee, and (b) federal and state income tax that should have been withheld from the employee's wages (46). According to IHRSA (64), many health clubs have had to reclassify independent contractors as employees after an audit. Misclassification of workers can cost an employer an average of $3,701.00 per worker in back taxes (64). In addition, employers risk having to pay back wages to independent contractors who were misclassified, if they worked more than 40 hours per week and were not paid overtime as an employee—a violation of the Fair Labor Standards Act (FLSA).

Of the three categories, behavioral control is an especially important factor that fitness managers and exercise professionals need to consider. If an employer directs or controls "how" the worker performs certain tasks, the worker would likely be classified as an employee. In *Donovan v. Unique Racquetball and Health Clubs, Inc.* (65), the court had to determine if "locker room attendants" and "front desk receptionists" were employees, or independent contractors as the defendants claimed (1). The court found that the defendant owner of the corporation was, "in active control and management of defendant corporation, regulated the employment of all persons employed… and thus an employer of said employees" (65, p. 79). The court ordered the defendants to pay almost $135,000 in compensation.

Exhibit 5-3: IRS Publication 1779, In Part*

Independent Contractor or Employee

Which are You?

The courts have considered many facts in deciding whether a worker is an independent contractor or an employee. These relevant facts fall into three main categories: behavioral control; financial control; and relationship of the parties.

Behavioral Control

These facts show whether there is a right to direct or control how the worker does the work. A worker is an employee when the business has the right to direct and control the worker. The business does not have to actually direct or control the way the work is done—as long as the employer has the right to direct and control the work. For example:

Instructions—if you receive extensive instructions on how work is to be done, this suggests that you are an employee. Instructions can cover a wide range of topics, for example:

- how, when, or where to do the work
- what tools or equipment to use
- what assistants to hire to help with the work
- where to purchase supplies and services

If you receive less extensive instructions about what should be done, but not how it should be done, you may be an independent contractor. For instance, instructions about time and place may be less important than directions on how the work is performed.

Training—if the business provides you with training about required procedures and methods, this indicates that the business wants the work done in a certain way, and this suggests that you may be an employee.

Financial Control

These facts show whether there is a right to direct or control the business part of the work. For example:

Significant Investment—if you have a significant investment in your work, you may be an independent contractor. While there is no precise dollar test, the investment must have substance. However, a significant investment is not necessary to be an independent contractor.

Expenses—if you are not reimbursed for some or all business expenses, then you may be an independent contractor, especially if your unreimbursed business expenses are high.

Opportunity for Profit or Loss—if you can realize a profit or incur a loss, this suggests that you are in business for yourself and that you may be an independent contractor.

Relationship of the Parties

These are facts that illustrate how the business and the worker perceive their relationship. For example:

Employee Benefits—if you receive benefits, such as insurance, pension, or paid leave, this is an indication that you may be an employee. If you do not receive benefits, however, you could be either an employee or an independent contractor.

Written Contracts—a written contract may show what both you and the business intend. This may be very significant if it is difficult, if not impossible, to determine status based on other facts.

---

*IRS Independent Contractor or Employee? Available at: https://www.irs.gov/pub/irs-pdf/p1779.pdf. Accessed December 11, 2018.

Vicarious and Direct Liability

Just as employers can be vicariously liable for the negligent acts of their employees and face direct liability claims such as negligent hiring of employees, so can employers who hire independent contractors. However, there are some differences. The general rule regarding vicarious liability is that an employer "who hires an independent contractor is not subject to vicarious liability for physical harm caused by the tortious conduct of the contractor" (66, p. 264). However, there are several exceptions to this general rule that are applicable to fitness facility employers. For example, an employer can be subject to vicarious liability for physical harm if the employer knows or should know that an activity that the contractor is hired to perform poses a particular risk and if the negligent conduct of the contractor was the cause of the harm (66). Obviously, exercise programs pose risks of injury, especially when programs are not deigned/delivered in a safe and effective manner.

An employer can also be vicariously liable when independent contractors appear to be employees or agents of the employer under certain circumstances. For example, when independent contractors provide programs and services at a fitness facility, but the facility does not divulge their status to participants and/or allows independent contractors to wear clothing with the facility's name and logo (1). Participants may believe that the independent contractors are employees and, thus, the employer can be held vicariously liable for the negligent acts of independent contractors based on a legal principle referred to as **ostensible agency.**

Courts will make the determination of the legal status of the worker in negligence lawsuits involving ostensible agents. For example, in *Layden v. Plante* (67), spotlight case in Chapter 7, the appellate court stated that the facility owner "may be held liable only if the trainer's negligence may be imputed under a theory of respondeat superior" (p. 462). The defendant owner claimed the personal fitness trainer was an independent contractor and, thus, there could be no vicarious liability. The court disagreed. To determine if the defendant trainer was an independent contractor, the court stated that this would require an "analysis of the extent of the fitness center's power to regulate the manner in which the trainer performed her work, and the parties' conflicting evidence poses factual questions as to this issue" (p. 462). This was the main reason for barring the motion for summary judgment of the defendant owner and the ruling in favor of the plaintiff. This case demonstrates the importance of behavioral control (i.e., controlling how a worker performs his/her job when determining worker status).

Direct liability is another concern of employers who hire independent contractors. As with hiring employees, employers also have a duty of care when hiring independent contractors to perform an activity (66). The employer's negligence can take various forms including "failure to use reasonable care to select a competent contractor; that is, a contractor who possesses the knowledge, skill, experience…to perform the work without creating unreasonable risk of injury" (66, p. 262). To help avoid direct liability claims, such as negligent hiring of independent contractors, employers will need to take a deep dive into the knowledge/skills of independent contractors before hiring them. Once hired, employers do not have behavioral control of them (e.g., cannot provide them training on how to perform the job). Employers, however, have control over how employees perform their jobs and can provide all types of training to help them properly perform job tasks. Given the wide variation of credentials that exist in the exercise profession, employers will need to fully understand the limitations of these credentials as described earlier, not only when hiring employees, but especially when hiring independent contractors.

Advantages and Disadvantages of Hiring Independent Contractors

There are many advantages to hiring independent contractors such as not having to pay payroll taxes and employee benefits as well as not having to spend time on training them on how to perform job tasks. There may even be a reduced risk of liability if the contractor's negligent conduct causes harm to a participant. However, there are many disadvantages as well, especially if they are misclassified or appear as employees/agents of the employer as discussed above. In addition, if an employer hires both employees and independent contractors, there will likely be inconsistencies in the design and delivery of programs/services to participants. For example, how a personal fitness trainer follows published

KEY POINT

Vicarious and direct liability issues as they apply to independent contractors need to be considered by employers prior to contracting with them. For example, if the employer misclassifies an employee as an independent contractor, the employer may have to pay back taxes and wages. In addition, if participants believe that the independent contractors are employees, the employer can be held vicariously liable for the negligent acts of independent contractors based on a legal principle referred to as **ostensible agency**.

safety standards and guidelines such as pre-activity screening procedures for each client may vary between employees who will be trained (or should be) to follow the facility's procedures and independent contractors who decide on their own on how to conduct screening procedures. Inconsistencies can lead to manager/supervisor frustrations, complaints from participants and staff members as well as create an increased risk of liability. Related to standards of practice, it may be difficult to defend in a court of law why inconsistencies existed within the same facility.

Vendors

Black's Law Dictionary defines a **vendor**, in part, as a "seller of goods or services" (62, p. 1079). There are thousands of vendors in the fitness industry who sell products and services. For example, there are many vendors who contract with businesses to provide all types of programs and services (e.g., employer-sponsored and hospital-based wellness programs including management of in-house fitness centers). There are also vendors who provide services such as personal fitness training, group exercise classes, and massage therapy. Fitness managers and exercise professionals need to consider many criteria before contracting with a vendor, including important legal/risk management criteria. For example, if the employees of the vendors will be providing programs and services for the fitness facility participants, a variety of inquires will need to be made regarding the credentials, insurance, and competence of the vendor's employees. As discussed

above regarding independent contractors, the vendor will likely be the party liable for any negligent acts of its own employees based on vicarious lability or direct liability. However, liability could also extend to a fitness facility, organization, or business that contracts with a vendor if they did not use reasonable care in selecting the vendor. See Exhibit 5-4 for criteria to consider when selecting a fitness and/or wellness vendor.

Interns

Students majoring in exercise science (or a related area) often complete a required internship (or other student work experiences) at various fitness and athletic facilities. Most often, these are unpaid internships. However, in some cases, certain fitness facilities (e.g. for-profit employers) may be required to pay interns in accordance with the FLSA. See Chapter 3 for more on the FLSA and interns.

Regarding legal liability issues, most internship sites and universities/colleges will require the intern to purchase his/her own professional liability insurance. Students can obtain such insurance as a membership benefit of a professional organization or a university/college can purchase blanket professional liability policy that will protect the school, faculty, and students for any negligence actions made against them. The blanket professional liability policy will likely be at a significantly lower premium rate/student than what a student would pay individually through a professional organization. It is important to realize that the internship site could also be liable for the negligent acts of an intern. Therefore, it would be wise to select the best qualified interns (have a structured selection process including an interview) and, most importantly, provide them with adequate training and supervision to help minimize liability.

Volunteers

Volunteers often provide various types of services in fitness facilities. The FLSA provides a definition of "volunteer" as well as regulations related to volunteers in public, non-profit, and for-profit entities. See Chapter 3 for more on the FLSA and volunteers. The federal Volunteer Protection Act (68) provides liability protection for volunteers. The major purpose of this liability

---

Exhibit 5-4: Criteria to Consider When Selecting a Fitness and/or Wellness Vendor *

1. Litigation history (e.g., describe current or previous legal claims or lawsuits against the vendor).

2. Audit history (e.g., describe current or previous audits by a federal, state, or county regulatory agency).

3. Written policies and procedures that demonstrate compliance with applicable federal, state, and local laws as well as published standards of practice. For example, given the prevalence of data breaches, how is the vendor complying with data breach laws?

4. Description of credentials and competence of all staff members, including degrees, certifications, licenses, and years of professional experience, as well as criminal background checks conducted prior to hiring.

5. Description of all staff trainings that are designed to help staff members comply with applicable laws and published standards of practice.

6. Verification that programs/services are based on best practices.

7. Description of the risk management advisory committee and/or medical advisory board and/or medical director.

8. Willingness to indemnify.

9. Verification of insurance (e.g., general and professional liability, workers' compensation, ratings of insurance providers).

10. Description of quality control procedures related to the safety and effectiveness of any equipment used or provided.

---

protection is to encourage individuals to volunteer their services in nonprofit and government entities. The Volunteer Protection Act states:

> …*no volunteer of a nonprofit organization or governmental entity shall be liable for harm caused by an act or omission of the volunteer on behalf of the organization or entity if—*
>
> *(1) the volunteer was acting within the scope of the volunteer's responsibilities in the nonprofit organization or governmental entity at the time of the act or omission;*
> *(2) if appropriate or required, the volunteer was properly licensed, certified, or authorized by the appropriate authorities for the activities or practice in the State in which the harm occurred, where the activities were or practice was undertaken within the scope of the volunteer's responsibilities in the nonprofit organization or governmental entity;*
> *(3) the harm was not caused by willful or criminal misconduct, gross negligence, reckless misconduct, or a conscious, flagrant indifference to the rights or safety of the individual harmed by the volunteer; and*

> *(4) the harm was not caused by the volunteer operating a motor vehicle, vessel, aircraft, or other vehicle for which the State requires the operator or the owner of the vehicle, craft, or vessel to—*
>
> > *(A) possess an operator's license; or*
> > *(B) maintain insurance* (68, p. 1)

This law provides liability protection only for the volunteer, not for the nonprofit or government entity. For example, a nonprofit or government entity could be vicariously liable for the negligent acts of a volunteer. Some states have similar laws that protect volunteers including certain states providing specific protection for those who volunteer in sport and recreation settings (69). A minority of states have charitable immunity statutes, in which a charitable organization may have some liability protections (e.g., liability is limited by capping the amount that may be awarded). Most states have abolished charitable immunity (70).

What About Entrepreneurs?

Exercise professionals sometimes want to start their own small business. It is recommended to first obtain several years of "high quality" professional work experience with an employer to help gain the needed knowledge, skills, and confidence to become an expert in the field as well as obtaining advanced credentials. It takes several years to become an expert in any profession. Entrepreneurs who are "true" experts are more likely to be successful. Entrepreneurs will need to make many important, informed decisions such as the type of business structure (e.g., sole proprietorship, partnership, limited liability company, corporation, etc.). Each structure will have advantages and disadvantages regarding taxes and legal liability. In addition, the exercise professional entrepreneur will need to become fully aware of the many legal liability exposures and risk management strategies that need to be implemented. The business owner is *the* risk management manager. If the entrepreneur will be hiring employees, there are many employment laws and regulations that will need to be followed. There is a lot to learn before starting a business. It may be wise to take academic courses in entrepreneurship, business law, etc. Some helpful resources are:

1. IRS Small Business and Self-Employed Tax Center: https://www.irs.gov/businesses/small-businesses-self-employed
2. U.S. Small Business Administration: https://www.sba.gov

General and Professional Liability Insurance

There are many types of insurance that fitness managers and exercise professionals should consider (e.g., general and professional liability, property, and cyber security). The following will describe "general" and "professional" liability insurance and how each can protect employers and employees from financial losses due to negligence (1). Other types of insurance are described in Chapter 10. As described in Chapter 1, if a defendant is found liable for negligence, the judge or jury can award the plaintiff various types of damages including (a) economic damages (e.g., medical expenses, loss wages), (b) non-economic damages (e.g., pain of suffering, loss of consortium), and (c) punitive damages for gross negligence (1). Insurance companies have a

duty to defend the insured (e.g., provide a lawyer to represent the exercise professional) and to indemnify for judgments up to the limits articulated in the policy. For example, if an exercise professional purchases a professional liability insurance policy, the limits might be $1 million per claim with a $3 million annual aggregate. As described in Chapter 2 (see Figure 2-2, Major Components for Each of the Four Risk Management Steps) liability insurance is an example of a **contractual transfer of risks** as is a waiver.

Both general liability and professional liability policies are needed to provide protection from ordinary negligence. A Commercial General Liability (CGL) policy provides general liability insurance and can protect fitness facilities from "ordinary" negligence (1) such as injuries from falls and other causes of injuries such as equipment malfunction. Like malpractice insurance for health care providers, a professional liability insurance policy protects exercise professionals and facilities from conduct that would be considered negligent (1). The following describes a case, *Jacob v. Grant Life Choices* (71, 72), which is an excellent case to demonstrate the need for professional liability insurance in addition to a CGL policy (1).

After a strenuous workout at the fitness center, Richard Jacob began to feel dizzy, faint, and light-headed in the locker room of the fitness center. Getz, the program director, asked Jacob a series of questions about how he was feeling, took his pulse and blood pressure, and performed a finger prick test to see if his blood sugar was low. His blood sugar was low, so Getz gave him some orange juice and a banana. Jacob left the fitness center but several hours later went to Riverside Hospital where he was diagnosed as having a heart attack.

Jacob filed a negligence lawsuit against four defendants: (a) employee Robert Getz, (b) Club Management, Inc. (CMI)—the management company (vendor) who managed Grant Life Choices Center (c) Grant Life Choices Center (the fitness facility), and (d) Grant Medical Center (hospital affiliated with the fitness center). Jacob claimed that Getz and CMI should have called 911 or obtained medical assistance, of some nature, at Grant Hospital Emergency Room or by calling a physician. The issue in this lawsuit was not about a duty to properly assist Jacob in a medical emergency, but "whether the nature of the services rendered or not rendered were professional services that fell within the exclusion of Meridian's insurance policy" (71, p. 2). Meridian, insurance provider for CMI, claimed that Getz's conduct was considered "professional" and, therefore, it did not have a duty to defend or indemnify CMI because the CGL policy specifically excluded professional services. The appellate court upheld the trial court's ruling that the conduct of Getz was not "professional" in nature—he was merely providing first aid—and, therefore, Meridian did have a duty to defend and indemnify CMI under the CGL policy. Once the insurance carrier's appeal of the trial court's ruling was finalized, the plaintiff's negligence lawsuit became active again (72). The defendants contended in their motion for summary judgment that the waiver of liability that the plaintiff signed barred his lawsuit. The trial court granted the motion of summary judgment which was upheld by the appellate court.

In addition to the *Jacob* case, the following cases, *Hanover v. Retrofitness* (73) and *York Insurance Company v. Houston Wellness Center* (spotlight case), demonstrate the need for fitness managers and exercise professionals to carefully review their insurance policies for any sections that contain exclusions. It is essential that the insurance policy covers all programs and services provided by the fitness facility.

In a 2017 case, *Hanover v. Retrofitness* (73), coverage for professional services was described in the Hanover Insurance Company policy in the lawsuit as well as policy exclusions. Six plaintiffs from several Retrofitness franchises (defendants) filed a class action complaint alleging that the defendants violated several New Jersey Acts including the Consumer Fraud Act and Health Clubs Services Act. Hanover Insurance claimed it had no duty to defend Retrofitness because the complaint did not state claims covered under the policy, only claims related to breaches of New Jersey consumer protection laws. The policy defined professional services as "those services… you perform for others for a fee" and defined a wrongful act as "any actual or alleged negligent act, error, omission, or misstatement committed in your professional

services" (p. 1). Regarding professional services coverage, the policy stated:

> *We will pay on your behalf those sums which you become legally obligated to pay as damages and claim expenses because of any claim made against you arising from a wrongful act in the rendering of professional services or failure to provide professional services by you.*

> *The following additional requirements and limitations shall apply to coverage…*
> a) *The wrongful act must have first occurred on or after the applicable retroactive date(s);*
> b) *You had no knowledge of facts which could have reasonably caused you to foresee a claim, or any knowledge of the claim, prior to the effective date of this policy; and,*
> c) *The claim must first be made and reported to us in writing during the policy period… and must arise from any wrongful act to which the policy applies (p. 1).*

The policy further stated: "We have the right to investigate and the exclusive right to defend any claim made under this policy…We are not obligated to defend any criminal investigation, criminal proceeding or prosecution against you. If a claim is not covered under this policy, we have no duty to defend it" (p. 1). The policy also contained an exclusion regarding claims arising out of "false advertising… unfair or deceptive business practices…including… violations of any local, state, or federal consumer protection laws" (p. 5).

The court ruled that Hanover was not obligated to defend Retrofitness given that the language in the policy was unambiguous and unequivocal as to the complaint (i.e., breaches of consumer protection laws). Regarding professional services, it appears that this policy would cover "negligent" acts but not gross negligence or criminal acts. Also, note the additional requirements and limitations regarding coverage for professional services. This case, again, demonstrates the importance for fitness managers and exercise professionals to carefully review their liability insurance policies and to consult with a competent lawyer if assistance is needed to interpret the coverages specified in the contract.

It is also important to realize, as demonstrated in *Hanover*, that the insurance provider has an obligation to the defend its clients, based on the terms of policy. For example, the liability insurance company would select a lawyer to defend its client (an exercise professional) who was named in the complaint. If the exercise professional does not have liability insurance, he/she would need to hire a lawyer at the time the summons is served.

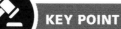

KEY POINT

In addition to purchasing general liability insurance, employers should provide professional liability insurance for employees who lead exercise programs such as personal fitness trainers, group exercise leaders, and others involved in instructing and supervising exercise programs. These policies need to be carefully reviewed for any exclusions. Exercise professionals who work for an employer that does not provide professional liability coverage need to obtain this coverage on their own.

SPOTLIGHT CASE

York Insurance Company v. Houston Wellness Center
583 S.E.2d 903 (Ga. Ct. App., 2003)

FACTS

Historical Facts:

After joining the Houston Wellness Center, Anne Vandalinda was instructed by one of Houston's employees on how to use the various exercise machines. At the time of her injury, she was using a machine that develops the triceps. She tried to release the machine using her arms, as instructed, but the machine improperly released causing an injury to her shoulder that later required surgery.

Procedural Facts:

Vandalinda filed a complaint alleging that her injury was due to improper instructions given to her by the employee. Houston Wellness Center claimed that York Insurance Company had a duty to defend and indemnify pursuant to the terms within the commercial general liability policy. However, York Insurance Company disagreed because of the following exclusion stated in the policy:

> This insurance does not apply to 'bodily injury,' 'property damage' or 'personal and advertising injury' arising out of the rendering of or failure to render any service, treatment, advice or instruction relating to physical fitness, including services or advice in connection with diet, cardio-vascular fitness, body building or physical training programs (pp. 904-905).

The trial court agreed with the Houston Wellness Center and denied the insurance company's motion for summary judgment. York Insurance company appealed the trial court's decision.

ISSUE

Did the trial court err when it denied the insurance company's motion for summary judgment?

COURT'S RULING

Yes, the trial court erred, and its ruling was reversed.

York Insurance Company continued...

COURT'S REASONING

The court stated, "An insurer's duty to defend is determined by comparing the allegations of the complaint with the provision of the policy" (p. 904). The allegations made by Vandalinda fall within the policy exclusion, specifically, "…rendering of or failure to render any service, treatment, advice or instruction relating to physical fitness…" (p. 905). The court also stated, "A term in an insurance policy that unambiguously and lawfully limits the insurer's liability may not be extended beyond what is fairly within its plain terms" and, therefore, York Insurance Company "was entitled to judgment as a matter of law because coverage was excluded for this loss" (p. 905).

Lessons Learned from *York Insurance Company:*

Legal

▶ An insurance company is free to determine the terms of its policies if such terms are not contrary to law.

▶ An insurance company is equally free to insure against certain risks while excluding others.

▶ An insurance company's duty to defend is determined by comparing the provisions within the policy and the allegations in the complaint.

Risk Management/Injury Prevention

▶ Fitness managers and exercise professionals need to consider having both general liability insurance and professional liability insurance coverages that provide protection for all types of programs and services offered.

▶ In consultation with legal and insurance experts, fitness managers and exercise professionals need to carefully review liability insurance policies for any exclusions that might be included.

▶ If a fitness facility plans to offer a new program/service or sponsor some type of event, consultation with legal and insurance experts is needed to help ensure adequate coverage is obtained.

DEVELOPMENT OF RISK MANAGEMENT STRATEGIES

 Assessment of Legal Liability Exposures → Development of Risk Management Strategies → Implementation of the Comprehensive Risk Management Plan → Evaluation of the Comprehensive Risk Management Plan

The preceding section identified many legal liability exposures related to employment issues with a special focus on the importance of hiring credentialed and competent personnel. The following risk management strategies can be developed to reduce these legal liability exposures, especially those related to vicarious and direct liability of an employer.

Risk Management Strategy #1: Comply with Current Federal, State, and Local Employment Laws (1).

Although many employment laws exist, this chapter and Chapter 3 cover some of these employment laws—statutory, administrative, and case law. Fitness managers and exercise professionals who have hiring and supervisory responsibilities need to become aware of these laws and regulations and comply with them. It is recommended they take a course in employment law, human resource management, and/or familiarize themselves with labor law resources provided by the federal government (45) and books such as *The Employer's Legal Handbook* (46). As employment issues arise, consultation with a competent lawyer is also needed.

2 **Risk Management Strategy #2:** Comply with Published Standards of Practice: Recommended Credentials for Fitness Managers, Exercise Professionals and Practitioners.

Almost all the standards of practice published by professional organizations, such as those listed in Chapter 4, have guidelines regarding the recommended credentials (e.g. education, certifications, etc.) for various exercise professionals. Fitness managers and exercise professionals need to refer to these publications for the specific, recommended credentials and then adopt these recommendations by listing them in job descriptions. Examples of education credentials include:

a) **Management Positions** (e.g., Fitness Manager, Program Director, Program Supervisor). The ACSM (74) recommends a 4-year degree in fitness, exercise science or health-related field and the MFA (75) recommends a bachelor's degree in exercise science or related area, master's degree preferred. The AACVPR (76) recommends a master's degree in an allied health field such as exercise physiology or licensure in a health care discipline such as registered nurse or physical therapist or both master's degree and licensure.

b) **Personal Fitness Trainers and Group Exercise Leaders.** The ACSM (74) recommends a 4-year degree in fitness, exercise science or related field with 2 years of college education in the field as the minimum and 2 years of college education in fitness, exercise science, dance or related field for group exercise leaders. The MFA (75) recommends a college certificate or associate degree in fitness/exercise science; bachelor's degree in exercise science or related field preferred for both personal fitness trainers and group exercise leaders.

c) **Fitness Instructors.** Instructors can be individuals such as fitness floor supervisors who provide instruction and supervision to participants while they are working out on their own in the facility. The ACSM (74) and MFA (75) education recommendations for fitness instructors are the same as indicated above for personal fitness trainers and group exercise leaders.

d) **Strength and Conditioning Coaches.** The NSCA (77) recommends a bachelor's degree

or master's degree in one or more of the topics under the Scientific Foundations domain in the CSCS examination content description or a related subject area.

Two resources may be helpful for employers to (a) find exercise professionals that have ACSM certifications (ACSM ProFinder—https://certification2.acsm. org/profinder), or (b) verify NCCA accredited certifications (US Registry of Exercise Professionals™— www.usreps.org).

3 **Risk Management Strategy #3:** Prepare Personnel Contracts in Consultation with a Competent Lawyer.

A variety of templates for personnel contracts (e.g., employees, independent contractors, vendors, volunteers) can be found on the Internet. However, it is best to have these and all contracts prepared by a competent lawyer. Whether to have employees review and sign an employment contract is something that needs to be discussed with legal counsel. State laws need to be reviewed regarding categories of employment relationships (e.g., contract employees and "at will" employees, as well as the advantages and disadvantages of having employees sign a contract). For example, a written employment contract will be enforceable regarding the terms stated in the contract such as how or why the employee can be terminated and any requirements that the employee must follow when terminating his/her employment such as 30 days' notice. Employment can be terminated by either party at any time for "at will" employees who do not sign an employment contract. However, termination cannot violate discrimination laws and regulations such as those described in Chapter 3. For more information on the (a) pros/cons of employment contacts, (b) typical content that goes in an employment contract, and (c) use of "at will" agreements, see a brief article titled: "Written Employment Contracts: Pros and Cons" (78).

Written contracts are needed for both independent contractors and vendors. Having a competent lawyer prepare these contracts is an absolute must. The terms (e.g., indemnity and hold harmless and proof of liability insurance clauses), need to be well-written and reflect applicable federal, state, and local laws. The terms should also be fully understood by the independent contractor and/or vendor signing the contract. For example, the language in these types of contracts may be difficult for exercise professionals to fully understand. It is essential that they understand all the terms including those that may have negative consequences for them, such as non-compete clauses. In cases where clarification of the terms is needed, it is recommended that exercise professionals consult with a lawyer who specializes in contract law, for assistance, prior to negotiating or signing the contract.

The contracts used for internships are usually prepared by the legal counsel's office at the academic institution. However, some internship sites (e.g., hospitals, large corporations) may have their own internship contracts. Legal counsel representing both parties will need to decide which contract to use and if any revisions are needed. It is also recommended to have volunteers sign a volunteer service agreement (79) that describes the volunteer's responsibilities. This will help clarify the services provided by the volunteer as well as the responsibilities of the supervisor of the volunteer(s) such as training/supervision.

Risk Management Strategy #4: Conduct Criminal Background Checks Before Employing Certain Personnel (1).

Employers often conduct various background checks such as work history, education, use of social media, and criminal records when hiring personnel. It is essential to follow federal, state, and local laws when conducting these background checks. For example, certain federal laws (80) prohibit discrimination based on race, color, national origin, sex, or religion; disability; genetic information (including family medical history); and age (40 or older). More information about these laws is covered in Chapter 3. Additional laws may also apply when conducting background checks such as the Fair Credit Reporting Act (FCRA) that requires providing a copy of the investigative report to the applicant if it is decided not to hire the applicant based on the findings in the report (46).

As stated above, employers, generally, are not held liable for the criminal acts (e.g., sexual assault) committed by their employees while performing job

responsibilities. Vicarious liability does not apply for conduct outside the scope of employment. However, employers can be held directly liable for civil claims such as negligent hiring, retention, and supervision of personnel. To minimize these types of claims, managers of fitness facilities that serve vulnerable populations, such as children, older adults, and people with disabilities should perform criminal background checks on all personnel who will be interacting with these individuals (1). In addition, criminal background checks should be considered for personnel who work closely with clients such as personal fitness trainers and massage therapists. Proper training upon hiring of all personnel regarding the facility's policies and procedures related to professional conduct and expectations as well as providing proper supervision is essential. Criminal background checks for volunteers who provide services in certain fitness programs may also be needed. For an example of such guidelines for volunteers, see The National Recreation and Parks Association (NRPA) guidelines (81).

Risk Management Strategy #5: Establish Interview Procedures to Help Ensure only Competent Personnel are Employed.

Several tasks are completed prior to conducting interviews with top candidates such as reviewing applications, reference checks, and verifying credentials. Various employment laws apply to these tasks as well as pre-employment inquiries such as questions asked in an interview. Questions related to marital status, national origin, arrests that did not lead to conviction, etc. cannot be asked (46). The focus of this risk management strategy will be preparing interview procedures that will help determine the depth of knowledge, skill, and competence that the candidate possesses to safely and effectively perform the job of an exercise professional. The questions for an exercise professional (or practitioner) who will be hired as a personal fitness trainer, group exercise leader, or fitness instructor will be different from an exercise professional who is pursuing a job with management and/or supervisory responsibilities.

Prior to the interview, it is best to provide candidates with a job description of the job for which they are applying as well as informing them that they will be required to teach a mock or demo exercise class or training session during the interview. This is recommended for all candidates who will have some type of teaching/training responsibilities. This will provide the employer with a general sense of the candidate's ability to properly teach/train. Interview questions should be prepared in advance and be the same for all candidates to help prevent any discrimination as well as to objectively evaluate the answers provided by each candidate. Questions to assess the candidate's level of exercise science knowledge/skills, especially those related to principles of safe exercise will be important to ask. For example, one question might be "explain what is meant by each of the following principles of safe exercise (e.g., progression, monitoring intensity, cool-down) and, then, describe how one would apply these when teaching/training participants. In addition to these types of questions, situational questions are also helpful to include. These questions get at situations that can arise while performing the job (e.g., for a personal fitness trainer: "if a client requests a break during a session, what would you do"?). For a group exercise leader: "if you notice a participant experiencing signs of overexertion, what would you do"? These types of questions will help discern the quality of experiences that candidates have had, as well as their judgment abilities.

For exercise professionals who are pursuing management or supervisory positions, several questions that assess their knowledge and skills in these areas will be important to ask. For professionals that will have oversight of the personal fitness training program or the group exercise program, questions could be created related to (a) the training they would provide for new hires, (b) procedures for conducting job performance appraisals, c) complaints from participants about a certain trainer/instructor, and (d) evaluation of the program at process and impact levels. Questions that assess their level of knowledge and skill in legal and risk management responsibilities are also important.

A careful selection of interview questions that can best determine the knowledge, skills, and competence of candidates is essential, especially given the variance in credentials (education, certification) that exist in the exercise profession. Not all academic programs and certifications are the same—the rigor involved to

obtain these credentials varies a great deal. It is up to the employer to take a deep dive in order to assess the credentials and the competence of prospective candidates. Immediately after each interview, the staff member(s) who conducted the interview should complete an evaluation form of the candidates interview performance. This evaluation form should be developed prior to the interviews and should be the same for all candidates. These consistent evaluations are helpful when selecting the best candidate for the job.

 Risk Management Strategy #6: Ensure that All Personnel have Liability Insurance Coverage (1).

Fitness facilities should ensure that their employees and volunteers have employer-provided liability insurance coverage that includes general liability insurance as well as professional liability insurance for those that provide professional services. Exercise professionals and professionals involved in wellness programs such as nutrition and stress management, should inquire as to whether their employer provides professional liability coverage for them and what kind of insurance is provided. If there is not adequate insurance, it would be wise for professionals to purchase their own professional liability coverage, which can be obtained at a reasonable rate as a member benefit through professional organizations. Independent contractors and vendors need to obtain and keep current their own professional liability insurance coverage and provide verification of such (1). The employers of contractors and vendors need to periodically request verification of insurances. This requirement should be specified in the independent contractor and vendor contracts. Student interns also need to provide verification of their professional liability insurance, which can be obtained by the insurance provider.

Liability insurance policies should be carefully reviewed for any exclusions. Failure to address any exclusions may result in the denial of insurance coverage and thus, expose the fitness facility to pay, potentially, large sums of money for legal expenses and damages awarded to a plaintiff. In addition, if any new program is offered or the facility decides to be an organizer or sponsor of a community event such as a triathlon, it is essential that the fitness manager consults with the facility's insurance provider to be sure the program or event is covered. If not, additional liability coverage may be needed. It is also essential that procedures, such as record-keeping, are in place to ensure that all liability insurance policies are kept current.

⑦ Risk Management Strategy #7: Inform Participants if Independent Contractors or Vendors Provide Programs and Services (1).

For fitness facilities that utilize independent contractors or vendors to provide programs and services, it is essential that participants are made aware of this through proper communication channels. For example, the facility can post signage in this regard and can include a section in the membership contract making this evident. It is important that these contractors do not appear as employees by wearing apparel with the facility's name and logo on it (1). It is wise to provide contractors an identifying "contractor" badge that they must always wear while in the facility (1). In addition, it may be helpful for participants, such as clients of personal fitness trainers who are independent contractors, to sign an agreement that they understand that the services are provided by an independent contractor. If steps like these are not taken, participants may believe the contractors are employees and, thus, the employer can be held vicariously liable for the negligent acts of independent contractors and vendors based on a legal principle referred to as ostensible agency.

⑧ Risk Management Strategy #8: Provide Training for Newly Hired Employees and Other Personnel.

Employers who fail to properly hire, train, and supervise employees as well as other personnel can be subject to both vicarious and direct liability. Although training and supervision are on-going job responsibilities of fitness managers and others in supervisory roles, this risk management strategy will focus on the initial training of newly hired employees to help them become competent employees. Because providing training to independent contractors would likely be exhibiting behavioral control, the training for

independent contractors would need to be quite limited. See Exhibit 5-3 above. Training is also needed for interns and volunteers which would be similar to the training that employees receive.

Training can be divided into two parts: (a) general training that all employees receive and (b) specific training or or on-the-job (OTJ) training regarding job tasks and responsibilities. In a large organization, the Human Resources (HR) department usually provides the general training for all newly hired employees which often covers the content in the Employee Handbook such as employee benefits, policies and procedures (e.g., sexual misconduct, harassment, discrimination, drug and alcohol abuse, social media, workplace privacy), and disciplinary actions for inappropriate conduct (46). With the assistance of legal and HR experts, it is recommended that small businesses, even with just a few employees, create their own employee handbooks. Templates available on the Internet as well as books such as this textbook are helpful resources to begin this process.

If there is no HR department, it will be the responsibility of the fitness manager (or other designated supervisor) to provide the general training. Given the rise in discrimination-type claims, as briefly discussed in Chapter 2 and described in more detail in Chapter 3, it is essential that all personnel receive training on discrimination laws, relevant policies and procedures of the facility, and expectations regarding professional conduct. Because requiring independent contractors to attend such a training may be exhibiting behavioral control, it might be best to include these types of responsibilities/expectations in the independent contractor's contract. Fitness managers and exercise professionals serving as supervisors often face challenges regarding inappropriate behavior of their employees. This "general" training will help mitigate these challenges and help create a professional environment. It is wise to have periodic, in-service trainings covering the content included in the general training to remind personnel of its importance.

OTJ Training for Exercise Professionals

Although all employees need OTJ training, the following discussion will focus on OTJ training for exercise professionals and practitioners. Before reading this section, it is recommended to review the information on OTJ training presented in Chapter 2. Staff training is an important component of a comprehensive risk management plan—if not the most important component. Many injuries and subsequent litigations could be prevented by providing high quality training programs that focus on participant safety. As stated in Chapter 2, fitness managers and other supervisors providing training programs need to possess excellent teaching skills and know how to apply the four P's of staff training—prepare, present, practice, and post-training follow-up. Facilities should have a "manager/supervisor" training manual that is used to train new managers/supervisors as well as those aspiring to serve in these roles. Content on pedagogy skills should be a section within this training manual. It cannot be assumed that someone, even with a degree in exercise science (or related area), is an effective teacher. In addition, training covering the content in the facility's Risk Management and Policies and Procedures Manual (RMPPM) is essential for all managers/supervisors.

Given the wide variety of academic, certification, and other educational preparation programs (e.g., personal trainer schools), employers cannot assume that new hires are competent or have ever taught a group or individual. Therefore, it is essential to train "all" new exercise professionals and practitioners (all five levels as shown in Figure 5-1), so they acquire a level of competence that helps ensure the safety of participants. For example, one personal fitness trainer, an exercise professional who possessed a master's degree in exercise science, stated she "had no idea how to work with older or sedentary people" and that "she realized many other

trainers were just as clueless" (82, p. 122). This same article published in *Women's Health* (82) referred to a survey of 2700 personal trainers in which two-thirds of them admitted that knew trainers they considered incompetent. In an article (83) that focused on jobs after retirement, one personal fitness trainer stated that after he retired, he wanted to pursue his passion for fitness and, thus, become a personal fitness trainer. He said that it was not hard to get a certification and that there were many online companies that could help. The same may be true for former collegiate and professional athletes who have a passion to pursue a career as an exercise professional. They may believe they have a lot of experience/expertise in exercise training but may not realize "how" to safely and effectively train the general population. OTJ training is the best way to address the potential lack of important knowledge and skills (or competence) of all newly hired employees.

Certainly, a training manual should be developed for each of the various types of employees such as full-time exercise professionals, personal fitness trainers, group exercise leaders, and fitness floor supervisors as well as others who provide programs/services such as massage therapists, health/wellness coaches, nutritionists, etc. Those who will be providing fitness programs and services will need both classroom training and practical training which is the focus of the following recommendations.

Classroom Training

Classroom training should cover the various content in the training manuals. However, classroom training should focus on and emphasize "safety" and risk management topics such as:

1. Principles of safe training and how to apply them in the design/delivery of exercise programs. Describe negligence cases to help understand why this is important.
2. Facility orientation for new participants—see Chapter 10 for the content covered in this orientation that new employees should know.
3. Scope of practice—see Chapter 7 for more on this topic.
4. Preparation of lesson plans that reflect safe/effective exercise programs and evaluation forms

KEY POINT

Given the wide variety of academic, certification, and other educational preparation programs (e.g., personal trainer schools), employers cannot assume that new hires are competent. Therefore, it is essential to train "all" newly hired exercise professionals and practitioners (all five levels as shown in Figure 5-1), so they acquire a level of competence that helps ensure the safety of participants.

completed after each class/training session and documentation of both—see Chapter 8 for more on this topic.

5. Relevant content from the facility's Risk Management and Policies and Procedures Manual (RMPPM) such as the Emergency Action Plans (EAPs) and policies/procedures related to sexual misconduct. Training involving "touching" participants is essential, e.g., how to first inform participants of the purpose of touching, asking the participant's permission, and respecting the participant's wishes/concerns.

6. Policies regarding ethical conduct of exercise professionals and practitioners such as following Codes of Ethical Conduct published by professional organizations. Short articles to review/discuss:

    a) 10 Ethical Issues Facing Health/Fitness Professionals (84)—a brief, but concise description of the following issues: business practices, supplements, professional boundaries, client confidentiality, conflict of interest, professional certifications, professional representation of skills, abilities and knowledge, intellectual property, medical advice, and professional education.

    b) Top Five Reasons to Make Fitness Safety Priority No. 1 (85)—describes why participant safety is the #1 legal and moral duty of exercise professionals.

7. Performance appraisal forms—these should be reviewed with new employees along with a description of how these will be used in their probationary period and on a needed and/or annual basis, thereafter. See Chapter 8 for more information on this topic and an example of a performance appraisal tool for group exercise leaders that can be adapted for personal fitness trainers.

8. Policies related to exercise equipment and facility issues, e.g., instruction on how to properly use the equipment and facility as well as areas within the facility that are off-limits for trainers to train clients.

9. Professional communication with participants, co-workers, and supervisors, e.g., policies regarding avoiding vulgar language or excessively loud or yelling voices as well as nonjudgmental language that can have a negative effect on par-

ticipants such as poor self-image (86) or feeling inferior or ashamed.

10. Safety culture—see Chapter 2 for more on this topic.

Practical Training

This area of training is essential, given that there are no requirements to have any practical training or assessment of practical skills in many exercise or fitness

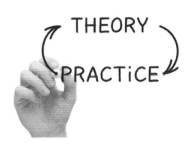

certifications. As described above, there is a link between the lack of practical skills and negligence claims/lawsuits. Fitness facility managers and supervisors can serve as "mentors" of new employees. Current employees can also serve as mentors. Mentors need to be credentialed employees who have demonstrated competence such as: (a) have received "exemplary" job performance evaluations evident of safe and effective teaching/training, (b) have obtained positive interactions with participants, and (c) have followed/supported the facility's policies and procedures. A new employee should work under the supervision of the mentor until he/she is ready to perform the job (e.g., personal fitness trainer, group exercise leader, fitness floor supervisor) on his/her own. One of the best ways to determine "readiness" is through a job performance appraisal or evaluation (see Chapter 8 for more on this topic). Once the new employee begins the job on his/her own for two-three weeks, it may be wise to conduct another job performance appraisal as a follow-up as well as to have participants submit evaluations of the new employee.

In addition to practical skills related to teaching and training, obtaining fitness testing skills will be important for those staff members who will be conducting fitness assessments. Even exercise professionals who have a degree in exercise science and have had an academic course in fitness testing may need to obtain additional training and practice in this area. For personal fitness trainers, who have never had to demonstrate their fitness testing skills to obtain a certification, training and practice will be absolutely needed in this area before conducting any assessments on participants. Some personal fitness training certifications have stated competencies in this area as part of the written examination content preparation, such as skill in selecting and administering cardiovascular fitness assessments (87). Perhaps knowledge of these competencies can be covered on a written examination, but skills such as accurately measuring resting and exercise blood pressures during a submaximal cardiovascular test or properly measuring skinfolds for a body composition test cannot be effectively assessed through written examinations.

Fitness testing skills take a great deal of practice on all types of individuals and populations (not just students in an exercise science program) to become proficient. Again, it is recommended for all new employees who will be conducting fitness assessments to work under a mentor until they have demonstrated proficient fitness testing skills. In addition to attaining practical skills to properly perform fitness assessments, there are many administrative procedures that need to be followed as described in *ACSM's Guidelines for Exercise Testing and Prescription* (88) and need to be included in the training.

Risk Management Strategy #9: Market and Advertise Only the Credentials that the Facility's Personnel Possess.

As demonstrated in *D'Amico v. LA Fitness*—spotlight case above—marketing or advertising credentials of personnel that are not truthful or deceptive may lead to violations of statutes such as unfair trade practices. If a facility states, in their advertising, that all personnel possess experience and expertise in providing fitness programs, then it will be important that the facility can back that up with evidence that the personnel have the credentials that support those claims. If the facility advertises that all their exercise professionals have a bachelor's degree in exercise science or that all personal fitness trainers and group exercise leaders have a current, accredited certification, then again, it will be important to provide supportive evidence of such in the event of a claim/lawsuit against the facility. As the court stated in *D'Amico*, such deceptive practices can mislead consumers and the misleading representation is likely to affect consumer decisions. Hiring only credentialed and competent exercise professionals will minimize negligent claims/lawsuits as

well as any violations of unfair trade practices such as deceptive advertising. Fitness managers can feel confident that their marketing and advertising of the facility's personnel credentials are truthfully conveyed. **Note:** It is also important that exercise professionals, when promoting themselves, do not exaggerate their credentials such as referring to themselves as a clinical exercise physiologist if they do not have the credentials to support that title. Not only is this unethical, but it could also result in a violation of certain "unfair trade practices" statutes as well as negligence.

Risk Management Strategy #10: Develop and Maintain Personnel Files to Provide Documentation of all Hiring, Training, and Supervision Procedures.

Hiring and training documents may provide evidence to help defend or refute negligence claims or lawsuits such as negligent hiring, training, and supervision. Fitness managers and others in supervisory roles need to develop a personnel file for each new employee and keep the file maintained (current) while the individual is employed and maybe longer such as the length of time as specified in the state's statute of limitations. There are a variety of documents that are kept in employee files such as application forms, job descriptions, tax forms, background checks, contracts/agreements, etc. (46). Other documents should also include: (a) job interview questions/answers and evaluations, (b) employee trainings attended/completed (initial and on-going), (c) performance appraisals (initial and on-going), (d) participant evaluations of the employee, (e) current credentials including exercise and first-aid/CPR/AED certifications, (f) continuing education courses completed, and (g) verification of current professional liability insurance if not provided by the employer. It is essential that procedures are established to help ensure that employee files are kept private, confidential, and secure. In addition to employee files, records related to all employee trainings should be retained as well as evaluations of the trainings completed by employees. These evaluations, that reflect a type of "process" evaluation, are essential to gather data to help improve the quality of future training programs.

RISK MANAGEMENT AUDIT
Hiring Credentialed and Competent Personnel

RISK MANAGEMENT (RM) STRATEGIES*	YES ✔	NO ✔
1. Comply with Current Federal, State, and Local Employment Laws.		
2. Comply with Published Standards of Practice: Recommended Credentials for Fitness Managers, Exercise Professionals and Practitioners.		
3. Prepare Personnel Contracts in Consultation with a Competent Lawyer.		
4. Conduct Criminal Background Checks Before Employing Certain Personnel.		
5. Establish Interview Procedures to Help Ensure only Competent Personnel are Employed.		
6. Ensure that All Personnel have Liability Insurance Coverage.		
7. Inform Participants if Independent Contractors or Vendors Provide Programs and Services.		
8. Provide Training for Newly Hired Employees and Other Personnel.		
9. Market and Advertise Only the Credentials that the Facility's Personnel Possess.		
10. Develop and Maintain Personnel Files to Provide Documentation of all Hiring, Training, and Supervision Procedures.		

*See the section above—Development of Risk Management Strategies -- for the recommendations associated with each risk management strategy and then, for each RM Strategy marked NO, create a list of action steps that need to be completed to meet the recommendations described in that RM strategy.

KEY TERMS

- Accreditation
- Competence
- Contractual Transfer of Risks
- Direct Liability
- Independent Contractor
- Job Task Analysis

- Licensure
- Ostensible Agency
- Respondeat Superior
- Statutory Certification
- Vendor
- Vicarious Liability

STUDY QUESTIONS

The Study Questions for Chapter 5 can be found on the Fitness Law Academy website (www.fitnesslawacademy.com) under Textbook. They are provided in a fillable format for convenience.

REFERENCES

1. Eickhoff-Shemek JM, Herbert DL, Connaughton DP. *Risk Management for Health/Fitness Professionals: Legal Issues and Strategies.* Baltimore, MD: Lippincott Williams & Wilkins, 2009.

2. Hirby J. What Percentage of Lawsuits Settle Before Trial? What are Some Statistics on Personal Injury Settlements? *The Law Dictionary—Featuring Black's Law Dictionary Free Online Legal Dictionary,* 2nd Ed. Available at: https://thelawdictionary.org/article/what-percentage-of-lawsuits-settle-before-trial-what-are-some-statistics-on-personal-injury-settlements. Accessed December 20, 2018.

3. Abbott AA. Fitness Professionals: Certified, Qualified and Justified. *The Exercise Standards and Malpractice Reporter,* 23(2), 98-101, 2009.

4. Craig A, Eickhoff-Shemek J. Educating and Training the Personal Fitness Trainer: A Pedagogical Approach. *ACSM's Health & Fitness Journal,* 13(2), 8-15, 2009.

5. Zabawa BJ, Eickhoff-Shemek JM. *Rule the Rules of Workplace Programs.* Chicago, IL: American Bar Association, 2017.

6. Find a Program. Commission on the Accreditation of Allied Health Education Programs, Available at: https://www.caahep.org/Students/Find-a-Program.aspx. Accessed February 3, 2020.

7. Accredited Programs. American Society of Exercise Physiologists. Available at: https://www.asep.org/professional-services/accredited-programs. Accessed February 3, 2020.

8. Performance Domains and Associated Competencies. Curriculum for Educational Programs in Exercise Sciences. Commission on the Accreditation of Allied Health Education Programs, Available at: https://www.caahep.org/CAAHEP/media/CAAHEP-Documents/ExerciseScience2017final.pdf; Standards and Guidelines for the Accreditation of Educational Programs in Exercise Physiology. Commission on the Accreditation of Allied Health Education Programs, Available at: https://www.caahep.org/CAAHEP/media/CAAHEP-Documents/Exercise-Physiology-FINAL-2019.pdf. Accessed February 3, 2020.

9. Standards for the Accreditation of Certification Programs. National Commission for Certifying Agencies. National Organization for Competency Assurance, Washington D.C., 2014; NCCA Standards Revision. Available at: https://www.credentialingexcellence.org/p/cm/ld/fid=66. Accessed February 6, 2020.

10. Feito Y. Certification Exam Changes. *ACSM's Health & Fitness Journal,* 22(4), 27-28, 2018.

11. ACSM Certified Exercise Physiologist® Exam Content Outline. Available at: https://www.acsm.org/docs/default-source/certification-documents/acsmep_examcontentoutline_2017.pdf. Accessed February 3, 2020.

12. Licensure Statutes and Information by State. Eat Right Pro. Academy of Nutrition and Dietetics. Available at: https://www.eatrightpro.org/advocacy/licensure/licensure-map. Accessed February 3, 2020.

13. Code of the District of Columbia. § 3–1209.08. Personal Fitness Trainer. Available at: https://code.dccouncil.us/dc/council/code/sections/3-1209.08.html. Accessed November 19, 2018.

14. Stromgren E. Bill Puts Personal Fitness Trainer Licensing on Hold in Washington, DC, *Club Industry.* September 23, 2015. Available at: https://www.clubindustry.com/profits/bill-puts-personal-fitness-trainer-licensing-hold-washington-dc, Accessed November 19, 2018.

15. Eickhoff-Shemek J, Herbert D. Is Licensure in Your Future? Issues to Consider, Part 2. *ACSM's Health & Fitness Journal,* 12(1), 36-38, 2008.

16. Herbert DL. New Jersey Reintroduces Personal Trainer Legislation. *The Exercise Standards and Malpractice Reporter,* 24(3), 37-41, 2010.

17. ACSM Exercise Professional Licensure Statement. Available at: https://www.acsm.org/get-stay-certified/policies-procedures/professional-licensure-statement. Accessed November 20, 2018.

18. National Center for Chronic Disease Prevention and Health Promotion. Centers for Disease Control and Prevention. About Chronic Diseases. Available at: https://www.cdc.gov/chronicdisease/about/index.htm. Accessed April 15, 2020.

19. Cohen A. It's Getting Personal, *Athletic Business,* 52-54, 56, 58, 60, July 2004.

20. Personal Trainer Accreditation. What is the IHRSA Board of Directors' Position on Personal Trainer Accreditation? IHRSA. Available at: https://www.ihrsa.org/industry-issues/personal-trainer-accreditation. Accessed February 3, 2020.

21. Registration. National Board of Fitness Examiners. Available at: http://www.nbfe.org/registration.html. Accessed November 21, 2018; Personal Communication, Dorette Nysewander, NBFE Director of Information, November 29, 2018.

22. Degree Requirements for the ACSM Exercise Physiologist Certification. Available at: https://www.acsm.org/get-stay-certified/get-certified/health-fitness-certifications/exercise-physiologist/degree-requirements-ep-c; ASEP Standards of Practice. Available at: https://www.asep.org/organization/practice. Accessed November 14, 2018.

23. NSCA Certification Handbook: Effective January 2018. Available at: https://www.nsca.com/globalassets/certification/certification-pdfs/certification-handbook_201805_web-2.pdf. Accessed February 3, 2020.

24. National Strength and Conditioning Association Announces Changes that will Advance the Strength and Conditioning Profession. July 12, 2018. Available at: https://www.nsca.com/media-room/press-releases/nsca-announces-changes-that-will-advance-the-strength-and-conditioning-profession. Accessed November 21, 2018.

25. All Certifications are Not Equal. SCCC Certification. Available at: http://www.cscca.org/certification/sccc. Accessed November 21, 2018.

26. Become an ACSM Certified Clinical Exercise Physiologist®. Are You Eligible? Available at: https://www.acsm.org/get-stay-certified/get-certified/cep. Accessed February 11, 2020.

27. How to Become a Certified Medical Exercise Specialist. American Council on Exercise. Available at: https://www.acefitness.org/fitness-certifications/certified-medical-exercise-specialist/how-to-become-a-medical-exercise-specialist.aspx. Accessed November 21, 2018.

28. AACVPR Professional Certification. Certified Cardiac Rehabilitation Professional: Available at: https://www.aacvpr.org/Certification/AACVPR-Professional-Certification. Accessed March 7, 2019.

29. Fitness Facility Director, Medical Fitness Director, Medical Fitness Association. Available at: http://www.medicalfitness.org/certifications/director-certification. Accessed February 3, 2020..

30. AACVPR Program Certification. Available at: http://www.aacvpr.org/Program-Certification. Accessed March 7, 2019.

31. Achieve the Medical Fitness Facility Certification. Available at: www.medicalfitness.org/certifications/facility-certification. Accessed March 7, 2019.

32. Learning by Doing Quotes. Goodreads. Available at: https://www.goodreads.com/quotes/tag/learning-by-doing. Accessed December 20, 2018.

33. Zenko Z, Ekkekakis P. Knowledge of Exercise Prescription Guidelines Among Certified Exercise Professionals. *The Journal of Strength and Conditioning Research,* 29(5), 1422-1432, 2015.

References continued...

34. Malek M. et al. Importance of Health Science Education for Personal Trainers. *NSCA Journal of Strength and Conditioning Research*, 16(1), 19-21, 2002.

35. Krosli K. Years of Experience Says Nothing about Your Offshore Competence. The Well Blog. Available at: https://blog.odfjellwellservices.com/years-of-experience-says-nothing-about-your-offshore-competence. Accessed February 3, 2020.

36. Strada-Gallup 2017 College Student Survey. Crisis of Confidence: Current College Students Do Not Feel Prepared for the Workforce, 2017. Available at:https://stradaeducation.gallup.com/reports/225161/2017-strada-gallup-college-student-survey.aspx. Accessed December 7, 2017.

37. Jaschik S. For Provosts, More Pressure on Tough Issues. *Inside Higher Ed*, January 23, 2019. Available at: https://www.insidehighered.com/news/survey/2019-inside-higher- ed-survey-chief-academic; Ledrman D. The Imperative to Improve College Learning. *Inside Higher Ed*, January 22, 2020. Available at: https://www.insidehighered.com/digital-learning/article/2020/01/22/imperative-improve-college-learning?utm_source=Inside+Higher+Ed&utm_campaign=acefbbbb33-DNU_2019_COPY_02&utm_medium=email&utm_term=0_1fcbc04421-acefbbbb33-197398701&mc_cid=acefbbbb33&mc_eid=75a7f3b682. Accessed February 6, 2020.

38. Tokic S. Rethinking Educational Malpractice: Are Educators Rock Stars? *Brigham Young University Education and Law Journal*, 105-133, 2014.

39. Boone T. The Role of ASEP and Changes in Academia. *Professionalism in Exercise Physiology Peponline.* American Society of Exercise Physiologists, 20(12), 1-7, 2017. Available at: https://www.asep.org/resources/pep-online. Accessed December 21, 2018.

40. Kwan BM, McGinnes HL, Ory MG, et al. RE-AIM in the Real World: Use of the RE-AIM Framework for Program Planning and Evaluation in Clinical and Community Settings. From: Front. Public Health, November 22, 2019. Available at: https://www.frontiersin.org/articles/10.3389/fpubh.2019.00345/full. Accessed February 3, 2020.

41. Jordan M, Wolever RQ, Lawson K, Moore, M. National Training and Education Standards for Health and Wellness Coaching: The Path to National Certification. *Global Advances in Health and Medicine,* 4(3), 46-56, 2015.

42. National Board for Health & Wellness Coaching. Exam Application. Available at: https://nbhwc.org/hwc-certifying-examination-application/. Accessed February 3, 2020.

43. Herbert DL, Ditmyer MM. Isn't It Time for Education & Evaluation of Hands-On Competence in Personal Training? *American Fitness*, 38-43, July/August 2014.

44. Certificate, Certification, or Both? What's Right for You? Institute for Credentialing Excellence. Available at: https://www.credentialingexcellence.org/page/certificate-vs-certification. Accessed February 4, 2020.

45. Labor Laws and Issues. Available at: https://www.usa.gov/labor-laws. Accessed December 21, 2018; U.S. Department of Labor. Available at: https://www.dol.gov. Accessed December 21, 2018.

46. Steingold FS. *The Employer's Legal Handbook: Manage Your Employees & Workplace Effectively*, 13th Ed. Berkeley, CA: Nolo Law for All, 2017.

47. *Baldi-Perry v. Kaifas and 360 Fitness Center, Inc.* Complaint. Index No. 2010-1927, Supreme Court, Erie County, New York. February 19, 2010.

48. *Bartlett v. Push to Walk,* No. 2:15-cv-7167-KM-JBC, 2018 WL 1726262 (D. N.J., 2018).

49. *Elena Myers Court v. Loews Philadelphia Hotel, Inc.,* No. 16-4848, 2017 WL 64064458 (D. Pa., 2017).

50. State Identification Bureau Listing. Federal Bureau of Investigation. Available at: https://www.fbi.gov/services/cjis/identity-history-summary-checks/state-identification-bureau-listing. Accessed December 12, 2018.

51. Identity History Summary Checks. Federal Bureau of Investigation. Available at: https://www.fbi.gov/services/cjis/identity-history-summary-checks/identity-history-summary-checks. Accessed December 12, 2018.

52. Mondics C. Penn State's Legal Spending on Sandusky Tops $250. *Athletic Business E-Newsletter.* January 9, 2017. Available at: https://www.athleticbusiness.com/civil-actions/penn-state-s-legal-spending-on-sandusky-tops-250k.html. Accessed December 20, 2018.

53. Bauer-Wolf J. Michigan State Settles Nassar Lawsuits for $500 Million. *Inside Higher Ed News.* May 17, 2018. Available at: https://www.insidehighered.com/news/2018/05/17/michigan-state-settles-nassar-survivors-half-billion-dollar-payout. Accessed December 20, 2018.

54. Levy M, Rubinkam M. Ex-Penn State Officials Sentenced in Sandusky Scandal. *Athletic Business E-Newsletter.* June 2017. Available at: https://www.athleticbusiness.com/law-policy/ex-penn-state-officials-sentenced-in-sandusky-scandal.html. Accessed December 20, 2018.

55. Clarke L. USA Gymnastics Files for Bankruptcy Amid Scandal. *Athletic Business E-Newsletter.* December 2018. Available at:https://www.athleticbusiness.com/governing-bodies/usa-gymnastics-files-for-bankruptcy-amid-scandal.html. Accessed December 20, 2018.

56. Protecting Young Victims from Sexual Abuse and Safe Sport Authorization Act of 2017. U.S. Center for Safesport. Available at: https://www.usef.org/forms-pubs/ZeXEaZoEt-k/fact-sheet-protecting-young-victims. Accessed December 20, 2018.

57. Hogshead-Maker N. How to Stop Sexual Abuse in Sports. *Athletic Business E-Newsletter.* January 2018. Available at: https://www.athleticbusiness.com/athlete-safety/how-to-stop-sexual-abuse-in-sports.html. Accessed January 4, 2019.

58. Sex Discrimination: Overview of the Law. U.S. Department of Education. Available at: https://www2.ed.gov/policy/rights/guid/ocr/sexoverview.html. Accessed December 20, 2018.

59. Steinbach P. Michigan State Takes Steps to Avoid Another Nassar. *Athletic Business E-Newsletter.* October 2018. Available at: https://www.athleticbusiness.com/athlete-safety/michigan-state-takes-steps-to-avoid-another-nassar.html. Accessed December 20, 2018.

60. Steinbach P. Ex-Coach Title IX Whistleblower Gets $100K Settlement. *Athletic Business E-Newsletter.* May 2019. Available at: https://www.athleticbusiness.com/civil-actions/ex-coach-title-ix-whistleblower-gets-100k-settlement.html. Accessed February 6, 2020.

61. The Whistleblower Protection Programs. U.S Department of Labor. Occupational Safety & Health Administration. Available at: https://www.whistleblowers.gov. Accessed December 20, 2018.

62. Black DC, Nolan JR, Nolan-Haley JM., et al. *Black's Law Dictionary*, 6th Ed. St. Paul, MN: West Publishing Company, 1991.

63. IRS Form SS-8. Determination of Worker Status for Purposes of Federal Employment Taxes and Income Tax Withholding. Available at: https://www.irs.gov/pub/irs-pdf/fss8.pdf. Accessed December 12, 2018.

64. Independent Contractors. An IHRSA Briefing Statement. Available at: https://www.ihrsa.org/publications/independent-contractors. Accessed December 21, 2018.

65. *Donovan v. Unique Racquetball and Health Clubs, Inc.,* 674 F. Supp. 77 (D. Ct., E.D. N.Y., 1987).

References continued...

66. *A Concise Restatement of Torts Third Edition.* Compiled by Bublick EM, Rogers JE. St. Paul, MN: American Law Institute Publishers, 2013.

67. *Layden v. Plante,* 957 N.Y.S.2d 458, 2012 LEXIS 9109 (N.Y. App. Div., 2012).

68. Volunteer Protection Act. 42 U.S.C.A. § 14503. Limitation on Liability for Volunteers, June 18, 1997.

69. Sharp LA, Moorman, AM, Claussen CL. *Sport Law: A Managerial Approach.* Scottsdale Arizona: Holcomb Hathaway, Publishers, 2007.

70. Immunity or Not? Charitable Tort Liability Limits in Modern Times. December 15, 2017. Wagenmaker & Oberly Blog. Available at: https://wagenmakerlaw.com/blog/immunity-or-not-charitable-tort-liability-limits-modern-times. Accessed February 5, 2020.

71. *Jacob v. Grant Life Choices,* No. 94APE10-1436, 1995 WL 390810 (Ohio Ct. App., 1995).

72. *Jacob v. Grant Life Choices,* No. 95APE12-1623, 1996 LEXIS 2313 (Ohio Ct. App., 1996).

73. *Hanover v. Retrofitness,* No. 16-1751-BRM-TJB, 2017 WL 4330366 (D. N.J., 2017).

74. *ACSM's Health/Fitness Facility Standards and Guidelines.* Sanders ME. (ed). 5th Ed. Champaign, IL: Human Kinetics, 2019.

75. *Medical Fitness Association's Standards & Guidelines for Medical Fitness Center Facilities,* Roy B. (ed.). 2nd Ed. Monterey, CA: Healthy Learning, 2013.

76. American Association for Cardiovascular and Pulmonary Rehabilitation (AACVPR). *Guidelines for Cardiac Rehabilitation and Secondary Prevention Programs.* Williams MA, Roitman JL (eds). 5th Ed. Champaign, IL: Human Kinetics, 2013.

77. NSCA Strength and Conditioning Professional Standards and Guidelines. *Strength and Conditioning Journal,* 39(6), 1-24, 2017. Available at: https://www.nsca.com/education/articles/nsca-strength-and-conditioning-professional-standards-and-guidelines/. Accessed November 5, 2018.

78. Written Employment Contracts: Pros and Cons. Know When You Should—and Should Not—Ask a New Employee to Sign a Written Employment Contract. Available at: https://www.nolo.com/legal-encyclopedia/written-employment-contracts-pros-cons-30193.html. Accessed January 3, 2019.

79. Sample Volunteer Service Agreement. Available at: https://www.nh.gov/dot/programs/scc/documents/SAMPLEVolunteerServiceAgreement-NHDOL10-28-101.pdf. Accessed January 3, 2019.

80. Background Checks: What Employers Need to Know. Joint Publication of the U.S. Equal Employment Opportunity Commission and the Federal Trade Commission. Available at: https://www.eeoc.gov/eeoc/publications/background_checks_employers.cfm. Accessed January 3, 2019.

81. National Recreation and Park Association Recommended Guidelines for Credentialing Volunteers. Available at: www.nrpa.org/uploadedFiles/nrpaorg/Membership/Endorsed_Business_Provider/NRPA%20recommended%20guidelines%20-%20Final(1).pdf. Accessed January 3, 2019.

82. McDowell D. Is Working Out the Newest Health Threat? Unqualified Personal Trainers Are Putting Your Life at Risk. Here's How to Protect Yourself from this Emerging National Exercise Epidemic. *Women's Health,* March 2009.

83. Great Second Careers. How They Did It—How You Can Too. *AARP Bulletin.* January/February 2018. Available at: https://www.aarp.org/work/career-change/info-2018/great-second-careers.html. Accessed January 7, 2019.

84. Peterson JA. 10 Ethical Issues Facing Health/Fitness Professionals. *ACSM's Health & Fitness Journal,* 14(3), 46, 2010.

85. Eickhoff-Shemek JM. Top Five Reasons to Make Fitness Safety Priority No. 1. *ACSM's Health & Fitness Journal,* 24(1), 37-38, 2020.

86. Anyaso HH. Fitness Instructors' Comments Shape Women's Body Satisfaction. December 13, 2018. Available at: https://news.northwestern.edu/stories/2018/december/fitness-instructors-comments-shape-womens-body-satisfaction. Accessed January 7, 2019.

87. ACSM Certified Personal Trainer® Job Task Analysis. Available at: https://www.acsm.org/docs/default-source/certification-documents/cpt/2017-acsm-cpt-jta-full-final-1.pdf?sfvrsn=dc02638a_10. Accessed January 8, 2019.

88. *ACSM's Guidelines for Exercise Testing and Prescription.* Riebe D. (ed). 10th Ed. Philadelphia, PA: Lippincott Williams & Wilkins, 2018.

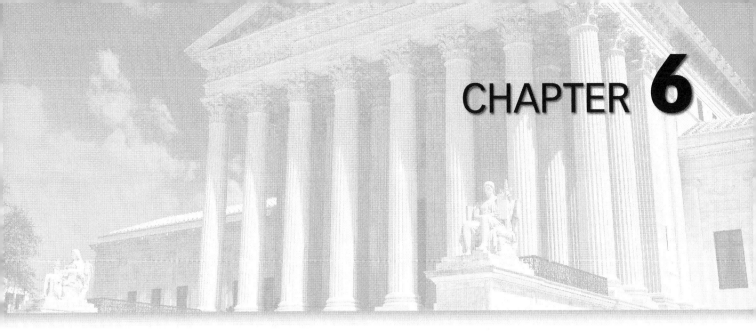

CHAPTER 6

Pre-Activity Health Screening and Fitness Testing

LEARNING OBJECTIVES

After reading this chapter fitness managers and exercise professionals will be able to:

1. Identify laws and regulations that are applicable to pre-activity screening and fitness testing (1).

2. Appreciate the importance of complying with pre-activity health screening and testing laws as well as standards and guidelines published by professional organizations (1).

3. Distinguish between self-guided screening and professionally-guided screening.

4. Develop and implement an efficient, professionally-guided pre-activity health screening process (1).

5. Explain the differences between pre-activity health screening and medical history questionnaires and how each should be applied in fitness settings.

6. Describe why exercise intensity levels should be listed on a medical clearance form.

7. Explain the need to obtain a medical history prior to fitness testing and exercise prescription from a legal liability perspective.

8. Distinguish between health-related fitness testing and clinical exercise testing.

9. Develop and implement a safe and effective health-related fitness testing program.

10. Explain the purpose of administering an informed consent prior to fitness testing and the various sections within an informed consent document.

11. Compare and contrast pain associated with an injury and muscle soreness.

12. Describe common negligence claims that have been made against exercise professionals and fitness facilities in cases

involving pre-activity health screening and fitness testing.

13. Define privacy, confidentiality, and security and explain their relevance to an individual's health-related information or protected health information (PHI).

14. List the knowledge and skills that need to be addressed in staff training programs that cover the facility's screening and testing procedures.

15. Describe the role of the facility's legal counsel, medical advisor, and/or risk management advisory committee regarding the development of screening and testing procedures.

16. Develop and implement 10 risk management strategies that will help minimize legal liability exposures associated with pre-activity health screening and fitness testing (1).

INTRODUCTION

This chapter focuses on the importance of fitness managers and exercise professionals to develop pre-activity health screening and health-related fitness testing procedures that are based on certain laws and regulations as well as standards of practice published by professional organizations. Background information is first provided for both screening and fitness testing followed by a list of steps describing how to properly develop and implement these procedures. Pre-activity health screening questionnaires are described along with an explanation of how these are distinct from medical history questionnaires. The need to obtain a medical history prior to fitness testing and exercise prescription is explained from a legal liability perspective. Several negligence lawsuits are described focusing on the types of negligence claims that can occur when exercise professionals failed to properly carry out screening and testing procedures. The chapter ends with a description of 10 risk management strategies that can be developed and implemented to minimize legal liability exposures associated with screening and testing.

PRE-ACTIVITY HEALTH SCREENING

According to the American Heart Association (AHA), cardiovascular disease (CVD) accounts for about one of every three deaths in the U.S. (2). The leading cause of cardiovascular death is coronary heart disease (CHD) at 43.2% followed by stroke (16.9%), high blood pressure (9.8%), heart failure (9.3%), diseases of the arteries (3.0%), and other cardiovascular diseases at 17.7% (2). As fitness managers and exercise professionals know, regular physical activity can help decrease the incidence of CVD. They also know that the risk of an exercise-related cardiovascular event is quite rare. However, vigorous exercise can increase the risk of sudden cardiac death (SCD) and acute myocardial infarction (AMI) in individuals with both occult and diagnosed CVD (3). Evidence also shows that vigorous exercise increases the risk of a cardiac event particularly among habitually sedentary individuals who have underlying cardiovascular disease (4). Therefore, mitigating these risks in susceptible individuals is important (3). For

more information on the exercise-related cardiovascular events, see the AHA scientific statement published in 2020 titled *Exercise-Related Acute Cardiovascular Events and Potential Deleterious Adaptations Following Long-Term Exercise Training: Placing the Risks Into Perspective—An Update* (5).

Although exercise is safe for most people and the many benefits of exercise outweigh the risks, exercise-related cardiac events (SCD and AMI) do occur in fitness facilities. A national study, conducted in 2014, found that 35% of fitness facilities had at least one cardiovascular emergency in the last five years (6). Fitness managers and exercise professionals need to be ready to respond to such emergencies as described in Chapter 11. They can minimize the risk of such medical emergencies by developing and implementing pre-activity health screening procedures. The major purposes of **pre-activity health screening** are to (a) identify new participants who may be at risk of an untoward event while participating in the facility's activities and, (b) obtain **medical clearance** for those participants at risk prior to their participation in the facility's activities and learn of any restrictions/limitations as indicated by their health care provider on the medical clearance form.

For 30 years, the pre-activity screening guidelines published in editions three through nine of *ACSM's Guidelines for Exercise Testing and Prescription* involved screening for (a) known cardiovascular, pulmonary and metabolic diseases, (b) signs/symptoms suggestive of disease, and (c) cardiovascular risk factors. Based on this health history information, individuals were classified into low, moderate, and high risk categories. Medical evaluation was recommended given the individual's risk category and exercise intensity. In the *ACSM's Guidelines for Exercise Testing and Prescription,* 10th edition (2018), the screening criteria were significantly changed (3). An article that described the rationale for the changes and an algorithm on how to apply the new criteria was published in 2015 (7). Generally, the revised screening criteria assess (a) activity level, (b) known disease (cardiovascular, metabolic and renal), and (c) signs/symptoms suggestive of disease. Identification of cardiovascular risk factors was eliminated. Instead of recommending medical evaluation based on the health history information, medical clearance is recommended. It is important to note that exercise professionals cannot recommend a medical evaluation—only the individual's health care provider can recommend a need for a medical examination, and, of course, perform the examination and determine what laboratory tests, etc. it should include. However, exercise professionals can recommend that an individual obtain medical clearance prior to participation in an exercise program. One of the major reasons for changing the screening criteria was because the previous criteria and recommended follow-up steps resulted in excessive physician referrals creating a potential barrier to exercise (7).

Pre-Activity Health Screening Standards and Guidelines

In addition to *ACSM's Guidelines for* Exercise *Testing and Prescription* (*ACSM's GETP*) that recommends preparticipation health screening (3), the *ACSM's Health/Fitness Facility Standards and Guidelines* (8) states "Facility operators shall offer a self-guided or professionally-guided exercise preparticipation health screening tool…to all new members and prospective users" (p. 4). Generally, with **self-guided screening,** participants are provided a screening tool (questionnaire) that they complete/interpret on their own and decide on their own to obtain medical clearance. With **professionally-guided screening**, participants complete a screening questionnaire, but the information is interpreted by an exercise professional (e.g., an individual with a degree in exercise science and professional certification) who determines if medical clearance is needed based on pre-determined criteria. Self-guided screening is best used in non-staff facilities such as hotel and apartment fitness centers or in facilities that do not hire exercise professionals. In these settings, a self-guided questionnaire can be posted within the facility. In facilities that employ exercise professionals, it is recommended to use professionally-guided screening.

Other professional organizations have also published pre-activity screening standards and guidelines such as: (a) the Medical Fitness Association (MFA) requires that medical fitness centers offer each new member an appropriate pre-activity screening process (9), (b) the National Strength and Conditioning Association (NSCA) requires health care provider screening and clearance for athletes in accordance with various standards/guidelines, regulations, and state statutes and for recreational activity programs, participants must undergo preparticipation

and clearance in accordance with AHA and ACSM recommendations (10), and (c) the American Association of Cardiovascular and Pulmonary Rehabilitation (AACVPR) states "each patient should undergo a careful medical evaluation and exercise test before participating in an outpatient cardiac rehabilitation/secondary prevention program" (11, p. 58). The two ACSM publications (3, 8) and the MFA publication (9) also have criteria that recommend medical clearance.

Pre-Activity Health Screening Research

In 2014, a national investigation of pre-activity health screening practices in fitness facilities was conducted (6, 12). The responses to a survey sent to ACSM-certified exercise physiologists (EP-Cs) provided both quantitative and qualitative data regarding these practices in the fitness facilities in which they worked. Regarding requiring new participants to complete a screening device, 73%, 24%, and 3% indicated yes, no, don't know, respectively. Those that indicated "yes" were asked the type of screening their facility conducted. These results showed that 26%, 43%, and 31% conducted self-guided, professionally-guided, both self-guided and professionally-guided, respectively. Most of the facilities (78%) that conducted professionally-guided screening required "at risk" individuals to obtain medical clearance.

Although the data from this national study (6, 12) indicated that 73% of all facilities had new participants complete a screening device, these percentages differed by type of setting as shown in Table 6-1. Commercial settings had the lowest percentage (40%) and hospital/clinical settings had the highest percentage (93%)

Table 6-1	Percentage of Fitness Facilities (by Setting) Requiring New Participants to Complete a Pre-Activity Screening Device (6, 12)
TYPE OF FITNESS SETTING	**PERCENTAGE**
Hospital/Clinical	93
Corporate	78
Government	67
University	56
Community	54
Commercial	40

indicating a high amount of variance in compliance rates regarding published, pre-activity screening standards/guidelines. It may be the hospital/clinical settings had a higher compliance rate because these settings are used to following various accreditation standards, such as the Joint Commission on the Accreditation of Healthcare Organizations (JCAHO). One possible explanation for the settings with lower compliance rates may be that the managers of these facilities were not aware of published standards that require and/or recommend screening. See Table 6-2. These data indicated that only about one-third of the managers were "very familiar" with the screening procedures in the two ACSM publications. It is likely that these managers may not be familiar with the many other published standards and guidelines either which, if true, is quite concerning. As described in Chapter 4, it is essential that fitness managers and exercise professionals be aware of and follow published standards of practice from both safety and legal perspectives.

Qualitative data from this national study (6, 12) were also relevant. Of the respondents indicating their facility did not require new participants to complete a screening device, a follow-up question as to why, generated the following responses:

a) Personal responsibility, i.e., members/participants are responsible for their own health and actions (36%)
b) Too time-consuming for staff (19%)
c) Facility or franchise policy (17%)
d) Barrier to participation (10%)
e) No need or purpose (9%)
f) Legal counsel advice (9%)

Although these may appear to be viable reasons, it is unlikely they would be considered effective legal defenses in a negligence lawsuit for not following the standard of care. It can only be speculated as to why legal counsel would advise against screening. Perhaps, they believe that there is less legal risk with less known about a new participant or do not believe that the facility staff members could properly carry out the screening procedures.

Survey participants were also asked about perceived challenges they had in carrying out their facility's screening procedures. The qualitative data from these responses were coded and then categorized into the following three major themes. Below each are examples of comments from respondents.

Member issues

▶ Clients not understanding the questions
▶ People do not understand the importance of it
▶ Many people are not totally honest on their forms

Medical clearance issues

▶ Some individuals do not want to go through the process of obtaining physician clearance prior to using the facility
▶ Some people do not come back/quit when informed they need to get medical clearance
▶ Dr. offices not responding to forms faxed regarding their patient's risk of exercise and any restrictions

Table 6-2	Level of Familiarity with ACSM's Published Pre-Activity Screening Procedures (12)				
ACSM CERTIFIED EXERCISE PHYSIOLOGISTS (N= 555)					
		VERY FAMILIAR	**FAMILIAR**	**SOMEWHAT FAMILIAR**	**NOT FAMILIAR**
ACSM's Health/Fitness Facility Standards and Guidelines		38%	35%	21%	6%
ACSM's Guidelines for Exercise Testing and Prescription		69%	26%	4%	1%
RATING BY ACSM CERTIFIED EXERCISE PHYSIOLOGISTS OF THEIR FACILITY MANAGER'S FAMILIARITY					
	VERY FAMILIAR	**FAMILIAR**	**SOMEWHAT FAMILIAR**	**NOT FAMILIAR**	**DON'T KNOW**
ACSM's Health/Fitness Facility Standards and Guidelines	26%	18%	19%	16%	21%
ACSM's Guidelines for Exercise Testing and Prescription	34%	19%	15%	14%	18%

Administrative/procedural issues

⟩ Lack of support from owners and managers who do not have an educational background in exercise science

⟩ Time is the biggest problem

⟩ No systems in place

These challenges can be addressed. See Risk Management Strategy #5. Often, published standards of practice indicate *what* to do but fall short on the *why* and *how*. To increase compliance with published standards of practice and applicable laws, fitness managers and exercise professionals need to learn not only the what, but the why and how, which is the focus of this textbook as discussed in Chapter 1.

Pre-Activity Health Screening Questionnaires

Several pre-activity screening questionnaires exist that fitness facilities can use. However, some facilities have opted to develop their own screening questionnaire. The results from the 2014 national study (6) showed that most facilities (53%) used a ready-made questionnaire such as the PAR-Q and 40% used a custom/in-house developed questionnaire. Although several examples or templates of pre-activity health screening questionnaires are available elsewhere (3, 8, 9) and on the Internet, two screening questionnaires will be described—the Physical Activity Readiness Questionnaire for Everyone (PAR-Q+) and the Pre-Activity Screening Questionnaire (PASQ).

The PAR-Q & You, developed by the Canadian Society for Exercise Physiology, has been updated to the PAR-Q+ and is available at www.eparmedx.com in both online and digital formats. The PAR-Q+ was developed using the AGREE process (described in Chapter 4) which requires an evidence-based approach such as conducting a systematic review of the literature. It contains seven "yes-no" questions. Individuals who answer "no" to all seven questions are provided recommendations regarding exercise intensity, consulting with an exercise professional, health changes, etc. Individuals who answer "yes" to any of the seven questions are directed to answer several follow-up questions that assess more specific medical conditions than the seven "yes-no" questions. Recommendations are provided for individuals who answer

KEY POINT

Data from a 2014 national study (6, 12) found that many fitness facilities were not having new participants complete a pre-activity health screening device as recommended or required by ACSM. The results of the same study also showed that only about one-third of fitness managers were "very familiar" with ACSM's pre-activity health screening guidelines (3) and standards (8). As described in Chapter 4, it is essential that fitness managers and exercise professionals be aware of and follow published standards of practice from both safety and legal perspectives.

"no" to all the follow-up questions as well as those who answered "yes" to one or more of the follow-up questions. Although the PAR-Q+ was designed to be a self-guided screening questionnaire, it can be used in professionally-guided screening programs. It would still be completed as designed. The only difference would be that an exercise professional would interpret the data obtained and determine if medical clearance is needed. Regarding medical clearance, the fitness manager, in consultation with the facility's medical advisor and/or risk management advisory committee, would need to establish the criteria that would warrant medical clearance. For example, anyone who answered "yes" to any the follow-up questions would need to obtain medical clearance.

The PASQ was developed after ACSM published its revised screening criteria in 2015 (7). It was based on the published algorithm (7) which provided direction on the follow-up steps for individuals who (a) do not participate in regular exercise, and (b) participate in regular exercise. An explanation of how the PASQ follows the criteria and medical clearance recommendations in the algorithm is provided elsewhere (13) and briefly described within Risk Management Strategy #5. A pilot study that investigated several factors related to implementing the PASQ was also described in this same article (13). Findings from the pilot study indicated that (a) the PASQ resulted in fewer physician referrals—one of the main goals for revising the ACSM criteria, and (b) both the participants who completed the PASQ and the staff members who administered the PASQ procedures indicated the process was easy and efficient. Additional forms to accompany the PASQ, a professionally-guided screening questionnaire, were also developed. These forms include a cover letter, an interpretation form, and a medical clearance form. All the PASQ forms are described within Risk Management Strategy #5 and can be found in this chapter's appendix. A self-guided PASQ that can be used in non-staffed facilities is also included in the appendix.

The ACSM algorithm provided medical clearance recommendations for moderate and vigorous intensity exercise, but not for high intensity exercise. This is a concerning limitation of the algorithm given that high intensity exercise, especially high intensity interval training (HIIT) is a popular trend in recent years (14). Some suggestions on how to address this limitation are provided within Risk Management Strategy #5.

Advantages and Disadvantages of the PAR-Q+ and PASQ

The PAR-Q+ was developed using evidenced-based best practice recommendations. The PASQ was developed based on the algorithm published by ACSM, which is also based on scientific evidence (7). The PAR-Q+ involves a lengthier completion process than the PASQ for individuals if they are directed to answer follow-up questions. The follow-up questions provide additional information about the individual's medical history (e.g., arthritis, cancer, stroke, respiratory disease, etc.). However, the PAR-Q+ does not include all nine signs and symptoms suggestive of cardiovascular, metabolic, and renal disease as does the ACSM algorithm and the PASQ. If the PAR-Q+ is used in professionally-guided screening, as described above, the medical history information obtained can be helpful when establishing the criteria for an appropriate fitness testing protocol and exercise prescription, along with any restrictions/limitations indicated on the medical clearance form completed by the individual's health care provider.

The PASQ does not contain these types of medical history questions because they were not included in the ACSM's algorithm criteria. However, the *ACSM's GETP* states that "exercise professionals are urged to be prudent in identifying those who may need medical clearance" (3, p. 44), meaning those with chronic conditions and other health challenges may need to obtain

clearance. In addition to the CVD statistics described earlier, about 50% of the U.S. adult population has at least one chronic condition with 25% having two more chronic conditions (15) and many are not metabolically healthy. Metabolic data (waist circumference, blood glucose, blood pressure, triglycerides, HDLs, and taking any related medication) from the National Health and Nutrition Examination Survey 2009-2016 (16), indicated that less than one-third of normal weight adults were metabolically healthy. For those that were overweight or obese, the prevalence of metabolically healthy adults decreased to 8.0% and 0.5%, respectively. Another source, the Centers for Disease Control and Prevention (CDC), provides the following data:

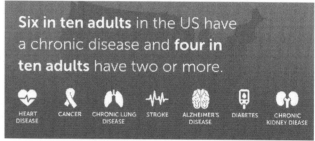

From: CDC. About Chronic Diseases. https://www.cdc.gov/chronicdisease/about/index.htm

Given the prevalence of chronic diseases and ACSM's recommendations, obtaining a medical history of individuals will be important before they begin participation in fitness testing and certain exercise programs.

Distinguishing Between Pre-Activity Health Screening and Medical History Questionnaires

A pre-activity health screening questionnaire would be offered to all new participants desiring to use the fitness facility and participate in the facility programs. The steps involved in a professionally-guided screening process are described below. However, if an individual wants to participate in the facility's fitness testing program, an individualized exercise program, or other "structured" programs in which exercise prescriptions are prepared, or should be prepared, such as exercise classes for persons with Parkinson's disease, it will be essential that exercise professionals obtain the **medical history** of these individuals.

As described in Chapter 4, exercise professionals have a responsibility to take special "safety" precautions based on the individual's medical conditions. For example, if

KEY POINT

A "medical history" questionnaire, which is different than a "pre-activity health screening" questionnaire, should be obtained to determine (a) a need for medical clearance prior to participation in fitness testing and preparation of individualized exercise prescriptions, and (b) what safety precautions are needed when conducting fitness testing and designing/delivering an exercise prescription given an individual's medical conditions. As described in Chapter 4 (see Exhibit 4-1), one factor that helps determine the standard of care of an exercise professional is the "type of participants"—meaning the exercise professional must be aware of the participant's medical conditions that may impose increased risks and know how to minimize those risks. In the spotlight and other cases described in this chapter, the failure of exercise professionals to obtain medical conditions were common negligence claims made by the plaintiffs.

someone is taking a beta blocker medication, has had recent surgery, has known neck/back problems, etc., it is essential that the exercise professional is aware of these conditions and any related restrictions/limitations indicated on the medical clearance form by the individual's health care provider. This allows the exercise professional to take the necessary safety precautions prior to conducting fitness testing and designing/delivering an exercise program. Therefore, it is necessary for fitness managers and exercise professionals to discuss this issue with their medical advisor and/or risk management advisory committee to determine (a) what additional medical history information is needed, and (b) the medical conditions that would warrant medical clearance prior to conducting fitness testing and/or establishing an appropriate exercise prescription? Examples/templates of various medical (or health) history questionnaires can be found on the Internet and in other resources. For example, the *Medical Fitness Association's Standards & Guidelines for Medical Fitness Center Facilities* (9) provides examples of pre-activity screening forms as well as health history forms that contain many more medical history questions than pre-activity health screening questionnaires. See Risk Management Strategy #6 for more information on this topic of obtaining a medical history.

Steps: Professionally-Guided Screening Process

Before the pre-activity screening process is administered, all participants need to be informed of the risks of physical activity. This can be completed by having participants read and sign a document that describes minor, major, and life-threatening risks including death. Examples of documents were provided in Chapter 4 such as an express assumption of risk (Exhibit 4-2), and an assumption of risk and waiver (Exhibit 4-3). This type of language also appears in an informed consent (see section titled "Risks" in Exhibit 6-2) and can be included in a membership agreement. The informed consent in Exhibit 6-2 is designed to be administered prior to fitness testing but it can be revised to be administered prior to participation in exercise activities. One way to inform participants of the risks in non-staffed facilities is to include a description of the risks in the self-guided screening form.

Various steps are involved in carrying out a professionally-guided pre-activity screening process. These include:

a) Inform participants of the purposes of pre-activity health screening. This can be done by providing participants with a cover letter that describes the purposes and the steps the process entails.

b) Have participants complete a pre-activity health screening questionnaire such as the PASQ.

c) Have an exercise professional interpret the data provided by the participant on the screening questionnaire, determine the need for medical clearance based on pre-established criteria, and document the interpretation and decision for medical clearance.

d) If medical clearance is needed, have the exercise professional provide the participant with the facility's medical clearance form that he/she can give to his/her physician or other health care provider for review and signature. This method is often quicker than mailing and/or faxing the clearance form to the physician's office and it does not create any potential privacy issues involving an individual's health information.

Note: Examples of forms that can be used to carry out the above steps are provided in this chapter's appendix.

e) Ensure that procedures are in place so that all the above documents are kept private, confidential, and secure as well as retained for a particular length of time (see Risk Management Strategy #10).

Fitness managers and exercise professionals need to consider obtaining the following from participants prior to their participation: (a) emergency contact information, (b) consent to receive medical care in an emergency, and (c) in some cases, a do-not-resuscitate order (DNR). Consultation with a competent lawyer is needed regarding DNRs because state statutes vary regarding DNRs. More information on DNRs is provided in Chapter 11. Regarding children, parents or legal guardians need to provide emergency contact information and give consent for their children to receive medical care in an emergency.

FITNESS TESTING

Once an individual completes the fitness facility's pre-activity health screening process, he/she is ready to participate in the facility's fitness testing program. Some facilities or exercise programs may require individuals to participate in certain fitness assessments before starting an exercise program, but most facilities provide fitness testing as an option for their participants. However, fitness testing should be done by exercise professionals who will be designing and delivering "individualized" exercise prescriptions such as personal fitness trainers and instructors of exercise classes for individuals with medical conditions. Screening data, medical history data, restrictions/limitations provided by the health care provider on the medical clearance form, and data obtained from fitness assessments are needed to develop a "safe" and "effective" exercise prescription.

There are two basic types of fitness testing (a) **health-related fitness testing**, and (b) **clinical exercise testing** (3). Health-related fitness tests are commonly conducted in fitness facilities and include assessments that measure cardiovascular endurance, muscle strength/endurance, flexibility, and body composition. The purposes of health-related fitness testing are:

- Collecting baseline data and educating participants about their present health-related fitness status…
- Providing data that are helpful in development of individualized exercise prescriptions to address all health/fitness components
- Collecting follow-up data that allow evaluation of progress…
- Motivating participants by establishing reasonable and attainable health/fitness goals (3, pp. 66-67).

A clinical exercise test, also referred to as a graded exercise test (GXT), is prescribed by physicians (or other health care providers) and are conducted in hospitals or clinical settings. Although there are several purposes for clinical exercise testing, the major purpose is to "diagnose" coronary artery disease (CAD). However, if a GXT is positive for CAD, additional diagnostic tests are conducted to confirm a CAD diagnosis. Because clinical exercise testing is not conducted in fitness facilities, legal liability and risk management issues associated with clinical exercise testing will not be the focus in this chapter. However, a couple case law examples are briefly described later in this chapter. Exercise professionals who would like to work as a clinical exercise test technologist will need extensive education and training in order to obtain the advanced knowledge and skills to perform these types of tests.

Steps: Health-Related Fitness Testing

Before health-related fitness testing services are provided, fitness managers and exercise professionals need to establish the steps that need to be followed. These include:

a) Obtain a medical history from participants. As stated above, the PASQ does not assess a variety of medical conditions that need to be determined before designing an individualized exercise program as well as conducting an individualized health-related fitness test. Medical clearance may be necessary after a medical history is completed by the participant. Also, fitness managers and exercise professionals along with their medical advisor and/or risk management advisory committee need to decide on the additional medical conditions that should be asked on a medical history form and, of those conditions, which ones would warrant medical clearance.

b) Establish the protocols that will be used. Exercise professionals will likely establish typical protocols for submaximal cardiovascular testing, muscle strength/endurance, flexibility, and body composition. However, alternative protocols will be needed for individuals who cannot complete a typical test due to health conditions and/or contraindications stated by their physician. It is recommended to work with a competent clinical exercise physiologist to assist in the decision-making regarding these alternative protocols. For example, if a participant is taking a beta-blocker medication, what adjustments need to be made to safely conduct/monitor a submaximal cardiovascular test or if a participant has back/neck problems, what modifications need to be made with any of the protocols?

c) Establish safety procedures (3) for conducting the fitness tests such as:

    a. Ensure a medical emergency action plan (EAP) is in place and staff are well-trained on how to properly carry it out

    b. Calibrate, inspect, maintain all testing equipment according to the manufacturer's specifications

    c. Provide participants with pre-test instructions

    d. Have participants read and sign an informed consent; Verbally explain each section of the informed consent—see Exhibit 6-2 below for an example

    e. Explain/demonstrate the tests to participants, e.g., for skinfolds, describe how each site is first measured/marked and how the caliper is used to take the skinfold measurement

    f. Explain the Rating of Perceived Exertion (RPE) chart and instructions to report any unusual symptoms, such as chest pain, during any of the tests

    g. Determine criteria for stopping a test

    h. Provide close supervision while all tests are being performed by participants, e.g., always observing participants for any unusual signs of fatigue

    i. Provide participants with post-test instructions

d) Provide a written test results report for participants that exercise professionals can use to describe and interpret the scores as well as explain errors/limitations of certain test results.

Should Fitness Facilities Conduct Maximal or Near-Maximal Cardiovascular Tests?

The general answer to this question is no. Given that many people within the general population are unfit (17) and have various medical conditions (15, 16), it is best to conduct only submaximal tests for safety reasons. Most submaximal protocols establish a maximal heart rate that should not be exceeded (e.g., 85% of an age-predicted formula). However, it is important to realize that even a submaximal test can quickly result in maximal or near maximal heart rates in some individuals. The same is true for field tests such as the Cooper 12-minute test and the Rockport One-Mile Fitness Walking Test (3), and step tests. See spotlight case, *Covenant Health System v. Barnett* (18), in which the plaintiff became fatigued only 2 minutes into a step test, lost her balance, and fell shattering her left wrist. For individuals that are sedentary or have certain medical conditions, it may be wise to modify the protocol prior to having them perform the test. For example, with the YMCA submaximal cycle ergometer test (3), if an individual has a heart rate of 80-89 beats per minute at the end of stage 1 (0.5 kg), the protocol indicates to move the workload to 2.0 kg for stage 2. This significant increase in workload can result in heart rates above the 85% age-predicted maximum quite quickly. Therefore, adjusting the protocol in advance to increase the stage 2 workload to 1.0 kg or 1.5 kg may be a safer approach versus an increase to 2.0 kg.

Exercise professionals need to follow recommendations regarding exercise intensity provided by a participant's health care provider on the medical clearance form. For example, the PASQ medical clearance form in this chapter's appendix, contains the following, in part, for the health care provider to complete:

Please check (√) the highest exercise intensity level your patient is cleared for and provide any other restrictions/limitations:

- ❏ Light (<57 to < 64% HR max)
- ❏ Moderate (64 to < 76% HR max)
- ❏ Vigorous (76 to < 96% HR max)
- ❏ Near Maximal to Maximal (≥ 96% HR max)

These intensity levels come from *ACSM's GETP* (3, p. 146). If the health care provider indicates

"moderate" intensity, then the exercise professional needs to follow this recommendation for both fitness testing and exercise prescription. As stated above, vigorous exercise increases the risk of a cardiac event particularly among habitually sedentary individuals with underlying CVD. (4). As shown above, high intensity (near maximal to maximal) is above vigorous intensity, so it is likely that an increased risk of a cardiac or other untoward event could be even greater with high intensity exercise than with vigorous intensity exercise.

ASSESSMENT OF LEGAL LIABILITY EXPOSURES

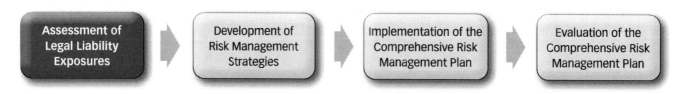

This section will discuss legal liability exposures associated with pre-activity health screening and fitness testing. Spotlight cases addressing these issues will be described along with summaries of other relevant cases. First, certain laws will be briefly described as they relate to screening and testing. These include the Health Insurance Portability and Accountability Act (HIPAA), Americans with Disabilities Act (ADA), Occupational Safety and Health Administration (OSHA) Bloodborne Pathogens Standard, Clinical Laboratory Improvement Amendments (CLIA), and Protection of Human Subjects. A detailed description of the HIPAA, ADA, and CLIA is presented in Chapter 3 along with risk management strategies that will help fitness managers and exercise professionals comply with them.

Editorial Note: The content in the following section titled "statutory and administrative laws" reflects content from Chapters 6 and 7 in Risk Management for Health/Fitness Professionals: Legal Issues and Strategies (1). The publisher transferred the rights to this textbook to the authors in 2017. Permission to reprint and revise/update this content was granted by the author of Chapters 6 and 7.

Statutory and Administrative Laws

Most fitness facilities are not considered "covered entities" under the HIPAA. Therefore, they would not need to comply with privacy, confidentiality, security provisions specified in this law related to **protected health information (PHI)**. These terms can be defined as follows:

Privacy is the right of an individual to enjoy freedom from intrusion…; the right to maintain control over certain personal information…

Confidentiality is the practice of permitting only certain authorized individuals to access information…

Security refers to the…safeguards used to control access and protect information from…disclosure to unauthorized person(s)… (19).

As described in Chapter 3, some employer-sponsored fitness/wellness and disease prevention programs may be subject to HIPAA regulations. For these programs, it will be essential that HIPAA provisions are implemented properly. Although most fitness facilities would not be subject to HIPAA violations, they could be subject to violations of state privacy laws as well as civil claims such as "breach of contract, intentional or negligent infliction of emotional distress, invasion of privacy, libel, slander or even disparagement" (20, p.

297). To minimize legal liability regarding health information that is collected by fitness facilities (e.g., participant data provided on screening, medical history, and medical clearance forms as well as fitness testing data), Herbert and Herbert (20) state that facilities should "adopt, as a matter of written policy, a statement which would help ensure the confidentiality of client health related information in the organization's possession" (p. 297). In addition to several legal liability reasons to keep an individual's health information private, confidential, and secure, there are ethical reasons. Major professional organizations provide a code of conduct (or ethical standards) for the members and certified individuals to follow which includes keeping an individual's health information confidential. It is also wise to inform participants that their health information is kept private, confidential and secure. See the PASQ cover letter in this chapter's appendix.

There is no reason for fitness facility staff members to disclose private health information of participants to anyone. Those who have a "need to know" would be the only exception. Examples include (a) the facility's fitness director shares an individual's health information with the exercise professional who will be designing and delivering the exercise program for that individual, and (b) a personal fitness trainer needs guidance from the facility's fitness director or clinical exercise physiologist to assist with the design/delivery of a safe and effective exercise program for an individual with a chronic condition. These discussions among exercise professionals need to occur in private and, of course, all health information forms (paper or electronic) need to be returned to their secure location and kept confidential.

Also, it is important that no individual health information is ever disclosed to a third party (including a participant's health care provider) without the written authorization of the individual. If an exercise professional wants to send a client's health information (e.g., health screening data, fitness testing data, progress reports) directly to the client's health care provider, the exercise professional should first have the client sign a **medical release**. Another option is for the exercise professional to prepare a report with the client's data/progress that the client can share with his/her health care provider at the next visit. If an exercise professional wants to obtain medical records of his/her client

KEY POINT

Although most fitness facilities would not be subject to HIPAA violations, they could be subject to violations of state privacy laws as well as various civil claims if an individual's protected health information (PHI) is not kept private, confidential, and secure. Fitness managers and exercise professionals need to adopt written policies and procedures that all fitness staff members must follow regarding keeping PHI private, confidential, and secure. The PHI includes information gathered on pre-activity health screening and medical history questionnaires, medical clearance forms, and reports with fitness testing scores.

such as graded exercise test (GXT) results, the client's health care provider will first have his/her patient sign a medical release that is HIPAA compliant. Another option is for the exercise professional to ask his/her client to obtain the medical records from his/her health care provider, and then have the client provide it to the exercise professional. See Chapter 3 for more information on medical releases and a form that is HIPAA compliant—Authorization for Release of Protected Health Information.

As described in Chapter 3, Title III of the ADA prohibits discrimination regarding programs and services offered by places of public accommodation and commercial facilities (21). For example, one of the 12 categories of places of public accommodation specified in Title III includes "a gymnasium, health spa, bowling alley, golf course, or other places of exercise or recreation" (21, p. 22). In an ADA discrimination lawsuit, the plaintiff will have to prove "1) that he or she is an individual with a disability; 2) that defendant is a place of public accommodation; and 3) that defendant denied him or her full and equal enjoyment of the goods, services, facilities or privileges offered by defendant on the basis of his or her disability" (22, p. 1342).

With reference to pre-activity health and medical history questionnaires, compliance with the ADA requires actions (decisions) to be neutral, non-discriminatory—meaning the criteria used to determine if medical clearance is needed must be the same for all individuals. Therefore, fitness managers and exercise professionals,

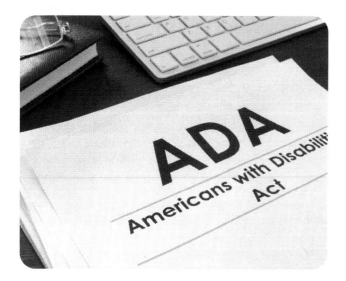

in consultation with their medical and legal advisors, need to carefully consider the medical clearance criteria. Also, if a health care provider indicates on the medical clearance form that his/her patient is not cleared to exercise at the fitness facility (see PASQ Medical Clearance Form in the appendix), the individual could still file an ADA (or other) discrimination lawsuit against the facility. See *Class v. Towson University* (22) described in Chapter 3. However, the recommendation from the health care provider would provide evidence to help defend the reason to deny participation.

Fitness managers and exercise professionals, along with assistance from their risk management advisory committee, need to develop a policy and procedures for participants who refuse to complete the facility's pre-activity health screening process. If it is decided to have a policy that excludes such individuals from joining the facility or participating in facility activities, the possibility of an ADA discrimination claim/lawsuit needs to be considered. Other discrimination claims/lawsuits, as described in Chapter 3, could also be made against the facility. Another option to consider is to have the individual sign a refusal form. See Exhibit 6-1 for an example of a refusal form. This form includes exculpatory language, so it is a waiver. As discussed in Chapter 4, waivers are unenforceable in some states, which is another factor to consider prior to having individuals sign a refusal form. Also related to the ADA is the ADA Final Rule issued by the Equal Employment Opportunity Commission (EEOC) in 2016 that applies only to employer-sponsored fitness/wellness programs.

There is a "notice" requirement when collecting health and medical history information as well as follow-up provisions to meet "promote health or prevent disease" requirements (23).

Biometric Screenings

Some fitness facilities offer biometric screenings that include blood tests to measure cholesterol and blood glucose as well as blood pressure tests. A blood test can be done using a fingerstick or a venous blood draw method. For both types of blood tests, fitness facilities need to comply with the requirements of OSHA's Bloodborne Pathogens Standard. See Chapter 11 for a description of this law and its requirements. In addition to this federal law, it is important to review the Clinical Laboratory Improvement Amendments (CLIA), which is described in Chapter 3. This law established quality standards for all laboratory testing including testing for the assessment of health regardless of where the test is performed. This regulation requires obtaining CLIA certification which is quite complex and costly. In some cases, such as performing fingerstick testing, a Certificate of Waiver can be obtained. In most cases, it would be best for fitness managers and exercise professionals to collaborate with a local hospital or clinic that already possesses the CLIA certification to provide such screenings. In addition, they should consult with their legal counsel regarding any applicable state or local laws regarding the qualification/credential requirements of individuals that can conduct these types of tests as well as any other related legal requirements.

Blood pressure screenings are common in fitness facilities. For example, they may be offered once per month as a service to participants. These screenings may be conducted by a credentialed and competent health care professional that the facility hires on a monthly basis or by exercise professionals who are employees of the facility. Exercise professionals with a degree in exercise science should possess adequate knowledge and skills to perform resting blood pressure tests. In fact, all exercise professionals who conduct cardiovascular fitness tests must have demonstrated skills in taking blood pressure because the protocols for even a submaximal cardiovascular test

Exhibit 6-1: Refusal to Participate in the Pre-Activity Health Screening Process*

To help ensure safe participation in fitness activities, most major professional fitness organizations have published standards and/or guidelines that require or recommend that health/fitness facilities and personnel have all participants complete a pre-activity health screening process prior to their beginning a fitness program. Therefore, to comply with these national standards and guidelines, _____ (name of health/fitness facility) ("Facility") has established a policy that requires all participants to complete its pre-activity health screening process. However, though not recommended, participants may refuse to participate in this process by reading and signing the following:

I _____ (name of participant) understand that Facility requires all participants to complete a pre-activity health screening process that includes: a) completing the Facility's pre-activity screening questionnaire, , and if indicated based upon the completion of that document b) obtaining medical clearance from my health care provider if deemed necessary by a qualified staff member of the Facility.

However, I have chosen not to participate in:
_____ Completing the Facility's pre-activity screening questionnaire
_____ Obtaining medical clearance from my health care provider

Risks associated with refusal to participate in the Facility's Pre-Activity Screening Process

The purpose of Pre-Activity Screening is to determine if an individual may participate in fitness testing and/or activity without examination and clearance by a health care provider. I understand and appreciate that there exists the possibility of adverse effects (risks) during fitness testing and/or activity. I have been informed that these potential adverse effects, though remote, include abnormal blood pressure, fainting, disorders of heart rhythm, stroke, and very rare instances of heart attack or even death. In addition, I understand that during participation in fitness testing and/or activity, I may experience musculoskeletal conditions or injuries such as fractured bones, muscle strains, muscle sprains, muscular fatigue, contusions, muscle soreness, joint injuries, torn muscles, heat-related illnesses, and back injuries. I understand that other risks not listed here, both minor and major, can also occur.

Benefits of participating in the Facility's Pre-Activity Screening Process

I understand that the benefits of participating in the Facility's Pre-Activity Screening Process are to reduce the chances of those risks occurring while I participate in fitness testing and/or activity and that screening is to help enhance my safety. I assert that my participation without screening is voluntary and that I knowingly assume all such risks.

Waiver/Release

My signature below indicates that I have been fully informed of, understand, and appreciate the benefits of completing the pre-activity health screening process as well as the potential risks of not completing the pre-activity screening process. In addition, my signature also indicates that I have executed a release and waiver document with the Facility which, among other things, contractually binds me and my estate not to bring any type of legal claim and/or lawsuit against the Facility and/or its staff members for among other things, the failure of the Facility and/or its staff to conduct any aspect of the pre-activity health screening process including Facility's request that I obtain medical clearance prior to participation. I also understand that this release/waiver gives up and relinquishes my right to institute a claim or lawsuit against the Facility and/or its staff members for a number of other acts and/or omissions, including those which could be classified as ordinary negligence. I hereby reaffirm my understanding and agreement to that release and waiver documents and to this statement.

This Agreement shall be interpreted according to the laws of the State of _____. If any part of this agreement should ever be determined by a court of final jurisdiction to be invalid, the remaining portions shall be deemed to be valid and enforceable.

_____   _____
Signature of Participant   Date

_____   _____
Signature of Staff Member   Date

*Reproduced and adapted with permission from David L. Herbert. Copyright 2019 by PRC Publications, Inc. Canton, Ohio. All other rights reserved. No form should be adopted without individualized legal advice and consultation.

require taking a resting blood pressure prior to the test and exercise blood pressures during the test. For blood pressure screenings conducted at fitness facilities, fitness managers and exercise professionals should consult with their medical and legal advisors regarding blood pressure screening procedures (e.g., record keeping, recommendations for participants who have measures outside the normal ranges, and if there are any state and local laws that might apply). The same would be true for fingerstick blood tests that are performed. And, of course, any health data collected needs to be kept private, confidential, and secure.

Protection of Human Subjects—Informed Consent

Sometimes exercise professionals who work in fitness facilities conduct research or collaborate with another organization to conduct research that involves human subjects. Informed consent is required by administrative law, 45 C.F.R. § 46—Protection of Human Subjects for individuals who participate in research projects. This law is quite complex and contains many parts. In general, this law requires that Institutional Review Boards (IRBs) approve the procedures of any study involving human subjects, including obtaining informed consent. Because many types of risks exist with participation in fitness testing and exercise programs, a written informed consent (versus implied consent) would, most likely, be required and would need to be approved by an IRB. Although obtaining IRB approval of the research procedures and informed consent is the responsibility of the principal investigator (PI), exercise professionals involved in the research need to understand the importance of their legal requirements to carry out the informed consent and other procedures properly.

In addition, informed consent is a legal requirement for clinical exercise testing as it is prior to other medical procedures conducted in hospitals and clinics. The failure to do so can result in either breach of contract or medical malpractice lawsuits, and in some cases, battery—an intentional tort (20). According to Herbert and Herbert (20), lawsuits have been filed against physicians, exercise technicians, and the health care organizations they represent for various reasons such as failing to administer a proper informed consent, stopping the test given the patient's signs/symptoms, and not following published standards of practice addressing clinical testing procedures. A couple cases involving clinical exercise testing procedures are briefly described later in this chapter—see Clinical Exercise Testing Cases.

Although informed consent is not a legal requirement prior to health-related fitness tests conducted in fitness facilities, it is highly recommended. See Exhibit 6-2 for an example of an informed consent for health-related fitness testing. An informed consent can also be prepared for other purposes. For example, some fitness facilities are using biometric technology such as having participants submit fingerprint data. Without first obtaining their consent, it can lead to a violation of state statutes that regulate the use of biometric data (24). More information on this topic is covered in Chapter 10.

The informed consent in Exhibit 6-2 has been used in the University of South Florida (USF) FIT program. This program, described elsewhere (13, 25), involves exercise science seniors paired up with an employee who they train throughout the fall semester as part of a required course. The students administer the informed consent prior to conducting the pre- and post-testing of the employee.

Note: *Informed consents do not contain exculpatory language.*

Case Law

This section will describe three spotlight cases—negligence lawsuits involving pre-activity health screening and fitness testing. The negligent claims in these cases included the failure to conduct pre-activity health screening and fitness testing/assessments (omission), but also improper fitness testing (commission), such as failing to follow protocols in a safe manner. Additional cases are briefly described after the spotlight cases. Examples of these types of negligence claims were evident in *Baldi-Perry* v. *Kaifas and 360 Fitness Center, Inc.* (26), described in Chapter 2 (see Exhibit 2-2). Numerous negligence claims were made against the trainer and the facility in this case including the following regarding screening and assessment failures:

Trainer

- ❯ Failing to perform a proper fitness evaluation of the plaintiff before devising an exercise routine
- ❯ Failing to consider the plaintiff's prior injuries and physical condition before preparing an exercise routine
- ❯ Failing to conduct a health risk appraisal
- ❯ Failing to identify the plaintiff as someone with an increased risk of injury
- ❯ Failing to evaluate the plaintiff's medical condition before preparing an exercise routine
- ❯ Failing to properly evaluate the plaintiff's exercise experience before creating an exercise routine
- ❯ Failing to warn the plaintiff about the risks of injury associated with her exercise routine (26, pp 6-8)

Facility

- ❯ Failing to have trainers who were certified and/or trained to conduct a proper pre-activity screening
- ❯ Failing to ensure that trainers performed a proper fitness evaluation of clients before devising an exercise routine
- ❯ Failing to have a medical liaison or medical advisory committee to assist in reviewing physical activity screenings and exercise plans
- ❯ Failing to ensure that trainers conducted a health risk appraisal
- ❯ Failing to have proper pre-activity screening tools in place for its trainers (26, pp. 9-10)

Spotlight Cases

The first spotlight case, *Rostai v. Neste Enterprises* (27), dealt with several issues but one of the primary issues was the personal fitness trainer's failure to assess Rostai's physical condition and cardiac risk factors. Perhaps, if this had been done, a much less intense workout would have been instructed by the trainer. An interesting aspect in this case was that the trial court sustained (approved) defendants' objection to a portion of a declaration made by expert witness Dr. Girandola (associate professor of Exercise Science at the University of Southern California) that stated "greater scrutiny should be exercised in monitoring

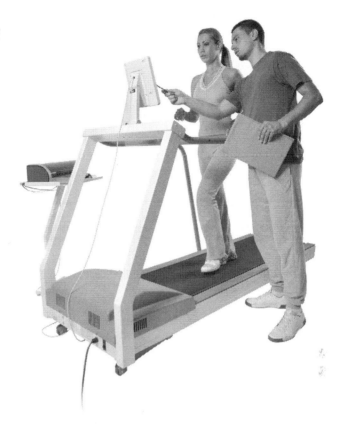

individuals at health and fitness clubs like Gold's Gym" and that "defendant Gold's Gym's acts and omissions also constituted a substantial factor in the cause of the plaintiffs heart attack" (27, pp. 418-419). The appellate court's response to this was that it was not relevant because whether a duty of care exists is an issue for the court to resolve. **Note:** Yes, courts determine duty in negligence cases, but most courts allow expert testimony to educate the court as to what the standard of care (or duty) was that the defendant owed to the plaintiff. If the court had viewed the expert's testimony as relevant, the expert witness might have shown that published standards of practice regarding pre-activity health screening were not followed as well as help the court understand the purposes of and safe approaches to exercise. Most exercise professionals would disagree with the court's statements such as a participant must engage in strenuous physical activity to improve fitness and appearance and that it is the "trainer's function ...to challenge the participant to work muscles to their limits" and "inherent in that process is the risk that the trainer will not accurately assess the participant's ability" (27, p. 417).

Exhibit 6-2: USF FIT Program — Informed Consent for Exercise Testing*

1. Purpose and Explanation of Tests

I hereby consent to voluntarily engage in various exercise tests to estimate my cardiovascular (aerobic) endurance, muscle strength/endurance, flexibility, and body composition. It is my understanding that the information obtained will help me evaluate future physical activities and sport activities in which I may engage. The tests will include:

- **Cardiovascular Endurance:** Submaximal Bike Test
- **Muscle Strength/Endurance:** Abdominal Curl-up (Crunch) Test; 1 RM for Upper Body Strength, 1 RM for Leg Strength
- **Flexibility:** Sit and Reach
- **Body Composition:** Bioelectrical Impedance Analysis (BIA); 3-site skin fold test; Waist-to-Hip Ratio; Body Weight and Height

Before I undergo the tests, I certify to the *USF Exercise Science FIT Program* that I am in good health and/or have had a physician's clearance if required by the FIT program. Further, I hereby represent and inform the program that I have completed the health history questionnaire presented to me by the instructor of the course and have provided correct responses to the questions as indicated on the history form. It is my understanding that I will be interviewed by my FIT student personal trainer prior to my undergoing the tests who will in the course of interviewing me determine if there are any reasons which would make it undesirable or unsafe for me to take the tests. Consequently, I understand that it is important that I provide complete and accurate responses to the interviewer and recognize that my failure to do so could lead to possible unnecessary injury to myself during the tests.

The cardiovascular endurance test I will undergo will be performed on a bicycle ergometer with the amount of effort gradually increasing. I understand that this text will not continue beyond 85% of my age-predicted maximal heart rate. As I understand it, the gradual increase in effort will continue until I feel and verbally report to my student personal trainer(s) any symptoms such as fatigue, shortness of breath, or chest discomfort which may appear. It is my understanding and I have been clearly advised that it is my right to request that a test be stopped at any point if I feel unusual discomfort or fatigue. I have been advised that I should immediately upon experiencing any such symptoms, or if I so choose, inform my student personal trainer(s) that I wish to stop the test at that or any other point. My wishes in this regard shall be absolutely carried out. It is further my understanding that during the test itself, my student personal trainer(s) will monitor my responses continuously and take frequent readings of blood pressure and my expressed feelings of effort.

The muscular strength tests I will undergo will assess dynamic muscular strength by means of a 1-Repetition Maximum bench press for upper body strength and 1-Repetition Maximum leg press for lower body strength (3). As I understand it, the 1-Repetition Maximum will be determined within four trials with rest periods of 3 to 5 minutes between trials. I have been advised that the test will begin with approximately 50%-70% of my perceived capacity and resistance will progressively increase by 2.5 to 20 kg until I have reached the maximum amount of resistance I can perform with correct speed and range of motion. An abdominal Curl-Up (Crunch) test (3) will also be performed to measure muscular endurance. I understand in this test I will perform as many curl-ups as I can in 1 minute.

The flexibility test that I will undergo will assess low back and hip joint flexibility. I have been advised that this test may be a better predictor of hamstring flexibility than low back flexibility and is limited in its ability to predict incidence of low back pain. I understand that the results of this test have relative importance to activities of daily living and sports performance. It is my understanding that I will perform two trials of this test, after a mild warm-up, and the highest score will be recorded.

The body composition tests that I will undergo will estimate my percentage of body mass that is fat tissue using a low-level electric current, calipers, height/weight, and circumference measures. I have been advised that the low-level electric current is low risk, noninvasive, and measures the impedance or resistance to the flow through the body fluids contained mainly in the lean and fat tissue. I understand that the calipers measure subcutaneous fat and the skinfold sites for men are chest, abdomen, and thigh. The skinfold sites for women are triceps, suprailiac, and thigh (3). I understand that my risk(s) for disease will be estimated by circumference measurements to be taken at the waist and hip and height and weight measurements that will be used to determine my body mass index.

Once the tests have been completed, but before I am released from the test area, I will be given special instructions about recognition of certain symptoms that may appear within 24 hours after the test. I agree to follow these instructions and promptly contact the program personnel or medical providers if such symptoms develop.

Exhibit 6-2 continued...

2. Risks

I understand and have been informed that there exists the possibility of adverse changes during the actual tests. I have been informed that these changes, though remote, include abnormal blood pressure, fainting, disorders of heart rhythm, stroke, and very rare instances of heart attack or even death. In addition, I understand that I may experience musculoskeletal conditions or injuries such as muscle strains, muscle sprains, muscular fatigue, contusions, post-testing muscle soreness, joint injuries, torn muscles, heat-related illnesses, and back injuries. I have been told that every effort will be made to minimize these occurrences by precautions and observations taken during the tests. I have also been informed that emergency equipment (First-Aid/AED) and personnel (AED/CPR/First-Aid certified) are readily available to deal with these unusual situations should they occur. Even though, I understand that there is a risk of injury, heart attack, stroke, or even death as a result of my performance of these tests, but knowing those risks, it is my desire to proceed to take the test as herein indicated.

3. Benefits to be expected and available Alternatives to the Exercise Testing Procedures

The results of these tests may or may not benefit me. Potential benefits relate mainly to my personal motives for taking the tests, that is, knowing my exercise capacity in relation to the general population, understanding my fitness for certain physical, recreational, and sport activities, planning my physical conditioning program, or evaluation of the effects of my recent physical activity habits. Although my cardiovascular endurance test might also be evaluated by alternative means, for example, a bench step test or an outdoor running test, such tests do not provide as accurate a fitness assessment as the bike test nor do these options allow equally effective monitoring of my responses. In addition, although the muscle strength/ endurance, flexibility, and body composition tests might also be evaluated by other means, the above tests were selected because they are common tests approved by the American College of Sports Medicine that can be completed within a reasonable amount of time.

4. Confidentiality and Use of Information

I have been informed that the information obtained in this exercise test will be treated as privileged and confidential to the extent possible by FIT and in accordance with permissible law and will consequently not be released or revealed to any person without my express written consent or pursuant to subpoena or court order. I do, however, agree to the use of any information for emergency medical treatment if needed. I also agree to the use for research or statistical purposes so long as the same does not provide facts that could lead to my identification. Any other information obtained, however, will be used only by the FIT program to evaluate my exercise status or needs.

5. Inquiries and Freedom of Consent

I have been given an opportunity to ask certain questions as to the procedures. Generally, these requests, which have been noted by my FIT student personal trainer and his /her response, are as follows:

_____

_____

I further understand that there are also other remote risks that may be associated with this procedure. Despite the fact that a complete accounting of all these remote risks has not been provided to me, I still desire to proceed with the test. I acknowledge that I have read this document in its entirety or that it has been read to me if I have been unable to read same. I consent to the rendition of all services and procedures as explained herein by all program personnel.

_____	_____
Participant's Signature	Date
_____	_____
Test Supervisor's (Student) Signature	Date
_____	_____
Course Professor's Signature	Date

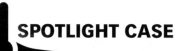
SPOTLIGHT CASE

Rostai v. Neste Enterprises, d/b/a Gold's Gym
41 Cal. Rptr. 3d 411 (Cal. Ct. App., 2006)

FACTS

Historical Facts:

The plaintiff, Masood Rostai, entered into a personal training agreement with trainer Jared Shoultz. Rostai was 46 years old, overweight and did not exercise. In the initial workout session, Shoultz instructed Rostai to exercise on a treadmill for 12-13 minutes at three to four miles per hour and then lift weights over his head on an incline bench (10 repetitions at 40 pounds and another set of 10 repetitions with slightly heavier weights). Rostai asked for a break but Shoultz said "later" and instructed him to perform 10 push-ups. Rosati again asked for a break informing Shoultz that he was very tired and out of breath. But Shoutlz said "don't be a (expletive) and first give me ten sit-ups" After completing the 10 sit-ups, Shoutz instructed Rostai to go back to the incline bench and repeat the lifting exercises but at the next heavier weight and at a faster tempo. After four-five repetitions, Rostai said he could not perform any more and stopped. After another expletive comment to the plaintiff, Shoultz had Rostai lay down on a mat and instructed him to lift both legs simultaneously. Rostai could only perform one leg lift and stopped but then Shoultz grabbed the plaintiff's legs and pushed them 10 to 12 times toward Rostai's head. At this point, the plaintiff began to experience chest pain and profuse sweating, so the workout stopped. The plaintiff told Shoultz he couldn't breathe and needed some water. After about five minutes, Rostai said, "Call 911, I think I am having a heart attack."

Procedural Facts:

In his negligent action, the plaintiff claimed the defendants Shoultz and Gold's Gym failed to adequately assess his health history, physical condition, and cardiac risk factors. Rostai also claimed that Shoultz knew he was not physically fit and was overweight but aggressively trained him in his first workout although he complained several times during the workout, he needed a break. The defendants moved for summary judgment asserting primary assumption of risk as their defense. The trial court granted the motion for summary judgment for the defendants and the plaintiff appealed contending that the doctrine of primary assumption of risk only applies to sports and not to fitness training.

ISSUE

Did the trial court properly grant the motion for summary judgment for the defendants based on the primary assumption of risk defense?

COURT'S RULING

Yes, the appellate court affirmed the trial court's decision agreeing with the defendants that the plaintiff assumed the risks.

COURT'S REASONING

The appellate court, citing previous California cases, concluded that primary assumption of risk is not limited to sports but also applies to any activities that contain elements of risk or danger. The court stated "Fitness training under the guidance of a personal trainer is such an activity. The obvious purpose of working out with a personal trainer is to improve physical fitness and appearance. In order to accomplish that goal, the participant must engage in strenuous physical activity. The risks inherent in that activity include physical distress in general and in particular muscle strains, sprains... not only in the obvious muscles such as those in the legs and arms, but also of less obvious muscles such as the heart... Eliminating that risk would alter the fundamental nature of the activity" (pp. 415-416).

Rostai continued...

In response to the plaintiff's claim that Shoultz failed to assess his physical condition and in particular his cardiac risk factors and challenged him to perform beyond his level of physical ability and fitness, the court stated: "That challenge, however, is the very purpose of fitness training, and is precisely the reason one would pay for the services of a personal trainer. Like the coach in other sports or physical activities, the personal trainer's role in physical fitness training is not only to instruct the participant in proper exercise techniques but also to develop a training program that requires the participant to stretch his or her current abilities…and challenge the participant to work muscles to their limits…Inherent In that process is the risk that the trainer will not accurately assess the participant's ability and the participant will be injured as a result" (p. 417).

Again, relying on previous California case law to support its decision, the appellate court stated that the doctrine of primary assumption of the risk "embodies a legal conclusion that there is 'no duty' on the part of the defendant to protect the plaintiff from a particular risk" (p. 419). However, the court did state that the evidence showed that defendant Shoultz did not accurately assess plaintiff's level of fitness and he may have interpreted plaintiff's complaints (e.g., tiredness, shortness of breath, profuse sweating) as usual signs of physical exertion rather than symptoms of a heart attack. However, because there was no evidence that Shoultz's conduct was intentional or reckless which would have increased the risks to Rostai, the court concluded there was no evidence that Shoultz breached any duty owed to the plaintiff.

Lessons Learned from *Rostai*

Legal

- Although the primary assumption of risk defense protected the defendants, the ruling and reasoning of this appellate court is likely not applicable in other jurisdictions where courts have ruled differently in similar cases involving negligent instruction of personal fitness trainers.

- As described in Chapter 4, the primary assumption of risk defense is generally an effective defense if the plaintiff knows and fully understands the risks inherent in the activity, which was not likely in this case given the plaintiff was a novice exerciser.

- The court stated the defendants would only have been liable if the trainer's conduct was reckless (gross negligence) or intentional.

- See Chapter 4 for a description of cases in which courts have distinguished between sport and fitness activities with regard to the primary assumption of risk defense.

Risk Management/Injury Prevention

- Personal fitness trainers must have the necessary knowledge and skills to safely and effectively train a client (i.e., know how to conduct pre-activity health screening and design/deliver an appropriate exercise program given the client's health/fitness status).

- Personal fitness trainers should not push their clients and should grant their requests for a break.

- Fitness managers need to properly hire, train, and supervise their fitness staff members.

- In addition to training regarding proper design/delivery of fitness programs, fitness managers also need to provide training on proper, professional communication with clients.

The following two spotlight cases, *Covenant Health System v. Barnett* (18) and *Howard v. Missouri Bone and Joint Center* (28), demonstrate the importance of properly administering fitness testing protocols according to standards of practice published by professional organizations and standards established by the facility. It is likely that the plaintiffs would have won in the *Covenant* case if they had filed a "health care liability" claim (medical malpractice claim) versus an ordinary negligence claim. The court provided evidence (i.e., guidelines published by the ACSM), to demonstrate how Covenant breached the standard of care applicable to health care providers. For example, the employees conducting the step test did not (a) possess the specialized knowledge and skills necessary to administer the test, and (b) properly supervise and terminate the test, as specified in the ACSM guidelines. It is also important to realize that cardiovascular fitness testing should never be done at a community heart symposium or health fair. It would be difficult to conduct pre-activity health screening, obtain medical clearance if needed, and tend to all the safety procedures as described above before fitness assessments should be done. A fitness booth or exhibit at such an event can provide educational materials and maybe some very simple tests such as height and weight (BMI) if done in private such as behind a screen if the participant gives consent.

In *Howard v. Missouri Bone and Joint Center* (28), the athletic trainer failed to (a) properly follow the clinic's initial evaluation protocol, (b) understand that a pop followed by a sharp pain may indicate an injury, and (c) provide proper instruction after the injury. Fitness managers and exercise professionals need to be sure all their fitness staff members understand the distinction between pain associated with muscle soreness or discomfort while exercising and pain associated with a possible injury. See Table 6-3. In another case, *Makris v. Scandinavian Health Spa, Inc.* (29), a personal fitness trainer told his client that the sharp pain in her neck that radiated own her arm while performing an exercise was due to muscle weakness. She believed her trainer and continued preforming the exercise. However, the pain was due to three herniated cervical disks. Not only was the trainer's instruction to continue improper, but so was his "diagnosis" of her pain which is outside the scope of practice of a personal fitness trainer. For more information on scope of practice, see Chapter 7.

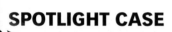

SPOTLIGHT CASE

Covenant Health System v. Barnett
342 S.W.3d. 226, 2011 LEXIS 3665 (Tex. App., 2011)

FACTS

Historical Facts:

The plaintiff, Linda Barnett, registered for free heart screenings offered at the Fifth Annual Heart Symposium sponsored by Covenant Health System. One of the screenings was a 3-minute step test. Barnett was instructed to step up and down on a 14-inch-high step and to keep time with the beat of a metronome that was set by a staff member. The step was placed close to the wall which forced her to lean back somewhat while stepping up, so she would not hit her head on the wall. About two minutes in, Barnett became fatigued and lost her balance while stepping up and down and came crashing down shattering her left wrist. No staff members supervised her while she performed the test. They were milling about and visiting with each other so there was no one there to coach or spot her during the test or to catch her when she fell or at least to break her fall.

Procedural Facts:

Linda Barnett and her husband, Robert Barnett, filed a lawsuit against Covenant Health System claiming they negligently failed to have anyone available to observe Linda as she performed the test and, if they had done so, the step

Covenant continued...

test could have been stopped by an employee when she became fatigued or an employee would have been close enough to have broken her fall, thus avoiding the serious injuries she sustained. Covenant Health System filed a motion to dismiss given that the Barnetts did not submit an expert report as required by Texas Law (Texas Civil Practice & Remedies Code § 74.351) when filing a health care liability (medical malpractice) claim. The Barnetts argued that the screening (step test) did not constitute medical treatment and, therefore, no expert report was required. The trial court denied Covenant's motion to dismiss and they appealed this decision.

ISSUE

Did the trial court err when ruling its denial of Covenant's motion to dismiss?

COURT'S RULING

Yes, the appellate court granted Covenant's motion to dismiss because the claim was constituted as a health care liability claim.

COURT'S REASONING

A definition of a health care liability claim is provided in the Texas statute as follows:

> A cause of action against a health care provider or physician for treatment, lack of treatment, or other claimed departure from accepted standards of medical care, or health care, or safety or professional or administrative services directly related to health care, which proximately results in injury to or death of a claimant, whether the claimant's claim or cause of action sounds in tort or contract (p. 230).

The Texas statute defines health care as "any act performed, or that should have been performed, by a health care provider for a patient during a patient's treatment" (p. 231), but it did not define treatment. Relying on previous case law decisions and other sources, the court defined treatment as including diagnosis and prevention. The court stated that the timed exercise test, as part of the heart symposium, was a form of treatment and, therefore, was within the statute's definition of health care.

Although the plaintiffs claimed that Covenant's employees were negligent by failing to properly supervise Barnett during the step test, they did not agree that their claim should be a health care claim. One of their reasons was that Covenant employees, not doctors or nurses (medical professionals) conducted the tests. However, the court disagreed stating that health care is not limited to the actions of doctors or nurses and that a "health care provider includes a hospital as well as its employee or agent acting in the course and scope of the employment or contractual relationship" (p. 233). According to the court, Covenant's personnel failed to watch Barnett's performance during the test which was a breach of the standard of care applicable to health care providers. In determining the standard of care, the court stated:

> The American College of Sports Medicine's guidelines anticipate that the person conducting the test will possess sufficient medical competence to evaluate the test participant and make the medical judgments inherent in the decision whether to continue the test. The existence and nature of such guidelines established by the health care community indicate that a judgment concerning Covenant's conduct of Linda Barnett's step test requires specialized knowledge, and ultimately support a conclusion the Barnetts' claims are based on a claimed departure from accepted standards of health care (p. 233).

Covenant continued...

The protocol on how to conduct a step test, published by the American College of Sports Medicine, was also included as evidence in this case as follows:

> The protocol calls for evaluation of the participant for risk factors commonly associated with coronary artery disease. According to the protocol, clearance for participation in the exercise testing rests largely in the evaluator's discretion. For example, the guidelines require the evaluator to determine the presence of "absolute" and "relative contraindications" to exercise testing, some of which are specified in two lists of medical terms. The guidelines also call for termination of the step test if the participant asks to stop, or on the occurrence of such events as angina or angina-like symptoms; a significant drop or an excessive rise in blood pressure; light-headedness, confusion, ataxia, pallor, cyanosis, nausea, or cold and clammy skin; failure of heart rate to increase with increased exercise intensity; physical or verbal manifestations of severe fatigue; and unusual or severe shortness of breath (p. 232).

Regarding the placement of the step too close to the wall, the court concluded that if this unsafe condition was also a cause of the Barnett's injury it too would constitute a health care liability claim.

Lessons Learned from *Covenant Health System*

Legal

- Health care liability claims must meet certain requirements as specified in state statutes and, thus, differ from ordinary negligence claims.

- Health care liability claims can involve the actions of doctors or nurses but can also apply to employees acting in the course and scope of employment of a health care provider (hospital) such as the employees in this case who were administering the step test.

- The actions/inactions of the employees overseeing the timed step test in this case constituted a departure of accepted standards of medical care as described in the exercise testing guidelines published by the American College of Sports Medicine.

Risk Management/Injury Prevention

- Avoid conducting cardiovascular (CV) fitness tests at events like health fairs because it is difficult to administer proper pre-activity screening and informed consent.

- Avoid conducting tests such as step tests in fitness settings because (a) it is difficult to properly monitor heart rate and blood pressure during the tests, and (b) these tests can quickly become fatiguing (or maximal/near maximal) as demonstrated in this case. Only submaximal CV testing should be conducted in non-clinical fitness settings.

- Follow published safety standards and guidelines related to the proper design and delivery of fitness tests.

- Develop policies and procedures regarding proper instruction and supervision before, during, and after all fitness tests.

- Have only well-trained, credentialed, and competent exercise professionals conduct fitness tests.

SPOTLIGHT CASE

Howard v. Missouri Bone and Joint Center
615 F.3d 991 (8th Cir., 2010)

FACTS

Historical Facts:

Alvin Howard, a college football player, went to Missouri Bone and Joint Center, Inc. (MBJC), an orthopedic and training clinic to improve his football skills after suffering an ankle injury. Kevin Templin, a certified athletic trainer employed by MBJC, had Howard complete an initial evaluation that did not include squat lifts as required in the MBJC's assessment protocol. Templin also did not ask Howard how long it had been since he exercised which was 12 weeks due to his ankle injury. During the second training session, Howard was instructed to complete a "pyramid" weight lifting technique in which he would lift progressively more weight but with fewer repetitions per set. While performing pyramid squat lifts, Howard immediately informed Templin he felt a pop and sharp pain in his lower back. Templin responded, "no pain, no gain" and to "push through it". Howard felt the pain increase significantly as he continued to finish the set. His pain level was at 6 when the injury occurred and increased to a level of 10 by the end of the set. Howard was then instructed by Templin to do some stretching and ride a stationary bike, neither of which relieved his pain. Howard was diagnosed with a herniated disc in his back which required surgery to repair and resulted in permanent damage to Howard's back.

Procedural Facts:

Howard, the plaintiff, brought a negligence action against the defendant MBJC claiming it was negligent in three aspects:

> (1) by failing to conduct a proper evaluation of Howard before designing a workout program; (2) by instructing Howard to continue to workout after being advised of his back pain during the workout; and (3) by failing to discontinue Howard's workout after being advised of his back pain (p. 994).

The jury returned a verdict in favor of Howard in the amount of $175,000. MBJC filed a motion of summary judgment as a matter of law or for new trial claiming that Howard failed to provide evidence that the alleged negligent acts caused the injury. The trial court (U.S. district court) overruled that motion and the defendant appealed to this court—U.S. Court of Appeals for the Eighth Circuit.

ISSUE

Did the trial court err when it overruled the defendant's motion for summary judgment?

COURT'S RULING

No, the appellate court upheld the trial court's ruling.

COURT'S REASONING

Relying on previous Missouri case law, the court stated that to establish a claim for negligence, the plaintiff must prove three elements: "(1) the existence of a duty on the part of the defendant to protect the plaintiff from injury, (2) a failure of the defendant to perform that duty, and (3) an injury proximately caused by the defendant's failure" (p. 966). The court also stated that there must be evidence to support the allegations, but an absolute certainty is not required when proving a causal connection between a defendant's negligent conduct and the plaintiff's injury. This causal connection was

Howard continued...

evident from the expert testimony of the physician that performed Howard's surgery and a certified athletic trainer who was the Director of Athletic Training at Simpson College.

The physician testified that Howard's injury was causally linked to the workout instructed by Templin and that the injury caused Howard significant pain and permanent damage to his back. The athletic trainer testified that Templin should have tested Howard on squat lifts in the evaluation and that "Templin's actions of telling Howard to continue lifting, even after Howard felt significant pain in his back, constituted a violation of the standard of care" (p. 995). In addition, Templin testified that he did not note when Howard worked out last and that this is important information to determine when designing a workout.

MBJC argued that there was no evidence that a proper evaluation would have somehow prevented Howard's injury, but the court disagreed stating that "Howard presented evidence that leads to the logical conclusion that if certain things had been properly done, certain results would not have occurred, and such results did occur" (p. 988), which was sufficient evidence to show causation. Therefore, the appellate court affirmed the district court's denial of MBJC's motion for summary judgment as a matter of law and held that that district court did not abuse its discretion by denying the defendants motion for a new trial.

Lessons Learned from *Howard*

Legal

▶ In a negligence lawsuit, the plaintiff must prove that the actions or inactions of the defendant *caused* the injury; the causal evidence does not need to be an absolute certainty but needs to be enough—the preponderance of the evidence.

▶ Testimony of expert witnesses can help establish the standards of care (or duties) owed to the plaintiff as well as any breaches of the standards of care.

▶ Employers, such as MBJC in this case, can be liable for the negligent conduct of their employees through a legal principle called respondeat superior.

Risk Management/Injury Prevention

▶ Follow fitness evaluations/assessments properly according to the facility's' protocol and published safety standards or guidelines.

▶ Train fitness staff members who lead exercise testing and training programs on the types of pain that can occur with exercise (e.g., pain associated with an injury and pain associated with general training such as muscle fatigue or soreness). A pop and sharp pain, as occurred in this case, would likely indicate an injury and the exercise should stop and follow-up care provided.

▶ Train fitness staff members to not use phrases like "no pain, no gain" (a myth of exercise) or to push through the pain. "Train, don't strain" is a better motto.

The "No Pain, No Gain" Myth of Exercise

The athletic trainer in *Howard* used this "no pain, no gain" slogan after his client felt a pop and sharp pain in his lower back—and then told him to push through it. Unfortunately, this long-time myth of exercise is still alive and well. As Dr. Len Kravitz, an internationally known and highly-respected exercise physiologist, states: "Any type of pain is a warning signal" (30, p. 166). Related to the no pain, no gain, myth is that many, even some exercise professionals, believe that feeling the "burn" while exercising or having continual and/or severe muscle soreness reflects a "great" workout. WRONG! As Dr. Len Kravitz also states: "None of the physiological mechanisms associated with 'the burn' have been demonstrated to have beneficial results for you" (30, p. 166). It would be best for exercise

Table 6-3	Soreness vs. Pain: How to Tell the Difference*	
	MUSCLE SORENESS	**PAIN**
Type of discomfort:	Tender when touching muscles, tired or burning feeling while exercising, minimal dull, tight and achy feeling at rest	Ache, sharp pain at rest or when exercising
Onset:	During exercise or 24-72 hours after activity	During exercise or within 24 hours of activity
Duration:	2-3 days	May linger if not addressed
Location:	Muscles	Muscles or joints
Improves with:	Stretching, following movement, and/or more movement, with appropriate rest and recovery	Ice, rest, and more movement, except in cases of significant injury
Worsens with:	Sitting still	Continued activity after appropriate rest and recovery
Appropriate action:	Get moving again, after appropriate rest and recovery, but consider a different activity before resuming the activity that led to soreness	Consult with medical professional if pain is extreme or lasts > 1-2 weeks

* "MoveForwardPT.com, the official consumer website of the American Physical Therapy Association ©2019". Available at: https://www.moveforwardpt.com/Resources/Detail/soreness-vs-pain-whats-difference. Accessed January 16, 2019. Reprinted with permission, American Physical Therapy Association.

professionals to refrain from using this slogan that perpetuates the myth and to also educate their participants as to why this is a myth of exercise. It would be wiser to use a slogan such as "train, don't strain" instead.

Additional Cases

In addition to negligent claims made by the plaintiffs in the above spotlight cases and in the *Baldi-Perry* case (26), the plaintiff in another spotlight case, *D'Amico v. L.A. Fitness* (31), claimed the defendants were negligent for failing to properly assess her fitness level. *D'Amico* is described in Chapter 5. Additional case law examples are briefly described in Table 6-4 that involve claims of negligent pre-activity health screening and/

or fitness assessments. Other negligent claims were also made in these cases.

Clinical Exercise Testing Cases

As stated above, various negligence or malpractice claims involving clinical exercise testing have been made against physicians, exercise technicians, and the health care organizations they represent. The following two cases briefly describe some of the issues that the courts addressed to determine if the defendants were negligent. In *Moore v. Jackson Cardiology Associates* (35), the plaintiff fell off the treadmill during a stress test that was supervised by nurses and a cardiologist. She claimed that as the treadmill sped up, she called for one of the nurses

Table 6-4	Additional Cases: Negligent Screening and Fitness Testing/Assessment Claims	
CASE	**INJURY**	**NEGLIGENT CLAIMS**
***Chai v. Sports & Fitness Clubs of America, Inc.* (32)**	Member who suffered a cardiopulmonary arrest while exercising	Failure to require prescreening of members, including assessment of member's fitness and health prior to his use of the facility
***L.A. Fitness International, LLC v. Julianna Tringali Mayer* (33)**	Death of a member from a cardiac arrest while using a stepping machine	Failure to properly screen the decedent's health history at the time he joined the club
***Proffitt v. Global Fitness Holdings, LLC, et al.* (34)**	Client hospitalized with exertional rhabdomyolysis resulting in permanent injures after first training session	Failure to assess the client's health/fitness status before his first training session

to stop the machine but none of them did and she fell. She also claimed the nurses were rude and would not help her get up. Moments later, the cardiologist evaluated her injures and determined she was fine, but she chose to not continue the test.

Two years and 10 months later, the plaintiff filed an ordinary negligence claim against Jackson Cardiology Associates seeking recovery for a knee injury she suffered from the fall off the treadmill. She claimed that the medical group failed to (a) maintain reasonably safe premises, and (b) warn her about the treadmill. A major issue in this case was if the stress test was considered a medical diagnostic test and if so, the claim should have been filed as a medical malpractice claim. In Mississippi where this case took place, a state statute requires that a medical malpractice action needs to be filed within two years of the injury. The statute also contains other requirements such as medical expert testimony. The plaintiff claimed it was not a medical malpractice claim, but the court agreed with the defendant that it was a medical malpractice claim because her injury arose out of the course of medical services. The court granted the defendant's motion for summary judgment because the plaintiff's action was not filed within the two-year statute of limitation required for a medical malpractice claim. The outcome of this case might have been different if the plaintiff had filed her lawsuit as a medical malpractice claim and within the two-year period. She might have been able to show that

KEY POINT

As demonstrated in the spotlight cases and other negligence lawsuits described, the failure to assess the medical conditions of participants prior to conducting fitness testing and/or designing and delivering exercise programs resulted in several negligence claims made against exercise professionals and fitness facilities. Improper administration of fitness tests also resulted in negligence claims in some of these lawsuits. If the exercise professionals in these cases had followed established best practices (i.e., properly obtained the medical conditions of their participants and knew what precautions to take given their medical conditions), the injuries and subsequent litigation would likely not have occurred.

the nurses and cardiologist failed to provide her proper instruction and supervision during the stress test.

In *Nosal-Tabor v. Sharp Chula Vista Medical Center* (36), Nosal-Tabor, a registered nurse who worked for Sharp Chula Vista Medical Center (Sharp), repeatedly refused to perform nurse-led stress tests. She made numerous complaints to Sharp's management that they had not adopted legally adequate Standardized Procedures to permit nurses to perform stress tests. After she continued to refuse to perform the nurse-led stress tests, she was disciplined and later terminated by Sharp. Nosal-Tabor filed a lawsuit against Sharp alleging wrongful termination claiming they violated several state codes including a section within the Labor Code which prohibits being discharged in retaliation for active opposition to unlawful company practices and policies. Sharp filed a motion for summary judgment in which the trial court granted, stating that plaintiff did not present any credible evidence that the Standardized Procedures were insufficient. Upon appeal, she claimed that the trial court erred in its ruling.

In its analysis, the appellate court reviewed the California Nursing Practice Act that includes a section that "permits nurses to perform certain functions that would otherwise be considered the practice of medicine, when such functions are performed pursuant to properly adopted standardized procedures" and "that standardized procedures shall be adopted pursuant to guidelines promulgated by the Board of Nursing and the Medical Board of California" (36, p. 1236). These guidelines require hospitals to develop standardized procedures before permitting registered nurses to perform standardized procedure functions and to provide evidence that the nurse meets the guideline's experience, training, and/or education requirements to perform such functions. After examining all the evidence in this case, the court ruled that Sharp's procedures for nurse-led cardiac stress testing failed to comply with the guidelines and that Sharp's retaliation against Nosal-Tabor was a violation of the Labor Code. Therefore, the court concluded that the trial court erred in granting summary judgment to Sharp.

As stated in *ACSM's GETP* (3), there has been a transition from clinical exercise tests being administered by physicians to nonphysicians such as nurses and other allied health professionals. Well-trained allied health professionals can safely administer such tests, but the overall supervision of the test remains the legal responsibility of the supervising physician. For more on this topic and the recommended knowledge

and skills needed to administer clinical exercise tests, see the *ACSM's GETP* (3). As demonstrated in *Nosal-Tabor*, hospitals and clinics need to be sure they are complying with any state and local laws applicable to clinical exercise testing requirements.

DEVELOPMENT OF RISK MANAGEMENT STRATEGIES

Assessment of Legal Liability Exposures → Development of Risk Management Strategies → Implementation of the Comprehensive Risk Management Plan → Evaluation of the Comprehensive Risk Management Plan

The preceding section identified many legal liability exposures related to pre-activity health screening and fitness testing. The following risk management strategies can be developed to reduce these legal liability exposures. In addition, descriptions of the risk management strategies related to pre-activity health screening address the screening challenges identified by exercise professionals in a 2014 national study (6, 12, 13)—member issues, medical clearance issues, and administrative/procedural issues. These risk management strategies are designed for fitness facilities that employ exercise professionals who can properly carry out professionally-guided screening. Non-staffed or unsupervised facilities (e.g., hotels, apartment complexes) should consider posting a self-guided screening questionnaire along with a document that informs participants of the inherent risks of exercise.

to their participation in the facility's activities. Certain documents such as membership agreements, informed consents, and waivers, are considered contracts and, thus, cannot be signed by minors. As described in Chapter 4, there are some states that allow parents/legal guardians to sign a waiver that might be enforceable. When a minor needs a medical procedure, the parents/legal guardians sign an informed consent. For youth sports and physical activity programs, children and their parents/legal guardians need to be informed of the risks inherent in the activity. See Chapter 4 that briefly describes an Agreement to Participate, which may not be considered a contract. Another reason for having participants sign such documents is that it will help refute negligence claims such as the failure to warn participants of the risk of injury.

① **Risk Management Strategy #1:** Have All New Participants Sign a Document Informing Them of the Inherent Risks of Exercise (1).

As described in Chapter 4, having participants read and sign a document that informs them of the inherent risks of exercise (i.e., minor, major, and life-threatening injuries, and death), may help strengthen the primary assumption of risk defense. This can be an effective defense when negligence claims/lawsuits occur. A variety of documents can contain this type of language such as a membership agreement, waiver, express assumption of risk, and informed consent. Facility guests should also sign a document that includes such language prior

② **Risk Management Strategy #2:** Comply with Federal, State, and Local Laws Regarding Pre-Activity Health Screening and Fitness Testing (1).

This chapter briefly described laws relevant to pre-activity health screening and fitness testing such as the ADA, HIPAA, OSHA's Bloodborne Pathogens Standard, CLIA, and 45 C.F.R. § 46—Protection of Human Subjects. Some of these laws are described in more detail in Chapter 3 regarding their application to fitness facilities and programs. The ADA and privacy laws are significant with regard to screening procedures and collection of individual health and fitness data. To avoid potential ADA discrimination claims (or other types of discrimination), a facility's screening procedures need to be the same for everyone (e.g., the criteria included on the screening form, the criteria used to require medical clearance, and any policies/procedures to refuse participation). Also, before a policy to refuse participation is implemented, no matter what the reason is, it needs to be carefully reviewed by the facility's legal counsel and/or risk management advisory committee. Although most fitness facilities would not be subject to the HIPAA because they would not be considered covered entities, it is still wise to comply with the privacy, confidentiality, and security provisions within this law regarding an individual's health-related information because state privacy laws might apply as well as certain civil claims. In addition, it is expected that exercise professionals follow codes of conduct or ethical standards published by professional organizations regarding confidentiality of individual health/fitness data.

3 **Risk Management Strategy #3:** Comply with Standards and Guidelines Published by Professional Organizations Regarding Pre-Activity Screening and Fitness Testing.

Some of the standards and/or guidelines published by professional organizations regarding screening were briefly described in this chapter, such as ACSM (3, 8), MFA (9), NSCA (10), and AACVPR (11). In addition, guidelines published by *ACSM's GETP* (3) regarding health-related fitness testing were also briefly described. These publications include many additional standards and/or guidelines regarding screening and testing than what was included in this chapter. As stated in Chapter 4, fitness managers and exercise professionals need to obtain these publications, especially those that are most relevant to their types of programs and facilities. It is important that the standards and guidelines related to screening and testing be incorporated into the facility's policies and procedures.

4 **Risk Management Strategy #4:** Have Only Credentialed and Competent Exercise Professionals Conduct Pre-Activity Health Screening and Fitness Testing Procedures (1).

Fitness managers or a designated exercise professional(s) need to assume the responsibility and oversight of the facility's pre-activity health screening process and

fitness testing program. Preferably, those with these responsibilities have a degree in exercise science (or related area), a professional exercise physiologist certification, and demonstrated knowledge/skills and experience in screening and testing. Fitness staff members who have not had adequate formal education that includes assessment of practical skills will need to be well-trained before assuming responsibilities in these areas. See Risk Management Strategy #9. Training of staff members on how to carry out the screening procedures with new participants is essential so that screening is performed properly and consistently. Training involving fitness testing will likely take a great deal of time. For example, to become proficient at submaximal cardiovascular testing and measuring skinfolds, it will take a great deal of practice, perhaps conducting tests on 50-100 individuals. Even those who have had an academic course and an accompanying lab in fitness testing may need additional fitness testing practice with the general population in order to gain proficiency. The exercise professional who has oversight of the fitness testing program will need to ensure that fitness staff members who are administering fitness tests have the knowledge/skills to do so.

5 **Risk Management Strategy #5:** Establish Efficient Pre-Activity Health Screening Procedures.

One of the reasons for not requiring new participants to complete pre-activity health screening was that it was too-time consuming for staff members (6, 12, 13). Therefore, developing time-efficient procedures can address this concern. Fitness managers and exercise professionals can select their own screening questionnaire and procedures in consultation with their medical advisor and/or risk management advisory committee. Once the procedures are finalized, they should be prepared in written form and included in the facility's' risk management policy and procedures manual. For this strategy, the PASQ (discussed above) and PASQ-related forms are described to provide an example of the steps that can be developed to carry out efficient screening procedures. Implementing the PASQ, that is based on ACSM's revised screening criteria (3), was shown to make the screening process easier, quicker for all parties compared to the screening criteria in previous editions of this publication (13). The PASQ and PASQ-related forms are found in this chapter's appendix and are described as follows.

PASQ Cover Letter

The PASQ Cover Letter informs new participants of the purposes of screening, the steps involved, the importance of medical clearance, and that their health-related information is kept private, confidential, and secure. When individuals are provided this information, they will understand why screening procedures are completed and appreciate the fact that the facility is following professional standards and guidelines. It is important that they understand that the process needs to be completed before they can begin exercising. However, they can begin by participating in the facility orientation as described in Chapter 10. Some individuals after reading this Cover Letter may refuse to complete the screening procedures. As described above, fitness managers and exercise professionals will need to consider what actions(s) to take when this occurs and any potential legal consequences that may exist. In consultation with the facility's legal counsel and/or risk management advisory committee, a policy decision will need to be made to either deny these individuals participation in the facility's activities or have them sign a refusal form such as the one in Exhibit 6-1. In the 2014 national study (6), 51%, 38%, and 11% of the facilities denied them participation, had them sign a refusal form, or some other approach, respectively.

PASQ—Professionally-Guided and PASQ Interpretation Form

The items in Sections 1-3 on the PASQ—Professionally-Guided are based on the criteria from the *ACSM's GETP* (3) and algorithm (3, 7). The questions in Section 1 determine the individual's current physical activity and current/desired intensity levels. In Section 2, the individual indicates if they have/had any diseases (i.e., cardiovascular, diabetes and kidney). The nine signs and symptoms listed in Section 3 are described in lay terms so that they are understandable. The statement and signature in Section 4 helps ensure that participants complete the questionnaire with accuracy and that they understand it is their responsibility to inform a staff member at the facility if their health status

changes at any time When this occurs, the screening process should be repeated. Some fitness facilities may have a policy that the screening is completed on annual basis (e.g., when a member is renewing his/her membership). However, an individual's health status can change at any time, so it is best to inform participants of their responsibility to inform a staff member when this occurs. The PASQ Interpretation Form is based on the medical clearance recommendations provided in the ACSM's algorithm (3, 7) and is completed by an exercise professional. This form serves as documentation of the interpretation and decision made regarding medical clearance.

PASQ Medical Clearance Form

For individuals who need to obtain medical clearance, it is wise to remind them of the purposes and benefits of medical clearance as described in the cover letter. Because it is unlikely that physicians or other health care providers will respond to such requests from an exercise professional in a timely fashion, it is best to have individuals take or send the medical clearance form (and a copy of their completed PASQ attached) directly to their health care provider. This approach does not require having the individual sign a "medical release" because the exercise professional is not disclosing protected health information to a third party. The short paragraph at the top of the PASQ Medical Clearance Form informs the health care provider of the purpose of the form and instructions for completion. For individuals who claim they do not have a health care provider, the facility can provide a list of physicians in the area that are accepting new patients. It is always best to have an exercise professional on duty during all operating hours who can administer these screening steps (review/interpret the screening questionnaire and make decisions regarding medical clearance) so there are minimal delays for a new participant.

Benefits of Establishing an Efficient Screening Process

Many of the pre-activity screening challenges described above (member, medical clearance, and administrative issues) expressed by ACSM certified exercise physiologists (6, 12, 13), will be addressed by following the above steps. After implementing these steps, one ACSM certified professional stated: "Establishing proper screening procedures had a positive impact on my business including (a) improved efficiency, (b) heightened credibility with my clients, and (c) enhanced collaborative communication with my client's health care providers" (37, p. 3). Another important benefit, especially from a legal liability perspective, is that screening forms serve as documentation and, thus, provide evidence that the screening process was completed properly, which will help refute any related negligence claims/lawsuits that might occur in the future.

Recommendations to Address "Missing" High Intensity Screening Guidelines

As stated above the ACSM algorithm provided medical clearance recommendations for moderate and vigorous intensity exercise, but not for high intensity exercise. This is an important issue to address, not only because high intensity exercise programs are very popular (14), but because many of the injuries and subsequent negligence lawsuits described throughout this text have involved high intensity exercise programs. Therefore, it is essential that fitness facilities that offer high intensity exercise programs take steps to help ensure that those who enroll in such programs can demonstrate that they can safely tolerate "vigorous" intensity exercise before participating in high intensity exercise. More information on high intensity exercise programs is covered in Chapter 8.

For individuals that need to obtain medical clearance, it will be important for exercise professionals to follow the intensity level indicated by the health care provider on the medical clearance form. For example, if the health care provider indicated "moderate" as the highest level of intensity for which his/her patient is cleared, it will be important that fitness testing protocols and exercise prescriptions do not exceed that level. For individuals that sign up for personal fitness training (or other structured exercise programs), the exercise professional can easily select/modify testing protocols or design/deliver exercise programs that do not exceed moderate intensity as well as teach their participants how to self-monitor intensity via heart rate and perceived exertion. Once individuals have achieved a level of fitness where they have demonstrated the ability to safely tolerate moderate intensity and are ready to move up to vigorous intensity, exercise professionals can have the participant obtain medical clearance again and include a progress report describing why the participant is ready to begin a vigorous exercise program. If the health care provider approves, the participant can then begin a vigorous intensity exercise program.

Exercise professionals can manage or monitor intensity levels for individuals enrolled in structured exercise programs. However, what about individuals that do not join a structured exercise program but have been directed by their health care provider not to exceed moderate or vigorous intensity? For these individuals, it would be best to have an exercise professional meet with the individual to explain exercise intensity (e.g., describe how to use the heart rate and perceived exertion charts posted in the facility) as well as many other principles of safe exercise such as signs and symptoms of overexertion. This meeting will also provide an opportunity to recommend certain programs such as beginner exercise classes offered by the facility and to explain why they should not exercise at intensity levels higher than what was recommended by their health care provider. They can be informed that when they feel ready to participate at a higher level of intensity, medical clearance to approve the higher intensity can be obtained at that time. Documentation of such a meeting and what was discussed, may be helpful from a legal liability perspective.

It may be wise for individuals, who want to enroll in a facility's high intensity exercise program, to first obtain medical clearance to be sure that their health care provider approves. Another approach would be to have the individual demonstrate that he/she can safely tolerate "vigorous" exercise and/or perform a fitness test to determine his/her fitness level. For example, if the individual is not in an "excellent" category of cardiorespiratory fitness, a high intensity program may be inappropriate.

Risk Management Strategy #6: Develop Procedures for Obtaining Medical History Information Prior to Fitness Testing and Exercise Prescription (1).

Some fitness facilities may opt to have one form for pre-activity screening purposes that includes, for example, the health-related screening criteria in ACSM's algorithm as well as additional medical history questions. Having one form and one set of criteria that is used to determine the need for medical clearance has its advantages. However, facilities that use the PASQ or PAR-Q+ (or similar questionnaires) need to realize that these are "pre-activity" health screening questionnaires. They would not be considered "medical history" questionnaires. Before conducting fitness testing and establishing an exercise prescription, the medical history of the individual needs to be obtained. As described in Chapter 4 (see Exhibit 4-1), one factor that determines the professional standard of care is the "type of participants"—meaning the exercise professional must be aware of the participant's medical conditions that may impose increased risks and know how to minimize those risks. There are several examples of negligence cases described in this text in which exercise professionals did not obtain a medical history of the participant or know what precautions to take to help minimize increased risks given their participant's medical condition(s). Therefore, obtaining a medical history is needed, especially in certain programs. A basic "pre-activity" health screening questionnaire would not be adequate.

If it is decided to use an existing medical history form, it should be reviewed and approved by the facility's medical advisor and/or risk management advisory committee. Facilities that choose to develop their own medical history form can do so with the assistance of the medical advisor and/or risk management advisory committee. The criteria that would warrant medical clearance will need to be determined. For example, there may be certain medical conditions such as cancer, high blood pressure, recent surgery, and certain medications that warrant medical clearance. Fitness managers and exercise professionals, in consultation with their medical advisor and/or risk management advisory committee, will need to decide the exercise programs for which a medical history should be obtained, such as fitness testing programs, individualized exercise programs (e.g., personal fitness training), special population exercise programs (e.g., prenatal fitness, senior fitness, fitness programs for individuals with Parkinson's disease, etc.). In addition, decisions will need

to be made regarding the necessary credentials and competence of exercise professionals who will be working with these types of programs/participants. More on this topic and scope of practice is covered in Chapter 7.

 Risk Management Strategy #7: Establish Pre-Activity Health Screening Procedures for Youth and Facility Guests (1).

"The pre-activity health screening procedures just described would apply to all adults—those who are 18 years of age (age of majority in most states) or older" (1, p. 169). Regarding procedures for youth, fitness managers and exercise professionals should refer to certain published standards of practice, such as YMCA (38) and NSCA (10), that recommend youth (minors that are 17 years of age or younger) be medically cleared prior to participation in sports and/or physical activities. For example, it may be recommended that a parent and/or guardian sign a form that "indicates the child has been properly screened and that no medical conditions exist that would preclude his/her participation in the sport or physical activities" (1, p. 169). Fitness managers and exercise professionals, with the assistance of their medical and legal advisors and/or risk management advisory committee, will need to decide if such a form is adequate (1). Because health problems (e.g., obesity, type 2 diabetes, and hypertension) among youth have increased in recent years, additional steps may be needed (1). For example, if the child has a medical condition, it may be necessary to obtain medical clearance from the child's health care provider.

Some fitness facilities may have a policy that guests are not allowed to use the facility. However, for facilities that welcome guests who desire to use the facility one time or a few times, it may not be practical for them to complete a formal, professionally-guided screening process that might involve obtaining medical clearance (1). It might be best to provide them with a self-guided screening form. For an example, see the appendix for the PASQ—Self-Guided. It is recommended that they sign a waiver and/or an express assumption of risk (1). See Chapter 4 for examples of each. The facility's legal counsel and risk management advisory committee should review such documents before they are implemented as well as a policy that does not allow guests to use the facility.

⑧ Risk Management Strategy #8: Develop a Comprehensive Fitness Testing Manual that Includes Testing Protocols and Safety Procedures.

The fitness manager or designated exercise professional who has oversight of the facility's fitness testing program should develop a comprehensive testing manual that will provide guidance for staff members involved with health-related fitness testing. The manual should describe how to carry out the steps described above (see Steps: Health-Related Fitness Testing) involving Medical History, Fitness Testing Protocols, Safety Procedures, and Fitness Test Results Report. Important decisions will need to be made regarding the protocols to include in the manual. A variety of resources exist that can be very helpful when making decisions on which protocols to include such as:

- *ACSM's Guidelines for Exercise Testing and Prescription* (10th ed., 2018)
- *ACSM's Health-Related Physical Fitness Testing Assessment Manual* (5th ed., 2017)
- *NSCA's Guide to Tests and Assessments* (2012)
- *ACE's Guide to Exercise Testing and Program Design* (2nd ed., 2007)
- *Senior Fitness Test Manual* (2nd ed., 2012)
- *Fitness Professional's Handbook*, (7th ed., 2017)

These resources describe how to properly carry out the protocols which is essential for several reasons such as enhanced accuracy and safety. A fitness facility may establish standard protocols for cardiovascular, muscle strength/endurance, flexibility, and body composition assessments to include in the fitness testing manual. However, alternative protocols or modifications of the standard protocols should also be included in the fitness testing manual. The standard protocols may not be appropriate for all individuals. Some fitness facilities may include protocols to measure posture, balance, functional fitness, etc. and if so, it will be important to include these protocols and how to properly carry them out in the fitness testing manual.

⑨ Risk Management Strategy #9: Create a Training Program for Staff Members Involved in the Pre-Activity Health Screening and Fitness Testing Procedures.

Once the pre-activity health screening procedures are finalized in written form and the fitness testing manual is complete, training of staff members involved in carrying out these tasks is essential. The fitness manager or the exercise professional, who has oversight of these screening and testing procedures, needs to develop a staff training program. For more information on staff training, e.g., preparing and delivering lesson plans, assessing outcomes of training programs, etc., see Chapter 2. Prior to training, it is best to have staff members review the written procedures such as the screening procedures in the risk management policy and procedures manual and the fitness testing procedures in the fitness testing manual. This will help staff members become somewhat familiar with these procedures prior to attending the required training. After the training is completed, it will be important to observe and assess if the staff members are carrying out the procedures properly. If not, re-training may be necessary.

Regarding fitness testing procedures, staff members should complete a practical test upon completion of the training program. The practical tests would include their ability to properly carry out the safety procedures, correctly perform the protocols, and provide proper interpretation and explanation of the fitness test results form. Those who cannot successfully pass the practical test should obtain more practice to develop these skills and work under a competent exercise professional who can provide additional training. Given the wide variety of credentials among exercise professionals as described in Chapter 5, it cannot be assumed that exercise professionals have the necessary knowledge and skills to conduct fitness testing. It is important to remember that certifications do not include any assessments of practical skills, which are essential from a legal liability perspective. Even those with a degree in exercise science (or related area) who likely had a fitness testing course in their academic program should complete the training program and take the practical test. Having fitness testing procedures that all exercise professionals follow provides a consistent and standardized approach.

10 **Risk Management Strategy #10:** Develop Systems to Keep All Participant Health Related Information Private, Confidential, and Secure (1).

As stated above, most fitness facilities would not be subject to the HIPAA because they are not considered covered entities. However, it is wise to comply with the privacy, confidentiality, and security provisions within this law regarding an individual's health-related information (or protected health information—PHI) because fitness facilities may be subject to violations of state privacy laws as well as certain civil claims if they fail to comply (1). The individual's health information would include, for example, the following documents: PASQ, PASQ Interpretation Form, Medical Clearance Form, and Fitness Test Results Report. A system that

includes written procedures on how these documents in both paper and electronic forms will be kept private, confidential, and secure should be developed and approved by the facility's risk management advisory committee (1). Fitness facility staff members involved in the pre-activity health screening process and fitness testing program should be required to attend training programs regarding these written procedures. It might be a good idea to have these staff members sign a document confirming their commitment to follow these written procedures.

In addition, all documents obtained in the pre-activity health screening process and the fitness testing program should be kept for the length of time that would be commensurate with the statute of limitations and in consultation with the facility's legal counsel (1). These include the protective legal documents obtained during the screening process and fitness testing program, such as a Refusal Form (Exhibit 6-1) and Informed Consent (Exhibit 6-2).

RISK MANAGEMENT AUDIT
Pre-Activity Health Screening and Fitness Testing

RISK MANAGEMENT (RM) STRATEGY*	YES ✔	NO ✔
1. Have All New Participants Sign a Document Informing Them of the Inherent Risks of Exercise.		
2. Comply with Federal, State, and Local Laws Regarding Pre-Activity Health Screening and Fitness Testing.		
3. Comply with Standards and Guidelines Published by Professional Organizations Regarding Pre-Activity Screening and Fitness Testing.		
4. Have Only Credentialed and Competent Exercise Professionals Conduct Pre-Activity Health Screening and Fitness Testing Procedures.		
5. Establish Efficient Pre-Activity Health Screening Procedures.		
6. Develop Procedures for Obtaining Medical History Information Prior to Fitness Testing and Exercise Prescription.		
7. Establish Pre-Activity Health Screening Procedures for Youth and Facility Guests.		
8. Develop a Comprehensive Fitness Testing Manual that Includes Testing Protocols and Safety Procedures.		
9. Create a Training Program for Staff Members Involved in the Pre-Activity Health Screening and Fitness Testing Procedures.		
10. Develop Systems to Keep All Participant Health-Related Information Private, Confidential, and Secure.		

*See the section above – Development of Risk Management Strategies—for the recommendations associated with each risk management strategy and then, for each RM Strategy marked NO, create a list of action steps that need to be completed to meet the recommendations described in that RM strategy.

KEY TERMS

- Clinical Exercise Testing
- Confidentiality
- Health-Related Fitness Testing
- Medical Clearance
- Medical History
- Medical Release

- Pre-Activity Health Screening
- Privacy
- Professionally-Guided Screening
- Protected Health Information (PHI)
- Security
- Self-Guided Screening

STUDY QUESTIONS

The Study Questions for Chapter 6 can be found on the Fitness Law Academy website (www.fitnesslawacademy.com) under Textbook. They are provided in a fillable format for convenience.

APPENDIX

This chapter's appendix follows the References.

REFERENCES

1. Eickhoff-Shemek JM, Herbert DL, Connaughton, DP. *Risk Management for Health/Fitness Professionals: Legal Issues and Strategies.* Baltimore, MD: Lippincott Williams & Wilkins, 2009.

2. Heart Disease and Stroke Statistics 2019 At-a Glance. American Heart Association. Available at: https://healthmetrics.heart.org/wp-content/uploads/2019/02/At-A-Glance-Heart-Disease-and-Stroke-Statistics-%E2%80%93 2019.pdf. Accessed April 5, 2020.

3. *ACSM's Guidelines for Exercise Testing and Prescription.* Riebe D. (ed). 10th Ed. Philadelphia, PA: Lippincott Williams & Wilkins, 2018.

4. Thompson PD, Franklin BA, Balady GJ, et al. Exercise and Acute Cardiovascular Events: Placing the Risks into Perspective. *Medicine & Science in Sports & Exercise,* 39(5), 886-897, 2007.

5. Franklin BA, Thompson PD, Al-Zaiti SS, et al. Exercise-Related Acute Cardiovascular Events and Potential Deleterious Adaptations Following Long-Term Exercise Training: Placing the Risks Into Perspective—An Update. *Circulation,* 141:e705-e736, 2020. Doi: 10.1161/CIR.0000000000000749. Available at: https://www.ahajournals.org/doi/10.1161/CIR.0000000000000749.

6. Craig AC, Eickhoff-Shemek JM. Adherence to ACSM's Pre-Activity Screening Procedures in Fitness Facilities: A National Investigation. *Journal of Physical Education and Sports Management,* 2(2), 120-137, 2015.

7. Riebe D, Franklin BA, Thompson PD, et al. Updating the American College of Sports Medicine's Recommendations for the Exercise Pre-Participation Health Screening Process. *Medicine & Science in Sports & Exercise,* 47(11), 2473-2479, 2015.

8. *ACSM's Health/Fitness Facility Standards and Guidelines.* Sanders ME. (ed). 5th Ed. Champaign, IL: Human Kinetics, 2019.

9. *Medical Fitness Association's Standards & Guidelines for Medical Fitness Center Facilities,* Roy B. (ed.). 2nd Ed. Monterey, CA: Healthy Learning, 2013.

10. NSCA Strength and Conditioning Professional Standards and Guidelines. *Strength and Conditioning Journal,* 39(6), 1-24, 2017. Available at: https://www.nsca.com/education/articles/nsca-strength-and-conditioning-professional-standards-and-guidelines/. Accessed November 5, 2018.

11. American Association for Cardiovascular and Pulmonary Rehabilitation (AACVPR). Guidelines for Cardiac Rehabilitation and Secondary Prevention Programs. Williams MA, Roitman JL (eds). 5th Ed. Champaign, IL: Human Kinetics, 2013.

12. Craig AC. A National Investigation of Pre-Activity Health Screening Procedures in Fitness Facilities: Perspectives for American College of Sports Medicine Certified Health Fitness Specialists. Doctoral Dissertation, University of South Florida, Tampa, FL. November 2014.

13. Eickhoff-Shemek JM, Craig AC. Putting the New ACSM's Pre-Activity Health Screening Guidelines into Practice. *ACSM's Health & Fitness Journal,* 21(3), 11-21, 2017.

14. Thompson WR. Worldwide Survey of Fitness Trends for 2019. *ACSM's Health & Fitness Journal,* 22(6), 10-17, 2019.

15. Ward BW, Schiller JS, Goodman RA. Multiple Chronic Conditions Among U.S. Adults: A 2012 Update. *Preventing Chronic Disease,* 11, E62, 2014. Available at: https://www.ncbi.nlm.nih.gov/pmc/articles/PMC3992293. Accessed January 25, 2019.

16. Araujo J, Cal J, Stevens J. Prevalence of Optimal Metabolic Health in American Adults: National Health and Nutrition Examination Survey 2009-2016. *Metabolic Syndrome and Related Disorders,* November 27, 2018. Available at: https://www.ncbi.nlm.nih.gov/pubmed/30484738. Accessed January 25, 2019.

17. Physical Activity Guidelines for Americans, 2d Ed. 2018. Available at: https://health.gov/paguidelines/secondedition/pdf/Physical_Activity_Guidelines_2nd_edition.pdf. Accessed February 9, 2019.

18. *Covenant Health System v. Barnett,* 342 S.W.3d. 226, 2011 LEXIS 3665 (Tex. App., 2011).

19. Blair SA. Implementing HIPAA. *ACSM's Health & Fitness Journal,* 7(5), 25-27, 2003.

20. Herbert DL, Herbert WG. *Legal Aspects of Preventive, Rehabilitative and Recreational Exercise* Programs, 4th Ed. Canton, OH: PRC Publishing, Inc., 2002.

21. American with Disabilities Act Title III Regulations. Part 36 Nondiscrimination on the Basis of Disability by Public Accommodations and Commercial Facilities. § 36.104 Definitions. January 17, 2017. Available at: https://www.ada.gov/regs2010/titleIII_2010/titleIII_2010_regulations.htm#a102. Accessed February 5, 2019.

22. *Class v. Towson University,* 118 F. Supp. 3d 833 (D. Md., 2015).

23. Zabawa BJ, Eickhoff-Shemek JM. *Rule the Rules of Workplace Wellness Programs.* Chicago, IL: ABA Publishing. 2017.

24. O'Malley M. Protecting Your Gym's Member Data in a Digital World: Informed Consent is Critical to Managing Personal Information Safely. *Club Business International.* July 2018, 106-107. Available at: http://pubs.ihrsa.org/CBI/2018/July2018/index.html. Accessed February 5, 2019.

25. Craig AC, Eickhoff-Shemek JM. Educating and Training the Personal Fitness Trainer: A Pedagogical Approach. *ACSM's Health & Fitness Journal,* 13(2), 8-15, 2009.

26. *Baldi-Perry v. Kaifas and 360 Fitness Center, Inc.* Complaint. Index No. 2010-1927, Supreme Court, Erie County, New York. February 19, 2010.

27. *Rostai v. Neste Enterprises,* d/b/a Gold'sGym, 41 Cal. Rptr. 3d 411 (Cal. Ct. App., 2006).

28. *Howard v. Missouri Bone and Joint Center,* 615 F.3d 991 (8th Cir., 2010).

29. *Makris v. Scandinavian Health Spa, Inc.,* No. 98 CA 193, 1999 LEXIS 4416 (Ohio Ct. App., 1999).

30. Kravitz L. *Anybody's Guide to Total* Fitness. 11th Ed. Dubuque, Iowa: Kendall Hunt Publishing, 2016.

31. *D'Amico v. LA Fitness,* 57 Conn. L. Rptr. 242, 2013 WL 6912912 (Conn. Super. Ct., 2013).

32. *Chai v. Sports & Fitness Clubs of America, Inc.,* Case No. 98-16053 CA (05). Analyzed In: Failure to Defibrillate Results in New Litigation. *The Exercise Standards and Malpractice Reporter,* 13(4), 55-56, 1999.

33. *L.A. Fitness International, LLC v. Mayer,* 980 So.2d. 550 (Fla. Dist. Ct. App., 2008).

34. *Proffitt v. Global Fitness Holdings, LLC, et al.* Analyzed In: Herbert, DL. New Lawsuit Against Personal Trainer and Facility in Kentucky—Rhabdomyolysis Alleged. *The Exercise, Sports and Medicine Standards & Malpractice Reporter,* 2(1), 3-10, 2013.

35. *Moore v. Jackson Cardiology Associates,* 192 So.3d 1050 (Miss. Ct. App., 2015).

36. *Nosal-Tabor v. Sharp Chula Medical Center,* 239 Cal.App.4th 1224 (Cal. Ct. App., 2015).

37. Topalian T. Risk Management Success Story. *Fitness Law Academy Newsletter,* 1(4), 3, 2018.

38. Safeguarding Health and Well-Being, Medical Advisory Committee Recommendations: A Resource Guide for YMCAs. Chicago, IL: YMCA of the USA, February 2011. Available at: http://safe-wise.com/downloads/MAC_2010a_Collection.pdf. Accessed November 5, 2018.

APPENDIX 6

NOTE: *These forms are available on the Fitness Law Academy website (www.fitnesslawacademy.com) under Textbook Resources along with Information and Instructions on their proper use.*

Form 6-1: PASQ Cover Letter

Dear Participant:

To increase the safety of our health/fitness programs and services as well as to comply with standards and/or guidelines established by major professional exercise/fitness organizations, we have all participants complete our Pre-Activity Health Screening process prior to participation. Step 1 in this process is to complete the attached PASQ, our health history questionnaire that will take you about 4-5 minutes. The major purpose of obtaining this information is to help us identify individuals who may be at risk for an adverse event during exercise and who have any medical conditions that may require medical clearance prior to participation in health/fitness activities.

 Once completed, it will be reviewed by one of our qualified staff members who will determine (using pre-established criteria) whether Step 2 (obtaining medical clearance) is necessary prior to your participation in our programs and services. Obtaining clearance from your physician may be a slight inconvenience and may delay your participation, but it is an important step that can help ensure your safety while participating in our programs/services.

Medical Clearance

If necessary, you will receive our Medical Clearance Form. Attached to it will be a copy of your completed PASQ. Please take this form to your physician and ask him/her to complete and sign it. If you have recently seen your physician, he/she may complete and sign the form without seeing you for a medical evaluation. However, if is been a while (or for other reasons), your physician may want you to make an appointment for a medical evaluation. Regular medical evaluations are important for a variety of reasons such as having certain medical screenings/tests (e.g., cholesterol, blood pressure, cancer) that may detect an underlying health problem or disease. Early detection can save your life.

Privacy-Confidentiality-Security

All information obtained in our Pre-Activity Health Screening process will be kept private, confidential, and secure. At no time will any of this information be shared with any unauthorized individuals and it will be stored in a secure location.

Thank you for your participation in our Pre-Activity Health Screening process. We appreciate your understanding of this important process prior to participation in our health/fitness activities, which is to help improve your safety.

Sincerely,

The Management at _____
　　　　　　　　　　　(Name of health/fitness facility)

Form 6-2: PASQ—Professionally-Guided

Instructions:
Please complete all four sections of this form. A staff member who is an exercise professional in our facility will review it and inform you if medical clearance is needed prior to engaging in physical activity.

Section 1 — Current Physical Activity
When answering the questions in this section, please note the following definitions:
- **Moderate Intensity:** An activity that causes noticeable increases in heart rate and breathing (e.g., brisk walking)
- **Vigorous Intensity:** An activity that causes substantial increases in heart rate and breathing (e.g., jogging)

Over the last three months, have you regularly performed physical activity for at least 30 minutes, three days/week at a moderate intensity level?
❑ No   ❑ Yes

If yes, which of the following best describes any vigorous intensity activity in your regular routine the last 3 months?
❑ I participate in some or all vigorous intensity activity
❑ None, but I want to begin some vigorous intensity activity
❑ None, and I want to continue moderate intensity activity

Section 2 — Medical Conditions
Please check the box (√) for any of the following medical conditions that you currently have or have had

❑ Heart attack
❑ Heart surgery
❑ Cardiac catheterization
❑ Coronary angioplasty (PTCA)
❑ Heart valve disease
❑ Heart failure
❑ Heart transplantation
❑ Congenital heart disease

❑ Abnormal heart rhythm
❑ Pacemaker/implantable cardiac defibrillator
❑ Peripheral vascular disease (PVD or PAD): disease affecting blood vessels in arms, hands, legs, and feet
❑ Cerebrovascular disease—stroke or TIA (transient ischemic attack)
❑ Type 1 or Type 2 diabetes
❑ Renal (kidney) disease

Section 3 — Signs or Symptoms
Please check the box (√) for any of the signs or symptoms that you have recently experienced.
❑ Pain, discomfort in the chest, neck, jaw or arms at rest or upon exertion
❑ Shortness of breath at rest or with mild exertion
❑ Dizziness or loss of consciousness during or shortly after exercise
❑ Shortness of breath occurring at rest or 2-5 hours after the onset of sleep
❑ Edema (swelling) in both ankles that is most evident at night or swelling in a limb
❑ An unpleasant awareness of forceful or rapid beating of the heart
❑ Pain in the legs or elsewhere while walking; often more severe when walking upstairs/uphill
❑ Known heart murmur
❑ Unusual fatigue or shortness of breath with usual activities

Section 4 — Acknowledgment, Follow-up, and Signature
I acknowledge that I have read this questionnaire in its entirety and have responded accurately, completely, and to the best of my knowledge. Any questions regarding the items on this questionnaire were answered to my satisfaction. Also, if my health status changes at any time, I understand that I am responsible to inform a staff member at this facility of any such changes. I also understand that the PASQ is not a substitution for a medical examination.

Please note: The authors of the PASQ assume no liability for individuals who participate in physical activity and/or complete the PASQ. If questions arise after completing the PASQ, seek the advice of your healthcare provider prior to physical activity

_____   _____
Participant's Name—Please Print   Participant's Signature

_____
Date

Copyright © 2020 by JoAnn M. Eickhoff-Shemek and Aaron C. Keese

Form 6-3: PASQ Interpretation Form

Participant's Name: _____

Medical Clearance Needed: ❏ No   ❏ Yes

If yes, Medical Clearance is needed for this participant for the following reason(s):

   ❏ Inactive **and** checked at least one item in either Section 2 or Section 3

   ❏ Active **and** checked at least one item in Section 2 **and** wants to begin in vigorous intensity activity

   ❏ Active **and** checked at least one item in Section 3

Copy of PASQ and Medical Clearance form given to participant on: _____
                                                                      Date

Completed/signed Medical Clearance form received: _____
                                                                      Date

Reviewed and Interpreted by: _____   _____
                                   Name of Exercise Professional   Date

Form 6-4: PASQ Medical Clearance Form

Your patient _____ (Name of Participant) would like to participate in the exercise/ fitness programs at _____ (Facility Name), a **non-clinical health/fitness facility** that provides a variety of exercise/fitness activities. To comply with pre-activity screening recommendations established by the American College of Sports Medicine, we have all participants complete a brief health history questionnaire (PASQ). Based on the responses to the PASQ (copy attached), your patient needs to obtain medical clearance prior to participating in our exercise/fitness programs. Once completed and signed by you, your patient can return this clearance form to me or you can fax it to me at _____ (secure fax number of fitness facility). If you have any questions, please feel free to contact me at _____. (phone number and e-mail address of exercise professional responsible for processing screening procedures).

Thank you,

_____

Name, credentials, and title of exercise professional staff member (e.g., John Smith, BS, ACSM EP-C, Fitness Director)

Please check (√) one of the following:

❏ Not cleared to exercise at this facility—should be referred to a clinically supervised exercise program
❏ Cleared to exercise at this facility

Please check (√) the highest exercise intensity level your patient is cleared for and provide any other restrictions/limitations

❏ Light (<57 to < 64% HR max)
❏ Moderate (64 to < 76% HR max)
❏ Vigorous (76 to < 96% HR max)
❏ Near Maximal to Maximal (> 96% HR max)

Restrictions/Limitations:

_____

_____

_____

_____   _____
Physician's Name (printed)   Physician's Signature

_____   _____
Phone number   Date

Form 6-5: PASQ—Self-Guided

Instructions:

Please complete this form and then refer to the Summary/Recommendations.

Please note: The authors of the PASQ assume no liability for individuals who participate in physical activity and/or complete the PASQ. If questions arise after completing the PASQ, seek the advice of your healthcare provider prior to physical activity. This PASQ is not a substitution for a medical examination.

Current Physical Activity

Over the last three months, have you regularly performed physical activity for at least 30 minutes, three days/week at a moderate intensity level?

> **Note:** Moderate intensity activity causes noticeable increases in heart rate and breathing such as walking at a brisk pace
> ❏ **Yes — Please proceed to page 2.**
> ❏ **No — Please complete the items below.**

Section 1 — Medical Conditions

Please check the box (√) for any of the following medical conditions that you have had or currently have.

❏ Heart attack
❏ Heart surgery
❏ Cardiac catheterization
❏ Coronary angioplasty (PTCA)
❏ Heart valve disease
❏ Heart failure
❏ Heart transplantation
❏ Congenital heart disease

❏ Abnormal heart rhythm
❏ Pacemaker/implantable cardiac defibrillator
❏ Peripheral vascular disease (PVD or PAD): disease affecting blood vessels in arms, hands, legs, and feet
❏ Cerebrovascular disease—stroke or TIA (transient ischemic attack)
❏ Renal (kidney) disease
❏ Type 1 or Type 2 Diabetes

Section 2 — Signs or Symptoms

Please check the box (√) for any of the signs/symptoms that you have recently experienced.

❏ Pain, discomfort in the chest, neck, jaw or arms at rest or upon exertion
❏ Shortness of breath at rest or with mild exertion
❏ Dizziness or loss of consciousness during or shortly after exercise
❏ Shortness of breath occurring at rest or 2-5 hours after the onset of sleep
❏ Edema (swelling) in both ankles that is most evident at night or swelling in a limb
❏ An unpleasant awareness of forceful or rapid beating of the heart
❏ Pain in the legs or elsewhere while walking; often more severe when walking upstairs/uphill
❏ Known heart murmur
❏ Unusual fatigue or shortness of breath with usual activities

Summary/Recommendations:

Did you check any of the items in Section 1 or in Section 2?

❏ **Yes** ⬇

- Medical clearance⁺ is recommended
- After obtaining medical clearance, begin with light* to moderate** intensity exercise and/or follow recommendations from healthcare provider

❏ **No** ⬇

- Medical clearance⁺ is not necessary
- Begin with light* to moderate** intensity exercise

⁺**Medical Clearance** — approval from a healthcare professional to engage in physical activity
***Light Intensity** — an activity that causes slight increases in heart rate and breathing
Moderate Intensity — an activity that causes noticeable increases in heart rate and breathing

Form 6-5 continued...

Physically Active Participants

Section 1 – Medical Conditions

Please check the box (√) for any of the following medical conditions that you have had or currently have.

- ❏ Heart attack
- ❏ Heart surgery
- ❏ Coronary angioplasty (PTCA)
- ❏ Heart valve disease
- ❏ Heart failure
- ❏ Heart transplantation
- ❏ Congenital heart disease
- ❏ Abnormal heart rhythm

- ❏ Pacemaker/implantable cardiac defibrillator
- ❏ Peripheral vascular disease (PVD or PAD): disease affecting blood vessels in arms, hands, legs, and feet
- ❏ Cerebrovascular disease—stroke or TIA (transient ischemic attack)
- ❏ Renal (liver) disease
- ❏ Type 1 or Type 2 diabetes

Section 2 — Signs or Symptoms

Please check the box (√) for any of the signs/symptoms that you have *recently* experienced.

- ❏ Pain, discomfort in the chest, neck, jaw or arms at rest or upon exertion
- ❏ Shortness of breath at rest or with mild exertion
- ❏ Dizziness or loss of consciousness during or shortly after exercise
- ❏ Shortness of breath occurring at rest or 2-5 hours after the onset of sleep
- ❏ Edema (swelling) in both ankles that is most evident at night or swelling in a limb
- ❏ An unpleasant awareness of forceful or rapid beating of the heart
- ❏ Pain in the legs or elsewhere while walking; often more severe when walking upstairs/uphill
- ❏ Known heart murmur
- ❏ Unusual fatigue or shortness of breath with usual activities

Summary/Recommendations:

1. Did you check any of the items in Section 1 or in Section 2?

❏ **No** ➡

- ⬧ Medical clearance[+] is not necessary
- ⬧ Continue with moderate* or vigorous** intensity exercise

2. Did you check any of the items in Section 1?

❏ **Yes** ➡

- ⬧ Medical clearance[+] is not necessary for continuing moderate* intensity exercise
- ⬧ Medical clearance[+] is recommended before engaging in vigorous** intensity exercise

3. Did you check any of the items in Section 2?

❏ **Yes** ➡

- ⬧ Medical clearance[+] is not necessary for continuing moderate* intensity exercise
- ⬧ Medical clearance[+] is recommended before engaging in vigorous** intensity exercise

[+]**Medical Clearance** — approval from a healthcare professional to engage in physical activity

***Moderate Intensity** — an activity that causes noticeable increases in heart rate and breathing

**Vigorous — an activity that causes substantial increases in heart rate and breathing

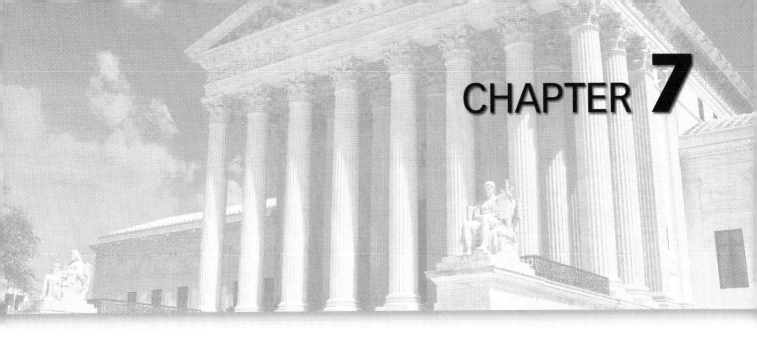

CHAPTER 7

Exercise Prescription and Scope of Practice

LEARNING OBJECTIVES

After reading this chapter fitness managers and exercise professionals will be able to:

1. Explain why exercise prescriptions need to be based on an individual's health/fitness status for safety and effectiveness.

2. Distinguish the 2018 Physical Activity Guidelines for Americans for (a) adults, and (b) adults with chronic health conditions and disabilities.

3. Describe the components of the FITT-VP principle and how they apply to an individualized exercise prescription.

4. Define "legal" scope of practice and "professional" scope of practice.

5. Explain the relationship between the professional standard of care and exercise prescription/scope of practice.

6. Describe three scenarios in which exercise professionals would be practicing outside their scope and the potential legal consequences of each.

7. Identify and summarize negligence lawsuits that involved improper exercise prescriptions designed/delivered by exercise professionals for apparently healthy individuals.

8. Describe the ADA and published standards of practice as they apply to proper exercise prescriptions for persons with disabilities.

9. Explain from a legal perspective, why it is essential that exercise professionals possess advanced knowledge and skills before prescribing exercise programs for clinical populations.

10. Describe the Exercise is Medicine® initiative and how it applies to exercise prescription and scope of practice.

11. Apply proper referral practices that can minimize legal liability associated with referrals.

12. Analyze the negligent conduct of exercise professionals in lawsuits involving plaintiffs with medical conditions.

13. List and describe steps to help ensure that exercise prescriptions for clinical populations will not be considered as medical treatment (e.g., the practice of medicine or the unauthorized practice of medicine).

14. Using case law examples, describe the potential legal consequences of providing an exercise prescription that crosses over the line into a licensed profession.

15. Develop and implement eight risk management strategies that will help minimize legal liability associated with exercise prescription and scope of practice.

INTRODUCTION

An exercise prescription needs to be designed and delivered based on the scope of practice of the exercise professional. This chapter describes the difference between legal scope of practice and professional scope of practice and how the **standard of care of a professional,** referred to as the **professional standard of care** in this textbook, applies to exercise prescriptions and scope of practice. Three scenarios are presented that describe situations that can lead to legal liability when an exercise professional practices outside his/her scope of practice. Spotlight cases and other cases are discussed to help demonstrate these legal liability exposures. The chapter ends with a description of eight risk management strategies that can be developed and implemented to minimize legal liability associated with exercise prescription and scope of practice.

The Health/Fitness Status of Americans

According to the *2018 Physical Activity Guidelines for Americans* (*2018 PA Guidelines*), there has been some improvement in physical activity among adults based on *Healthy People 2020* data (1). However, much more improvement is needed. For example, only 26 percent of men, 19 percent women, and 20 percent of adolescents report sufficient activity to meet the relevant aerobic and muscle-strengthening guidelines (1).

Negative Consequences of Physical Inactivity

Back in 2009, well-known exercise physiology epidemiologist, Dr. Steven Blair, stated that physical inactivity was the biggest public health problem of the 21st century (2). Based on cardiorespiratory fitness (CRF) data determined from maximal exercise tests with more than 40,000 men and nearly 13,000 women, low CRF accounted for substantially more deaths when compared with other risk factors such as obesity, smoking, high cholesterol, and diabetes. Figure 7-1 demonstrates how physical inactivity can lead to risk factors/medical conditions, chronic diseases, and premature death. As previously described in Chapter 6, 60% of the U.S. adult population has at least one chronic disease with 40% having two or more chronic

diseases (3, 4) and many are not metabolically healthy (5). These data along with increasing health care costs, demonstrate the need for more Americans to become physically active. Chronic diseases such as heart disease, cancer, and diabetes and their underlying causes (e.g., inactivity, obesity) affect nearly half the population and account for 75% of the U.S. health care spending or $1.5 trillion annually (6).

As health care costs continue to rise each year, so do the costs of prescription medications. In 2016, these costs increased almost 9% which was the fourth consecutive year of annual increases above 8%—much higher than the Consumer Price Index which increased 2.1% in 2016 (7). Nearly three in five Americans take a prescription drug (8). Between 2000 and 2012, the percentage of people taking five or more prescription drugs nearly doubled from 8% to 15% (8). Many of these drugs are prescribed for conditions (e.g., high cholesterol, hypertension, thinning bones, anxiety/depression, chronic pain, insomnia, and heartburn) often caused by an unhealthy lifestyle. In addition to the high costs, many drugs can have negative side effects with some shown to even have safety risks. In a 2017 article published in the *Journal of the American Medical Association,* a study found about one-third of all Food and Drug Administration (FDA) approved drugs had safety risks (9).

One way to decrease the high costs and negative effects of prescribed drugs is to decrease the reliance on them by treating conditions caused by lifestyle.

Figure 7-1: Negative Health Consequences of Physical Inactivity

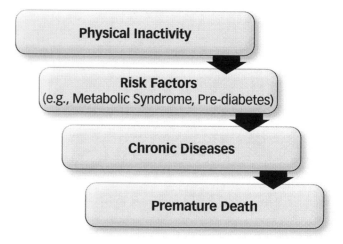

Through the Exercise is Medicine® (EIM) initiative, health care providers are encouraged to prescribe exercise instead of medications for some of their patients. More information on EIM is described below under Assessment of Legal Liability Exposures. Regular physical activity, along with other healthy lifestyle choices, can help individuals get off their prescribed drugs or reduce their dosage (in consultation with their health care provider). For example, one individual, who was on 16 prescribed medications, had his medications reduced to one over-the-counter drug and one prescribed drug after participating in the Ornish Lifestyle Medicine program (10) that focuses on physical activity, nutrition, stress management, and love/support (11).

Health/Fitness Status and Exercise Prescription

The "one size fits all" approach to exercise prescription is not feasible. As shown in Figure 7-2, the health/fitness status of Americans can vary tremendously—many are in varying degrees of poor health and varying degrees of good health. Therefore, exercise professionals, no matter what type of setting they work in, will need to establish individual exercise prescriptions for all types of individuals along this continuum. For example, a safe and effective exercise prescription needs to be different for a (a) cardiac patient who has just completed cardiac rehabilitation, (b) hip replacement

patient who just completed physical therapy, (c) sedentary person who is low risk, or (d)

The *2018 PA Guidelines* document includes general physical activity guidelines for various groups of Americans including (a) adults, and (b) for adults with chronic health conditions and disabilities (1) as presented in Exhibit 7-1. There are not many differences between the two sets of guidelines other than the last guideline for adults with chronic conditions and disabilities. It is important to realize that these guidelines reflect the desired activity levels to be achieved/maintained and do not reflect "individualized" exercise prescriptions.

As described in Chapter 6, prior to establishing an "individualized" exercise prescription, the exercise professional needs to obtain the individual's medical history and medical clearance if needed, conduct an appropriate fitness assessment, and then design a "safe" and "effective" program tailored to that individual based on the data obtained. These data also need to include any feedback from the individual's health care provider on the medical clearance form (see Chapter 6 appendix for an example) regarding any restrictions/limitations and exercise intensity level.

The FITT principle is often used when establishing an exercise prescription as follows: F = Frequency, I = Intensity, T = Time, and T = Type. In recent years, the FITT principle has been expanded to **FITT-VP principle** where V = Volume (the total volume or amount

Figure 7-2: The Poor Health to Good Health Continuum of Americans

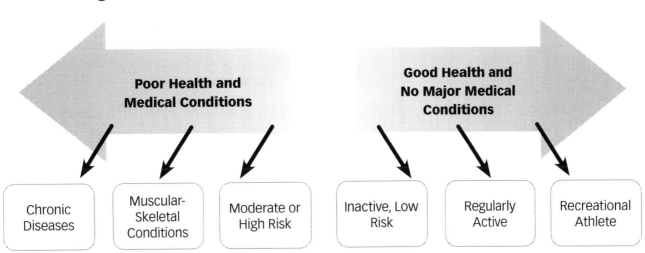

Exhibit 7-1: 2018 Physical Activity Guidelines

Adults (1, p. 8)

- Adults should move more and sit less throughout the day. Some physical activity is better than none. Adults who sit less and do any amount of moderate-to-vigorous physical activity gain some health benefits. *

- For substantial health benefits, adults should do at least 150 minutes (2 hours and 30 minutes) to 300 minutes (5 hours) a week of moderate-intensity, or 75 minutes (1 hour and 15 minutes) to 150 minutes (2 hours and 30 minutes) a week of vigorous-intensity aerobic physical activity, or an equivalent combination of moderate- and vigorous-intensity aerobic activity. Preferably, aerobic activity should be spread throughout the week.

- Additional health benefits are gained by engaging in physical activity beyond the equivalent of 300 minutes (5 hours) of moderate-intensity physical activity a week.

- Adults should also do muscle-strengthening activities of moderate or greater intensity that involve all major muscle groups on 2 or more days a week, as these activities provide additional health benefits.

---

*The *2008 PA Guidelines* stated that 10-minute blocks of activity were needed to achieve health benefits. However, that is no longer the case. The 2018 document describes research showing that physical active throughout the day has health benefits. The goal is to sit less and move regularly throughout the day.

Adults with Chronic Health Conditions and Disabilities (1, pp. 9-10)

- Adults with chronic conditions or disabilities, who are able, should do at least 150 minutes (2 hours and 30 minutes) to 300 minutes (5 hours) a week of moderate-intensity, or 75 minutes (1 hour and 15 minutes) to 150 minutes (2 hours and 30 minutes) a week of vigorous-intensity aerobic physical activity, or an equivalent combination of moderate- and vigorous-intensity aerobic activity. Preferably, aerobic activity should be spread throughout the week.

- Adults with chronic conditions or disabilities, who are able, should also do muscle-strengthening activities of moderate or greater intensity and that involve all major muscle groups on 2 or more days a week, as these activities provide additional health benefits.

- When adults with chronic conditions or disabilities are not able to meet the above key guidelines, they should engage in regular physical activity according to their abilities and should avoid inactivity.

- Adults with chronic conditions or symptoms should be under the care of a health care provider. People with chronic conditions can consult a health care professional or physical activity specialist about the types and amounts of activity appropriate for their abilities and chronic conditions.

---

of exercise), and P = Progression (advancement of the exercise program) (12). Each of these components are important to consider for the exercise prescription to be "reasonably safe" for the individual and, thus, are important from a legal liability perspective. Below, under Assessment of Legal Liability Exposures, are descriptions of negligence lawsuits in which the exercise professional did not properly apply one or more of these components when designing/delivering the exercise prescription. For example, the intensity was too high, the volume was too much, the type of exercise was unsafe, or progression was not properly applied, given the individual's health/fitness status.

Legal Scope of Practice Versus Professional Scope of Practice

Legal scope of practice is defined within the context of licensed healthcare professions such as:

Scope of practice is defined as the activities that an individual health care practitioner is permitted to perform within a specific profession. Those activities should be based on appropriate education, training, and experience. Scope of practice is established by the practice act of the specific practitioner's board, and the rules adopted pursuant to that act (13 p. 8).

The legal scope of practice is defined in state statutes for other licensed professionals, such as lawyers, counselors, barbers, and massage therapists. However, it is important to understand that **professional scope of practice** is applicable to all professions and vocations that require special knowledge, skills, and training—not only licensed professionals. All non-licensed professionals, such as exercise professionals, should practice within their education, training, experience, and practical skills to stay within their professional scope of practice. The legal scope of practice is not applicable to exercise professionals except for licensed clinical exercise physiologists in Louisiana. See Chapter 5 for more information on licensure. Under Assessment of Legal Liability Exposures, three scenarios are presented in which exercise professionals would be practicing outside their scope. The first two scenarios reflect professional scope of practice and the third scenario reflects legal scope of practice. Case law examples are described to help clarify and understand how these three scenarios are applied from a legal perspective.

Some professional organizations provide descriptions that appear to delineate the professional scope of practice for their various levels of certification. It is unlikely that courts will refer to these descriptions to determine if an exercise professional breached his/her duty or the professional standard of care. The factors that courts will use are described below under the professional standard of care. However, if someone is practicing dietetics without a license, the legal scope of practice, as specified in the licensing statute, will be reviewed by state licensing boards and/or courts to determine if the individual's conduct is in violation of the statute.

See Exhibit 7-2 for the National Strength and Conditioning Association (NSCA) and American College of Sports Medicine (ACSM) certification job descriptions, in part, and note the similarities and differences. In addition to these brief descriptions, the professional scope of

---

Exhibit 7-2: Brief Job Descriptions for ACSM and NSCA Certifications*

Personal Fitness Trainer—NSCA and ACSM
NSCA-Certified Personal Trainers (NSCA-CPT®) are health/fitness professionals who, using an individualized approach, assess, motivate, educate and train clients…They design safe and effective exercise programs…and respond appropriately in emergency situations… (15).

The ACSM Certified Personal Trainer (ACSM-CPT®), possessing a high school diploma or GED at minimum, works primarily with apparently healthy individuals to enhance fitness…The ACSM-CPT® conducts basic preparticipation health screenings… and fitness assessments… (16).

ACSM Exercise Physiologist
ACSM Certified Exercise Physiologists® are fitness professionals with a minimum of a bachelor's degree in exercise science qualified to pursue a career in university, corporate, commercial, hospital, and community settings…ACSM-EPs not only conduct complete physical assessments—they also interpret the results… (17).

ACSM Clinical Exercise Physiologist
The ACSM Certified Clinical Exercise Physiologist®… with a minimum of a bachelor's degree in exercise science…and 1,200 hours of clinical hands-on experience or a master's degree in clinical exercise physiology and 600 hours of hands-on clinical experience. CSM-CEPs® utilize prescribed exercise, basic health behavior interventions and promote physical activity for individuals with chronic diseases… (18)

NSCA Certified Special Population Specialist
Certified Special Population Specialists® (CSPS®) are fitness professionals who, using an individualized approach, assess, motivate, educate, and train special population clients of all ages regarding their health and fitness needs, preventively, and in collaboration with healthcare professionals… (19.)

*Descriptions provided are "in part." For the full descriptions, see the NSCA and ACSM websites listed in the references.

practice is also reflected in the domains and competencies associated with the varying levels of certification. Certification domains and competencies, discussed in Chapter 5, provide much more detail than the job descriptions. Although these certification job descriptions and competencies reflect professional scopes of practice, they are not always adhered to in practice. For example, as demonstrated in the negligence lawsuits described in this textbook, there are exercise professionals designing/delivering exercise programs for clinical populations who do not possess the necessary credentials and/or competencies.

These exercise professionals who do not have the necessary background in clinical exercise are, likely, practicing outside their professional scope when designing/delivering exercise programs for clinical populations. As described in Chapter 4, they will be unable to meet the standard of care required and, thus, subject themselves to negligence claims and lawsuits. For example, in the spotlight case below, *Bartlett v. Push to Walk* (14), the court stated that fitness facilities that serve clinical populations "may impose particular duties that an ordinary health club would not have…What would constitute ordinary negligence would differ as between an ordinary health club and a facility like Push to Walk"

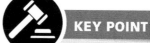

KEY POINT

It is important to distinguish *legal scope of practice* and *professional scope of practice*. For example, if an exercise professional appears to be practicing dietetics without a license, the legal scope of practice as specified in the licensing statute will be reviewed by state licensing boards and/or courts to determine if the professional's conduct is in violation of the statute.

The professional scope of practice is applicable to all professions and vocations that require special knowledge, skills, and training—not only licensed professionals. All non-licensed exercise professionals (e.g., personal fitness trainers, exercise physiologists, clinical exercise physiologists) should practice within their education, training, experience, and practical skills to stay within their professional scope of practice and to minimize negligence claims and lawsuits.

(p. 7). In other words, facilities that serve clinical populations may be obligated to have qualified professionals who can meet the standard of care required to properly and safely serve such populations.

ASSESSMENT OF LEGAL LIABILITY EXPOSURES

 Assessment of Legal Liability Exposures → Development of Risk Management Strategies → Implementation of the Comprehensive Risk Management Plan → Evaluation of the Comprehensive Risk Management Plan

Legal liability exposures associated with exercise prescription and scope of practice are primarily negligence related. However, conduct that is outside one's scope of practice can also lead to criminal charges if the conduct crosses over into a profession that is regulated by state licensing statutes. As demonstrated in Figure 7-3, there are three scenarios in which practicing outside one's scope can lead to legal liability for exercise professionals. The failure of exercise professionals to practice within their scope leads to negligence claims and lawsuits more often than criminal charges. There appears to be more case law involving the first two scenarios (negligence)

than the third scenario (criminal charges). Each of these three scenarios are described in more detail below. But first, it will be important to review the **professional standard of care** to which exercise professionals will likely be held when negligence claims/lawsuits are filed against them as described in Chapter 4.

Professional Standard of Care: Exercise Prescription and Scope of Practice

One expert witness stated, "there is no professional standard of care in the personal training industry" (20, p. 5).

Perhaps this perspective is based on the premise that licensure does not exist for personal fitness trainers or any exercise professionals for that matter (except in Louisiana for clinical exercise physiologists). However, the *Restatement of Law Third, Torts* states "If an actor has skills or knowledge that exceed those possessed by most others, these skills or knowledge are circumstances to be taken into account in determining whether the actor has behaved as a reasonably careful person" (21, pp. 82-83). Negligence, in the context of the exercise profession, can be defined as failing to do what a reasonable prudent exercise professional would have done or doing something that a reasonable prudent exercise professional would not have done, under the same or similar circumstances (22). There are three important points to understand regarding the professional standard of care in the context of exercise prescription and scope of practice as follows:

a) Exercise professionals, no matter what their job title is, should possess knowledge and skills that exceed those of the lay public. In fact, participants expect them to have special knowledge and skills in exercise science and to stay current with the literature, best practices, etc. If not, why would there even be a need for exercise professionals? Therefore, exercise professionals will be held to a different standard of care (a professional standard of care) than the lay public in which a reasonable standard of care is expected as described in Chapter 4.

b) The behavior (actions/inactions) of exercise professionals will be what is judged by the courts more so than the credentials they possess (i.e., did they behave as a reasonable prudent professional would have given the circumstances or situational factors). Obviously, an exercise professional who is well-educated and possesses the necessary knowledge and skills will be less likely to behave in an inappropriate manner because they know how to prescribe safe and effective exercise programs and how to stay within their scope of practice.

c) Situational factors help determine the professional standard of care as follows: (1) nature of the

Figure 7-3: Three Scenarios that Can Lead to Conduct Outside the Scope of Practice of an Exercise Professional and the Potential Legal Consequences

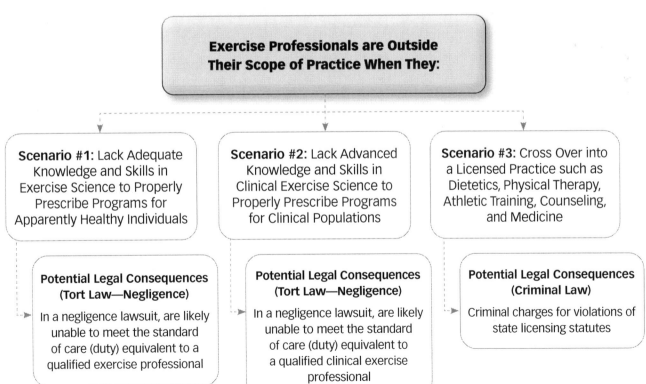

activity, (2) types of participants, (3) environmental conditions. See Exhibit 4-1 in Chapter 4 where each of these is explained in more detail.

» If the nature of the activity is complex or difficult, it inherently increases the risk of injury. Exercise professionals who teach complex/difficult activities should be well-experienced in these activities. They need to fully understand how to apply important safety precautions to reduce the risk of injury and only teach them to participants who are "ready" for such advanced activities.

» Exercise professionals need to be aware of individual factors regarding the types of their participants (i.e., an increased risk of injury can exist given an individual's health and fitness status). Examples:

a. For a person with Parkinson's disease, what are the increased risks of injury and what precautions are necessary to minimize those risks in the design and delivery of an exercise prescription?

b. For a person who has been sedentary but otherwise apparently healthy, what are the increased risks if they begin with a vigorous-high intensity exercise program?

» Exercise professionals also need to take precautions to minimize risks associated with environmental conditions, such as heat/humidity and floor surfaces.

These three important points regarding the professional standard of care are often reflected in the testimony that expert witnesses provide in negligence lawsuits involving exercise professionals and fitness facilities. They will give their opinions regarding the knowledge/skills and behavior of the defendants (e.g., exercise professional, fitness manager) as well as any of the three situational factors that might be relevant.

SCOPE OF PRACTICE SCENARIO #1: EXERCISE PROFESSIONALS LACKING ADEQUATE KNOWLEDGE AND SKILLS

Several spotlight and other cases described throughout this textbook involved apparently healthy individuals who were injured because of **improper exercise prescription** (i.e., the exercise professional had the participant (a) perform an unsafe exercise, or (b) perform exercise at an intensity level that the participant was unable to safely tolerate). See Figure 7-4. Exercise professionals need to understand that prescribing unsafe or high intensity exercises can create an increased risk of injury. Related to improper exercise prescription is improper instruction such as failing to teach how to perform an exercise correctly or safely use a piece of exercise equipment. Cases related to improper instruction are described in Chapters 8 and 9.

Spotlight Cases: Improper Exercise Prescriptions Involving Apparently Healthy Individuals

Table 7-1 includes a brief summary of spotlight cases in this textbook that dealt with improper exercise

Figure 7-4: Types of Improper Exercise Prescriptions for Apparently Healthy Participants

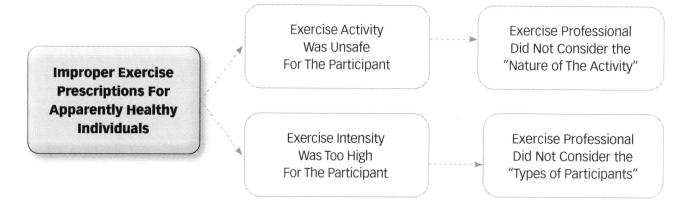

Table 7-1	Spotlight Cases Involving Apparently Healthy Individuals: Type of Improper Exercise Prescriptions	
SPOTLIGHT CASE (CHAPTER)	**CAUSE AND TYPE OF INJURY**	**TYPE OF IMPROPER PRESCRIPTION**
Evans v. Fitness Sport Clubs, LLC (4)	Personal fitness trainer had 62-year old client perform suicide and backward runs—client fell and fractured both wrists.	Unsafe exercise
Santana v. Women's Workout and Weight Loss Centers, Inc. (4)	Group exercise leader had participants perform combined stepping and upper body strengthening exercises participant fell and fractured her ankle.	Unsafe exercise
D'Amico v. L.A. Fitness (5)	Personal fitness trainer had client perform an intensive exercise—client suffered serious injuries to her arm and shoulder.	Intensity level too high
Rostai v. Neste Enterprises, d/b/a Gold's Gym (6)	Personal fitness trainer had inactive, overweight client perform heavy lifting exercises—client suffered a heart attack.	Intensity level too high
Vaid v. Equinox (8)	Personal fitness trainer had client perform rowing machine exercise at an intensity level that was excessive—client had a massive stroke.	Intensity level too high
Butler v. Seville et al. (9)	Personal fitness trainer had 62-year old client perform standing exercise on an upside down BOSU ball—client fell and fractured her wrist and hip.	Unsafe exercise

prescriptions causing injuries to apparently healthy individuals. Four additional cases (*Hinkel, Mellon, Proffitt,* and *Mimms*) are described below. In these cases, the exercise professionals did not consider two of the three situational factors (nature of the activity, type of participants) when prescribing the exercise activity. See Figure 7-4. It is evident from these cases that the exercise professionals did not possess adequate knowledge and skills to safely prescribe exercise for apparently healthy participants (i.e., they did not fully understand the risks associated with the exercises that they were prescribing). For example, well-educated and trained exercise professionals know that prescribing certain stepping/hopping exercises can increase the risk for a fall and prescribing high intensity exercise can increase the risk of exertional rhabdomyolysis. Individuals who do not possess the necessary knowledge and skills to practice as an exercise professional should either stop working as an exercise professional or obtain the formal education and practical training needed to do so. If they continue to practice as an exercise professional without obtaining adequate knowledge and skills, they are practicing outside their scope and subject themselves and their employers to negligence claims and lawsuits.

Additional Cases: Improper Exercise Prescriptions Involving Apparently Healthy Individuals

Hinkel v. Gavin Pardoe & Gold's Gym—Intensity Level Too High

In this case (23), Melinda Hinkel, client of personal fitness trainer Gavin Pardoe, suffered a rupture of the C5 disc in her neck requiring two surgeries. She claimed her injury was caused by Pardoe putting too much weight on a piece of exercise equipment and had her continue the exercise without realizing she had sustained a serious injury. The trial court granted summary judgment in favor of the defendants and the appellate court affirmed based on the waiver signed by Hinkel. However, there were two dissenting justices that believed the waiver was invalid because it contravenes public policy to enforce such provisions (exculpatory clauses) in the context of a contract for personal training services and because the terms of the waiver did not clearly apply to personal training services. They stated that they would agree with the court's conclusion regarding the waiver if Hinkel had been injured while working out on her own or in a group fitness program. However, she paid a significant amount of money for her training sessions and "in choosing to work with a personal trainer, a client presumably relies on the health and safety training of the trainer who holds him or herself out as an expert in the field. Indeed, a novice trainee would understandably rely on the expertise of a trainer to avoid the inherent risk of personal injury in using exercise equipment and machines" (p. 751).

Mellon v. Crunch—Unsafe Exercise

In this case (24), the plaintiff, Nell Mellon, was injured while under the direction of personal fitness trainer, Gavin Umeh. Umeh testified that he was a professional personal trainer and prior to being employed by Crunch, he had been employed by three other facilities as a personal trainer. He testified that he was certified by the American Council on Exercise and completed several programs with Equinox's Fitness Training Institute as well as Crunch's requirement to undergo personal training continuing education. In Mellon's second training session with Umeh, he had her perform an exercise "which consisted of having one foot on top of a rectangular bench approximately 2-3 feet high, having the other foot on the ground and hopping in order to switch feet" (p. 2). In her first attempt, "her left foot became caught under the bench causing her to fall backwards. She threw her hands behind her back to catch herself and fractured both wrists" (p. 2). One of the several negligent claims she made against the defendants was that Umeh pushed her beyond her physical abilities. An expert for the plaintiff stated that Umeh departed from accepted personal training practices and the departures directly resulted in the plaintiff's injury. The expert also stated that the exercise "was too advanced based on the height of the bench… that the height of the bench increased her risk of injury, and a safer method would have been to practice the exercise without elevation or on an apparatus with lower elevation" (p. 7). The court denied the defendant's motion of summary judgment. Although the personal fitness trainer in this case was an experienced trainer and possessed certain credentials, he did not appear to be competent.

Proffitt v. Global Fitness Holdings, LLC, et al.—Intensity Level Too High

In this case (25), personal fitness trainer Jared Ashcroft had his client, Vince Proffitt, perform several strenuous, squat-type exercises for about 40 to 45 minutes in the first training session. During the exercises he became very fatigued and "lost the ability to raise himself from a squatting position, and repeatedly fell to the floor" (p. 4). Despite obvious signs/symptoms of overexertion and requests by Proffitt to stop, Ashcroft had him continue with the exercises. For many hours after the session, Proffitt experienced extreme pain and fatigue and after 38 hours he noticed his urine was dark brown. He went to the emergency room where he was diagnosed and hospitalized with exertional rhabdomyolysis resulting in permanent injuries including 30% loss of muscle tissue in both quadriceps muscles. The case was settled out of court (26).

Mimms v. Ruthless Training Concepts, LLC—Intensity Level Too High

This case (27) is like the *Proffitt* case in that the exercise prescription involved high intensity exercise before the participant was ready (conditioned) to safely tolerate high intensity levels. In his first workout under the direction of a fitness trainer Javier Lopez, Mimms participated in a CrossFit workout that included continuous strenuous leg exercises—burpees, thrusts, and squats—in a short time period of 20 minutes. Although Mimms voiced his fatigue level, he continued to follow Mr. Lopez's direction to continue the exercises. Two days later Mimms experienced severe pain and dark colored urine. He was hospitalized and diagnosed with several injuries including exertional rhabdomyolysis, lumbosacral spine strain, and strain of the bilateral quadriceps resulting in surgery and permanent disability. In his lawsuit, he sought $500,000 in compensatory damages for negligence and $350,000 in punitive damages for gross negligence. He was awarded $300,000. An expert witness for the plaintiff with a Ph.D. in exercise physiology stated that Mimms should have been warned about the risk of developing rhabdomyolysis and an assessment of his fitness level should have been done prior to the training session. The expert also stated that because Mimms was a novice, care should have been taken that he did not overexert himself (i.e., the intensity could have been reduced by having him perform fewer repetitions and sets as well as including adequate rest periods). Part of the evidence included the ACSM position paper—*Progression Models in Resistance Training for Healthy Adults* that provides safety recommendations such as rest periods.

KEY POINT

In the negligence lawsuits described under Scope of Practice Scenario #1, it was apparent that the individuals who were practicing as exercise professionals did not first obtain adequate knowledge and skills needed to design/deliver safe and effective exercise prescriptions. Without adequate knowledge/skills, it is likely they did not realize what the scope of practice of an exercise professional entails.

Vigorous-to-High Intensity Exercise Programs

Credentialed and competent exercise professionals know the varying levels of exercise intensity as follows: Light (<57 to <64% HR max), Moderate (64 to < 76% HR max), Vigorous (76 to < 96% HR max), and Near Maximal to Maximal (> 96% HR max) (28, p. 146). Near maximal to maximal means "high" intensity in this context. However, sometimes in the literature, vigorous intensity has also been referred to as high intensity. Exercise professionals understand that intensity is relative to the individual's level of fitness. For example, less fit people will require a higher level of effort. They will experience increased exertion to the cardiovascular and musculoskeletal systems more so than fit people when performing the same exercise intensity level. In addition, exercise professionals know that having low-fit individuals or beginners perform vigorous and/or high intensity exercise can increase their risk of injury. As demonstrated in the above negligence lawsuits, exercise programs that were too intense for the plaintiffs led to all types of injuries such as musculoskeletal, cardiovascular, and exertional rhabdomyolysis even among apparently healthy adults. More information on this topic is covered in Chapter 8 along with describing the distinction between High Intensity Training (HIT) and High Intensity Interval Training (HIIT) from safety and legal liability perspectives.

SCOPE OF PRACTICE SCENARIO #2: EXERCISE PROFESSIONALS LACKING ADVANCED KNOWLEDGE AND SKILLS

As described in Chapter 3, Title III of the Americans with Disabilities Act (ADA) prohibits discrimination regarding programs and services offered by places of public accommodation and commercial facilities (29). For example, one of the 12 categories of places of public accommodation specified in Title III includes "a gymnasium, health spa, bowling alley, golf course, or other places of exercise or recreation" (29, p. 22). In an ADA discrimination lawsuit, the plaintiff will have to prove "1) that he or she is an individual with a disability; 2) that defendant is a place of public accommodation; and 3) that defendant denied him or her full and equal enjoyment of the goods, services, facilities or privileges offered by defendant on the basis of his or her disability" (30, p. 1342). Therefore, it is essential that fitness managers and exercise professionals provide services for those with disabilities, which may include those with chronic medical conditions (see the ADA's definition of disability in Chapter 3).

Exercise Prescription and the Americans with Disabilities Act (ADA)

As explained above, prescribing exercise programs for these individuals requires advanced knowledge and skills in order to meet the professional standard of care. Several certifications were listed in Chapter 5 that required academic coursework and/or practical experience in clinical exercise. Additional certifications are described later under Development of Risk Management Strategies. Given the high percentage of Americans with at least one chronic medical condition (60% as previously stated) and one in five Americans (53 million) having a disability (31), it is imperative that fitness facilities employ exercise professionals who possess the credentials and competence to safely design and deliver programs for these individuals. This is important, not to just comply with the ADA but also, to serve these populations that could achieve numerous health/fitness benefits from a properly prescribed exercise program. According to *Healthy People 2020*, only 36.5% of persons with disabilities are meeting physical activity objectives whereas 58.5% of persons without disabilities are meeting physical activity objectives (32). Exercise is Medicine® (EIM), described below after the spotlight cases, is one initiative that can help increase physical activity participation among these individuals.

Professional Standards of Practice Regarding the ADA

Standards and guidelines published by professional organizations do not specifically address scope of practice from legal and professional perspectives. However, several professional organizations have published various standards and guidelines that address Title III of the ADA that require the provision of programs/services for persons with disabilities. For example, the ACSM (33) has a guideline that facilities should consider providing an array of activity options to serve the physical, emotional, and personal preferences of each user. The NSCA (34) has a standard requiring compliance with federal, state, and local laws that address equal opportunity and access. The International Health, Racquet & Sportsclub Association (IHRSA) (35) has a standard that requires compliance with local, state, and federal discrimination laws (i.e., membership is open to persons of all races... and physical disabilities). The Medical Fitness Association (MFA) (36) has a guideline recommending facilities to provide programs for persons with chronic medical conditions and another guideline that recommends clinical fitness staff members, who provide programs for individuals representing clinical/special populations, to have additional credentials (e.g., degree, certification, and experience related to clinical exercise).

Spotlight Cases

The following three spotlight cases describe injuries that occurred, primarily, because the exercise professional did not appear to have the advanced knowledge and skills to safely design and deliver an exercise program for individuals with medical conditions.

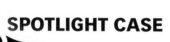

SPOTLIGHT CASE

Levy v. Town Sports International, Inc.
101 A.D.3d 519, 2012 LEXIS 8543 (N.Y. App. Div., 2012)

FACTS

Historical Facts:

During a training session, personal trainer Franklin Lee, employed by Town Sports International, Inc. (TSI), instructed Gayle Levy to perform a series of jump repetitions on a BOSU ball. Lee knew that Levy had osteoporosis. After successfully completing the exercise a few times, Levy lost her balance and fell fracturing her wrist which required surgery to have a plate and screws inserted into her wrist. In prior training sessions with Lee, Levy testified that she used the BOSU ball in prior workouts. When Levy joined the gym, she signed a membership agreement that included a waiver of liability for any injury sustained on TSI's premises.

Procedural Facts:

Levy, the plaintiff, filed a personal injury lawsuit against the defendant TSI. The defendant filed a motion of summary judgment asserting that Levy assumed the risks associated with the workout. The trial court granted the motion. However, Levy appealed this decision arguing that she did not assume the risks because when Lee had her perform the jump repetitions on the BOSU ball, he increased the amount of risks ordinarily associated with the activity.

ISSUE

Did the trial court err when it granted the motion of summary judgment in favor of the defendant based on the primary assumption of risk defense?

COURT'S RULING

Yes, the appellate court reversed the trial court's ruling.

Levi continued...

COURT'S REASONING

Citing previous case law (*Mathis v. New York Health Club,* 261 A.D.2d 345 and *Corrigan v. Musclemakers,* Inc. 258 A.D.2d 861), the court stated that "entitlement to judgment…based on an assumption of risk defense, raised triable issues of fact that warrant denial of the motion" (p. 519). These issues included:

> "whether the trainer, knowing that plaintiff had osteoporosis and had recently had surgery, unreasonably increased the risk of harm to plaintiff by recommending that she perform an advanced exercise with multiple repetitions; whether the trainer was in a proper position to help guard against plaintiff falling during the exercise; whether plaintiff voluntarily assumed the risks or was following the trainer's expert advice and encouragement while attempting to complete the exercise" (p. 519).

The trial court ruled that Levy assumed the risks because she had exercised with the BOSU ball on prior occasions and, therefore, understood and appreciated the risks associated with using a BOSU ball and voluntarily chose to perform the BOSU ball exercise. Regarding the trainer being in a better position to catch Levy if needed, the trial court stated this was irrelevant because the risk was open and obvious. The appellate court obviously did not agree with this analysis of the trial court. It appears from the appellate court's ruling that the major reason why Levy did not assume the risks is because the trainer increased the risk of harm by instructing her to perform advanced exercises, especially given her health condition.

At trial, Levy argued that the waiver of liability that she signed in her membership agreement was unenforceable under the New York General Obligations Law § 5-326. The trial and appellate courts did not address this issue.

Lessons Learned from *Levy*

Legal

▶ The primary assumption of risk doctrine negates any duty on part of the defendant to safeguard individuals from inherent risks associated with participation in sport and recreation activities if the individual is aware of the risks, has an appreciation of the risks, and voluntarily assumes the risks.

▶ The primary assumption of risk defense generally is not an effective defense when a defendant (e.g., a fitness instructor leading/teaching exercises) increases the inherent risks above those ordinarily associated with the activity. See also *Corrigan* and *Santana* cases in Chapter 4.

▶ When the primary assumption of risk defense is ineffective, the defendant(s) will likely be found liable unless some other defense might be effective in protecting the defendants such as a waiver.

Risk Management/Injury Prevention

▶ Know, understand, and apply the precautions that need to be taken when leading/teaching exercises to individuals with medical conditions (e.g., in this case, the trainer should have known that a fall could lead to a fracture, and he easily could have had the client perform a different exercise that could achieve the same benefit without the risk of a fall).

▶ For fitness staff members who are unaware of these precautions, it is best that they refer these individuals to an exercise professional who is aware of these precautions.

▶ Avoid jumping exercises onto balls (or other devices) until the individual is ready (e.g., has acquired the necessary balance and skill to perform the exercise safely) and, in some cases, never have individuals perform this type of exercise because the risk of injury outweighs any benefit.

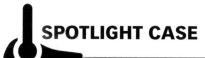

SPOTLIGHT CASE

Bartlett v. Push to Walk
No. 2:15-cv-7167-KM-JBC, 2018 WL 1726262 (D. N.J., 2018)

FACTS

Historical Facts:

Caleb Bartlett, a 36-year-old quadriplegic, attended Push to Walk, a specialized gym for people with spinal cord and neurological disorders, to seek personal training. Prior to beginning the training program, he signed a waiver. Mr. Bartlett had been in a wheelchair for eighteen years and suffered from low bone density, muscle atrophy, digestive problems, and had a goal to lose weight. Barlett worked with trainer Tiffany Warren who had a bachelor's degree in exercise science, four years of experience at Push to Walk, and ACSM personal trainer certification. After completing both on-the-job observational hours and on-the-job "hands-on" hours at Push to Walk, Warren began working as a neuroexercise trainer. She did not receive any formal training to become a neuroexercise trainer.

About six months prior to his injury, Bartlett requested to change trainers. He became uncomfortable with Warren because he did not believe that she understood spinal cord injury and other conditions that can arise with a spinal cord injury, especially autonomic dysreflexia. He also felt that Warren did not respect his years of experience in a wheelchair and what his limitations were. An employee at Push to Walk attempted to arrange for a new trainer but that did not happen before the day of Bartlett's injury, May 22, 2014.

On the day of the injury, Warren expressed that she would like him to try a "kneeling" technique, to which Bartlett expressed his concerns because he had never been in that position before, although he was willing to give it a try. Warren learned this technique from another trainer at Push to Pull, not by reading any materials regarding this technique with respect to persons with spinal cord injuries. But she informed Bartlett that this technique had helped other clients improve their balance and that she was not concerned about any risk at all given his progression after working out at Push to Pull for over a year. According to Bartlett, he made it very clear to Warren that he was not comfortable with the exercise because he had not knelt in over 20 years but did not want to be chicken and was willing to try. She reassured him that he could stop if he felt uncomfortable. Other employees assisted Warren to help Bartlett perform the exercise. According to Bartlett, the employees:

> rotated me over onto my stomach, which was already uncomfortable because I had not laid on my stomach in ten years, and when you do that with a spinal cord injury, … it's very painful and very uncomfortable. You're then pulled into a kneeling position backwards …. They grab you from behind by the hips and literally pull you back upward up in a kneeling position, and immediately when I was on my knees, it was much worse than when I was in the standing frame. I was lightheaded. There was some stronger dysreflexic symptoms. I knew that this was not a good situation. I could tell that they did not have control of my body, just because of my size, and I needed to lay down. I did not feel well and I asked them to put me down, and they did, and when I laid down, I was tingling, I was lightheaded and I was nauseous (p. 3).

Warren then told Bartlett that she would like him to perform the exercise one more time. He told her that he did not think that was a good idea, but he went ahead and tried it again. During the exercise, his hips buckled to the left and he fell forward to his right and his hips went to the left. Bartlett experienced several symptoms after this incident including early symptoms of dysreflexia. He was lightheaded, nauseous, and had pain shooting up his right side (he thought due to a possible cracked rib). He was unable to complete his training session that day which always ended with riding the electrical stimulation bicycle.

Bartlett continued...

Following the incident, Mr. Bartlett went to the hospital. He did not have any cracked ribs, but his oxygen levels were low and was still experiencing pain, so he remained in the hospital for monitoring. Soon after being discharged from the hospital, Bartlett noticed his right knee and leg began to swell. Instructed by his doctor, he went to the hospital emergency room. The doctors determined that Bartlett had a fractured leg for at least three weeks and that it had started to mend in the fractured position. Surgery to repair would be too dangerous given his spinal cord injury. Bartlett claims that the injury has prevented him from participating in electronic stimulation and other types of physical therapy that have helped him in the past.

Procedural Facts:

On September 29, 2015, the plaintiff filed a complaint against the defendant on two counts: negligence in providing services and the negligent hiring of defendant Tiffany Warren. The defendants filed a motion for summary judgment, to which the plaintiff opposed and, in addition, requested to file an amended complaint that added a cause of action for gross negligence. The court granted the plaintiff's request to file an amended complaint and terminated the motion for summary judgment. On September 16, 2016, the plaintiff filed an amended complaint that added the cause of gross negligence and the defendants again filed a motion for summary judgment claiming they were entitled to summary judgment because of the waiver that Bartlett signed and the charitable immunity act.

ISSUE

Did the court grant the motion for summary judgment in favor of the defendants in reference to the three counts in the plaintiff's complaint: 1) negligence, 2) negligent hiring, and 3) gross negligence.

COURT'S RULING

Yes and no. Summary judgment was granted for the defendants on the first two counts, but it was denied on the third count.

COURT'S REASONING

Regarding count one, Bartlett claimed that the waiver was unenforceable on public policy grounds. The court stated that an exculpatory agreement does not violate public policy and will be enforced if:

(1) it does not adversely affect the public interest;

(2) the exculpated party is not under a legal duty to perform;

(3) it does not involve a public utility or common carrier; or

(4) the contract does not grow out of unequal bargaining power or is otherwise unconscionable (p. 6).

After analyzing all four factors and relying on previous New Jersey cases such as *Stelluti v. Casapenn Enterprises, LLC* (spotlight case in Chapter 4), the court concluded that the exculpatory waiver clause was enforceable. Regarding a legal duty to perform, the court stated that:

> Here, defendants surely had a duty of care. That duty is not unlimited, however…When it comes to physical activities in the nature of sports…injuries are not an unexpected, unforeseeable result of such strenuous activity…Such physical activities require the participant to assume some risk because injury is a common and inherent aspect of the activity…the standard of care due to individuals who participate in recreational sports should not be based on a standard of ordinary negligence but on the heightened standard of recklessness or intent to harm (p. 6).

In other words, the court made no distinction between recreational sports (contact and noncontact sports) and physical activity/exercise programs regarding the standard of care (i.e., the primary assumption of risk defense is an effective defense for injuries due to ordinary negligence but not for reckless or intentional conduct). However, the

Bartlett continued...

court did indicate that programs like Push to Walk that serve injured individuals "may impose particular duties that an ordinary health club would not have...What would constitute ordinary negligence would differ as between an ordinary health club and a facility like Push to Walk" (p. 7). However, using the analysis in the *Stelluti* case, the court concluded that the waiver signed by Bartlett was compatible with public policy by New Jersey courts.

Regarding count two, the court stated: "New Jersey courts recognize the tort of negligent hiring where the employer either knew or should have known that the employee was violent or aggressive, or that the employee might engage in injurious conduct toward third persons" (p. 8). Because Warren did not commit any intentional acts (e.g., false imprisonment, assault, battery, intentional infliction of emotional distress), Push to Walk cannot be held liable for negligent hiring.

The court denied summary judgment for count three, gross negligence. The court distinguished ordinary negligence, gross negligence, and willful/wanton or reckless conduct as follows:

> ...negligence is the failure to exercise ordinary or reasonable care that leads to a natural and probable injury, gross negligence is the failure to exercise slight care or diligence. Although gross negligence is something more than inattention or mistaken judgment, it does not require willful or wanton misconduct or recklessness (p. 8).

Citing New Jersey's model jury instructions, the court referred to gross negligence as "a person's conduct where an act or failure to act creates an unreasonable risk of harm to another person because of the person's failure to exercise slight care or diligence" (p. 9). Warren's conduct was grossly negligent when she knew that Bartlett's first attempt at kneeling did not go well and then pressed him to try it again a second time and the injury resulted.

The waiver was an effective defense protecting the defendants for counts one and two (ordinary negligence) but not for count three, gross negligence. Regarding the charitable immunity doctrine, it would only bar an action for ordinary negligence, not gross negligence, based on a New Jersey statute (N.J. Stat. Ann § 2A:53A-7) in which a charity (e.g., nonprofit organization such as Push to Walk) is not immune from gross negligence, willful/wanton acts or intentional acts. The ordinary negligence claims were already dismissed based on the waiver and because the charitable immunity defense would not apply to gross negligence, it would not be an effective defense for count three.

Lessons Learned from *Bartlett*

Legal

- Waivers in New Jersey are an effective defense for ordinary negligence but not for gross negligence.

- Based on this court's analysis, there is no distinction between sports/recreation activities and fitness/exercise activities regarding the primary assumption of risk defense. Other courts (see Chapter 4) have made this distinction indicating that when risks are increased over and above the inherent risks in fitness/exercise activities, the assumption of risk defense is ineffective whereas with sports/recreation activities, increased inherent risks are common and, thus, the defense would apply.

- Fitness facilities that provide exercise programs for vulnerable populations such as those with medical conditions, may have particular duties (i.e., a different standard of care, perhaps) than an ordinary health club would have.

- Some states, such as New Jersey, distinguish gross negligence and willful/wanton or reckless conduct. Other states do not—they are considered the same.

- New Jersey courts recognize the tort of negligent hiring if the employer knew or should have known that the employee might engage in injurious conduct toward third persons.

- Charitable immunity state statutes may provide some protections for fitness facilities that are nonprofit organizations. However, most states have abolished these statutes as described in Chapter 5.

Bartlett continued...

Risk Management/Injury Prevention

- ◆ Fitness managers and exercise professionals need to realize that exercise programs for individuals with medical conditions should only be designed and delivered by exercise professionals with advanced formal education regarding the medical condition(s). On-the-job training is important, but formal education is also needed.

- ◆ To prevent claims of gross negligence, exercise professionals need to honor and respect the requests of the participant (e.g., when the participant expresses a concern about his/her ability to perform an exercise safely or when a request to stop is made).

- ◆ Titles of exercise professionals, such as "neuroexercise trainer" in this case, need to be carefully determined. Program participants may believe that this title reflects that the trainer has had advanced formal education (e.g., graduate coursework) in neuro exercise above and beyond an undergraduate degree in exercise science or a personal training certification. Deceptive advertising/promotion of staff members' credentials can lead to litigation, as in *D'Amico v. LA Fitness* (spotlight case in Chapter 5).

- ◆ Fitness managers have a responsibility to properly hire, train, and supervise employees as described in Chapter 5.

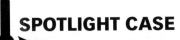

SPOTLIGHT CASE

Layden v. Plante
957 N.Y.S.2d 458, 2012 LEXIS 9109 (N.Y. App. Div., 2012)

FACTS

Historical Facts:

The plaintiff, Diane A. Layden, participated in a personal training program at No Limits Fitness owed by Deborah Greenfield. Prior to beginning the personal training sessions, Layden notified her certified personal trainer, Angela Plante, of her medical history of back problems and a herniated disc. Plante instructed and supervised Layden in a program of weight lifting. A couple days later, Layden used the written instructions provided by Plante to repeat the program on her own without supervision. While performing one of the exercises, a Smith squat, the plaintiff experienced lower back pain which ultimately resulted in a surgical procedure to correct two herniated discs with fragments.

Procedural Facts:

The plaintiff and her spouse filed a complaint against the defendant personal trainer for improper supervision and instruction and against the defendant owner for "failing to provide a safe place with properly trained staff and also upon the doctrine of respondeat superior given the trainer's acts as an agent or employee" (p. 460). Each defendant filed a motion for summary judgment, and each was granted by the court primarily based on the primary assumption of risk doctrine. The court stated that the "plaintiff's own testimony established that she had previously participated in weight-lifting exercise programs—including a prior program designed by the trainer—and that she knew that back injuries are an inherent risk of such activities" and, therefore, the "plaintiff knew of the risks, appreciated their nature and voluntarily assumed them" (p. 461). The plaintiffs appealed.

ISSUE

Did the court err when it granted the motions for summary judgment in favor of the defendants?

Layden continued...

COURT'S RULING

Yes, the motions for summary judgment were reversed by the appellate court.

COURT'S REASONING

Citing previous case law, the appellate court stated that the "doctrine of assumption of risk provides that a person who voluntarily participates in recreational or athletic activities is deemed to consent to the commonly appreciated risks inherent in that activity…However, a participant does not assume risks resulting from a dangerous condition over and above the usual dangers inherent in the activity" (p. 460). Based on the testimony of two expert personal trainers, the court indicated that the "plaintiffs raised triable issues of fact as to whether the trainer's direction to perform the Smith squat, her allegedly improper instructions, or both, served to unreasonably increase the risk to which plaintiff was exposed" (p. 461). Both experts opined that the Smith squat, even if properly performed, is a contraindicated exercise for someone with a herniated disc because it causes "direct vertical loading of the spinal column and places extreme stress on the lower back" (p. 461).

The experts also testified that the trainer did not provide proper instruction to the plaintiff on how to perform the Smith squat. In contrast to the expert testimony, the trainer testified that whether the Smith squat is dangerous for a person with a back injury will depend on the form used by the exerciser. She also testified that she did not warn the plaintiff that the exercise posed any risk to her back.

Regarding the liability of the owner Greenfield, the appellate court stated that Greenfield "may be held liable only if the trainer's negligence may be imputed under a theory of respondeat superior" (p. 462). However, Greenfield contended that there was no derivative liability because the trainer was an independent contractor. To determine if the defendant trainer was an independent contractor, the court stated that this would require an "analysis of the extent of the fitness center's power to regulate the manner in which the trainer performed her work, and the parties' conflicting evidence poses factual questions as to this issue" (p. 462). This was main reason for the barring the motion for summary judgment of the defendant owner. The plaintiff also signed a waiver, but the language did not clearly state the negligence or fault of the fitness center employees or agents and, thus, was unenforceable. However, even if the exculpatory language had been properly written to protect the defendants from their own negligent conduct, it still would not have been enforceable based on New York General Obligations Law § 5-326 that prohibits waivers.

Note: Two judges that disagreed with the majority's opinion stated in their dissent that the plaintiff did assume the risks. She asked the trainer to teach her a new program after three months of training. While performing the new Smith squat exercise, the plaintiff did not experience any discomfort but did experience some mild back pain afterwards and the next day. The dissenting judges said the plaintiff was well aware of her back condition and that weight-lifting could further injure her back, but nevertheless returned to perform the exercise on her own.

Lessons Learned from *Layden*

Legal

- The primary assumption of risk defense may not be an effective defense when defendants increase risks over and above the inherent risks. (See Chapter 4 for more on this defense).

- Expert witnesses can help educate the court as to the duty owed to the plaintiff and if the defendants breached that duty.

- Employers can be vicariously liable for the negligent acts of their employees under the doctrine of respondent superior, but generally not for the negligent conduct of independent contractors.

- Employers who hire independent contractors may not have liability protections if the employer regulates the way independent contractors perform their work as they do with employees. (See Chapter 5 for more on this topic).

Layden continued...

Risk Management/Injury Prevention

▶ Fitness managers and exercise professionals cannot assume that a "certified" personal fitness trainer is competent. An in-depth assessment of their knowledge and skills is needed prior to hiring.

▶ Because employers do not have behavioral control of independent contractors, an in-depth determination of their knowledge and skills is needed prior to hiring.

▶ Fitness staff members, such as personal fitness trainers who train participants with medical conditions, need to possess advanced knowledge and skills to fully understand the precautions that might be necessary when designing/delivering an exercise program.

KEY POINT

The ADA requires fitness facilities to serve populations with disabilities, including those those with physical limitations and chronic illnesses. Therefore, it is essential to employ exercise professionals with advanced knowledge and skills who can safely and effectively design/deliver exercise programs for these populations. This will help minimize liability associated with discrimination (e.g., meet the requirements of the ADA) and civil liability associated with negligence (e.g., an exercise professional with advanced knowledge and skills will likely be able to meet a certain standard of care that the courts might require).

Note: It is important to realize that professionals with advanced knowledge and skills in clinical exercise (e.g., clinical exercise physiologists) may not always possess the needed expertise to work with certain individuals, given there are so many types of medical conditions with varying degrees of severity. In these situations, it would be best to refer the individual to a professional who possesses the needed expertise or work closely with the participant's health care provider(s) who could provide assistance and guidance.

Exercise Prescription and Exercise is Medicine®

Exercise is Medicine® (EIM), a collaborative effort co-launched by the ACSM and the American Medical Association, began in the United States in 2007 and has expanded into a worldwide health initiative managed by ACSM. EIM encourages physicians and other health care providers to (a) assess and record physical activity (PA) as a vital sign during patient visits, (b)

provide brief advice/exercise prescription or referral to a certified exercise professional or allied health professional (37). An effective strategy to assess the PA levels at every patient visit is to embed a Physical Activity Vital Sign (PAVS) into electronic health records. Common vital signs are blood pressure, pulse rate, respiration, temperature, and height/weight. Adding PA can be achieved by asking questions such as:

1. On average, how many days a week do you perform physical activity or exercise?
2. On average, how many total minutes of physical activity or exercise do you perform on those days?
3. Describe the intensity of your physical activity or exercise: light…moderate…vigorous (38, p. 210).

For patients meeting the *2018 PA Guidelines* (1), the physician (or other health care provider) might say something like "good job, keep it up" and for a patient with high blood pressure and a PAVS score of zero, the physician might say "before I start you on a medication, why don't you try walking briskly for 30 minutes each day to lower your blood pressure. If that does not work, then we will ty a medication" (39, p. 226). This approach follows the 5 A's to facilitate behavior change—ask, advise, assess, assist, and arrange (38).

PAVS has been implemented successfully in several healthcare systems. For example, Kaiser Permanente in Southern California captured PAVS on 85% of eligible patients (38). One of the challenges of EIM is that only 6% of U.S. medical schools have core curricula regarding physical activity and exercise (38). A recommended medical school curricula on physical activity has been developed (38), but it will take time and a concerted effort for medical schools to adopt these curricula.

Even if physicians have the educational background to provide exercise prescription/counseling, there are other challenges they face when implementing EIM. For example, time demands to prepare an exercise prescription or provide PA counseling, inadequate reimbursement codes, and their lack of connections/partnerships with the community fitness facilities/programs (40). Given these challenges, one of the EIM recommendations is for physicians or other health care providers to refer their patients to a credentialed exercise professional or to a community fitness facility or program that employs credentialed exercise professionals. However, this proposes another challenge for physicians. How do they go about making a proper referral given that exercise professionals are not licensed, and the credentials vary tremendously among exercise professionals? Physicians are accustomed to making referrals to licensed professionals such as physical therapists and medical specialists (e.g., cardiologists), but they also know it is essential they take some precautions prior to making such referrals.

Legal Liability for Improper Referral

Physicians can be liable for medical malpractice if they knew (or should have known) that the health care provider to whom they referred their patients was incompetent (41). They may also face liability if the clinic or medical facility to which they referred their patients was unaccredited or improperly staffed (41). Therefore, physicians are expected to exercise due care (e.g., investigate health care providers and facilities) prior to making referrals. Improper referrals do not only apply to physicians, but all professionals including exercise professionals. Before exercise professionals make a referral, they should use the same due care to help avoid professional liability claims or possible ethics violations (41). If physicians and other professionals exercise this due care, it can reduce their liability associated with referrals (42). In addition, the referral needs to be acceptable to all three parties—the referring physician, the receiving health care provider, and the patient. Therefore, it is necessary for the referring physician to ensure the receiving health care provider, or exercise professional will accept the patient before the referral (42).

Given these **proper referral practices**, physicians, who make referrals to exercise professionals

KEY POINT

The Exercise is Medicine® initiative involves physicians and other health care providers referring their patients to qualified exercise professionals. To minimize legal liability associated with referrals, it is important that they utilize proper referral practices. These same practices also apply to exercise professionals when they make referrals.

as recommended with the EIM initiative, will need to exercise the same due care to help prevent negligent referral claims/lawsuits. Because the exercise profession is self-regulated versus government-regulated through licensure, physicians may be hesitant to make referrals to exercise professionals unless they personally know them and are aware of their credentials/competence. It is unlikely that physicians will take the time to conduct the necessary research to seek out credentialed and competent exercise professionals and/or credible fitness facilities/programs in the community. It is also unlikely that they will be familiar with all the credentialing issues that exist in the exercise profession as presented in Chapter 5. Therefore, it would be wise for fitness managers and exercise professionals to proactively develop relationships with various medical clinics in their communities.

Obtaining Physician Referrals

A first step may be to actively involve the fitness facility's medical advisor or advisory committee to help develop a strategic plan to establish these relationships (e.g., how to set up meetings with local medical clinics, the content to be presented at the meetings, and follow-up steps). It will be important to describe and distinguish the knowledge and skills of an exercise physiologist and clinical exercise physiologist. Physicians may not understand how these are different from physical therapy, other allied professions, and personal fitness training. See Exhibit 7-3 for brief descriptions provided by the U.S. Bureau of Labor Statistics. The second "exercise physiologist" description is perhaps more reflective of a clinical exercise physiologist than the first one.

Medical fitness facilities that have developed these trusting relationships have resulted in successful physician

---

Exhibit 7-3: U.S. Bureau of Labor Statistics: 2018 Standard Occupational Classification System*

Exercise Physiologists (29-1128): Assess, plan, or implement fitness programs that include exercise or physical activities such as those designed to improve cardiorespiratory function, body composition, muscular strength, muscular endurance, or flexibility.

Excludes "Physical Therapists" (29-1123), "Athletic Trainers" (29-9091), and "Exercise Trainers and Group Fitness Instructors" (39-9031).

Illustrative examples: *Applied Exercise Physiologist, Clinical Exercise Physiologist, Kinesiotherapist*

Exercise Trainers and Group Fitness Instructors (39-9031): Instruct or coach groups or individuals in exercise activities for the primary purpose of personal fitness. Demonstrate techniques and form, observe participants, and explain to them corrective measures necessary to improve their skills. Develop and implement individualized approaches to exercise.

Illustrative examples: *Aerobics Instructor, Personal Trainer, Yoga Instructor*

U.S. Bureau of Labor Statistics: Occupational Outlook Handbook**

Exercise physiologists develop fitness and exercise programs that help patients recover from chronic diseases and improve cardiovascular function, body composition, and flexibility

*https://www.bls.gov/soc/2018/major_groups.htm#31-0000
**https://www.bls.gov/ooh/healthcare/exercise-physiologists.htm

---

referrals (43). Employing credentialed and competent exercise professionals who can properly design/deliver exercise programs is one of the main reasons for their success as well as demonstrating the positive health outcomes the patients have achieved. Fitness managers and exercise professionals, who work in non-medical fitness facilities, can follow a similar model if they want to promote the EIM initiative and have physicians refer their patients to their fitness programs/facilities. However, it will be essential they employ credentialed and competent exercise physiologists. The EIM website (http://exerciseismedicine.org) has excellent resources for both health care providers and exercise professionals.

Medical fitness facilities directly affiliated with a health system may have some additional advantages in implementing the EIM initiative and physician referrals. The exercise professionals and medical directors who have oversight of these fitness facilities have been able to arrange physician referrals through the health system's electronic medical records (EMRs) or electronic health records (EHRs). For example, in one medical fitness facility, the facility's exercise professionals received physician referrals through the EMRs and also used the

EMRs to maintain two-way communication (discussed below) between themselves and the referring physicians (J. Hannan, PhD, personal communication, April 22, 2019). Given the direct referral, medical clearance was not needed. Even though the exercise professionals had access to the patient's EMR, they still had the patient complete a medical history questionnaire. The data from the medical history was used to develop and implement the exercise prescription more so than the patient's EMR. However, because of their access to the EMRs, the exercise professionals had to complete the health system's HIPAA training program and meet other related requirements. It is also important to note that the physicians were well-informed of the credentials/competence of the exercise professionals who worked in the medical facility prior to making the referrals. Physicians were encouraged to make referrals to the fitness program as well as other lifestyle medicine programs offered within the health system.

Physicians who worked outside the health system could also refer their patients to this medical fitness facility. They faxed the referral over to the fitness facility, the patient completed the medical history questionnaire, and then the two-way communication was maintained by fax communications. Of course, the medical fitness facility needed to ensure they had a "secure" fax machine. With outside referrals, the exercise professionals—employees of the health system's medical fitness facility—did not have access to the EMRs of those patients.

Clinical exercise physiologists working in hospital rehabilitation programs (e.g., cardiac and pulmonary) would likely have authorization to access a patient's EMR. However, exercise professionals working in most community settings would not be able to obtain authorization to access an individual's EMR. If certain medical records are needed, the patient needs to first sign a HIPAA authorization to disclose health information form before a physician or other health care provider can release them (see Chapter 3 for more on HIPAA and a sample authorization release form).

The EIM Credential and Exercise Prescription

As shown in Figure 7-5, exercise prescriptions can be designed for both prevention and treatment of chronic diseases. Exercise is an essential component of treatment for many chronic diseases. Exercise helps control the disease, prevent further progression of disease, and in some cases, reverse the disease. As described above, exercise professionals who design/deliver exercise programs for individuals with chronic diseases and/or disabilities need to possess advanced knowledge and skills. If they do not, they may subject themselves to negligence lawsuits as did the exercise professionals in the three spotlight cases—*Levy, Bartlett,* and *Layden.* For example, the exercise professional in *Bartlett* possessed a bachelor's degree in exercise science and was an ACSM

Figure 7-5: Exercise Prescription for Prevention and Treatment

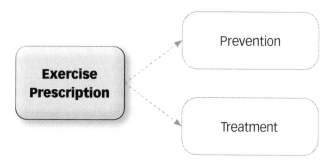

certified personal trainer. She did not appear to possess the advanced credentials or competence needed to work with participants like Mr. Bartlett. The court ruled that her conduct, which caused the plaintiff's injury, was not only negligent but grossly negligent.

To help address some of the credentialing issues regarding exercise prescription for clinical populations, the EIM credential was created. There are three levels as follows:

- Levels 1 & 2: These credentialed exercise professionals may work with individuals who are healthy or who have health-related issues but have been cleared by their physicians for exercise.
- Level 3: These credentialed exercise professionals may work with patients who require clinical support and monitoring (44).

The requirements (45) vary among the three levels. For example, EIM Level 1 does not require a degree, only a NCCA or ANSI/ISO-accredited fitness certification such as the ACSM personal trainer certification and completion of the EIM credential online course (a course in which 5.0 CECs can be earned). EIM Level 2 requires a bachelor's degree in Exercise Science, Exercise Physiology or Kinesiology and a NCCA or ANSI/ISO-accredited fitness professional certification such as the ACSM exercise physiologist certification and completion of the EIM credential online course. Individuals seeking EIM Levels 1 and 2 may be exempt from the online course if certain other requirements are met. EIM Level 3 requires an approved master's degree in Exercise Science, Exercise Physiology or Kinesiology or approved bachelor's degree in the same areas with 4,000 hours of clinical exercise experience and a NCCA or ANSI/ISO-accredited clinical exercise certification (e.g., ACSM clinical exercise physiologist certification).

Like most exercise credentials as described in Chapter 5, EIM credentials Levels 1 and 2 do not require any assessment of an individual's practical skills, but Level 3 does require clinical experience. For EIM Level 2 that requires a bachelor's degree, individuals may have had academic coursework in which practical skills were included and assessed. However, the extent of the practical skills, especially skills related to designing/delivering exercise prescriptions for individuals who have health-related issues and are medically-cleared, would likely be unknown to employers even in CAAHEP undergraduate accredited programs. Utilizing the ACSM screening criteria as described in Chapter 6, these "medically-cleared" individuals could be people with heart disease, diabetes, etc.

For individuals with the EIM Level 1, it is likely that even less will be known about their knowledge and skills to design/deliver exercise programs for people with health-related issues. Many of these individuals may have only completed an online accredited personal training certification examination and the EIM online course. Therefore, an in-depth assessment of the credentials and competence of individuals with the EIM Level 1 credential is needed. It may be that they need to obtain formal education and practical training before they even lead exercise programs for apparently healthy individuals. As described above and demonstrated in the case law examples, they will not be able to meet the standard of care without having the necessary knowledge and skills and, thus, subject themselves and their employers to legal liability. Therefore, an in-depth assessment of the credentials/competence of individuals with the EIM Level 1 credential is needed.

Below under Development of Risk Management Strategies, it is recommended that fitness facilities hire at least one clinical exercise physiologist with advanced credentials and competence who could provide oversight of the facility's programs for clinical populations as well as provide guidance and training to exercise professionals with the EIM Level 2 credential who may be leading these programs. It can be argued that exercise professionals, with a bachelor's degree in the field and a professional certification (e.g., ACSM EP, ASEP EP, ACE Medical Exercise Specialist described in Chapter 5), should be qualified to design and deliver safe and effective exercise programs for clinical populations. However, a deeper dive into their clinical knowledge and skills may be necessary. If they completed only one academic course in clinical exercise or special populations (as required to sit for the ACSM and ASEP EP certification examinations described in Chapter 5), this may not be adequate. They may need to complete additional or advanced coursework (or other advanced training) in clinical exercise that includes practical training and experience.

The need for advanced credentials and competence to work with clinical populations is evident from a systematic review completed by Warburton et al. (46).

This comprehensive review of the literature concluded with seven recommendations. Recommendations #3 and #4 are as follows:

#3—Qualified exercise professionals should possess…core competencies for work with prominent higher risk conditions (15 core competencies are listed with one of these addressing the need for comprehensive knowledge to safely and effectively design/implement exercise prescriptions for persons with chronic disease, functional limitations and disabilities).

#4—The qualifications for an exercise professional should include completion of an undergraduate degree in the exercise sciences and the passing of rigorous, independent, national written and practical exams demonstrating competency to work with at-risk populations (46, pp. S252, S253).

Related to recommendation #4, Warburton et al. (46) stated that the evidence is clear. Exercise professionals must demonstrate knowledge and skills regarding the absolute and relative contraindications to exercise for varied populations and "simply completing a general undergraduate degree in exercise science is an insufficient qualification for work with clinical populations" (p. 260).

Views related to this topic were expressed by Dr. William Herbert (47) who has more than 45 years of professional experience which includes the development and evaluation of clinical exercise services as well as serving as an expert witness in exercise injury litigation. He states that because physical activity will soon be considered an integral component of medical care, it will increase employment opportunities for exercise professionals who want to specialize in designing and delivering exercise programs for individuals with medical conditions. However, it is unknown if credentialed and competent clinical exercise physiologists will be the primary providers of these services. The direct involvement of physicians and health care systems will require exercise professionals to provide evidence of their knowledge and skills to provide safe and effective exercise prescriptions for clinical populations. Given the exercise profession is not government regulated through licensure, physicians may be more inclined to refer their patients to licensed professionals who may or may not be qualified. In addition, exercise professionals in community settings may be enticed to serve clinical populations to increase their clientele but may not have the advanced credentials and competence to do so. Given these circumstances, Dr. Herbert states that there is an "increased exposure of the 'medicalized' exercise client to greater chances of physical activity related injury and death. And, such events inevitably would increase risks of personal injury litigation affecting not only exercise providers, but also legal actions against referring physicians and community health care systems" (p. 86).

KEY POINT

The spotlight cases described under Scope of Practice Scenario #2 demonstrated the importance of exercise professionals having advanced knowledge and skills to design/deliver safe and effective exercise prescriptions for clinical populations. The research by Warburton et al. (46) and the views of Herbert (47) also support why this is so important. A deep dive into the credentials and competence is needed to determine if an exercise professional is truly prepared to work with clinical populations.

Exercise Prescription for Treatment: Legal Issues to Consider

As discussed in the next section (Scope of Practice Scenario #3), exercise professionals should never "diagnose or treat" a medical condition, which could be considered crossing over into the practice of medicine. To avoid this possibility, there are several strategies to consider. First, if an individual is experiencing any type of pain, the exercise professional should be able to determine if the pain might be due to an underlying medical condition or if it is typical pain/discomfort associated with exercise or a new exercise? See Table 6-3 in Chapter 6 for action steps to take. Obviously, exercise professionals should never attempt to diagnose or treat a medical problem or communicate in a manner that could be interpreted as a diagnosis/treatment. For example, saying something like the following to a participant would be inappropriate—"You have osteoarthritis in your shoulder, and I can prescribe an exercise program that will help treat your arthritis". Rather, if a person is suffering from shoulder pain that does not subside after a week or two, referral to his/her physician is needed. Then, communicate with the physician (or other health care provider) in designing a proper exercise program.

Second, after medical clearance is obtained for someone with a medical condition(s), it is good idea to maintain **two-way communication** with the participant's primary care physician (PCP) or other health care providers. See Figure 7-6. Other health care providers include, for example, physical therapists or clinical exercise physiologists working in cardiac rehabilitation programs. After patients complete physical therapy or cardiac rehabilitation, they are often encouraged to continue their exercise in community fitness facilities. It would be helpful for exercise professionals working in community facilities to obtain pertinent information (via proper authorization) about the individual's physical therapy or cardiac rehabilitation exercise program (e.g., any contraindications, current levels of fitness, etc.) and maintain two-way communication with these health care providers too, when needed, as the participant progresses in the community program. It is also a good idea to inform these PCPs and other health care providers that the facility has a medical advisor and/or committee that helps provide oversight of clinical exercise programs and has a clinical exercise physiologist on staff, if applicable. All these strategies can be effective to help avoid exercise prescriptions that might be construed to be "treating" a medical condition. In addition, establishing these professional relationships (a) helps the participant be successful, (b) enhances the credibility of the exercise profession, and (c) increases future referrals from PCPs and health care providers.

Technology applications, such as mobile apps and wearable technology, promise to be an efficient way in which everyone involved in the care of the patient can stay connected. However, as described in Chapter 3, privacy issues and possible FDA regulations need to be addressed.

Figure 7-6: Two-Way Communication Between the Exercise Professional and PCP

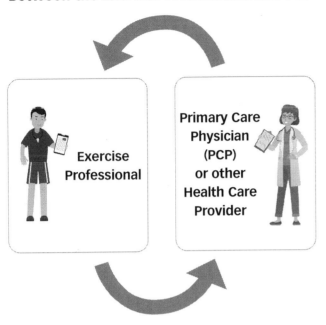

Waivers (Releases of Liability) and Clinical Exercise Prescriptions

When a physician refers a patient for physical therapy or cardiac rehabilitation, the health insurance provider reimburses the clinic/program for the medical services provided based on the provisions established in the patient's health care plan. The patient does not pay or pays a small percentage of the costs for the services. Because these services are considered medical treatments, the patient would not sign a waiver. As described in Chapter 4, a waiver would likely be unenforceable for these services just as they are for virtually all other medical services. Rather, an informed consent is likely signed by the patient.

Community fitness programs/services are not reimbursed by insurance providers as are physical therapy and cardiac rehabilitation services. However, some health insurance providers offer an incentive program that reimburses individuals $20/month if they workout so many times per month (48) or reimburses them for a portion of their annual fitness center membership fee such as $150-$250. Older adults, 65+, who are on certain Medicare plans, can take advantage of programs such as Silver-Sneakers. They can locate a community fitness center that provides discounts for memberships and/or programs for SilverSneakers participants. Because these community

programs/services are not considered medical treatments such as physical therapy and cardiac rehabilitation, participants can sign a waiver, at least in states where they are enforceable. For example, in the *Bartlett* spotlight case above, the waiver protected the defendants (for ordinary negligence, not gross negligence) for a community fitness program for individuals with disabilities.

SCOPE OF PRACTICE SCENARIO #3: EXERCISE PROFESSIONALS CROSSING OVER INTO A LICENSED PROFESSION

It is important that an exercise professional's conduct does not cross over into the practice of a licensed profession because it "can lead to criminal charges for practicing medicine (or some other allied health profession) without a license or the unauthorized practice of medicine (or some allied health profession)" (49, p. 192). The criminal charges vary by state. In Florida, a state statute titled Unlicensed Practice of a Health Care Profession (50), provides the criminal penalties for violating a statute that relates to the practice of any licensed health care profession (see Exhibit 7-4 for a brief summary of this statute). In addition to potential criminal charges, an exercise professional could also face civil claims if their conduct or advice causes harm. For example, if a personal trainer informs a client to take a certain supplement and that supplement causes harm, the trainer and his/her employer could face a negligence lawsuit as well as demonstrated in *Capati v. Crunch Fitness* (51, 52).

Many fitness managers and exercise professionals are familiar with the *Capati* case (51, 52). In this case, a personal fitness trainer advised his client, Mrs. Capati who took hypertension medication, to take a variety of nutritional supplements including some that contained ephedra. The trainer probably did not realize that the combination of hypertension medication and ephedra can be lethal. One day, while exercising at the Club, Mrs. Capati became very ill and later died of a brain hemorrhage (stroke) at the hospital. Her husband filed a $320 million wrongful death claim against the defendants—the trainer, the Club, and a variety of other defendants including Vitamin Shoppe Industries. The case was settled out of court for over $4 million with

---

Exhibit 7-4: Violation of State Licensing Statutes: Brief Summary of Criminal Penalties*

Cease and desist notice: Issued by the state department or appropriate regulatory board within the department when there is probable cause a person who is not licensed has violated any provision specified in the statute. The penalty shall be a fine of not less than $500 nor more than $5,000 as established by rule of the department. Each day that the unlicensed profession continues after issuance of a notice to cease and desist constitutes a separate violation.

3rd degree felony: The practice, attempt to practice, or offer to practice a health care profession without an active, valid Florida license. The minimum penalty is a fine of $1,000 and a minimum mandatory period of incarceration of 1 year.

2nd degree felony: The practice results in serious bodily injury. The minimum penalty is a fine of $1,000 and a minimum mandatory period of incarceration of 1 year.

1st degree misdemeanor: The practice, attempt to practice, or offer to practice a health care profession with an inactive or delinquent license for any period of time up to 12 months. The minimum penalty is imprisonment of 30 days and a fine of $500. For 12 months or more it is a 3rd degree felony.

* Unlicensed Practice of a Health Care Profession. Fla Stat. § 456.065 (2001).

---

the trainer and Club being liable for $1,750,000 and the other defendants being liable for the remaining amount.

Exercise professionals need to realize that nutritional advice that may seem benign (e.g., recommending a supplement) might lead to harm. If faced with a negligence lawsuit, exercise professionals cannot claim, as a legal defense, that they did not know about the harmful consequences of the nutritional advice they provided. Several viable, legal defenses to refute negligence lawsuits do exist but ignorance or lack of knowledge is not one of them. It also is important to realize that licensed dietitians conduct different health screenings than exercise professionals. For example, they screen for all types of medical conditions and they also know the specific nutritional needs for individuals with chronic diseases and medical conditions.

Legal Scope of Practice: Nutrition

State licensing statutes define the legal scope of practice for each licensed profession. For example, see Exhibit 7-5 for the scope of practice definition for the practice of dietetics in Ohio. The state of Ohio also provides a statute entitled General Nonmedical Nutritional Information that defines the type of nutritional information that non-licensed dietitians can provide, also shown in Exhibit 7-5. Exercise professionals should not have

their participants complete an "individual" nutrition assessment and then provide follow-up dietary recommendations based on the assessment or provide any type of individualized nutritional advice such as recommending a certain diet or supplement. This could be considered practicing dietetics without a license in Ohio as well as the majority of states that require licensure to practice dietetics. There are two states with no state regulation—Arizona and Michigan. In these states, anyone can practice dietetics. Other states have licensure of title only or certification of Registered Dietitian Nutritionists (e.g., statutory certification) or title protection with no state regulation (53).

It is best for exercise professionals to provide only "general" nonmedical nutritional information such as the five items shown in Exhibit 7-5. Another way to help determine the nutrition scope of practice for exercise professionals is to review the competencies such as those provided for ACSM certifications. For example, the competencies related to nutrition/weight management for the ACSM certified personal trainer and exercise physiologist all begin with *knowledge of* such as knowledge of the Dietary Guidelines for Americans (16). None of them begin with *skill in* such as skill in conducting nutritional assessments. Therefore, it is within their scope to provide "general" nutrition education. Many exercise professionals who have had academic coursework in nutrition or who have obtained a certification in nutrition

---

Exhibit 7-5: Ohio Scope of Practice Statutes: Licensed Dietitians and Non-Licensed Dietitians, In Part

Licensed Dietitians*

"Practice of dietetics" means any of the following:

1. Nutritional assessment to determine nutritional needs and to recommend appropriate nutritional intake, including enteral and parenteral nutrition;

2. Nutritional counseling or education as components of preventive, curative, and restorative health care;

3. Development, administration, evaluation, and consultation regarding nutritional care standards.

Non-Licensed Dietitians**

"General nonmedical nutritional information" means information on any of the following:

1. Principles of good nutrition and food preparation;

2. Foods to be included in the normal daily diet;

3. Essential nutrients needed by the human body and recommended amounts of those nutrients;

4. Foods and supplements that are good sources of essential nutrients;

5. The actions of nutrients on the human body and the effects of nutrient deficiency and nutrient excess.

---

*Ohio R.C. § 4759.01 (March 20, 2013)
**Ohio R.C. § 4762.01 (March 22, 2013)

---

may believe that they have the knowledge and skills to provide "individual" nutritional education or advice, but this, likely, would be outside their scope of practice. However, if the nutrition education obtained through an academic course and/or certification is of high quality (e.g., based on empirical research), exercise professionals can share all types of general nonmedical nutritional information with participants. Given there is so much inaccurate dietary information on the Internet and elsewhere, exercise professionals can help their participants become aware of this misinformation and direct them to reliable and credible resources. Another option that some fitness managers have implemented is to hire a registered dietitian nutritionist (RDN) as an independent contractor or employee. Exercise professionals can refer their participants to the RDN who can provide "individualized" nutritional advice.

Licensing Reform

On June 30, 2020, Florida's governor signed into law the Occupational Freedom and Opportunity Act (HB 1193) that loosens or abolishes occupational licensing regulations across 30 professions. For example, barbers and cosmetologists, licensed in other states, can practice their trades in Florida without having to get re-licensed. Regarding those who provide wellness recommendations and nutrition advice, the following was added to subsection (1) of F.S.A. § 468.505 Exemptions; Exceptions.

Nothing in this part may be construed as prohibiting or restricting the practice, services, or activities of:

Any person who provides information, wellness recommendations, or advice concerning nutrition, or who markets food, food materials, or dietary supplements for remuneration, if such person does not provide such services to a person under the direct care and supervision of a medical doctor for a disease or medical condition requiring nutrition intervention, not including obesity or weight loss, and does not represent himself or herself as a dietitian, licensed dietitian, registered dietitian, nutritionist, licensed nutritionist, nutrition counselor, or licensed nutrition counselor, or use any word, letter, symbol, or insignia indicating or implying that he or she is a dietitian, nutritionist, or nutrition counselor (pp. 16-17).

Licensing reform bills are also occurring in other states. In consultation with legal counsel, fitness managers and exercise professionals should stay abreast of these bills. It appears from this Florida law, that exercise professionals and health/wellness coaches in Florida can provide individual nutrition advice to clients for a fee except for certain individuals and they must be careful of how they represent themselves.

Legal Scope of Practice: Additional Licensed Professions

In addition to practicing dietetics without a license as described above, there are several other licensed professions in which exercise professionals can cross over if they are not careful. Some of these are medicine, physical therapy, athletic training, counseling, and chiropractic medicine. As stated previously, the "legal" scope of practice for licensed professionals is defined in the state licensing statute. It will be important for exercise professionals to stay away from certain practices defined in these statutes (e.g., manual therapy, electrical stimulation, and traction that are performed by physical therapists and counseling for personal problems such as financial, drugs/alcohol, and relationships performed by licensed counselors). Participants may believe that the exercise professionals that work in a fitness facility are medical professionals and, therefore, can diagnose and treat physical or psychological problems. Fitness managers and exercise professionals need to provide training for all staff members on how to properly handle these situations when they arise and how to make referrals when needed. (See Risk Management Strategy #7).

Although the legal scope of practice is defined in the licensing statute, there may be some cross over with the "professional" scope of practice among professions. For example, exercises prescribed by physical therapists and athletic trainers may be the same type of exercises that exercise professionals may prescribe such

as exercises to increase core strength. Some of the academic coursework and knowledge/skills obtained may be the same across professions as well. The key for exercise professionals is to stay away from practices that fall within the domain of a licensed professional. The following case examples demonstrate this importance.

Legal Scope of Practice: Case Examples

There are not a lot of cases involving criminal charges against exercise professionals for violating state licensing laws. Negligence claims/lawsuits are much more common. However, based on blogs and other sources, it is evident that some exercise professionals are providing individualized dietary advice such as prescribing certain supplements and diagnosing and treating pain. It may be that state licensing boards are issuing a cease and desist notice (or something similar) when they become aware of such violations. If the individual then stops his/her unauthorized practice, the licensing board would likely not pursue criminal charges such as a felony or misdemeanor. The first case, *Ohio Board of Dietetics v. Brown*, involves an individual who violated the Ohio state statute (briefly described above in Exhibit 7-5). The second case, *Cooksey v. Futrell*, involves an individual who, allegedly, violated an administrative code according to the North Carolina Board of Dietetics/Nutrition. The third case, *Sosa-Gaines v. Capital Fitness Inc.*, is a negligence lawsuit but involves a personal fitness trainer who, allegedly, was practicing chiropractic medicine.

Editorial Note: *The content describing the following Ohio Board of Dietetics v. Brown case reflects content taken from Chapter 7 in Risk Management for Health/ Fitness Professionals: Legal Issues and Strategies (49). The publisher transferred the rights to this textbook to the authors in 2017. Permission to reprint and revise this content was granted by the author of Chapter 7.*

Ohio Board of Dietetics v. Brown

In this case (54), the defendant: (a) performed nutritional assessments and recommended nutritional supplements to individuals, (b) engaged in nutritional counseling and education for the purpose of treating specific complaints and ailments of individuals, and (c) represented himself as a nutritionist, registered nutritionist, doctor of nutrition and/or as a Ph.D. or M.D. The appellate court upheld the trial court's ruling allowing the Board's (Ohio Board of Dietetics) request for an injunction (a court order) against the defendant because as the trial court stated:

1. the defendant was not licensed to practice dietetics in the state of Ohio;
2. defendant was engaged in the practice of dietetics as defined in R.C. 4759.01(A);
3. defendant's activities were not protected by the Free Exercise Clause of the First Amendment to the United States Constitution, and;
4. until defendant "obtains a license, he is barred from engaging in nutritional counseling or assessments of any other activity set forth in R.C. 4759.02(A) (pp. 246-247).

Interestingly, the defendant in this case attempted to excuse his unlawful activities by calling himself a "nutritionist" versus a dietician. However, the appellate court stated, "the acts defendant performs are more important than his title and since he does not possess a license to provide nutritional counseling and assessments, defendants acts are in violation of R.C. 4759.02(A)" (p. 248). This ruling has application to exercise professionals as well. Though titles of exercise professionals should be commensurate with job duties and responsibilities, a title a person gives himself/herself will probably not be a factor in determining if there was a violation of a state statute (unless titles are clearly defined by statute as to who can use them) or practicing outside one's scope of practice in a civil claim. It will be the conduct of exercise professionals that courts will use to make these types of determinations.

Cooksey v. Futrell

In this case (55), Cooksey started a website called Diabetes Warrior (www.diabetes-warrior.net) that provided various types of "free" nutrition information. He also offered a fee-based service called Diabetes Support Life-Coaching in which he charged a fee for individualized nutritional advice. The Executive Director of the North Carolina's State Board informed him that the "life-coaching" part of his website needed to be taken down because these services constituted practicing dietetics without a license, a violation of the North Carolina's Dietetics/Nutrition Practice Act, in part, as follows:

The Act prohibits any unlicensed person from engaging in "the practice of dietetics/nutrition," N.C. Gen.Stat. § 90–365(1), which is defined as "the integration and application of principles derived from the science of nutrition, biochemistry, physiology, food, and management and from behavioral and social sciences to achieve and maintain a healthy status" ... "The primary function of dietetic/nutrition practice is the provision of nutrition care services."... (p. 230).

In addition, Cooksey was informed that his website violated a state administrative code that states "Any person, whether residing in this state or not, who by use of electronic or other medium performs any of the acts described as the practice of dietetics/nutrition, but is not licensed ... shall be deemed by the [State] Board as being engaged in the practice of dietetics/nutrition and subject to the enforcement provisions available to the Board" (p. 231).

The Executive Director of the State Board told Cooksey that the Board has statutory authority to seek an injunction to prevent the unlicensed practice of dietetics. Cooksey complied with the request to take down the part of his website where he offered life-coaching services stating he feared civil and criminal actions against him. The Complaint Committee of the State Board reviewed his website and reported back to Cooksey with comments in red indicating areas of concern. Cooksey posted this document on his website (56). Cooksey did not contact the State Board after he received the red-pen review; rather he altered his website. The Executive Director then informed Cooksey that "it appears that you have remained in substantial compliance with the requirements…of the North Carolina General Statutes. Therefore…, the Board is closing this complaint. As with all complaints, the Board reserves the right to continue to monitor this situation" (55, p. 232).

Interestingly, Cooksey then filed an action alleging the North Carolina Board violated his First Amendment rights by causing him to self-censor certain speech on his Internet website where he offered both free and fee-based dietary advice. The United States District Court dismissed this action. Cooksey appealed. The appellate court reviewed the "standing" and "ripeness" requirements of the First Amendment to determine if the actions of the State Board constituted an injury-in-fact. It disagreed with the

Appellee's (State Board's) arguments that Cooksey had not been injured for "standing" purposes and that his claims are not "ripe" given the State Board had taken no action against Cooksey. However, the appellate court stated that "the injuries in this case—a chilling of speech and threat of prosecution—were caused directly by the actions of the State Board" (55, p. 238). The appellate court added:

> *None of the State Board's statements, however, indicate that Cooksey is free from the "threat of penalty." ...To the contrary, the last communication from the State Board to Cooksey specifically stated otherwise... ("As with all complaints, the Board reserves the right to continue to monitor this situation."). Cooksey desires a clarification of the conduct that [he] can engage in without such a threat* (p. 241).

Therefore, the appellate court concluded that "the district court's order dismissing Cooksey's complaint is vacated, and this case is remanded for consideration on the merits" (p. 241).

Sosa-Gaines v. Capital Fitness Inc.

During a personal training session, trainer Don Myles instructed Gabriela Sosa-Gaines "to lie on her stomach, take a deep breath, and exhale, whereupon the trainer forcibly pressed down on her spine" (p. 4) causing an injury to her spine. The plaintiff (Sosa-Gaines) alleged in her complaint (57) that the defendants (Myles and Capital Fitness) breached their duty by the following acts/omissions:

1. forcibly pressing on her spine with great force sufficient to injure;
2. placing her in a position where force on her spine was sufficient to injure;
3. instructing and directing her to exhale and forcibly pressing on her spine with force sufficient to injure;
4. repeatedly pressing on her spine;
5. failing to inform, warn, and obtain consent before applying force to her spine;
6. failing to inform warn, and obtain consent before forcibly pressing on her spine;
7. performing a "chiropractive type of adjustment maneuver" on her spine; and

8. otherwise being negligent in providing personal training services (pp. 4-5).

The jury returned a verdict for the defendants and the plaintiff appealed. The appellate court addressed several procedural issues in this case, but issues related to the plaintiff's argument that the trainer had acted as an unlicensed chiropractor physician are relevant.

Sosa-Gaines had signed a membership agreement as well as a personal training agreement in which both contained exculpatory language. The personal trainer agreement also included the following, in part:

> *Member covenants, represents and warrants that member has not received, is not receiving and shall not receive any medical advice from company or its agents or independent contractors... Member acknowledges that company is not a licensee, medical care provider and does not and will not offer medical advice* (57, pp. 8-9).

In her motions, the plaintiff claimed that the defendants violated this part of the agreement because the trainer had acted as an unlicensed chiropractor physician. The defendants filed an opposing motion for summary judgment, but the trial court denied the motions of both parties. The appellate court stated that whether the plaintiff's alleged injury would be covered by the language in the agreement was a question of fact. They stated that "even if the issue was a question of law, plaintiff failed to introduce expert testimony to establish that anything the trainer did amounted to a chiropractor maneuver" (p. 23).

The plaintiff did not disclose any witnesses before the trial that "(1) practices chiropractic medicine, (2) can establish the standard of care for chiropractic medicine; (3) can establish that the trainer's action constituted a chiropractic maneuver specifically reserved to the practice of chiropractic medicine. Plaintiff also did not disclose a personal training expert to opine that the trainer exceeded the scope of his training" (57, pp. 22-23). The trainer testified that he had been certified for more than 20 years and that he had been trained and qualified to perform the "mild adjustment" he did on the plaintiff. He also stated that he had performed this pressure on the backs of other clients many times that never caused injury. Whether the plaintiff suffered an injury caused by the action of the trainer also was questioned. Although she complained about stabbing pain in her back after the training session, she also admitted that she had suffered a back injury at work four years earlier. Experts for the plaintiff, her treating physician and an orthopedic surgeon, as well as a defendant's expert witness (a physician), all concluded there were no signs of injury from medical examinations and tests. The appellate court affirmed the trial court's verdict.

Several lessons can be learned from the above three cases:

a) A job title that an exercise professional uses (unless protected by statute) will not determine if there was a violation of state licensing laws—the "conduct" of the exercise professional will be what is judged.

b) Exercise professionals should not assume that the outcome in the North Carolina case will be the same in other cases. However, given state licensing reform bills, such as the one in Florida that was passed in June 2020 (described above), there may be fewer state licensing boards threatening individuals who provide individual nutrition advice for a fee. This law will likely help prevent cases such as the case involving a CrossFit trainer and health coach who was fined $750 for the unlicensed practice of dietetics for providing individualized dietary advice in Florida (58). She challenged the fine in federal court (11th U.S. Circuit Court of Appeals). This case was pending at the time this chapter was written.

Note: Even though this Florida law may allow trainers/ coaches to provide individual nutrition advice without the risk of criminal penalties, they still can face negligence claims/lawsuits if their nutrition advice harms someone.

c) Exercise professionals should not assume it is in within their scope of practice to perform back pressure maneuvers (or other similar movements performed by licensed professionals) based on the outcome in *Sosa-Gaines*. Although this personal fitness trainer indicated he had been trained to perform such a maneuver, that does not necessarily mean it is within the scope of practice of a trainer.

If there is ever a question of certain practices (e.g., exercises, advice/recommendations) that might cross over the line into a licensed practice, fitness managers and exercise professionals can check with their state's regulatory departments or agencies and their legal counsel, in advance of providing such services, to help clarify what is permissible and what is not.

KEY POINT

The cases described under Scope of Practice Scenario #3 demonstrate how the conduct of an exercise professional can cross over into the practice of a licensed profession that can then lead to criminal charges associated with violations of state licensing statutes. If there is ever a question of certain practices (e.g., exercises, advice/recommendations) that might cross over the line into a licensed practice, fitness managers and exercise professionals can check with their state's regulatory departments or agencies and their legal counsel.

Licensed Health Care Professionals: Should They Practice as Exercise Professionals?

Because there is no government regulation of the exercise profession, anyone can work as an exercise professional. However, individuals need to understand their vulnerability to civil claims (negligence) as well as criminal charges as described above. Sometimes, licensed health care professionals desire to work as exercise professionals which would be outside their normal "legal" scope of practice but, perhaps, within their "professional" scope of practice. For example, physical therapists and athletic trainers both have extensive backgrounds in the exercise sciences from their academic coursework and professional experiences. However, it would still be best for these licensed professionals (and any others) to obtain a degree in exercise science and/or a "professional" certification such as the exercise physiologist certification offered by ACSM and ASEP (described in Chapter 5) before working as an exercise professional. They may not realize that their professional background/experiences might not have prepared them for designing and delivering all types of exercise programs. For example, athletic trainers are knowledgeable and skilled in prescribing pre-hab and rehab exercise programs for athletes. However, they may have little or no background/experience in designing and delivering programs for apparently healthy and clinical populations. Obviously, they will need to fully understand that an exercise prescription for an elite athlete versus an adult with a medical condition will be very different for both safety and legal liability reasons.

In addition, physical therapists and athletic trainers may not be familiar with the many published standards of practice in the exercise profession (e.g., *ACSM's Health/Fitness Facility Standards and Guidelines*) that they will need to follow, especially if they own or manage a facility (e.g., athletic trainers who open a personal training studio or physical therapists who open their clinic and sell memberships to the general population who can use the clinic during non-clinic hours or offer exercise programs for the general public at their clinic). As owners or managers of a fitness facility, they have numerous responsibilities including legal/risk management responsibilities as described throughout this textbook. They need to realize that their liability insurance that protects them while working as a licensed professional may not cover them while working as an exercise professional or manager/owner of a facility.

It is also important that professionals, such as physical therapists and athletic trainers, keep their licensed practice separate from their practice as an exercise professional. This became a major legal problem for a physical therapist in *United States v. Faux* (59). Danielle Faux, a licensed physical therapist in Connecticut, was also a part owner of a gym located in the same building as her physical therapy practice. She was a participating provider for the Medicare program as well as Anthem Blue Cross Blue Shield and Aetna health care plans. At times, Faux would refer some of her patients to personal fitness trainers at the gym. The clients would either purchase the personal trainer package through the gym or pay Faux for the sessions and then Faux would pay the trainer directly. Of course, only physical therapy sessions are covered by Medicare and the health care plans, not personal training sessions provided by unlicensed trainers. Around June of 2010 one of the trainers, who worked extensively with Faux, informed agents of the Federal Bureau of Investigation (FBI) and the U.S. Department of Health and Human Services, Office of the Inspector General (HHSOIG) that

"Faux was engaging in a scheme to defraud Medicare and private insurance companies by billing personal training sessions as physical therapy services provided by a licensed physical therapist" (p. 4).

The government began an investigation into Faux's business and billing practices and found that she was, fraudulently, billing personal training sessions as physical therapy sessions. The grand jury issued indictments charging Faux with numerous violations. In February 2014, "the grand jury issued an indictment charging Faux with forty-six counts of healthcare fraud, in violation of *18 U.S.C. § 1347*, and one count of obstruction of a federal audit, in violation of *18 U.S.C. § 1516*" (59, p. 4). In April 2016, "the grand jury returned a superseding indictment charging Faux with fifty counts of healthcare fraud, for falsely billing personal training sessions as physical therapy services on fifty separate occasions" (pp. 4-5) as well as several other charges such as submitting false records designed to conceal healthcare fraud and false statements on tax returns. Faux filed several motions in which the trial court denied but the court also indicated that her motions to suppress evidence and suppress statements would be addressed at a separate ruling. In this separate ruling (60), the court denied her motion to suppress evidence but granted her motion to suppress statements. However, the U.S. Court of Appeals (61) ruled that her statements (made in her home while a search warrant was being executed) should not have been suppressed. The court concluded by stating "we vacate and remand for further proceedings consistent with this opinion" (61, p. 130).

This case is especially relevant for exercise professionals who work in facilities in which physical therapy services are also offered, which is becoming more common in recent years. There are many benefits to these types of arrangements such as referrals and two-way communications as described above. However, it is important that all parties ensure that the services are kept separate so that no laws are violated.

Scope of Practice: Health and Wellness Coaches

Exercise professionals also, often, work as health and wellness coaches. There is no government regulation through licensure but there are numerous certifications, many of which offer an online preparation program and online certification examination. As with almost all fitness certifications, many do not require an assessment of practical skills. However, the National Board for Health & Wellness Coaching (NBHWC), described in Chapter 5, requires both formal education and practical experience from an approved program prior to sitting for the certification examination. One of the competencies under domain III states: Health and wellness coaches practice in accordance with accepted professional standards and within the limits of their scope of practice (62). Health and wellness coaches provide individual education and motivation to help their clients improve their health behaviors but do not provide, for example, individualized exercise prescriptions and/or nutrition advice, which would be outside their scope of practice.

Providing general information regarding the U.S. Physical Activity Guidelines (1) and the Dietary Guidelines for Americans (63) would be within their scope of practice. Exercise professionals may have additional knowledge in the area of exercise they can share with clients as a health and wellness coach. However, it will be best to keep these practices (exercise professional and health/wellness coach) separate. It would be difficult to design/deliver a safe and effective exercise program for a client you do not meet with in person. Health and wellness coaching services are often offered over the Internet and by telephone and, therefore, have certain limitations. Legal liability issues associated with online personal fitness training are covered in Chapter 8.

DEVELOPMENT OF RISK MANAGEMENT STRATEGIES

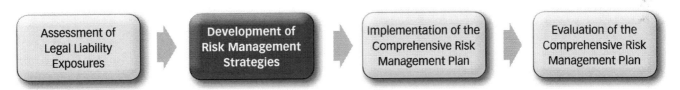

Many legal liability exposures related to exercise prescription and scope of practice were described in the preceding section. The following risk management strategies can be developed and implemented to minimize these legal liability exposures. This is an important area of risk management due to the many negligence lawsuits that have occurred related to improper exercise prescriptions given the individual's health/fitness status. It also is essential for those fitness facilities who want to become involved with the Exercise is Medicine® initiative and market to clientele with medical conditions.

1 **Risk Management Strategy #1:** Comply with Federal, State, and Local Laws as well as Published Standards of Practice to Help Prevent Disability Discrimination Litigation.

As described in Chapter 2, discrimination lawsuits involving fitness facilities appear to be increasing. Although there are various types of discrimination lawsuits as presented in Chapter 3, this risk management strategy will focus on the importance of complying

with the ADA. Related state and local laws may also apply to fitness facilities and fitness managers should consult with their legal counsel regarding these laws. As described above, Title III of the ADA prohibits discrimination regarding programs and services offered by places of public accommodation and commercial facilities (e.g., most fitness facilities). Prohibiting discrimination is also specified in standards and guidelines published by professional organizations. Therefore, it is essential that fitness facilities provide programs/services to individuals with disabilities, which not only includes individuals with certain physical and mental disabilities (e.g., use a wheelchair, have Down Syndrome) but also includes individuals with various chronic medical conditions.

To meet this obligation and to minimize legal liability, it will be necessary to employ exercise professionals who have advanced knowledge and skills to safely and effectively design/deliver exercise prescriptions for these clinical populations. In addition to hiring at least one clinical exercise physiologist (see Risk Management Strategy #3), it is recommended to have exercise professionals with certifications such as the Certified Inclusive Fitness Trainer (CIFT) offered by ACSM and the National Center on Health, Physical Activity and Disability (NCHPAD). Although this certification does not require a degree or any practical experience (64), it would be best for fitness facilities to have exercise professionals who possess both a degree and hands-on practical experience as well as the CIFT credential. Employing exercise professionals that have the necessary credentials and competence to design/deliver safe and effective programs for persons with disabilities not only demonstrates a sincere commitment to serve these individuals, but the credentials and competence of these professionals can be described in marketing and other strategies to help reach these populations.

The NCHPAD website (https://www.nchpad.org) is a valuable resource for fitness managers and exercise professionals. It provides numerous resources, videos, and informative articles. For example, a set of fact sheets are provided for more than 40 different disabilities and health conditions that include considerations for physical activity and overall health (65). Another set of numerous fact sheets describe various techniques, modes, methods, adaptations, etc. that can be used when working with individuals with a variety of disabilities and health conditions (66). Fitness managers and exercise professionals are encouraged to use the many resources on the NCHPAD website and to subscribe to their free monthly newsletter. Another valuable "free" resource is also available—*Removing Barriers to Health Clubs and Fitness Facilities: A Guide for Accommodating All Members Including People with Disabilities and Older Adults* (67).

Fitness managers and exercise professionals need to provide training for all staff members. In one study (68), very few fitness professionals had received training in providing services to individuals with disabilities. Fitness managers can bring in local experts (e.g., physical therapists, recreation therapists, educators with adapted physical education expertise) who can provide in-service trainings for exercise professionals and other staff members to help them understand the needs of and interacting with people with disabilities. Often, fitness facilities do not offer a welcoming environment for people with disabilities, which is a barrier to increasing physical activity among persons with disabilities.

2 **Risk Management Strategy #2:** Establish Scope of Practice Policies for All Exercise Professionals Who Design and Deliver Individual Exercise Prescriptions for Apparently Healthy and Clinical Populations.

The credentials and competence among exercise professionals who work in a typical fitness facility can vary significantly as described in Chapter 5. Therefore, it is essential that fitness managers establish a written scope of practice policy that describes the population(s) that each exercise professional can work with that reflects these varying backgrounds. For example, a policy for the exercise professional (or exercise practitioner) that only possesses an accredited certification in personal fitness training (e.g., has not received formal education and practical training) may be that these employees only design/deliver exercise prescriptions for apparently healthy individuals such as those who, after completing pre-activity screening, do not need to obtain medical clearance. Obviously, these professionals need to have the knowledge and skills to properly design and deliver programs for apparently healthy individuals. If not, they are practicing outside their scope and subject themselves and their employers to legal liability as demonstrated in the negligence cases described above under Scope of Practice Scenario #1. As described in Chapter 5 (see Risk Management Strategy #8), employers should provide a comprehensive training program (classroom and practical training) for employees before they begin their jobs because they cannot assume that possessing an accredited certification means that they will be competent exercise professionals.

An example of another policy may be that only exercise professionals with a degree in the field and a professional certification (e.g., ACSM or ASEP exercise physiologist) will design/deliver individual exercise prescriptions for persons with medical conditions or older adults and who teach classes designed for these individuals (e.g., exercise classes for persons with Parkinson's disease or older adults). These are individuals, who after obtaining pre-activity screening data, will likely need to obtain medical clearance. Many of these professionals should possess the knowledge and skills to incorporate the recommendations and/or limitations provided by the individual's physician, specified on the clearance form. They should also have the knowledge and skills to obtain medical history data (as described in Chapter 6) that is used to design/deliver a proper fitness testing protocol and exercise prescription. However, some of these professionals may not possess the advanced knowledge/skills needed to work with clinical populations as demonstrated in the spotlight cases described above under Scope of Practice Scenario #2. However, they could acquire the advanced knowledge/skills through additional education and certifications. For example, they could take graduate level academic courses in clinical exercise and/or obtain clinical certifications offered by ACSM, ACE, AACVPR, and NSCA as described in Chapter 5. Other clinical certifications can also be considered such as CIFT described above, the Medical Exercise Specialist offered by the Medical Exercise Training Institute (69) and the Certified Cancer Exercise Trainer offered by the ACSM and the American Cancer Society (70). There are educational programs and/or certifications in the area of senior fitness provided by organizations such as the American Senior Fitness Association and ACE. The eligibility requirements vary with these certifications but, as with almost all certifications, none of them require passing a practical examination so there are limitations to consider. For fitness managers, the MFA offers a Medical Fitness Facility Director certification and the Medical Exercise Training Institute offers a Medical Exercise Program Director certification.

Fitness managers in consultation with their medical advisor and/or risk management advisory committee should make these determinations regarding scope of practice policies versus relying solely on scope of practice descriptions provided by professional organizations as described above. Applying only these descriptions to develop scope of practice policies may not minimize legal liability exposures for the exercise professionals and employers. For example, as described in the *Bartlett* spotlight case above, courts may require a certain standard of care for fitness facilities that offer programs for clinical populations which means exercise professionals need advanced knowledge and skills to work with these populations.

Fitness managers should reflect these scope of practice policies in the job descriptions of the various positions and, perhaps, consider referring to those without a degree in the field as "exercise practitioners" versus "exercise professionals" leaving the title of exercise professional for only those with a degree in the field. For example, list titles such as personal fitness trainer practitioner and personal fitness trainer professional on the job descriptions. Fitness managers may want to have some flexibility with their scope of practice policies to allow for exceptions in some cases. For example, there may be individuals without a degree who could, with additional quality education, training, and practical experiences, be quite competent in working with clinical populations. This is a judgment call that needs to be carefully considered but could be a possibility, especially, if the facility hires a clinical exercise physiologist who can provide oversight of individual clinical exercise prescriptions and clinical exercise classes.

Written scope of practice policies relating to the importance of not crossing over the line into a licensed profession need to be established. For example, a policy such as all exercise professionals provide only general, nonmedical nutrition information using credible resources. They do not provide individualized nutritional advice that includes recommending nutritional supplements or diets. Similar policies can be developed for other licensed professions. As with all policies, the facility's risk management advisory committee or legal counsel should be involved in forming the scope of practice policies to help ensure they reflect the law and any relevant published standards of practice.

③ Risk Management Strategy #3: Hire at Least One Clinical Exercise Physiologist Who Can Provide Oversight of Individual Clinical Exercise Prescriptions and Exercise Classes for Clinical Populations.

There are several reasons to consider hiring at least one clinical exercise physiologist (e.g., a professional who possesses the credentials commensurate with ACSM Certified Clinical Exercise Physiologist) from a variety of perspectives including:

a) Many members and participants of fitness facilities will likely have chronic diseases given the statistics described at the beginning of this chapter. For example, 60% of adults have at least one chronic medical condition and 40% have two or more chronic conditions (3). Therefore, special expertise is needed to provide safe/effective programs for these individuals to meet the professional standard of care and minimize legal liability as demonstrated in the spotlight cases in this chapter.

b) An exercise professional with a degree in exercise science may not possess the advanced knowledge and skills needed to prescribe individual clinical exercise prescriptions and teach exercise classes for clinical populations. However, clinical exercise physiologists can serve as mentors for these exercise professionals and help provide them with the education and practical experiences to attain the advanced knowledge and skills needed. They can also provide oversight and assistance to these professionals in the design/delivery of clinical exercise programs serving as a resource when situations or questions arise. Given their advanced knowledge and skill, they may also be able to develop, in consultation with the individual's health care provider, "targeted exercise prescriptions" that can ameliorate the negative effects of a disease and/or medications treating the disease. In other words, a more sophisticated and effective prescription. One of the major responsibilities of a clinical exercise physiologist serving in this role is to provide education. Therefore, he/she needs to possess excellent pedagogy skills as described in Chapter 2.

c) For fitness facilities that want to participate in initiatives such as the Exercise is Medicine® initiative, it is important to realize that physicians and health care providers will only want to refer their patients to fitness facilities that employ credentialed/competent exercise professionals as well as meet other standards such as having a medical advisor or advisory committee. Employing a clinical exercise physiologist who has oversight of the facility's clinical programs will be a real plus in this regard. The clinical exercise physiologist can serve as the staff liaison with the medical advisor or advisory committee to establish a strategic plan to implement EIM as well as policies and procedures related to the facility's clinical exercise programs.

④ Risk Management Strategy #4: Comply with Published Standards of Practice Addressing General Principles of Exercise and Exercise Prescriptions for Apparently Healthy and Clinical Populations.

As described in Chapter 4, many professional organizations have published standards of practice (e.g., standards, guidelines, and position stands) that address various safety issues. This risk management strategy will, briefly, describe a few of these standards of practice that focus on (a) general principles of safe exercise, and (b) exercise prescriptions for apparently healthy adults and those with chronic illnesses. As demonstrated in some of the negligence lawsuits described in this chapter and throughout this textbook, the defendants (exercise professionals) failed to follow basic, safe principles of exercise (e.g., warm-up, cool-down, proper progression, monitoring intensity, and signs/symptoms of overexertion). In addition to incorporating these safe principles of exercise into the design and delivery of exercise programs, it is essential for exercise professionals to teach their participants the "what, how, and why" regarding these principles so they understand their importance and can properly apply them into their lifelong exercise program.

As demonstrated in the negligence cases described in this chapter and throughout this textbook, exercise prescriptions need to reflect the professional standard of care and take into consideration the nature of the activity, the types of participants, and environmental factors. This is important for both apparently healthy individuals (see the negligence cases described under Scope of Practice Scenario #1) and individuals with chronic conditions (see the spotlight cases under Scope of Practice Scenario #2).

Regarding general principles of safe exercise, the *ACSM's Guidelines for Exercise Testing and Prescription* (28) contains an entire chapter devoted to general principles of exercise prescription and the second edition of the *Physical Activity Guidelines for Americans* (1) provides the following:

Key Guidelines for Safe Physical Activity: To do physical activity safely and reduce risk of injuries and other adverse events, people should:

- Understand the risks, yet be confident that physical activity can be safe for almost everyone.
- Choose types of physical activity that are appropriate for their current fitness level and health goals, because some activities are safer than others.
- Increase physical activity gradually over time to meet key guidelines or health goals. Inactive people should "start low and go slow"

by starting with lower intensity activities and gradually increasing how often and how long activities are done.

- Protect themselves by using appropriate gear and sports equipment, choosing safe environments, following rules and policies, and making sensible choices about when, where, and how to be active.

- Be under the care of a health care provider if they have chronic conditions or symptoms. People with chronic conditions and symptoms can consult a health care professional or physical activity specialist about the types and amounts of activity appropriate for them (1, p. 10).

The ACSM has published several standards of practice addressing exercise prescriptions for apparently healthy and clinical populations. For example, two position stands focus on healthy adults: (a) Quantity and Quality of Exercise for Developing and Maintaining Cardiorespiratory, Musculoskeletal, and Neuromotor Fitness in Apparently Healthy Adults: Guidance for Prescribing Exercise (71), and (b) Progression Models in Resistance Training for Healthy Adults (72). The *ACSM's Guidelines for Exercise Testing and Prescription* (28) also contains several chapters addressing exercise prescription for apparently healthy individuals and those with chronic diseases.

Several position stands have also been published by ACSM and many other professional organizations regarding exercise prescriptions for clinical or special populations (e.g., hypertension, diabetes, and older adults). It is impossible to describe all the published standards of practice addressing exercise prescriptions published by professional organizations. As described in Chapter 4, a valuable resource to use to become familiar with these published standards of practice is *Physical Activity and Health Guidelines: Recommendations for Various Ages, Fitness Levels, and Conditions from 57 Authoritative Sources* (73). This resource briefly describes and cites many physical activity recommendations, published by authoritative sources, for various age groups/populations and those with chronic illnesses. For example, age groups/populations include infants, toddlers, school-age children, pregnant and postpartum women, older adults, and those with chronic illnesses including:

- Cancer
- Hypertension and cardiovascular disease
- Arthritis and osteoporosis
- Diabetes
- Neuromuscular disorders
- Asthma

An exercise professional establishing an exercise prescription for someone with diabetes can easily access and read a brief summary of the published guidelines regarding exercise and diabetes. Examples of brief summaries are guidelines published by the American Diabetes Association, ACSM, ACE, and the International Society for Pediatric and Adolescent Diabetes. An exercise professional who is establishing an exercise prescription or teaching an exercise class for pregnant and postpartum women can review published guidelines by organizations such as the American College of Obstetricians and Gynecologists (ACOG).

It is, again, important to remind fitness managers and exercise professionals to follow these published standards of practice because they can be considered as evidence to help courts determine duty in negligence lawsuits. Some of these published standards of practice, especially those covering clinical content, require technical background in clinical exercise to fully understand and properly apply them. This is another reason to have only exercise professionals, with advanced knowledge and skills in clinical exercise, design and deliver exercise programs for individuals with chronic illnesses and medical conditions.

⑤ Risk Management Strategy #5: Utilize Professional Resources to Properly Design and Deliver Exercise Prescriptions for Individuals with Medical Conditions.

In addition to standards of practice (e.g., standards, guidelines, and position stands) published by professional organizations, additional resources like textbooks provide helpful information regarding the design and delivery of safe and effective clinical exercise prescriptions and fitness classes. The following is a list of a few of these resources.

a) *ACSM's Clinical Exercise Physiology* (74)
b) *ACSM's Exercise Management for Persons with Chronic Diseases and Disabilities* (75)
c) *NSCA's Essentials of Training Special Populations* (76)

d) *Fitness Instructor's Handbook* (77)
e) *Clinical Exercise Physiology* (78)
f) *EIM Exercise Pro Action Guide* (79)

Numerous other resources are listed on government and professional organization websites. Because there is so much misinformation about exercise for healthy adults and those with chronic illnesses on the Internet and elsewhere, it is essential that exercise professionals only utilize resources from credible sources and help their participants do the same.

 Risk Management Strategy #6: Develop Procedures to Help Ensure Exercise Prescriptions are Not Considered Medical Treatment.

Diagnosis and "treatment" of a disease reflect the legal scope of practice of physicians and other licensed health care providers. However, as previously described, exercise prescriptions are designed to help "prevent" and "treat" disease. Exercise is an effective treatment to help (a) control a disease, (b) prevent further progression of a disease, and (c) in some cases, eliminate a disease or medical condition. Exercise professionals, who design and deliver clinical exercise programs, are involved in the treatment of the disease. Therefore, it is wise to take steps to help prevent possible criminal charges related to the unauthorized practice of medicine or practicing medicine without a license (or some other health care licensed profession). These steps include:

a) Have a medical advisor or medical advisory committee who can provide guidance related to exercise programs for clinical populations.

b) Have at least one employed clinical exercise physiologist who can provide oversight and education for those exercise professionals who design/deliver exercise prescriptions and teach exercise classes for clinical populations. This will help ensure safe/effective programs are implemented and that published standards of practice related to clinical exercise programs are followed.

c) Establish two-way communications between the exercise professional and the participant's physician and other health care providers. For example, the physician may provide recommendations/limitations on the medical clearance form

(see Chapter 6 appendix for an example form) and perhaps provide a written exercise prescription for the exercise professional to follow. An example prescription form is on the EIM website (80). The exercise professional can then provide the physician with a progress report such as the one provided on the EIM website (81). This progress report can be given to the participant who can share it with his/her physician at the next patient visit. If it is sent directly to the physician, it is best to first obtain authorization from the participant to prevent any violations of privacy laws as described in Chapters 3 and 6.

The overall goal is to demonstrate that the clinical exercise programs reflect a joint effort. It is not the purpose or the intent of the exercise professional to treat the disease by himself/herself but, instead, to work with the participant's physician (or other health care providers) regarding the initial and on-going design of the patient's exercise program. These steps also demonstrate that the fitness facility managers have made a concerted effort to provide high quality (safe and effective) programs that reflect published standards of practice related to exercise programs for clinical populations. Following these published standards of practice help demonstrate that the clinical exercise prescriptions/classes are within the exercise professional's scope of practice.

Like the term "treatment," terms such as "prescription" and "counseling" also reflect the legal scope of practice of licensed health care providers. Some fitness programs have avoided using these terms and have substituted terms such as "exercise program" and "education", respectively. However, licensing boards and courts will likely consider the purpose/intent and conduct of the professional more so than the term used when investigating violations of licensing statutes.

Risk Management Strategy #7: Provide Scope of Practice Training for All Exercise Professionals and Other Personnel.

Of all the risk management strategies described here, this is one of the most important. Training is needed in four areas: (a) the facility's policy on scope of practice—described above under Risk Management Strategy #2, (b) education regarding the distinction between "professional" scope of practice and "legal" scope of practice and their connection with civil and criminal law, (c) educational resources for exercise professionals to read in preparation of in-service trainings on scope of practice, and (d) in-service trainings with a practical scope of practice learning activity. The facility's scope of practice policy can be shared with candidates in job interviews as well upon hiring during new employee orientation. It will be important they understand the reasons for the policy and the importance of following it. For the second area, distinguishing legal and professional scope of practice, the information and legal cases in this chapter under Scope of Practice Scenario's #1, #2, and #3 can be reviewed and discussed during in-service trainings.

Regarding the third area of training, in addition to the information provided and resources cited in this chapter, there are several educational resources that can help exercise professionals obtain an in-depth understanding of scope of practice. For example, an article by Dr. Anthony Abbott titled *Scope of Practice* (82) provides an overview of scope of practice and describes specific situations in which an exercise professional may be practicing medicine, physical therapy, and dietetics. The author also cautions exercise professionals regarding recommending supplements to participants. Because exercise professionals often provide nutrition information to their participants, scope of practice training in this area is essential.

Scope of Practice Training: Nutrition and Nutritional Supplements

The following two articles are educational resources for exercise professionals working in fitness and athletic programs, respectively, that can be reviewed prior to in-service trainings addressing nutrition scope of practice.

- *Drawing the Line: Understanding the Scope of Practice Among Registered Dietitian Nutritionists and Exercise Professionals* (83)— this article provides an overview distinguishing the roles of the RDN and exercise professional regarding nutrition as well as describes scenarios of negative health consequences that can occur when an exercise professional recommends a participant take a dietary supplement or make certain dietary changes.

- *Bridging the Performance Gap: Interdisciplinary Collaboration with Sports Dietitians* (84)—this article provides an overview of the role of the RDN and Certified Specialist in Sports Dietetics (CSSD) regarding the nutritional needs of athletes. It also distinguishes the educational background and scope of practice of the RDN/CSSD with many of the "nutritionist" sport certifications such as the one offered through the International Society of Sport Nutrition.

In-service trainings should also address scope of practice issues related to nutritional supplements. In 2013, an article in *Forbes* (85) stated that the nutritional supplement group (vitamins, minerals, and supplements or VMS) is one of the fastest growing industries in the world. Nutritional supplements alone produced about $32 billion in revenue in 2012 and by 2021 over $60 billion is projected (85). It has been reported that about 50% of the U.S. population consumes dietary supplements and with athletes, this percentage is higher (86). Exercise professionals need to be well-educated on the topic of nutritional supplements and understand why it is important to not recommend supplements to their participants from both scope of practice and safety perspectives. However, they can provide general information about nutritional supplements using credible resources.

Participants may believe that the FDA conducts a premarket safety review of dietary supplements but they do not. Therefore, there is no legal requirement to help ensure the supplement is safe (e.g., contains no prohibited substances) or that the supplement's claims are true. However, the FDA has recalled numerous supplements with potentially harmful ingredients including:

- more than 40 products marketed for weight loss
- more than 70 products marketed for sexual enhancement
- more than 80 products marketed for body building (87)

There are third party agencies that certify dietary supplements, but each establishes their own quality assurance program with varying testing components, so they are not 100% reliable. Strategies to improve these quality assurance programs have been suggested (88). There are several refereed journal articles regarding the safety of nutritional supplements that can be discussed during in-service trainings. A couple of these are *Risky Business: Dietary Supplement Use by Athletes* (86) and *Stimulant-Containing Energy Drinks: What You Need to Know* (89). The following government resources may also be helpful: (a) Office of Dietary Supplements (https://ods.od.nih.gov), (b) National Center for Complementary and Integrative Health—Dietary and Herbal Supplements and (https://nccih.nih.gov/health/supplements), and (c) Dietary Supplements for Athletes (https://www.nutrition.gov/dietary-supplements/dietary-supplements-athletes).

The fourth area of scope of practice training focuses on practical application of the scope of practice policies. Participants often believe that exercise professionals can answer medical questions, diagnose and treat various ailments, provide counseling for personal problems, and can give dietary advice and recommendations on dietary supplements. When participants bring up these types of topics, it is essential that exercise professionals know how to properly address these issues to avoid crossing over the line into a licensed profession. Therefore, interpersonal communication skills are essential.

One effective teaching strategy to help develop practical skills related to interpersonal communication would be role-playing. Prior to the training, have the exercise staff members submit a list of questions and issues (e.g., medical, nutrition, personal problems) their participants often ask or want to discuss with them. Assign staff members into pairs with one playing the role of the exercise professional and the other playing the role of the participant. Each pair role plays (e.g., one asks one of the nutrition questions on the list and the other answers, in front of the entire group). Then, the entire group critiques the responses of the exercise professional to evaluate if his/her response was consistent with the facility's scope of practice policy. If it was not, have the members of the group share answers that would properly reflect the policy. The leader of the training would then provide feedback and clarify the responses that reflect proper application of the policy. The role-playing continues until all pairs have had an opportunity to participate. An outcome of this training should be that the exercise staff members know how to effectively communicate and interact with participants. For example, regarding nutrition education, do they fully understand how to provide "general non-medical nutrition education" when answering questions and when certain questions warrant a referral to an RDN? If the fitness facility employs an RDN, it will be important that staff members know the procedures for making the referral. Procedures for making referrals to licensed professionals in the community need to take into consideration certain factors as described earlier under Legal Liability for Improper Referral.

The four areas of training also need to be provided for other facility personnel, not just the exercise professionals. For example, all employees who may be interacting with participants including fitness floor supervisors, health/wellness coaches, and front desk staff. As described in Chapter 5, employers cannot exhibit a great deal of behavioral control of independent contractors, such as requiring they attend employee trainings. However, it can, perhaps, be stated in their contract that they are expected to follow the facility's policies such as the scope of practice policies. As described previously, legal counsel needs to be involved in the preparation of all contracts.

⑧ Risk Management Strategy #8: Develop Policies and Procedures to Keep all Written and Oral Communications Regarding an Individual's Exercise Prescription Private, Confidential, and Secure.

Although most fitness facilities are not subject to the HIPAA privacy and security provisions because they are not considered covered entities, there may be state and local privacy laws that do apply. Professional codes of conduct also specify the importance of keeping an individual's health/fitness information confidential. Because exercise prescriptions, progress reports, etc. all contain an individual's health/fitness data, it will be important that these written and/or electronic documents are kept private, confidential, and secure. It will also be important that exercise professionals and other personnel do not orally discuss an individual's exercise prescription or progress in the open area where the conversation might be overheard by others. For example, if the facility's clinical exercise physiologist is providing guidance to an exercise professional regarding the exercise prescription for a certain participant, this conversation should be conducted in a private office. These policies and procedures should also be covered in the in-service trainings for staff members.

RISK MANAGEMENT AUDIT
Exercise Prescription and Scope of Practice

RISK MANAGEMENT (RM) STRATEGY*	YES ✔	NO ✔
1. Comply with Federal, State, and Local Laws as well as Published Standards of Practice to Help Prevent Disability Discrimination Litigation.		
2. Establish Scope of Practice Policies for All Exercise Professionals Who Design and Deliver Individual Exercise Prescriptions for Apparently Healthy and Clinical Populations.		
3. Hire at Least One Clinical Exercise Physiologist Who Can Provide Oversight of Individual Clinical Exercise Prescriptions and Exercise Classes for Clinical Populations.		
4. Comply with Published Standards of Practice Addressing General Principles of Exercise and Exercise Prescriptions for Apparently Healthy and Clinical Populations.		
5. Utilize Professional Resources to Properly Design and Deliver Exercise Prescriptions for Individuals with Medical Conditions.		
6. Develop Procedures to Help Ensure Exercise Prescriptions are Not Considered Medical Treatment.		
7. Provide Scope of Practice Training for All Exercise Professionals and Other Personnel.		
8. Develop Policies and Procedures to Keep all Written and Oral Communications Regarding an Individual's Exercise Prescription Private, Confidential, and Secure.		

*See the section above—Development of Risk Management Strategies—for the recommendations associated with each risk management strategy and then, for each RM Strategy marked NO, create a list of action steps that need to be completed to meet the recommendations described in that RM strategy.

KEY TERMS

- Exercise is Medicine®
- FITT-VP Principle
- Improper Exercise Prescription
- Injunction
- Legal Scope of Practice
- Professional Scope of Practice

- Professional Standard of Care
- Proper Referral Practices
- Safe and Effective Exercise Prescription
- Standard of Care of a Professional
- Two-Way Communication

STUDY QUESTIONS

The Study Questions for Chapter 7 can be found on the Fitness Law Academy website (www.fitnesslawacademy.com) under Textbook. They are provided in a fillable format for convenience.

REFERENCES

1. Physical Activity Guidelines for Americans, 2nd ed. 2018. Available at: https://health.gov/paguidelines/second-edition/pdf/Physical_Activity_Guidelines_2nd_edition.pdf. Accessed March 27, 2019.

2. Blair SN. Physical Inactivity: The Biggest Public Health Problem of the 21st Century. *British Journal of Sports Medicine,* 43(1), 1-2, 2009.

3. National Center for Chronic Disease Prevention and Health Promotion. Centers for Disease Control and Prevention. About Chronic Diseases. Available at: https://www.cdc.gov/chronicdisease/about/index.htm. Accessed April 15, 2020.

4. Buttorff C, Ruder T, Bauman M. Multiple Chronic Conditions in the United States. Rand Corporation, 2017. Available at: https://www.rand.org/content/dam/rand/pubs/tools/TL200/TL221/RAND_TL221.pdf. Accessed April 15, 2019.

5. Araujo J, Cal J, Stevens J. Prevalence of Optimal Metabolic Health in American Adults: National Health and Nutrition Examination Survey 2009-2016. *Metabolic Syndrome and Related Disorders*, November 27, 2018. Available at: https://www.ncbi.nlm.nih.gov/pubmed/30484738. Accessed January 25, 2019.

6. Value of Prevention. Partnership for Prevention. Partnership to Fight Chronic Disease. Available at: http://prevent.org/data/files/initiatives/valueofprevention%28pfpandpfcd%29.pdf. Accessed April 9, 2019.

7. Prescription Drug Prices Continue to Climb, Soaring 8.77% in Latest Truveris NDI Report. Available at: https://www.prnewswire.com/news-releases/prescription-drug-prices-continue-to-climb-soaring-877-in-latest-truveris-ndi-report-300454774.html. Accessed April 9, 2019.

8. Kantor ED, Rehm CD, Hass JS, et al. Trends in Prescription Drug Use among Adults in the United States from 1999–2012. *Journal of the American Medical Association,* 314 (17), 1818-1831, 2015.

9. Downing NS, Shah ND, Aminawung JA, et al. Postmarket Safety Events Among Novel Therapeutics Approved by the US Food and Drug Administration Between 2001 and 2010, *Journal of the American Medical Association,* 317(18), 1854-1863, 2017.

10. Langreth R. Just Say No. *Forbes,* November 29, 2004. Available at: https://ahrp.org/just-say-no-forbes. Accessed April 9, 2018.

11. Ornish Lifestyle Program. Available at: https://www.ornish.com. Accessed April 9, 2019.

12. Bushman BA. Determining the I (Intensity) for the FITT-VP Aerobic Exercise Prescription. *ACSM's Health & Fitness Journal,* 18(3), 4-7, 2014.

13. Federation of State Medical Boards. *Assessing Scope of Practice in Health Care Delivery: Critical Questions in Assuring Public Access and Safety,* 2005. Available at: http://www.fsmb.org/siteassets/advocacy/policies/assessing-scope-of-practice-in-health-care-delivery.pdf. Accessed April 11, 2019.

14. *Bartlett v. Push to Walk*, No. 2:15-cv-7167-KM-JBC, 2018 WL 1726262 (D. N.J., 2018)

15. Become a NSCA-Certified Personal Trainer (NSCA-CPT). Available at: https://www.nsca.com/certification/nsca-cpt. Accessed February 10, 2020..

16. ACSM Certified Personal Trainer®. Job Description. Available at: https://www.acsm.org/docs/default-source/certification-documents/acsmcpt_examcontentoutline_2017.pdf. Accessed February 10, 2020.

17. Become an ACSM Certified Exercise Physiologist®. Available at: https://www.acsm.org/get-stay-certified/get-certified/health-fitness-certifications/exercise-physiologist. Accessed February 10, 2020/

18. Become as ACSM Certified Clinical Exercise Physiologist®. Available at: https://www.acsm.org/get-stay-certified/get-certified/cep. Accessed February 10, 2020.

19. NSCA Certification Overview. Certified Special Population Specialist. Available at: https://www.nsca.com/certification/certification-overview. Accessed February 10, 2020.

20. *Vaid v. Equinox*, CV136019426, 2016 LEXIS 828 (Conn. Super. Ct., 2016).

21. *A Concise Restatement of Torts Third Edition*. Compiled by: Bublick EM, Rogers JE. St. Paul, MN: American Law Institute, 2013.

22. Dougherty NJ, Goldberger AS, Carpenter LJ. *Sport, Physical Activity, and the Law*. 3rd Ed. Champaign, IL: Sagamore Publishing, 2007.

23. *Hinkel v. Gavin Pardoe & Gold's Gym*, 133 A.3d 738, 2016 LEXIS 32 (Pa. Super. Ct., 2016).

24. *Mellon v. Crunch*, 934 N.Y.S.2d 35, 2011 LEXIS 3379 (N.Y. Misc., 2011).

25. *Proffitt v. Global Fitness Holdings, LLC, et al.* In: Herbert DL. New Lawsuit Against Personal Trainer and Facility in Kentucky—Rhabdomyolysis Alleged. *The Exercise, Sports and Sports Medicine Standards & Malpractice Reporter,* 2(1), 1, 3-10, 2013.

26. Rhabdomyolysis Lawsuit in Kentucky Settled. *The Exercise, Sports and Sports Medicine Standards & Malpractice Reporter,* 2(4), 58, 2013.

27. *Mimms v. Ruthless Training Concepts, LLC,* Amended Complaint and Plaintiff's Designation of Expert Witnesses, No. 78584 (Cir. Ct. of Prince William County, VA, 2008); Jury Awards $300,000 in Gym Lawsuit. *Virginia Lawyers Weekly*. October 9, 2008. Available at: https://valawyersweekly.com/2008/10/09/jury-awards-300000-in-gym-lawsuit/. Accessed February 16, 2020.

28. *ACSM's Guidelines for Exercise Testing and Prescription.* Riebe D. (ed). 10th Ed. Philadelphia, PA: Lippincott Williams & Wilkins, 2018.

29. American with Disabilities Act Title III Regulations. Part 36 Nondiscrimination on the Basis of Disability by Public Accommodations and Commercial Facilities. § 36.104 Definitions. January 17, 2017. Available at: https://www.ada.gov/regs2010/titleIII_2010/titleIII_2010_regulations.htm#a102. Accessed February 5, 2019.

30. *Larsen v. Carnival Corp. Inc.*, 242 F. Supp. 2d 1333 (S.D. Fla., 2003).

31. CDC: 53 Million Adults in the US Live with a Disability. Centers for Disease Control and Prevention. Available at: https://www.cdc.gov/media/releases/2015/p0730-us-disability.html.Accessed April 17, 2019.

32. *Healthy People 2020*. Physical Activity Objectives. Available at: https://www.healthypeople.gov/2020/data-search/Search-the-Data#objid=5069. Accessed May 14, 2019.

33. *ACSM's Health/Fitness Facility Standards and Guidelines.* Sanders ME. (ed.) 5th Ed. Champaign, IL: Human Kinetics, 2019.

34. NSCA Strength and Conditioning Professional Standards and Guidelines. *Strength and Conditioning Journal,* 39(6), 1-24, 2017. Available at: https://www.nsca.com/education/articles/nsca-strength-and-conditioning-professional-standards-and-guidelines/. Accessed November 5, 2018.

35. IHRSA Club Membership Standards. In: *IHRSA's Guide to Club Membership & Conduct.* 3rd Ed. Boston, MA: International Health, Racquet & Sportsclub Association, 2005. Available at: http://download.ihrsa.org/pubs/club_membership_conduct.pdf. Accessed November 5, 2018.

36. *Medical Fitness Association's Standards & Guidelines for Medical Fitness Center Facilities,* Roy B. (ed.). 2nd Ed. Monterey, CA: Healthy Learning, 2013.

37. Health Care. Exercise is Medicine®: A Standard in the Clinical Setting. Available at: https://www.exerciseismedicine.org/support_page.php/healthcare. Accessed April 18, 2019.

References continued...

38. Sallis RE, Matuszak JM, Baggish AL, et al. Call to Action on Making Physical Activity Assessment and Prescription a Medical Standard of Care. *Current Sports Medicine Reports,* 15(3), 207-214, 2016.

39. Sallis RE. Exercise in the Treatment of Chronic Disease: An Underfilled Prescription. *Current Sports Medicine Reports,* 16(4), 225-226, 2017.

40. Bowen PG, Mankowski RT, Harper SA, et al. Exercise Is Medicine as a Vital Sign: Challenges and Opportunities. *Translation Journal of the ACSM,* 4(1), 1-7, 2018.

41. Can You be Held Liable for a Negligent Referral? Legal Match. Available at: https://www.legalmatch.com/law-library/article/can-you-be-held-liable-for-a-negligent-referral.html. Accessed April 18, 2019.

42. Liability for Improperly Managed Referrals. The LSU Medical and Public Health Law Site, April 19, 2009. Available at: https://biotech.law.lsu.edu/map/LiabilityforImproperlyManagedReferrals.html. Accessed April 18, 2019.

43. Lynch DJ. Involving the Physician in Medical Fitness: A Must for Success. *ACSM's Health & Fitness Journal,* 10(3), 29-30, 2006.

44. ACSM Exercise is Medicine® Credential. Available at: https://www.acsm.org/get-stay-certified/get-certified/specialization/eim-credential. Accessed April 19, 2019.

45. EIM Credential Eligibility. Available at: https://www.acsm.org/get-stay-certified/get-certified/specialization/eim-credential/eim-eligibility. Accessed April 19, 2019.

46. Warburton D. Bredin S. Charlesworth S., et al. Evidence-Based Risk Recommendations for Best Practices in the Training of Qualified Exercise Professionals Working with Clinical Populations. Applied Physiology, Nutrition, and Metabolism, 36, S232-S265, 2011.

47. Herbert WG. Forces Driving Change in the U.S. Exercise Industry Today: A Final Word. The Exercise, Sports and Sports Medicine Standards & Malpractice Reporter, 5(6), 85-89, 2016.

48. Berg A. Minnesota Grad Students May Lose Fitness Benefits. *Athletic Business E-Newsletter.* May 2, 2019. Available at: https://www.athleticbusiness.com/governing-bodies/minnesota-grad-students-may-lose-fitness-benefits.html. Accessed May 7, 2019.

49. Eickhoff-Shemek JM, Herbert DL, Connaughton, DP. *Risk Management for Health/Fitness Professionals: Legal Issues and Strategies.* Baltimore, MD: Lippincott Williams & Wilkins, 2009.

50. Unlicensed Practice of a Health Care Profession. Fla Stat. § 456.065, 2001.

51. Herbert DL. $320 Million Lawsuit Filed Against Health Club. *The Exercise Standards and Malpractice Reporter,* 13(3), 33,36, 1999.

52. Wrongful Death Case of Anne Marie Capati Settled for Excess of $4 Million. *The Exercise Standards and Malpractice Reporter,* 20(3), 36, 2006.

53. Licensure Statutes and Information by State. Academy of Nutrition and Dietetics. Available at: https://www.eatrightpro.org/advocacy/licensure/licensure-map. Accessed February 10, 2020.

54. *Ohio Board of Dietetics v. Brown,* 83 Ohio App. 3rd 242, 1993 LEXIS 88 (Ohio Ct. App., 1993).

55. *Cooksey v. Futrell,* 721 F.3d 226 (4th Cir., 2018).

56. Website Review-Cooksey. Available at: https://www.diabetes-warrior.net/wp-content/uploads/2012/01/Website_Review_Cooksey_Jan._2012.pdf. Accessed May 8, 2019.

57. *Sosa-Gaines v. Capital Fitness Inc.,* No. 2-17-1035, 2019 LEXIS 111 (Ill. App. Ct. 2d., 2019).

58. Florida Enacts Occupational Freedom and Opportunity Act. CrossFit. July 2, 2020. Available at: https://www.crossfit.com/battles/florida-nutrition-bill-state. Accessed July 3, 2020.

59. *United States v. Faux,* No. 3:14-cr-28(SRU), 2015 LEXIS 31527 (D. Conn., 2015).

60. *United States v. Faux,* 94 F. Supp. 3d 258, 2015 LEXIS 37051 (D. Conn., 2015).

61. *United States v. Faux,* 828 F.3d 130, 2016 LEXIS 12577 (2nd Cir., 2016).

62. National Board for Health & Wellness Coaching. Health and Wellness Coaching Job Task Analysis Findings. Available at: https://nbhwc.org/wp-content/uploads/2019/04/FINAL-JTA-4_15_19.pdf. Accessed May 13, 2019.

63. Dietary Guidelines for Americans 2015-2020 Eighth Edition. Office of Disease Prevention and Health Promotion. Available at: https://health.gov/dietaryguidelines/2015/guidelines/. Accessed May 13, 2019.

64. ACSM/NCHPAD Certified Inclusive Fitness Trainer. Available at: https://www.acsm.org/get-stay-certified/get-certified/specialization/cift. Accessed May 14, 2019.

65. Disability/Condition. National Center on Health, Physical Activity and Disability. Available at: https://www.nchpad.org/Articles/7/Disability~Condition. Accessed May 14, 2019.

66. Exercise and Fitness. National Center on Health, Physical Activity and Disability. Available at: https://www.nchpad.org/Articles/9/Exercise~and~Fitness. Accessed May 14, 2019.

67. *Removing Barriers to Health Clubs and Fitness Facilities: A Guide for Accommodating All Members Including People with Disabilities and Older Adults.* North Carolina Office on Disability and Health, 2008. Available at: https://fpg.unc.edu/sites/fpg.unc.edu/files/resources/other-resources/NCODH_RemovingBarriersToHealthClubs.pdf. Accessed May 14, 2019.

68. Johnson MJ, Stoelzle HY, Finco KL, et al. ADA Compliance and Accessibility of Fitness Facilities in Western Wisconsin. *Topics in Spinal Cord Injury Rehabilitation,* 18(4), 340-353, 2012.

69. Medical Exercise Specialist. Medical Exercise Training Institute http://www.medicalexercisespecialist.com. Accessed May 15, 2019.

70. ACSM/ACS Certified Cancer Exercise Trainer. Available at: https://www.acsm.org/get-stay-certified/get-certified/specialization/cet. Accessed May 15, 2019.

71. Garber CE, Blissmer B. Deschenes MR, et al. ACSM Position Stand. Quantity and Quality of Exercise for Developing and Maintaining Cardiorespiratory, Musculoskeletal, and Neuromotor Fitness in Apparently Healthy Adults: Guidance for Prescribing Exercise. Medicine & Science in Sports & Exercise, 43(7), 1334-1359, 2011.

72. ACSM Position Stand. Progression Models in Resistance Training for Healthy Adults. *Medicine & Science in Sports & Exercise,* 41(3), 687-708, 2009.

73. Rahl RL. *Physical Activity and Health Guidelines: Recommendations for Various Ages, Fitness Levels, and Conditions from 57 Authoritative Sources.* Champaign, IL: Human Kinetics, 2010.

74. Thompson WR. (ed.). *ACSM's Clinical Exercise Physiology.* Philadelphia, PA: Wolters Kluwer, 2019.

75. Moore GE, Durstine JL, Painter PL. *ACSM's Exercise Management for Persons with Chronic Diseases and Disabilities.* Champaign, IL: Human Kinetics, 2016.

76. Jacobs PL (ed.). *NSCA's Essentials of Training Special Populations.* Colorado Springs, CO: National Strength and Conditioning Association. Available at: https://www.nsca.com/store/product-detail/INV/9780736083300/9780736083300. Accessed May 16, 2019.

77. Howley ET, Thompson DL. (eds). *Fitness Instructor's Handbook.* (7th Ed.). Champaign, IL: Human Kinetics, 2017.

78. Ehrman J, Gordon P, Visich P. et al. *Clinical Exercise Physiology.* (4th Ed.). Champaign, IL: Human Kinetics, 2019.

References *continued...*

79. EIM Exercise Pro Action Guide. Resources for Exercise Professionals. Available at: https://www.exerciseismedicine.org/support_page.php/exercise-professionals. Accessed May 22, 2019.

80. Health Care Providers Action Guide. Exercise is Medicine®—Rx Form. Available at: https://www.exerciseismedicine.org/assets/page_documents/Exercise%20is%20Medicine%20Rx%20form_fillable.pdf. Accessed May 17, 2019.

81. Health Care Providers Action Guide. Patient Fitness Progress Report (for exercise professionals). Available at: https://www.exerciseismedicine.org/assets/page_documents/EIM%20patient%20fitness%20progress%20report.pdf. Accessed May 17, 2019.

82. Kruskall LJ, Manore MM, Eickhoff-Shemek JM, et al. Drawing the Line: Understanding the Scope of Practice Among Registered Dietitian Nutritionists and Exercise Professionals. *ACSM's Health & Fitness Journal,* 21(1), 23-32, 2017.

83. Abbott AA. Scope of Practice. *ACSM's Health & Fitness Journal,* 22(5), 51-55, 2018.

84. Potter S. Boyd JM. Bridging the Performance Gap: Interdisciplinary Collaboration with Sports Dietitians. *Strength and Conditioning Journal,* 39(4), 4-9, 2017.

85. Lariviere D. Nutritional Supplements Flexing Muscles as Growth Industry. Available at: https://www.forbes.com/sites/davidlariviere/2013/04/18/nutritional-supplements-flexing-their-muscles-as-growth-industry/#142d-6ca98845. Accessed May 21, 2019.

86. Rosenbloom C, Murray B. Risky Business: Dietary Supplement Use by Athletes. *Nutrition Today,* 50(5) 240-246, 2015.

87. Beware of Fraudulent Dietary Supplements. Available at: https://www.fda.gov/consumers/consumer-updates/beware-fraudulent-dietary-supplements. Accessed May 21, 2019.

88. Eichner AK, Coyles J, Fedoruk M, et al. Essential Features of Third-Party Certification Programs for Dietary Supplements: A Consensus Statement. *Current Sports Medicine Reports,* 18(5), 178-182, 2019.

89. Higgins JP, Babu KM, Deuster PA, et al. Stimulant-Containing Energy Drinks: What You Need to Know. *ACSM's Health & Fitness Journal,* 22(3), 17-21, 2018.

CHAPTER 8

Instruction and Supervision

LEARNING OBJECTIVES

After reading this chapter, fitness managers and exercise professionals will be able to:

1. Realize that improper instruction and supervision is the most common allegation of negligence.

2. Define specific, general, and transitional supervision and describe how each is utilized in various exercise programs and services (1).

3. Describe the causes of exertional rhabdomyolysis (ER) and negligence lawsuits involving ER injuries that have occurred in various exercise programs.

4. Distinguish between high intensity training (HIT) and high-intensity interval training (HIIT) from an injury risk and legal liability perspective.

5. Explain precautions that exercise professionals need to consider when instructing and supervising HIIT programs.

6. List and describe negligence lawsuits involving improper instruction and supervision in each of the following programs: (a) personal fitness training, (b) group exercise, (c) youth exercise, (d) strength and conditioning, (e) clinical exercise, (f) first responder/military exercise.

7. Appreciate the many potential legal liability exposures that exist with non-traditional personal fitness training (i.e., Internet, home, and outdoor training).

8. Discuss the legal and risk management "lessons learned" provided in each of the four spotlight cases and how these lessons learned can be applied to a fitness facility's risk management plan.

9. Using case law examples, describe why there is a need for education and training regarding the prevention and recognition of exertional heat injuries among strength and condition coaches in athletic programs.

10. Define sovereign immunity and explain its application in cases involving injuries occurring in first responder and military physical training programs.

11. Describe how providing proper instruction and supervision protects exercise professionals from legal liability as well as employers from vicarious liability.

12. Explain the potential legal protections provided to exercise professionals and fitness facilities by offering beginner-level exercise programs.

13. Describe how negligence claims/lawsuits regarding improper instruction/supervision can be minimized by fitness managers who (a) have exercise professionals prepare written lesson plans, and (b) offer a continuing education program focusing on safe instruction.

14. Develop and utilize a performance appraisal tool that can be effective in assessing and improving the instructional skills of exercise professionals as well as minimize direct liability of employers.

15. Identify and comply with various standards of practice published by professional organizations regarding instruction and supervision (1).

16. Develop and implement eight risk management strategies that will be effective in minimizing injuries and subsequent litigation related to improper instruction and supervision (1).

INTRODUCTION

As described in Chapter 4, fitness managers and exercise professionals have a duty to provide reasonably safe programs and services for the participants they serve. Several risk management strategies need to be developed and implemented to carry out this duty. One important strategy is to provide proper instruction and supervision. Numerous injuries and subsequent lawsuits are due to negligent instruction and supervision as demonstrated in spotlight and other cases described throughout this textbook. The late legal scholar, Betty van der Smissen, stated that the "lack of or inadequate supervision is the most common allegation of negligence" (2, p. 163). She defined supervision as specific, general, and transitional as described below. Experienced expert witnesses, Harvey Voris and Dr. Marc Rabinoff (3) and Dr. Anthony Abbott (4) have also indicated that negligence lawsuits frequently involve improper instruction and supervision such as when an exercise professional has a participant perform exercises that are unsafe or too intense, given the participant's health/fitness status. Due to the popularity of high intensity exercise programs, this chapter will address injuries associated with these programs and provide risk management strategies on how to minimize these injuries and subsequent litigation.

This chapter describes four spotlight cases and other negligence cases in which exercise professionals failed to provide proper instruction and supervision in various exercise programs including personal fitness training, group exercise, youth, strength and conditioning, and clinical exercise as well as programs for first responders and military personnel. Additional cases addressing improper instruction/supervision involving exercise equipment are described in Chapter 9 (Exercise Equipment Safety) with a special focus on strength training equipment injuries and negligent instruction. The general instruction that should be provided for all new participants is addressed in Chapter 10 under Facility Orientation. This chapter ends with a description of eight risk management strategies that can be developed and implemented to minimize legal liability associated with instruction and supervision.

Instruction and Supervision Defined

Editorial Note: *The content in this section, instruction and supervision defined, reflects content from Chapter 8 in* Risk Management for Health/Fitness Professionals: Legal Issues and Strategies *(1). The publisher transferred the rights to this textbook to the authors in 2017. Permission to reprint and revise/update this content was granted by the author of Chapter 8.*

Betty van der Smissen classified supervision into three categories—specific, general, and transitional (2). **Specific supervision** means that the supervisor is "directly" with an individual or small group and involves an "instructional" format. In fitness facilities, this would typically include personal fitness training, group exercise classes, and the initial orientation/instruction to new participants on the proper use of the equipment and facility. From a legal perspective, specific supervision should provide the participant an opportunity to gain knowledge of the activity, an understanding of one's own capabilities, and an appreciation of the potential injuries that can occur so that he/she can assume the inherent risks of the activity (2). Once this is achieved, the supervision of the participant can move to transitional and then general categories.

It is important to realize that specific supervision "is not a function of the activity but of the individual participating," meaning that the "determinant of likelihood of injury is directly related to the participant's skill capability, physical and mental condition to do the activity, and knowledge/understanding/appreciation of the activity itself" (2, p. 170). For example, participants who have medical conditions (e.g., high blood pressure, diabetes, pregnancy, etc.) should be provided adequate specific supervision (instruction) that includes knowledge, understanding, and appreciation of any specific risks that may exist and any special precautions they should take, given their individual medical condition.

General supervision involves a supervisor who has the responsibility for overseeing an activity going on in the facility (2). An example of someone who provides general supervision would be a fitness floor supervisor or anyone else who has responsibilities to supervise facilities such as the locker rooms, saunas, racquetball courts, and childcare areas. There are two dimensions of general supervision, individual-oriented and group behaviors-oriented (2). An example of individual-oriented supervision would be observing participants, to see that they are properly using the exercise equipment and facility. Group behaviors-oriented supervision involves watching the behaviors of participants (e.g., being sure participants are following the fitness center's policies and procedures) and observing and taking appropriate action if any dangerous conditions occur such as if a piece of equipment breaks down.

Transitional supervision involves changing from specific to general and back, perhaps several times during any supervisory session (2). An example of this would be when a staff member has taught a small group of new participants how to use certain exercise equipment during the facility's orientation program (specific supervision) and then has them exercise on their own while providing general supervision. At times during the general supervision, the staff member may individually and directly help (or re-teach) a participant an exercise, then go back to general supervision of all participants. This also happens when fitness floor supervisors who provide general supervision may at times, need to transition to specific supervision (e.g., when they notice a participant misusing the equipment and offer correct instruction).

ASSESSMENT OF LEGAL LIABILITY EXPOSURES

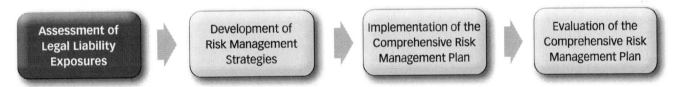

Assessment of Legal Liability Exposures → Development of Risk Management Strategies → Implementation of the Comprehensive Risk Management Plan → Evaluation of the Comprehensive Risk Management Plan

Two of the four spotlight cases described below deal with serious injuries associated with high intensity exercise programs, one involving a massive stroke and the other a heat injury death. Additional cases in this chapter describe another serious injury also associated with high intensity programs—**exertional rhabdomyolysis**. Given the popularity of high intensity exercise programs, it is essential that fitness managers and exercise professionals learn about the injury risks associated with these programs and how to prevent them from occurring. Background information regarding these potential injuries is first provided with a special focus on exertional rhabdomyolysis. Following this discussion, several negligence cases are described that involved improper instruction and supervision in various exercise programs.

High Intensity Exercise Injuries

As previously described in Chapter 6, a 2007 ACSM and American Heart Association (AHA) Joint Position Paper concluded that "compelling evidence indicates that the vigorous exercise acutely increases the risk of cardiovascular events among...adults with both occult and diagnosed heart disease...particularly among habitually sedentary persons" (5, p. 890). An updated version of this paper, published in 2020 by the AHA (6), had a similar conclusion stating, "vigorous physical activity, particularly when performed by unfit individuals, can acutely increase the risk of sudden cardiac death and acute myocardial infarction in susceptible people" (p. e705). If vigorous intensity exercise (77-95% HR max) can increase risks, it can be assumed that high intensity exercise (> 96% HR max) may further increase these risks. Exercise professionals know these risks are clearly foreseeable and, thus, need to take precautions to help prevent them. For example, one of the recommendations to reduce cardiovascular events in the ACSM/AHA joint position paper was to encourage adults "to develop gradually progressive exercise regimens" (5, p. 893). In addition to cardiac events, high intensity exercise programs have been associated with heat injuries and deaths as well as various musculoskeletal injuries. Many exertional rhabdomyolysis injuries have also occurred from participation in high intensity exercise programs.

Exertional Rhabdomyolysis: A Historical Perspective

Exertional rhabdomyolysis (ER) has been a long-time, foreseeable risk associated with high intensity exercise and/or extreme conditioning programs, such as programs with little or no recovery periods. Several articles published in medical journals in the 70s and 80s described the link between extreme exercise and exertional rhabdomyolysis. One of the first negligence cases involving an ER injury involved a 23-year old medical student who was required to run an 8-minute mile as a class experiment. This case, *Turner v. Rush Medical College*, described in Chapter 4, occurred in 1989. The *Mimms v. Ruthless Training Concepts, LLC* and *Proffitt v. Global Fitness Holdings, LLC, et al.* cases described in Chapter 7 occurred in 2008 and 2013, respectively. Additional cases, *Moore v. Willis Independent School District* in 2000 and *Pineda v. Town Sports*

KEY POINT

What is Exertional Rhabdomyolysis (ER)?

ER occurs from strenuous exercise that leads to a breakdown of skeletal muscle resulting in a protein (myoglobin) being released into the bloodstream (8). Excess myoglobin can lead to kidney damage and in severe cases, kidney failure. Severe muscle damage can also lead to **compartment syndrome**—a swelling of the affected muscle tissue that can cause muscle necrosis (death). Early signs/symptoms include excessive muscle soreness and dark brown urine. To diagnose ER, a urine analysis is needed along with a blood test to determine levels of creatine phosphokinase (CPK)—an enzyme associated with muscle damage.

As demonstrated in the negligence cases described in this chapter and in other chapters, ER can occur in all types of (a) high intensity exercise programs (e.g., body weight/resistance and cardiovascular) and (b) populations (e.g., general population and elite athletes).

International, Inc. in 2009, involved high intensity exercise resulting in exertional rhabdomyolysis (7). From these cases and additional cases described later, it is evident that any type of exercise (e.g., body weight/resistance activities, cardiovascular, or various combinations) that are high intensity may lead to ER.

In 2005, CrossFit expressly acknowledged the risk of ER associated with its high intensity exercise programs in two published articles (7). One of these articles described five reported cases of ER resulting from CrossFit workouts (9). A warning, confirming the link between CrossFit and ER, was included in the article about this potentially lethal risk. The rapid growth of CrossFit worldwide in the 2000s and beyond created a hot topic of debate among exercise professionals and the CrossFit community. Although this debate focused on safety concerns with CrossFit training, it also increased the awareness among exercise professionals and the lay public regarding the connection between extreme exercise programs and ER. During this time, CrossFit and other extreme conditioning programs (ECPs) such as P90X and Insanity became increasingly popular among military and athletic conditioning programs.

Given the rising popularity of ECPs in military and civilian communities, the authors of a 2011 article (10) stated injuries from ECPs including ER are reportedly occurring at increasing rates. They stated that these programs appear to violate accepted standards for safety and that solutions to reduce these injury risks are of paramount importance. One recommendation of the many listed in this article was to "introduce ECPs to new participants gradually with a specific progression (acclimation) to exercise intensity, duration, and advanced exercises" (10, p. 387). Regarding the increases in the frequency of ER among collegiate athletes, the authors of a 2012 article (11) stated that "workouts that are too novel, too much, too soon, or too intense (or a combination of these) have a strong connection to exertional rhabdomyolysis. Introducing full-intensity workouts too quickly is especially high risk" (p. 478). This article, prepared by authors representing 12 different organizations, provided a list of several recommendations. The first two recommendations focus on the prevention of ER: (1) acclimatize progressively for utmost safety, and (2) introduce new conditioning activities gradually (11).

The major purpose of these two articles, published in professional journals, was to increase the awareness of this potentially life-threatening condition and provide recommendations for exercise professionals on how to prevent the serious risks associated with high intensity or extreme conditioning programs (ECPs). Additional articles to increase the awareness of ER were also published in various journals between 2003 and 2013 such as *Medicine & Science in Sports & Exercise* (12), *Strength and Conditioning Journal* (13), *Journal of Physical Education, Recreation & Dance* (14), and *IDEA Fitness Journal* (15). This topic of ECPs has also been presented at various professional conferences. For example, the lead author of the 2011 paper, Dr. Michael Bergeron, gave a presentation titled: Extreme Conditioning Programs—Are They Worth the Risk? at the ACSM Health & Fitness Summit in 2013 (16).

By 2013, ample published, scientific evidence showed that high intensity exercise programs or ECPs can lead to ER, especially if the exercise regimen was too novel, too much, too soon, or too intense. Although numerous efforts have been made to help ensure that exercise professionals were well-informed of this clearly "foreseeable" ER risk, individuals are still being diagnosed with ER after participation in high intensity exercise programs led by exercise professionals. Why? There may be several reasons, but the likely ones are: (a) some exercise professionals leading these programs lack adequate knowledge and skills to design/deliver a program incorporating important safety principles of exercise such as progression, and (b) some fitness/athletic managers are not making a concerted effort to help ensure their employees possess the necessary knowledge and practical skills to properly teach, train, and/or coach. They also have likely not focused on their responsibility to create a safety culture and professional environment.

Interestingly, the strength and conditioning coaches in the University of Iowa case, that occurred in 2011 and is described later, claimed they did not know about ER. This lack of knowledge (or ignorance) is not a legal defense. Even if they did not know about ER, they should have known about the importance of applying safe principles of exercise such as progression, intensity, overload, etc. in the design and delivery of an exercise program before working as an exercise professional.

These basic principles have been covered in all quality academic and certification preparation programs for decades. If applied properly, the risk of ER would not exist or would be significantly reduced. It is important to point out, however, that the risk of ER, as well as other injuries such as heat injuries, can be increased in individuals who take certain medications or have certain medical conditions. See the *UCF Athletics Association v. Plancher* spotlight case. For these individuals, exercise professionals need to be aware of additional precautions that need to be considered when designing and delivering exercise programs. This is one of the main reasons to obtain medical histories as described in Chapter 6.

Exercise professionals that instruct a low-fit person or a beginner (or even an athlete) to perform a high intensity workout on their first day of exercise or training are, clearly, failing to meet the standard of care of a reasonable, prudent, exercise professional. Even after the 2012 publication addressing serious risks associated with collegiate conditioning programs, athletes are still being diagnosed and hospitalized with ER that could have been prevented. Negligence lawsuits that have resulted in some of these cases are described later. The ER cases continue into 2019—seven years after the 2012 publication. For example, in January 2019, 12 collegiate women soccer players were diagnosed with ER after participation in an extreme conditioning program led by the strength and conditioning coach at the University of Houston (17).

Distinguishing Between HIT and HIIT

It is important to distinguish between **high intensity training** (HIT) or ECPs and **high-intensity interval training** (HIIT) from safety and legal liability perspectives. The injuries that occurred in the high-intensity exercise cases, described later in this chapter, resulted primarily from "sustained" high intensity exercise (HIT), such as continuous high intensity exercise with little or no recovery intervals, and not from high-intensity interval training (HIIT) that incorporates recovery intervals. The HIT injuries occurred with both body weight/resistance and cardiovascular activities, indicating the type of activity made no difference regarding the risk of injuries. In recent years, HIIT programs have become popular and have been rated a top fitness trend (18). Although the injury risk is lower in HIIT than HIT programs, injuries have occurred.

An Internet search using terms "HIIT and injuries" will generate several articles describing the increased risks of injuries associated with HIIT. For example, a study published in 2019 (19) investigated injury data from the National Electronic Injury Surveillance System (NEISS) related to exercises such as burpees, push-ups, and lunges and exercise equipment such as barbells, kettle bells, and boxes. The authors stated that these types of activities were representative of HIIT programs. From 2007 through 2016, there were almost four million injuries resulting from these types of exercises with the most common being musculoskeletal injuries of the lower extremity (35.3%) followed by trunk injuries (25%). The authors also compared the number of injuries between 2007 and 2011 with the number of injuries between 2012 and 2016 and found an increase of 144%. They concluded that as the popularity of high intensity programs increased so did the number of injuries.

Note: *Given the type of musculoskeletal injuries reported in this study (19), it may be that the injuries were due to improper instruction, the inability of the individuals to safely perform the exercises, and/or the failure to incorporate adequate rest intervals. Injury risks increase with certain exercises that are (a) advanced or difficult for individuals who have not attained the necessary skill, strength, and balance to perform them properly, and/or (b) contraindicated for individuals with medical conditions.*

Precautions for HIIT Programs

A key safety feature of HIIT is the recovery interval which, most often, is an active recovery period performed at a light-moderate intensity level. High-volume exercises without adequate recovery intervals can

"prompt early fatigue, additional oxidative stress, less resistance to subsequent exercise strain, greater perception of effort, and unsafe movement execution leading to acute injury..." (10, p. 384). To help ensure the safety of individuals participating in a body weight/resistance HIIT program, it is essential to first determine if they can properly and safely perform the exercises. Certain body weight/resistance exercises require precise technique and/or considerable skill, balance, and strength for them to be safely executed. For individuals participating in cardiovascular HIIT programs, it will be important to first determine if they have safely progressed to a continuous "moderate-vigorous" intensity level of exercise. Therefore, in addition to obtaining a medical history (and medical clearance if needed), exercise professionals will need to make these determinations prior to instructing HIIT programs. Of course, the HIIT program must be individually designed. If the HIIT program is taught in a group exercise class, not all participants should have the exact same prescription for the high-intensity interval, and the recovery interval may vary as well. There are a variety of methods in designing the exercise (work) and recovery intervals with HIIT programs (20, 21, 22). Exhibit 8-1 provides a description of HIIT from the 2018 Physical Activity Guidelines.

HIIT—Not for Everyone

Aerobic HIIT studies have shown to improve health/fitness variables often superior to traditional continuous moderate-intensity exercise (20, 21, 24). Because less time is needed to achieve these benefits compared to an exercise program that follows the 2018 Physical Activity Guidelines, it can be an attractive option for certain individuals. However, some individuals may not enjoy exercising at high-intensity levels and, therefore, may not adhere to a HIIT program (22). In addition, a HIIT program would not be appropriate for a novice or sedentary person, given the increased risk

---

Exhibit 8-1: HIIT Description from the 2018 Physical Activity Guidelines

High-Intensity Interval Training (HIIT) is a form of interval training that consists of alternating short periods of maximal-effort exercise with less intense recovery periods. There are no universally accepted lengths for the maximal-effort period, the recovery period, or the ratio of the two; no universally accepted number of cycles per session or the entire duration of the session; and no precise relative intensity at which the maximal-effort component should be performed (23, p. 60).

of injury. It would be wise to first assess an individual's readiness for both body weight/resistance and cardiovascular HIIT programs. However, as with almost all exercise programs, HIIT can be modified or tailored to meet individual needs. Interestingly, HIIT programs have been safely implemented, even with clinical populations, e.g., cardiac patients in cardiac rehabilitation programs (25). Dalleck (25) describes some of these studies and provides various safety precautions for exercise professionals to follow. However, according to an AHA paper published in 2020 (6), additional studies are needed to assess the safety, compliance, morbidity, and mortality after HIIT before it can be widely adopted in patients with known or suspected CAD, especially in unsupervised, non-medical settings.

NEGLIGENCE CASES: IMPROPER INSTRUCTION AND SUPERVISION

This section describes four spotlight cases and other negligence cases that demonstrate the importance of providing safe instruction and supervision. In most of these cases, it was evident that the trainers/instructors/coaches did not have adequate knowledge and skills to properly perform their teaching and/or training responsibilities. To minimize injury and subsequent litigation, it is essential that fitness/athletic managers and exercise professionals follow the risk management strategies described in Chapter 5 such as providing on-the-job training as well as implement the eight risk management strategies at the end of this chapter. Spotlight and other negligence cases are described for each of the following types of exercise programs as well as related legal liability issues.

a) Personal Fitness Training
b) Group Exercise
c) Youth Exercise
d) Strength and Conditioning
e) Clinical Exercise
f) First Responder and Military

Personal Fitness Training Programs

Several spotlight and other negligence cases involving improper instruction and supervision of personal

fitness trainers are presented throughout this textbook. These reflect a small sample of the many cases that exist. See Table 8-1 for a list of the spotlight cases. The spotlight case below, *Vaid v. Equinox*, describes serious injuries that occurred to a physician caused by the negligent instruction and supervision of the physician's personal fitness trainer. The jury awarded the plaintiff $14,500,000, which far exceeds the damages awarded in most cases involving exercise professionals and their employers.

Table 8-1	Spotlight Cases: Negligent Instruction/Supervision Claims Made by Clients Against Their Personal Fitness Trainers

CASE	CHAPTER
Corrigan v. Musclemakers, Inc.	4
Evans v. Fitness & Sport Clubs, LLC	4
Stelluti v. Casapenn Enterprises, LLC	4
D'Amico v. LA Fitness	5
Rostai v. Neste Enterprises	6
Levy v. Town Sports International, Inc.	7
Bartlett v. Push to Walk	7
Layden v. Plante	7
Butler v. Seville et al.	9

Non-Traditional Personal Fitness Training

With the growth of **non-traditional personal fitness training** programs (i.e., training conducted outside a fitness facility), it is important that personal fitness trainers consider the potential legal liability issues they face before beginning non-traditional forms of training such as (a) Internet training, (b) home training in either the trainer's home or in the client's home, and (c) outdoor training in areas such as public parks. Some of the legal liability issues associated with each of these are briefly described. It is important to realize that the potential legal duties of personal fitness trainers do not go away with non-traditional personal fitness training programs. As described in Chapter 4, personal fitness trainers have a duty to provide reasonably safe exercise programs for their clients. In addition, it is likely that the trainer will be held to a **professional standard of care** and, thus, needs to take precautions regarding potential risks related to

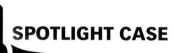

SPOTLIGHT CASE

Vaid v. Equinox
CV136019426, 2016 LEXIS 828 (Conn. Super. Ct., 2016)

FACTS

Historical Facts:

While exercising on a Concept2 rowing machine under the supervision of personal fitness trainer Joseph Dominguez, Dr. Chetan Vaid suffered a carotid artery dissection. A few hours later at the hospital Dr. Vaid suffered a massive stroke, which caused the loss of 40 percent of his brain and permanent injuries resulting in significant interference with his medical practice and enjoyment of life. Dominguez, allegedly, did not provide proper instruction to Dr. Vaid, an inexperienced user of the rowing machine (i.e., the damper setting was too high and he did not instruct him on proper form).

Procedural Facts:

The complaint filed by the plaintiffs alleged negligence against the trainer, Equinox Old Track Road, the owner of a fitness facility in Greenwich Connecticut, and Equinox Holdings, Inc., the parent company for "vicarious liability, negligent retention and supervision, and recklessness, as well as loss of consortium against all defendants" (p. 1). The plaintiffs made several claims against the defendants' managers including that they knew that Dominguez used training methods that were too aggressive but still allowed him to work as a personal fitness trainer. (Herbert). The plaintiffs listed 18 negligence claims against Dominguez in their complaint including:

- He failed to adequately instruct Vaid on the proper and safe technique for rowing;

- He failed to adequately monitor Vaid during Vaid's use of the rowing equipment;

- He instructed Vaid to continue exercising even through Vaid reported he was not feeling well (Herbert, p. 37).

At trial, the jury returned a verdict of $14,500,000 in favor of the plaintiffs that was reduced $10,875,000 based on a finding of twenty-five percent comparative negligence by Dr. Vaid. The defendants filed a motion to set aside (reverse or vacate) the verdict based on the following five grounds:

1. The court improperly permitted Jonathan Near, a rowing coach, to offer expert testimony about the standard of care applicable to a personal trainer when giving instruction on a rowing machine;

2. The court improperly admitted evidence of the handling and destruction of the notes of Mr. Dominguez's supervisor, Patrick Freeman;

3. The court improperly charged the jury as to negligence, permitting the use of either a professional or a layman's standard of care;

4. The evidence did not support the verdict as to causation; and

5. The evidence did not support the verdict as to foreseeability of Dr. Vaid's injuries (p. 2).

ISSUE

Did the court agree with the five grounds submitted by the defendants in their motion to set aside the verdict?

COURT'S RULING

No. The court denied the defendants' motion to set aside the verdict in its entirety.

COURT'S REASONING

The court provided their reasoning for denying all five grounds, but three (the first, fourth, and fifth) are discussed here. Regarding the first ground, the defendants claimed that Mr. Near was not qualified to provide an opinion as to the standard

Vaid continued...

of care for a personal trainer on the use of a rowing machine because he had not worked as a personal trainer in a gym. However, he had taught hundreds of novices and athletes in the proper use of the Concept2 rowing machine. He testified that the proper setting on the rowing machine should have been much lower than the setting used by Dominguez and that Equinox was negligent because it did not instruct Dominguez on how to use the machine properly. The defendants relied on medical and legal malpractice cases dealing with expert testimony in which statute provisions require the standard of care testimony be provided by a similar health care provider. However, the court stated that the defendants were mistaken to conceive this case in the context of medical or legal malpractice. In addition, an expert for the defendant testified that there was no professional standard of care in the personal training industry. Mr. Near's testimony was supported by another expert, a certified personal trainer, gym owner, and author of a best practices manual. This expert also testified that the defendants were negligent in their instructions to Dr. Vaid and training of Dominguez. In addition, the Concept2 manuals were admitted as evidence which specified settings dramatically at odds with those used by Dominguez.

Regarding the fourth ground, the court found that there was sufficient evidence to support the jury's finding that the defendants' negligence "was the cause in fact and proximate cause of the injuries claimed by plaintiffs" (p. 11). The defendants referred to one of their expert witnesses that testified there was no minimum threshold of exertion to cause a dissection of the carotid artery (e.g., a sneeze may be sufficient). However, the defendants did not refer to their other expert witnesses who were all medical professionals. One indicated that the rowing machine activity "probably did…cause the carotid dissection" and the other three testified "that the extension of the neck caused by the use of rowing machine as instructed by Mr. Dominguez could cause such a dissection" (p. 11). Given this expert testimony, the court stated that the jury could reasonably have concluded that Dr. Vaid's injuries were caused by the defendants' negligence.

For the fifth ground, the defendants claimed that the risk of a stroke arising from the improper use of the rowing machine was not foreseeable. Evidence submitted showed that stroke is a risk of exercise and that persons inexperienced with the use of rowing machines were especially at risk. Medical experts for the plaintiffs testified that "excessive exercise, especially with bad form, can cause serious injury" and "that neck injury was a foreseeable risk on a rowing machine, especially if the damper setting was too high" (p. 13). Citing previous cases, the court stated, "The inquiry fundamental to all proximate cause questions is whether the harm which occurred was of the same general nature as the foreseeable risk created by the defendant's negligence . . . This does not mean that you must find that Mr. Dominguez actually foresaw the probability of the exact harm that Plaintiffs allege befell Dr. Vaid" (pp. 12-13). Therefore, the proof submitted at trial was adequate in supporting the jury's finding regarding foreseeability as to the type of harm suffered by Dr. Vaid.

Herbert DL. $14.5 Million Verdict in Personal Training Case. *The Exercise, Sports and Sports Medicine Standards & Malpractice Reporter*, 5(5), 33, 35-41, 2016.

Lessons Learned from *Vaid*

Legal

- Expert testimony strongly demonstrated causation and foreseeability in this case to help the court determine the negligence of the defendants.

- Expert testimony in medical malpractice cases must meet certain statutory provisions regarding the standard of care testimony (i.e., experts must be a similar health care provider).

- This case was not a medical malpractice case, but the court stated that experts must "possess knowledge beyond the ken of an average juror that would be of assistance in the fact-finding function" (p. 5). The court ruled that Mr. Near met these qualifications and, thus, admitted his evidence.

- Medical malpractice pertains to the negligence of medical professionals and negligence can apply to any professional including exercise professionals.

- The expert witness for the defendants who testified that there was no professional standard of care in the personal training industry was incorrect. See Chapter 4 regarding the professional standard of care.

Vaid continued...

> ‣ The content in exercise equipment manuals can be admitted into evidence as the manuals for the Concept2 rower were in this case.
>
> **Risk Management/Injury Prevention**
> ‣ Personal fitness trainers need to be properly credentialed and competent.
>
> ‣ Fitness managers/supervisors need to recognize that formal education and training are needed for all personal fitness trainers with a focus on assessment of practical skills upon hiring.
>
> ‣ Fitness managers/supervisors need to conduct regular performance evaluations of personal fitness trainers during the probation period and on a regular basis thereafter.
>
> ‣ Direct supervision of personal fitness trainers is needed to help ensure they are providing quality (safe and effective) exercise programs.
>
> ‣ Specifications in all exercise equipment owners' manuals need to be followed including the proper instruction that is to be provided to novices.

the nature of the activity, type of participants, and the environment (26). The professional scope of practice as described in Chapter 7 also applies. Remember, if a client is harmed by following the instruction or advice of his/her trainer, the trainer can be held liable for the injury.

Internet/Live Online Training

Internet training is often delivered using live (real-time, synchronous) platforms such as Skype, FaceTime, and Zoom as well as trainer-client communications by email and phone. Although Internet personal fitness training has been around for many years, it became more prevalent given the COVID-19 epidemic in 2020 when fitness facilities were required to close. There are many potential legal liability exposures that personal trainers need to realize and discuss with their attorney before beginning Internet training. Being able to meet the professional standard of care will be challenging. For example, it will be difficult to conduct a proper fitness assessment, provide direct instruction/supervision to correct improper execution of an exercise or monitor intensity, provide emergency care, etc. For additional challenges and limitations with Internet training, see an article titled "Online Impersonal Training Risk Versus Benefit" written by Dr. Anthony Abbott (27).

Effective communication can also be a challenge. For example, if the client misunderstood something the trainer said, it could be problematic for the trainer if the misunderstanding led to a client's injury. Documentation of each training session including advice/instruction provided to

the client is recommended along with the client signing a summary of such advice/instruction immediately after each session. See Risk Management Strategy #4 below regarding the preparation of lesson plans and lesson plan evaluations. Extra safety precautions should be considered when preparing lesson plans such as avoiding complex/difficult exercises and high-intensity exercise routines.

Privacy of the client's protected health information (PHI) such as medical history data is an issue to be addressed given that cyberspace security is a continual risk. The Health Insurance Portability and Accountability Act (HIPAA) would, likely, not apply for most personal fitness training programs. However, state privacy and data breach notification laws may be applicable. Internet personal fitness trainers should ensure they are using a secure server and may need to purchase cyber liability insurance.

Home Training

Establishing a home gym has advantages but personal fitness trainers need to consider not only legal liability risks associated with instruction and supervision but also with maintenance of the property and exercise equipment. In *Zehnder v. Dutton* (28), Amy Zehnder, while at the home of Jay Dutton, fell to the ground while using a pull-up bar. She suffered serious injury to her thoracic and cervical spine. She alleged that Dutton was negligent in one or more of the following ways:

    a) For installing the pull-up bar in a manner that was inconsistent with the manufacturer's instructions for installation;

b) For installing the pull-up bar in a manner that the defendant knew was not safe;

c) For allowing the plaintiff to use the pull-up bar despite knowledge that it was not properly installed consistent with the manufacturer's instructions; and

d) For failing to warn the plaintiff that the pull-up bar, as installed on the I–Beam, was unsafe (28, p. 5).

The trial court ruled in favor of Dutton based on procedural issues and the appellate court upheld the trial court's ruling. This case raises issues related to proper inspection, maintenance and installation of exercise equipment as discussed in Chapter 9. In a typical fitness facility, this responsibility lies with the management or designated staff members and not, necessarily, with personal fitness trainers. However, trainers managing a gym in their home need to realize the many legal duties associated with managing a fitness facility and programs as presented throughout this textbook. They also need to be aware of any zoning laws or subdivision restrictions that might prohibit this type of home business.

Providing personal fitness training in the client's home also creates various liability exposures regarding instruction/supervision as well as exercise equipment. The trainer may be using some of his/her own equipment as well as equipment owed by the client, but who is responsible for inspection, maintenance, etc. involving the client's equipment?

Outdoor Training

It is common these days to see personal fitness trainers (and other exercise professionals such as group exercise leaders) leading exercise programs in outdoor places like city parks. Many of the legal liability issues described for home personal training also apply to outdoor training. It is important to realize that some cities/counties/districts prohibit such activities provided by private parties or they may require the purchase of a permit.

Individualized Legal Consultation: A Must for Non-Traditional Training

Note: *The following is not only applicable to personal fitness trainers, but to all exercise professionals including group*

exercise leaders and strength and conditioning coaches who lead non-traditional exercise programs (Internet/live online, home, and outdoor) for their participants.

The need for legal consultation is described throughout this textbook for traditional fitness facilities and programs. However, given the different types of legal liability exposures that exist with non traditional training, it is essential to obtain individualized legal advice before offering any of these types of programs. The following are some of the issues to discuss with legal counsel:

◆ **Protective Legal Documents**

It is likely that the many limitations associated with each type of non-traditional training will need to be specified in the waiver or other legal protective document such as an express assumption of risk. For example, inability to provide emergency care with Internet training and possible limited emergency care with home-based and outdoor training. Regarding waivers, state laws vary so this needs to be addressed for those who provide Internet training across state lines as well as the fact that waivers are unenforceable in some states (see Chapter 4). The administration of the protective legal document, such as how it is explained to the participant and how it is signed/submitted, also needs to be addressed.

◆ **Applicable Laws**

There are likely several laws that may be applicable such as state privacy and data breach notification laws for Internet training, zoning laws for home-based training, and city/county ordinances that may prohibit or require a permit for outdoor exercise programs in parks. If using music, copyright laws need to be addressed.

◆ **Insurance**

All exercise professionals should have professional liability insurance. It will be important to ensure that the policy covers non-traditional training. These policies often have exclusions, so it is essential they be carefully reviewed, perhaps, in consultation with legal counsel. Additional insurance needs should be considered such as cyber security insurance for Internet training and any other possible insurance needs for home and outdoor training programs.

▶ Documentation

In most non-traditional programs, if an injury and subsequent lawsuit occur, there will likely be no fact witnesses who could testify as to what happened. It will be the exercise professional's word against the injured participant, which may make it more difficult for the professional to defend. Risk management strategies such as having and keeping documentation (e.g., lesson plans, communications, etc.) should be discussed with legal counsel.

KEY POINT

Exercise professionals who teach non-traditional exercise programs (e.g., Internet, home, outdoor) for their participants must seek legal counsel to address the different types of legal liability exposures that exist compared to those that exist in a typical fitness facility. Potential legal duties do not go away with non-traditional training programs. Examples of issues to discuss with legal counsel are protective legal documents, applicable laws, insurance, and documentation.

On-demand Virtual Exercise Programs that Anyone can Access for Free or Purchase: Exercise professionals involved in the development and/or delivery of on-demand or video-taped/pre-recorded exercise programs that "anyone" can access for free or purchase may not face the same type of legal liability exposures that exercise professionals who are actively engaged in the design and delivery of programs for "their" participants. However, certain duties may exist. These should be discussed with legal counsel along with any laws (e.g., music copyright laws) that might be applicable as well as the need for any documents such as a terms agreement or disclaimer statement that is read and agreed to prior to accessing the virtual program.

Group Exercise Programs

Almost all fitness facilities offer a variety of group exercise classes. Many negligence cases have occurred involving negligent instruction/supervision in all types of group exercise classes. Examples were presented in Chapter 4 as spotlight cases, such as *Santana v. Women's*

Workout and Weight Loss Centers, Inc. (step aerobics injury) and *Stelluti v. Casapaenn Enterprises, LLC* (indoor cycling injury) or briefly described, such as *Tadmor v. New York Jiu Jitsu, Inc.* (martial arts injury). This section focuses on injuries and negligence lawsuits involving a group exercise program that has become increasingly popular in recent years—indoor cycling.

Injuries and lawsuits involving other popular group exercise programs such as yoga and bootcamp are also discussed. Many of the injuries are due to these programs being offered at high intensity or advanced levels. A need to offer beginning level classes and having well-trained and competent instructors can help minimize these injuries and subsequent litigation. See Key Point at the end of this section.

Indoor Cycling Injuries and Lawsuits

The *Scheck v. Soul Cycle* spotlight case is like the *Stelluti* case in that the instructor did not teach the participant, a novice, on how to properly use the bike. Injuries suffered by the plaintiffs in these two indoor cycling classes were musculoskeletal injuries. However, many ER injuries have also occurred. Research has shown that indoor cycling is considered a vigorous-high intensity exercise program. See Table 8-2 for a brief description of studies that investigated the physiological demands of a typical indoor cycling class. However, as with almost any exercise program, it can be taught at lower levels of intensity to meet the needs of individuals based on their health/fitness status—if the instructor knows how to properly teach and monitor intensity levels for these individuals while teaching the class. Unfortunately, as discussed next, many cases of ER have occurred in indoor-cycling classes due to improper instruction, especially for first-time participants.

In a study published in the *American Journal of Medicine* in 2016 titled "Freebie Rhabdomyolysis: A Public Health Concern. Spin Class-Induced Rhabdomyolysis", the authors describe three cases involving two women aged 33 and a 20-year-old man who were all diagnosed with ER after their first spin class (33). The authors stated that a total of 46 ER cases had been reported with 42 of these cases occurring following the first spin class. They also stated that "spinning must be considered an intense exercise mode and a risk for rhabdomyolysis in

Table 8-2	Investigations of the Physiological Demands of Indoor Cycling, 2007-2013
STUDY TITLE—YEAR PUBLISHED	**STUDY CONCLUSIONS**
Quantification of Spinning® Bike Performance During a Standard 50-minute class—2007 (29)	"Analysis of individual performances showed that they were compatible with physical exercise that ranged from moderate-to-heavy to very heavy, the latter conditions prevailing. The results show that this type of fitness activity has a high impact on cardiovascular function and suggest it is not suitable for unfit or sedentary individuals…" (p. 421)
Physiological Responses During Indoor Cycling—2008 (30)	"Data suggest that indoor cycling must be considered a high-intensity exercise mode of exercise training" (p. 1236) and "there is good evidence that unaccustomed high-intensity exercise may contribute to the triggering of acute myocardial infarction…those wishing to lead indoor cycling classes should make sure that they have conducted appropriate pre-exercise screening" (p. 1240).
Heart Rate and Overall Perceived Exertion During Spinning® Cycle Indoor Session in Novice Adults—2010 (31)	"The intensity during indoor cycling class in novice adults ranged from moderate-to-hard values. These data suggest that indoor cycling must be considered a high-intensity exercise mode for novice adults" (p. 238).
Exercise Intensity and Validity of the Ratings of Perceived Exertion (Borg and OMNI scales) in an Indoor Cycling Session—2013 (32)	"It can be concluded that indoor cycling elicits effort of high intensity which could be inappropriate for some participants" (p. 93).

the untrained individual" (p. 485). They concluded that the "only way to prevent rhabdomyolysis from spinning is to have safety guidelines set up. Beginners need to know how to gradually increase the time and cadence on the indoor cycle…Participants need to be informed of the risks of rhabdomyolysis" (p. 486).

After this study was published, the *New York Times* did a follow-up story titled "As Workouts Intensify, a Harmful Side Effect Grows More Common" (34). This story focused on a woman who suffered ER after a grueling spin class. An interesting outcome of this *New York Times* was the 827 comments submitted by the readers. The comments were both positive and negative, with some reflecting a good understanding of exercise safety principles such as progression and overload and others complaining about instructors continually pushing their riders to exercise harder. One reader commented: "Seems like if you're paying for an exercise class you can expect the instructor to know something about exercise. They should be held accountable".

It is unknown how many ER or other injuries have resulted in negligence claims/lawsuits against indoor cycling instructors and fitness facilities. One case involving ER, *Horowitz v. Luxury Hotels International of Puerto Rico, Inc.,* is briefly describe below. In another case, *Wallis v. Brainard Baptist Church* (35), a man collapsed and died after participating in an indoor cycling class in a facility owned by the church. The main issue in this case was the failure to use the automated external defibrillator (AED) that was onsite at the facility. In another case, briefly described in Chapter 10, *Levine v. GBG, Inc.* (36), the plaintiff claimed that the unreasonably high and dangerous volume caused acoustic trauma and injury to his inner ear and associated nervous system. Interestingly, many of the comments from the *New York Times* story were complaints about the loud music in indoor cycling classes.

In *Horowitz v. Luxury Hotels International of Puerto Rico, Inc.,* (37) the plaintiff, Damond Horowitz, participated in a 45-minute spinning class the day after he had checked into the Ritz-Carlton Hotel. Luxury Hotels operates and manages the fitness center at the hotel. On the following day, Horowitz informed Ritz Carlton personnel that he suffered from soreness and had difficulty walking. An on-call physician treated Horowitz at his hotel room. Later that evening, he visited a hospital emergency room and discharged himself against the advice of the attending physician. He claims he suffered ER from his participation in the spinning class and continues to endure bilateral weakness, bilateral intermittent pain, and bilateral discomfort. He seeks $1,250,000 in economic damages from Luxury Hotels and made the following negligence claims against them because:

a) they never screened him to assess his suitability or level of expertise in spinning;

b) they never informed him of any of the risks to which he was about to be exposed, including the very serious risk (as a first-time spinner) of rhabdomyolysis;

c) even though he had never previously engaged in any spinning at all, they placed him in a non-beginner class along with much more advanced spinners;

d) they placed him in a 45-minute class, which was 50 percent longer in duration than the 30-minute limit which spinning provides and that professionals had been cautioned and urged to adhere to for first-time spinners (37, p. 284).

The defendant filed a motion for summary judgment based on several factors related to the admissibility of expert testimony and documents regarding industry standards. The court denied this motion and dates were set for the pretrial conference and trial.

SPOTLIGHT CASE

Scheck v. Soul Cycle
No. 104046/10, 2012 LEXIS 3719 (N.Y. Misc., 2012)

FACTS

Historical Facts:

While both Mr. and Mrs. Scheck were participating in their first indoor cycling class at Soul Cycle, Mr. Scheck was injured. About five or ten minutes into the class, the instructor of the class, Marybeth Regan, told the class to stand up for the next exercise. In doing so, Mr. Scheck stated that the machine grabbed his right leg and pulled it around and that the pedals kept revolving all while his feet were strapped in. He heard a "pop" and felt an intense pain. He was taken to the hospital by ambulance, where it was discovered that he had torn the quadriceps muscle in his right leg.

The couple was instructed to arrive 15 minutes prior to the class so a staff member could explain everything carefully so nothing would go wrong. After arriving at the facility, an employee, who was not instructing the class, approached the couple to ask about their indoor cycling experience. When the couple noted that neither of them have participated in such a class, the employee suggested they sit in the back of the class in order to watch what everyone was doing. The employee adjusted Mr. Scheck's seat for him and showed him where the brake on the bike was located but did not provide instructions on how to use the brake. Noticing Mr. Scheck was not wearing proper shoes, she instructed him to go get a pair of bike shoes from the front desk, which he did.

After this very brief introduction of the class by the employee, the instructor Marybeth helped Mrs. Scheck get her bike ready for the class. She spent a lot of time with her and provided her instructions on how to use the resistance, where the emergency brake is, and assured her that there is no need to keep up with anyone else. However, she does not recall providing Mr. Scheck with the same instructions. She did recall that she "always asks beginners to raise their hand so she can keep an eye on them…but does not recall if Mr. Scheck raised his hand or, if he did, whether she saw him" (p. 8).

Madison Warren, the front desk associate who was working on the day the incident occurred, testified that when purchasing classes online as Mrs. Scheck did, someone can purchase more than one class, or classes for more than one person. It is required, however, that the person making the purchase must check a box indicating he/she has seen the waiver before completing the transaction. A hard copy of the waiver is at the front desk for each participant to sign upon arrival, however, she was not sure if the Schecks were each handed a copy of the waiver when they arrived.

Ms. Warren also testified that "the instructor teaches to the skill level of the class…and instructors usually warn beginners not to get up out of the saddle" (p. 7). In addition, she testified that the "Soul Cycle training manual requires that new

Scheck continued...

spinners be given certain preliminary instructions that apparently were not provided to Mr. Scheck" (p. 15). The facility did not keep a log of who trains each new participant.

Procedural Facts:
Mr. Scheck, and his wife Mrs. Scheck, filed a complaint against the defendant Soul Cycle for improper instruction and supervision on how to use the equipment. Mr. Scheck claimed that the danger of this activity was not readily apparent and was increased by the defendant's actions. In its motion for summary judgment, Soul Cycle contended that the complaint should be dismissed "because Mr. Scheck, by voluntarily participating in Soul Cycle's spin class assumed the risks inherent to the participation of that recreational activity, thereby relieving…any duty to prevent the type of accident he complains of" (p. 3).

ISSUE
Was the doctrine of primary assumption of risk an effective defense to protect the defendant Soul Cycle?

COURT'S RULING
No, the court found that the plaintiff did not assume the risks inherent in participating in a spin class. The defendant's motion for summary judgment was denied.

COURT'S REASONING
Citing previous case law regarding the primary assumption of risk doctrine, the court stated "A participant in a sporting activity is held to have consented to the risks inherent in it if the risks of the activity are fully comprehended or perfectly obvious and that participants…have consented, by their participation, to those injury-causing events which are known, apparent or reasonably foreseeable consequences of the participation" (p. 15). However, the court indicated that the use of a gym facility is not participation in a sporting event and that the level of experience of the plaintiff must be considered. Mr. Scheck was a neophyte.

In addition, the court stated that "A participant in a recreational activity will not be deemed to have assumed unreasonably increased risks…the defendant has a duty to make the conditions as safe as they appear to be…Thus, when measuring the defendant's duty to a plaintiff, the risks undertaken by the plaintiff also have to be considered…" (p. 14). The court concluded that the "Plaintiff has raised triable issues of fact whether the activity he agreed to participate in was safe as appeared to be and whether he assumed the risks which he was subjected to…There are also triable issues of fact whether the defendants properly instructed him in how to use the equipment" (p. 16-17).

Lessons Learned from *Scheck*

Legal
- The primary assumption of risk defense was not an effective defense for the defendant in this case because the indoor cycling activity was not a sporting activity and the plaintiff was a novice and, thus, did not fully understand and appreciate the inherent risks.

- The failure to instruct the plaintiff and follow the instructions for beginners in the Soul Cycle manual created a situation that increased the risks over and above those inherent in the activity (unreasonably increased risks).

- Because it was unclear if the plaintiff signed the waiver, it was not an issue in this case that the court addressed. If the plaintiff did sign the waiver, it might have been an effective defense, except this case occurred in New York which has a statute that prohibits health club waivers.

Risk Management/Injury Prevention
- Novices, especially when participating in an activity that is complex regarding its safety, need to be formally instructed on how to perform the activity prior to participation. In addition, immediately after or during the

Scheck continued...

instruction, the instructor should observe the novices performing the activity to help ensure they understand how to apply the safety instructions properly. Offering beginner indoor cycling classes also is a wise approach.

▶ For activities that require quite a bit of instruction prior to participation, it would be best for facilities to have a document that includes a checklist of all the items that the instructor needs to cover for novices, and have the novices sign it acknowledging they have received the instruction. The instructor also signs and dates the document. This may serve as evidence to help strengthen the primary assumption of risk defense and prevent claims related to negligent instruction.

▶ Instructors should encourage beginners to participate in the front of the class, not in the back as in this case, so they can clearly observe and supervise the beginners. The instructor in this case just informed beginners to raise their hand. She did not know if the plaintiff raised his hand, perhaps because he was in the back of the room.

▶ Procedures need to be in place regarding the administration of a Waiver and Assumption of Risk document, which did not appear to occur in this case. For example, each participant needs to read and sign the document. See Chapter 4 for more information on protective legal documents.

Additional Group Exercise Programs: Injuries and Lawsuits

Based on recent studies, there appears to be an increase in the number of injuries or a high number of injuries in group exercise programs such as yoga, boot camp, and Zumba®. A brief description of some of these studies are described along with some examples of negligence cases involving these programs and Pilates and kickboxing programs.

Yoga. A study published in the *Orthopaedic Journal of Sports Medicine* (38) investigated the number and type of yoga injuries between 2001 and 2014. Using NEISS data (injury data collected by hospital emergency department visits), the authors found that there were 29,590 yoga-related injuries during this time period. The trunk was the most frequent injured (46.6%) with sprain/strain accounting for the majority of the diagnoses. The overall injury rate almost doubled, increasing from 9.55 per 100,000 participants in 2001 to 17.01 per 100,000 participants in 2014. It was greatest in those 65 years and older (57.9/100,000). The authors explain that the higher injury rate among older adults could be due to biological changes such as reduced muscle mass, flexibility, and strength. However, because there was an increase in the number of injuries in all age groups, the authors explain that the lack of qualified instructors is, likely, a potential cause. With the increase in yoga popularity, there has been an increase in the number of certified yoga instructors. The authors state that there is a potential lack of proper education, even for certified instructors, citing other studies indicating certified training programs do not prepare instructors on how to prevent injury. The authors conclude that yoga has many health benefits but to help prevent injuries, individuals need to consult with their physician, participate in classes taught by well-qualified instructors, and not engage in poses that are beyond their physical limitations.

A similar study was conducted in Victoria, Australia (38a). This study found a 375% increase in the number of yoga-related injury cases from July 2009 to June 2016. Most cases involved females between 20 and 39 years old with the most common injuries being dislocations/sprains/strains followed by fractures. The author recommended future nationwide research and an investigation into risk management strategies of yoga service providers to minimize injury risks.

Note: *Given the increased popularity in hot yoga (Bikram yoga) and its potential increased risk of injuries, fitness managers and exercise professionals need to be aware of specific precautions that need to be in place prior to offering these classes—see an article (39) published by the American Council on Exercise on this topic.*

Yoga Case: *In* Webster v. Claremont Yoga *(40), the plaintiff, Amalia Webster, claimed that her yoga instructor Kurt Bumiller, injured her several times during the class. "He placed a belt around her waist and right leg to help her position her right leg over her left, which plaintiff claimed was painful. He pushed down on her lower back while* *she was in a 'cow position,' which plaintiff claimed hurt her knee. Plaintiff contended that while she was lying on her back, Bumiller twisted her neck to both sides three times, which she asserted caused her pain" (p. 286) and a neck injury.*

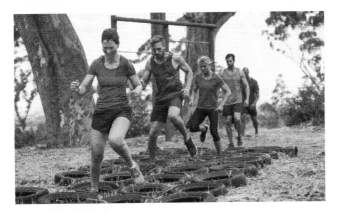

Boot Camp. Boot camp classes mimic military-style training programs and often include advanced or intense exercises such as squat thrusts and sprints as well as exercises performed with equipment such as tractor tires, anchor ropes, wood blocks, and kettle bells. In an article titled Beware of Boot Camp Fitness Classes (41), orthopedic surgeon, Ty E. Richardson who has treated dozens of patients with boot camp injuries, provides insight regarding these injuries. His worst injury occurred to a 30-year-old woman who fell off a wood block while performing jumps. She fractured her elbow requiring surgery resulting in loss of motion in that arm. He also has treated injuries such as meniscal tears, rotator cuff tears, Achilles tendon ruptures, lumbar strains, wrist fractures, and stress fractures in the foot. He stated that many of the injuries are due to improper execution (i.e., individuals do not have advanced motor skills to safely execute them). The classes need to address individual abilities but often have no screening process, health review, or medical history. "You simply sign a waiver and start throwing around some truck tires" (p. 3). He provides several recommendations including finding a class that is well supervised and addresses individual fitness levels.

Boot Camp Case: *In* Burgos v. Active Health and Fitness Club *(42), the plaintiff, Jeannette Burgos in her $2.5 million lawsuit filed against the defendants (the gym, instructor Emil Paolucci*

and his Hard Bodies Extreme Fitness program) was severely injured when a 400-pound tire fell on her foot crushing her ankle. She alleged that the defendants should have known of the dangerous conditions associated with exercises using very heavy tires and overcrowding of their classes.

Zumba®. Zumba® is a popular program with about 14 million participants in 150 countries (43). Based on one study (43), one in four participants experienced injuries with the knees being most common injury site (44%) followed by the ankles (14%) and shoulders (14%). The authors concluded that there is a need to improve Zumba® routines, instructor training, and counseling from health care providers to reduce the risk of injuries.

Pilates and Kickboxing. The following two cases describe injuries incurred in Pilates and kickboxing classes.

Pilates case: *In* Marchese v. Gamble *(44), the plaintiff, Frank Marchese, alleged that he was injured at a Pilates studio (PHIT Pilates Studio) while engaged in exercise under the supervision of the defendant, Erin Gamble. He claimed, "that his injuries were caused by Gamble's negligence in that she failed to properly set up exercise equipment, failed to make sure that the equipment was safe and secure and failed to properly supervise and assist" (p. 1) him when using the equipment.*

Kickboxing case: *In* Honeycutt v. Meridian Sports Club *(45), the plaintiff, Tanya Honeycutt in her first kickboxing class, claimed she was injured when her instructor, Hakeem Alexander, assisted her in performing a roundhouse kick. While attempting to guide her through the movement, "Alexander held on to Honeycutt's right leg, with her left leg locked and planted on the floor. Alexander told Honeycutt to rotate, open her hips, and turn her planted foot outward to allow for a pivot before the kicking maneuver. When she rotated her left knee, she felt a pop and the knee gave out. She suffered a ruptured ACL which required physical therapy, surgery, and four months of rehabilitation" (p. 255).*

KEY POINT

Legal Liability Reasons for Offering Beginner-Level Classes

Given the increased popularity in group exercise classes that are considered high intensity and/or advanced (e.g., indoor cycling, yoga, boot camp), it would be best for fitness facilities to offer beginner-level classes. Many of the injuries described in these group exercise classes involved instructors having novices perform exercises beyond their abilities.

In his analysis of the *Honeycutt* case (kickboxing case), attorney and Professor John Wolohan (46) stated that activity providers "need to separate students into appropriate class levels. Not only are beginner students at greater risk of injury when put into classes designed for intermediate or advanced students, such action also places the club at risk for liability" (p. 19). He also states that instructors who fail to properly instruct beginners, it is likely that courts will find the instructor and club not only negligent, but potentially grossly negligent.

In addition, as explained by legal scholar van der Smissen (2), specific supervision (instruction) provides the participant an opportunity to gain knowledge of the activity, an understanding of one's own capabilities, and an appreciation of the potential injuries so that he/she can assume the inherent risks of the activity. Providing proper instruction and adequate experience for beginners, as well as documentation of such, can strengthen the primary assumption of risk defense for defendants.

Youth Exercise Programs

Many fitness facilities offer exercise programs for youth. It is essential that these programs are **developmentally appropriate** and are instructed and supervised by exercise professionals that are well-educated and trained. Developmentally appropriate programs based on age are generally provided in the 2018 Physical Activity Guidelines as shown in Exhibit 8-2. However, for more specific information, exercise professionals should refer to resources such as *Developmental Physical Education for All Children: Theory into Practice* (47). This book addresses proper program design/delivery for all ages as well as for children who have health risks and

disabilities. An ACSM book, *Essentials of Youth Fitness*, published by Human Kinetics in 2020, is also recommended. Authors are Faigenbaum, Lloyd, and Oliver.

In the spotlight case, *Lotz v. The Claremont Group*, the instruction and supervision provided for the youth activity was improper for a variety of reasons. The appellate court stated that neither the waiver defense nor the primary assumption of risk defense protected the defendants. The conduct of the youth instructor (a) was considered grossly negligent, and (b) increased the risks of injury beyond those inherent in the activity

In addition to developmentally appropriate activities led by credentialed and competent instructors, fitness facilities need to follow various published standards of practice (e.g., standards, guidelines, position papers)

Exhibit 8-2: Key 2018 Physical Activities Guidelines for Children*

Preschool-Aged Children

▶ Preschool-aged children (ages 3 through 5 years) should be physically active throughout the day to enhance growth and development.

▶ Adult caregivers of preschool-aged children should encourage active play that includes a variety of activity types.

Children and Adolescents

▶ It is important to provide young people opportunities and encouragement to participate in physical activities that are appropriate for their age, that are enjoyable, and that offer variety.

▶ Children and adolescents ages 6 through 17 years should do 60 minutes (1 hour) or more of moderate-to-vigorous physical activity daily:
  - Aerobic: Most of the 60 minutes or more per day should be either moderate- or vigorous-intensity aerobic physical activity and should include vigorous-intensity physical activity on at least 3 days a week.
  - Muscle-strengthening: As part of their 60 minutes or more of daily physical activity, children and adolescents should include muscle-strengthening physical activity on at least 3 days a week.
  - Bone-strengthening: As part of their 60 minutes or more of daily physical activity, children and adolescents should include bone-strengthening physical activity on at least 3 days a week.

*23, pp. 47-48

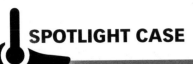

SPOTLIGHT CASE

Lotz v. Claremont Club
No. B242399, 2013 LEXIS 5748 (Cal. Ct. App., 2013)

FACTS

Historical Facts:

Upon joining the Claremont Club, Thomas Lotz completed a family membership information form and signed a Membership Agreement as well as a Waiver of Liability, Assumption of Risk and Indemnity Agreement that contained a provision stating: "This agreement constitutes my sole and only agreement respecting release, waiver of liability, assumption of risk, and indemnity concerning my involvement in The Claremont Club…I, for myself, my spouse…hereby release, waive, discharge, and covenant not to sue The Claremont Club…for liability from any and all claims including the negligence of the Claremont Club, resulting in damages or personal injury…" (p. 4). Although the waiver identified certain activities provided at the Club, it did not include dodgeball. The family membership was for himself, his wife Deborah, and their two children.

When checking her 10-year-old son, Nicholas, into the Club's childcare InZone program, Deborah was not informed that her son might be playing dodgeball as part of the InZone activities. However, Qasem, an 18-year-old employee of the Club, took the children to a racquetball court to play dodgeball. He had never worked in the InZone program nor had the Club provided him any training to work with or supervise children. During the game, anywhere between three and six rubber balls were being thrown at one time. About 20 minutes into the game, Qasem threw a ball hard and fast toward Nicholas hitting him in the face. His head was slammed into the wall behind him leaving tooth marks on the wall. Nicholas suffered multiple dental injuries. Qasem was disciplined for violating the Club's childcare policies and a policy that supervisors do not participate in dodgeball games with children.

Procedural Facts:

In their complaint, the plaintiffs alleged both negligence and gross negligence on part of the Club by: "a. hiring, employing, training, entrusting, instructing, and supervising defendant Adam Qasem; b. failing to adequately protect children under the care of defendant Adam Qasem; c. participating in a game of dodge ball in an unreasonably forceful and dangerous manner so as to endanger the health, safety, and welfare of children placed by their parents into the care of the defendants" (p. 8). The Club moved for summary judgment based on the waiver and the primary assumption of risk defenses.

The trial court granted summary judgment in favor of defendants. The trial court ruled that a release signed by Nicholas's father barred the plaintiffs' claims and there was no evidence showing the Club's conduct amounted to gross negligence. The court further ruled the primary assumption of risk doctrine barred the plaintiffs' claims. The plaintiffs appealed.

ISSUE

Did the trial court err when it granted summary judgment in favor of the defendants?

COURT'S RULING

Yes. The appellate court reversed and remanded with directions for the trial court to vacate (dismiss) its order to grant summary judgment to the defendants and to enter a new order to deny summary judgment.

COURT'S REASONING

Regarding the waiver, the appellants (plaintiffs) demonstrated a triable issue of fact as to whether the language within the waiver contemplated the type of injuries suffered by Nicholas. According to the Club's written policies, dodgeball was not among the activities permitted to be played on the Club's racquetball courts, nor were Deborah or Thomas informed that Nicholas would be playing dodgeball. Furthermore, the club maintained a policy to preclude supervisors from engaging in dodgeball games with children. At a minimum, evidence of the employee's conduct violated the Club's written policy

Lotz continued...

concerning the use of the racquetball court, participating in the game, and lack of supervision of the game. Based on this evidence, the appellants raised a triable issue of fact as to whether the waiver would be void against public policy since the waiver did not clearly and explicitly release the club from liability for Nicholas's injuries. Citing previous case law regarding ambiguity of the waiver, the court stated, "if a release is ambiguous, and it is not clear the parties contemplated redistributing the risk causing the plaintiffs injury, then the contractual ambiguity should be construed against the drafter, voiding the purported release" (p. 24).

Regarding gross negligence, the court stated that gross negligence could be found on the "basis of the Club's failure to address the repeated violations of its own policy prohibiting dodgeball on the racquetball courts, failure to implement rules or policies designed to protect those playing dodgeball and failure to provide any training to individuals assigned to supervise the children in its childcare program" (pp. 28-29). The appellants offered expert opinion that "the injury to Nicholas Lotz occurred during an extreme departure from what must be considered as the ordinary standard of conduct when children are playing dodgeball and are supposed to be...supervised" (p. 28). The court concluded that triable issues existed as to whether the conduct of the defendants was grossly negligent and, therefore, outside the scope of any release in the waiver.

Regarding the primary assumption of risk doctrine, the court stated that Nicholas could not assume the risk of being hit in the head with the ball. Although being hit with a ball is one of the objectives of dodgeball and hence an inherent risk, the defendants increased that risk in numerous ways (e.g., the Club's failures described in the previous paragraph). Citing previous case law, the court stated, "it is well established that defendants have a duty to use due care not to increase the risks to a participant over and above those inherent in the sport" (p. 29). The defendants argued that their conduct might have increased the severity of Nicholas's injuries as opposed to increasing the risk of injury. However, the court disagreed stating that the severity of the injury is not applicable to the primary assumption of risk doctrine when a defendant increases the risks beyond those inherent in the sport.

Lessons Learned from *Lotz*

Legal

- Waivers need to be carefully written as demonstrated in this case in which the activity of dodgeball was not included in the waiver making it ambiguous and unenforceable.

- As the court ruled in this case, a waiver will not protect defendants from their own gross negligence.

- Fitness facilities that repeatedly fail to follow their own policies can be faced with gross negligence claims.

- Based on this court's ruling, the primary assumption of risk defense is ineffective when a defendant increases the risks of injury to a participant over and above those risks that are inherent in the activity.

- Although not an issue raised in this case, in most states parents/guardians cannot sign a waiver on behalf of their children.

Risk Management/Injury Prevention

- Youth activities need to be instructed and properly supervised by well-trained and mature adults.

- Youth activities that increase the risk of injury over and above the risks inherent in the activity should be avoided.

- Safety policies need to be in place for all youth activities and well-communicated to all children and their parents/guardians prior to participation.

- There are many alternative activities to dodgeball that are safer for children. However, if a fitness center is going to offer dodgeball, several safety measures need to be established (e.g., use a softer ball other than a rubber ball and adopt rules published by professional organizations).

- Be sure parents/guardians are informed of the types of activities in which their children will be participating in a childcare program or other structured activities.

regarding youth programs. The resource by Rahl (48), recommended in previous chapters, describes these publications for infants/toddlers and school-aged children such as those published by American Academy of Pediatricians, U.S. Department of Health and Human Services, and National Association of Sport and Physical Education. Other organizations have also published standards of practice for youth exercise programs such as the YMCA, NSCA, ACSM, AFAA, MFA, and IHRSA.

Childcare Facilities

Before offering childcare, it will be necessary to determine if there are any local or state laws that regulate childcare services provided in a fitness facility. For example, there are states that grant licensure exemptions for childcare facilities that provide short term care and when the parent is located on the premises (49). Fitness managers need to realize the importance of providing proper instruction and supervision in their childcare facilities. In *Lyle v. 24 Hour Fitness* (50), a four-year-old child fractured her elbow, requiring substantial medical treatment, when she fell off the playscape in the childcare area called Kids Club. The mother of the child, who was exercising in the facility at the time, was not notified until she picked up her child about 50 minutes after the incident. The mother, Jada Lyle, brought the following claims against the defendant facility: (a) negligence (vicarious liability claim due to the negligent conduct of the childcare supervisors), and (b) negligent training and supervision of the childcare staff members (direct liability claims). The court granted the defendant's motion for summary judgment for the direct liability claims but denied it for the vicarious liability claim. Lyle was unable to show that the direct liability claims such as the negligent training of the childcare staff members, were the cause of her daughter's injury. The defendant argued that it provided an extensive formal training for employees who supervise the Kids Club program. However, the testimony of an expert witness for the plaintiff, a specialist in child safety, is relevant for all fitness managers and supervisors that provide employee training which included the following:

Training is not just "sit and get." It's not just, "go to a computer program and punch through the buttons until it says you passed." Training is knowledge that

people who are caring for children can understand the expectations and do what they are expected to do. Training is not a thing that you pass, it's a level of competency that typically involves ... actual hands-on observation and coaching as needed so that a supervisor knows there's a level of mastery (p. 5).

Staff training, covered in Chapters 2 and 5, includes the Four Ps—prepare, present, practice, and post-training follow-up. It is essential that managers and supervisors leading staff training programs conduct post-training follow-up to assess whether their staff members have gained the necessary competency to safely and effectively perform their jobs.

Youth Sports Programs

It is beyond the scope of this textbook to cover injury and legal liability issues related to youth sports. However, a brief discussion of some helpful resources is provided for fitness facilities that offer youth sports programs. Unfortunately, the participation in youth sports has declined in recent years. Although there are a variety reasons for the decline, high costs and poor coaching have been listed as top reasons (51). Only about one-third of coaches are trained in core competencies and safety/injury prevention (51). Many injuries such as overuse injuries, heat injuries, etc. can be prevented with proper coaching (i.e., proper instruction and supervision). In a comprehensive article—Overuse Injuries in Youth Sport: Legal and Social Responsibilities (52)—the authors state: "Overuse injuries are increasingly prevalent within youth sports, can lead to lifelong disabilities, and are almost entirely preventable" (p. 151). They argue that policies need to be enacted to educate parents, coaches, schools, and organizations about overuse injuries. Various organizations are working toward enhancing the safety of youth sports. A few of these are:

a) **Safe Stars**—a collaborative initiative between the Program for Injury Prevention in Youth Sports at Vanderbilt University and the Tennessee Department of Health. Teams can earn bronze, silver, and gold safety ratings for meeting certain safety standards. (https://www.tn.gov/health/health-program-areas/fhw/vipp/safe-stars-initiative.html)

b) **Youth Sports Safety Alliance**—convened by the National Athletic Trainers' Association (NATA) in 2009 with the goal to make America's sports programs safer for young adults. It created a National Action Plan to meet this goal. (https://youthsportssafetyalliance.org).

c) **The National Youth Sports Health & Safety Institute**—an organization that partners with Sanford Health and ACSM. Its mission is to advance and disseminate the latest research and evidence-based education, recommendations and policy to enhance the experience, development, health and safety of our youth in sports. (http://nyshsi.org).

Note: *The YMCA has been providing youth sport programs for many years. They have established many safety recommendations (53) regarding youth sports that might be helpful for other organizations offering youth sports.*

Strength and Conditioning Programs

Exertional heat illness and exertional rhabdomyolysis are well known serious injuries that can occur while participating in sport conditioning programs. Even though many believe these injuries are preventable by following important safety procedures, they are still occurring. Some of these injuries have resulted in death or permanent disability and costly litigations. This discussion will describe some of the lawsuits that collegiate athletes (or their family members) have made against the strength and conditioning coaches and other athletic personnel as well as the academic institutions. In the following spotlight case, Ereck Plancher was a football player at the University of Central Florida (UCF). The medical records at UCF showed that Ereck had sickle cell trait, but unfortunately precautions were not taken during an intense workout. Proper precautions would have helped minimize his increased risk of injuries, especially those associated with intense workouts in hot environments. In addition, proper emergency procedures were not carried out. Following the *UCF Athletics Association v. Plancher* case, additional heat injury cases are described as well as cases involving exertional rhabdomyolysis.

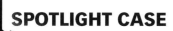 **SPOTLIGHT CASE**

UCF Athletics Association v. Plancher
121 So.3d 1097 (Fla. Dist. Ct. App., 2013)

FACTS

Historical Facts:

University of Central Florida (UCF) football player, Ereck Plancher, died while participating in a series of conditioning drills. During a workout of intense mat drills, Ereck Plancher experienced several signs and symptoms of overexertion including a loss of balance resulting in a collapse. Instead of properly addressing these signs and symptoms, the coaches allegedly responded by making him stand up and complete the drills. The coaches observed his deteriorating condition. At the conclusion of the drills, Ereck collapsed a second time and died (Herbert).

Prior to playing football, all UCF football players were required to sign an agreement entitled UCFAA INC. SPORTS MEDICINE DEPARTMENT Medical Examination & Authorization Waiver. Ereck Plancher signed this waiver that, in part, included the following:

"...Because of the aforementioned dangers of participating in any athletic activity, I recognize the importance of following all instructions of the coaching staff, strength and conditioning staff, and/or Sports Medicine Department. Furthermore, I understand that the possibility of injury, including catastrophic injury, does exist even though proper rules and techniques are followed to the fullest...

UCF Athletic Association continued...

> In consideration of the University of Central Florida Athletic Association, Inc. permitting me to participate in intercollegiate athletics and to engage in all activities and travel related to my sport, I hereby voluntarily assume all risks associated with participation and agree to exonerate, save harmless and release the University of Central Florida Athletic Association, Inc., its agents, servants, trustees, and employees from any and all liability, any medical expenses not covered by the University of Central Florida Athletic Association's athletics medical insurance coverage…" (pp. 1100-1101).

Procedural Facts:

The parents of Ereck Plancher filed a wrongful death lawsuit against the University of Central Florida Board of Trustees and the UCF Athletics Association (UCFAA) making numerous negligence claims such as:

- Failing to provide proper supervisors during the mat drills who should recognize when a player is in physical distress;
- Failure of training staff to appropriately administer medical assistance…in a timely manner;
- Failing to provide its players with known sickle cell trait with proper access to water…pursuant NCCA guidelines (Herbert, p. 1).

At trial, the Orange County, Florida medical examiner and three experts hired by the Plancher family attorneys testified that Plancher died from complications of sickle cell trait, but UCF officials contended that it was a heart ailment that caused his death. Evidence from four UCF players recalled the strenuous workout and testified that Plancher struggled throughout the workout. One of these players indicated that the workout was "punishment" for coming back from spring vacation out of shape (Ereck Plancher Appeal to be Heard).

The jury awarded the Planchers damages in the amount of $10 million. UCFAA appealed claiming that the trial court erred when it denied UCFAA's motion for summary judgment based on the waiver that Ereck Plancher signed, and when it entered summary judgment against UCFAA on the issue of limited sovereign immunity.

ISSUES

Did the trial court err on the issues related to (A) the waiver, and (B) limited sovereign immunity?

COURT'S RULING

(A) No. The appellate court agreed with the trial court on the issue of the waiver indicating that it did not absolve the defendants from their own negligence.

(B) Yes. The appellate court reversed the trial court's ruling regarding sovereign immunity stating that the UCFAA was entitled to limited sovereign immunity.

COURT'S REASONING

Regarding the waiver, the appellate court agreed with the trial court stating that the exculpatory clause "did not expressly inform Ereck that he would be contracting away his right to sue UCFAA for its own negligence" (p.1101). According to the appellate court, the ambiguous language alone would be enough to find the clause unenforceable, but the language within the waiver could also "have easily led Ereck to believe that UCFAA would be supervising his training and instructing him properly (non-negligently), and that he was only being asked to sign the exculpatory clause to cover injuries inherent in the sport" (p. 1102).

According to a Florida statute on limited sovereign immunity, "the state and its agencies and subdivisions are liable for tort claims in the same manner and to the same extent as a private individual under like circumstance, but the liability shall not include punitive damages…Additionally, neither the state nor its agencies are liable to pay a claim or judgment by any one person that exceeds $200,000" (§ 768.28(5). Fla. Stat.). UCFAA, a private corporation, was

UCF Athletic Association continued...

created by UCF in 2003 as a University direct-support organization to administer the UCF's athletic department. In its motion for summary judgment, UCFAA claimed that it was subject to UCF's governance and operational control. Therefore, the sovereign immunity protection that UCF receives should also be extended to UCFAA. According to the appellate court, "the key factor in determining whether a private corporation is an instrumentality of the state for sovereign immunity purposes is the level of governmental control over the performance and day-to-day operations of the corporation" (p. 1106). The trial court ruled that UCFAA had not been substantially controlled by UCF, but after reviewing the evidence, the appellate court concluded that UCFAA functions as an instrumentality of UCF and is entitled to limited sovereign immunity. Therefore, the appellate court ruled that the judgment against UCFAA shall be reduced to $200,000.

The Planchers sought a review of the appellate court's ruling. In its review, the Florida Supreme Court (*Plancher v. UCF Athletics Association, Inc., et al.,* 175 So.3d 724) agreed with the appellate court's holding that UCFAA was entitled to limited sovereign immunity. However, the Supreme Court indicated rather than requiring a reduction of judgment as stated by the appellate court, "we remand for entry of judgment corresponding to the jury's award of damages but limiting UCFAA's liability to $200,000..." and that the "Planchers must look to the Legislature to collect any amount awarded above the statutory cap" (p. 729).

Herbert DL. One Football Player's Wrongful Death Suit Settled and Another Filed. *The Sports, Parks & Recreation Law Reporter,* 23(1), 1, 4-5, 2009.

Ereck Plancher Appeal to be Heard. Associated Press, August 13, 2014. Available at: https://www.espn.com/college-football/story/_/id/11348583/central-florida-knights-case-involving-ereck-plancher-reviewed-florida-supreme-court. Accessed June 6, 2019.

Lessons Learned from *UCF Athletics Association*

Legal

▶ For a waiver to be enforceable, the exculpatory clause must be explicitly written, e.g., it must contain language that clearly and unambiguously absolves the defendants of their own negligence.

▶ Most states have sovereign immunity statutes that limit the amount that state agencies pay in damages. Their main purpose is to protect taxpayers.

▶ Although plaintiffs can seek additional compensation above the limits stated in the sovereign immunity statutes from their state legislatures, it is rarely approved.

Risk Management/Injury Prevention

▶ Strength and conditioning coaches need to be properly credentialed and competent in order to design and deliver safe conditioning programs for their athletes.

▶ Strength and conditioning coaches need to know the medical conditions of their athletes and take necessary precautions accordingly. Note: In this case, there was conflicting evidence as to whether Ereck Plancher had been informed that he had sickle cell trait and if the coaches knew he had sickle cell trait. However, UCF did know—it was documented in Ereck's medical records.

▶ Athletes with sickle cell trait are at greater risk for heat, dehydration, and other injuries. Therefore, taking precautions (e.g., closely monitoring exercise intensity and environmental conditions, providing adequate rest periods and access to water) to prevent such injuries are essential.

▶ Strength and conditioning coaches need to be well-informed of the sickle cell trait guidelines published by the National Collegiate Athletic Association (NCAA), the National Athletic Trainers' Association (NATA), and other professional organizations.

▶ A written emergency action plan is needed, and strength and conditioning coaches need to be well-trained on how to properly carry out the plan.

Heat Injury Cases

Although heat injuries can occur with participation in a variety of sports, they appear to be more common among football athletes. According to the National Center for Catastrophic Sport Injury Research (54), there were 148 football players between 1960 through 2018 who died from heat stroke. Between 1995 and 2018 "64 football players have died from heat stroke (47 high school, 13 college, 2 professional, and 2 organized youth). Ninety percent of recorded heat stroke deaths occurred during practice" (54, p. 16). The following two case examples (Lee and McNair) describe a heat injury suffered by a basketball player and a heat stroke death of a football player.

In *Lee v. Louisiana Board of Trustees for State Colleges* (55), it was reported that Grambling State University (GSU) in Louisiana offered Jacobee Lee a full basketball scholarship. He arrived at the program on August 12, 2009 which was three days after the required August 9th report date. On August 14th, members of the team participated in a 45-minute unofficial weight-lifting workout with coaching staff members present. After this workout, assistant basketball coach Stephen Portland told Lee and seven other players they had to run around the university campus (four to four and a half miles) because they had reported late for the fall semester. They had to finish the run, called the Tiger Mix, in 40 minutes or would need to complete it on another day. Coach Portland followed the runners in golf cart. No fluids were available on the golf cart "although it was over 90 degrees" and "no athletic trainers or medical personnel were present as they did not know about the run" (p. 181). Lee's teammate Henry White and Lee both passed out in the gym after completing the run. Both White and Lee were transported to the hospital by ambulance. White died several days later as a result of the severity of the heatstroke he suffered (see *Williams v. Board of Super's of University of Louisiana System*, 135 So.3d 804) and Lee was diagnosed with elevated creatine phosphokinase (CPK), heat exhaustion and mild rhabdomyolysis.

Lee went back to GSU after his discharge from the hospital but did not rejoin the team. He did poorly academically and withdrew from GSU in 2010. In February 2010, Lee was again hospitalized a few days after playing in an independent basketball tournament with a fever and CPK levels of 7955. The rheumatologist who treated Lee believed the heat injury (heat stroke according to his testimony) he suffered back in August of 2009 caused him to suffer permanent irreversible damage to his skeletal muscles and exercise tolerance, which would limit his future job opportunities. In August of 2010, Lee filed a Petition for Damages against the Board of Supervisors of the University of Louisiana System for personal injuries and damages as the result of the negligent conduct of the defendants. After a seven-day trial in March 2016, the jury awarded Lee $2,529,229 in damages as follows:

Past and future physical pain and suffering . . $200,000.00
Past and future mental pain and suffering . $1,000,000.00
Past medical expenses. $15,229.00
Future medical expenses $24,000.00
Past lost wages $90,000.00
Loss of earning capacity $600,000.00
Loss of enjoyment of life. $600,000.00

Total = $2,529.229.00 (55, p. 183)

In April 2016, Lee and the defendants filed proposed judgments. In February of 2017, the trial court ruled that items 1, 2, 6, and 7 above were all collectively subject to the state's $500,000 limitations on general damages (i.e., Louisiana Governmental Governmental Claims Act (LSA-R.S. 13:5101) that addresses **sovereign immunity** for substantive tort liability against the state, a state agency, or a political ubdivision of the state). Therefore, total damages came to $629,229.00 ($500,000 plus items 3, 4, and 5 above). Upon appeal, the First Circuit Court of Appeals in Louisiana upheld the damages awarded and added the costs of the appeal.

Several experts testified in this case, including the head strength and conditioning coach at GSU between 2008 and 2012. He stated that no one discussed with him the Tiger Mix, and, if he had been aware of it, he would have advised against it. He testified that the "Tiger Mix was a blatant disregard for athletic rules and regulations and National Collegiate Athletic Association (NCAA) policies. He stated that pursuant to NCAA bylaws, structured activities are not allowed before the first day of academics in a school year" (55, p. 187). He also stated that "athletes, especially freshman athletes, want to please their coaches and will do whatever is asked of them…" (p. 187).

In an article titled, "College Pays for Coach Who Used Exertion as Punishment" (56), author Kristi Schoepfer-Bochicchio, J.D., described the *Lee* case. She provided a compelling opinion regarding the harmful impacts of excessive physical activity, especially when combined with the impacts of heat. She states "the death of White and the sustained harm suffered by Lee should have been a clear example that student-athletes are exposed to significant physical risks when coaches implement extreme practice measures. Yet, using extreme physical activity as punishment is a coaching strategy that remains commonplace, despite the incidence rate of harm to student-athletes" (p. 25). Her opinion is "spot on" given that Lee's injury occurred in 2009 and that heat injury deaths have occurred since then including the death of Jordan McNair in 2018.

Jordan McNair Case. As a member of the University of Maryland's football team, Jordan McNair participated in the first summer organized workout on May 29, 2018. Sadly, it was his last workout—he died 15 days later from complications due to heat stroke. The University conducted independent investigations that resulted in two reports: (a) An Independent Evaluation of Procedures and Protocols Related to the June 2018 Death of a University of Maryland Football Student-Athlete (57), and (b) Report to the University System of Maryland of an Independent Investigation of the University of Maryland Football Program (58). The major purpose of the second investigation was to determine if the culture of the football program was as "toxic" as alleged in media reports. For example, an investigation by ESPN referred to a pattern of abuses by the Maryland coaching staff toward players and referred to the program as having a toxic culture (59). On August 14, 2018, before these reports were completed, Maryland President Wallace D. Loh stated that the university "accepts legal and moral responsibility for the mistakes that our training staff made on that fateful workout day of May 29, which of course led subsequently to his death" (60).

The first report described Jordan's McNair's injury and the actions and/or inactions of the coaches, trainers, and athletes. During an intense workout of running 110-yard wind sprints, McNair showed signs of exhaustion. A gap of 34 minutes occurred before he was taken off the field. The athletic trainers did not follow several emergency procedures including not immersing him in cold water. They did administer ice packs in an attempt to cool him down. He displayed symptoms for over an hour before EMS was called and there was an additional half hour before he was admitted to the hospital.

The second report (58) discussed several findings and recommendations. One of the findings was that Rick Court, the head strength and conditioning coach, "on too many occasions, acted in a manner inconsistent with the University's values and basic principles of respect for others" (p. 7). Although interviews with student-athletes and employees had positive things to say about Mr. Court, there were many comments about his abusive behavior (e.g., his words became "attacking" in nature). "This included challenging a player's manhood and hurling homophobic slurs (which Mr. Court denies but was recounted by many). Additionally, Mr. Court would attempt to humiliate players in front of their teammates by throwing food, weights, and on one occasion a trash can full of vomit…" (p. 8). In August of 2018, before this report was released, the University announced the removal of Mr. Court, but Court also resigned with a settlement (60). Another finding in this report described the failures of the head football coach DJ Durkin and the athletic department. The report found that "both Mr. Durkin and leadership in the Athletics Department share responsibility for the failure to supervise Mr. Court" (p. 8). In addition to Rick Court, several other individuals were also fired including DJ Durkin and two athletic trainers (61).

In April 2019, the University of Maryland announced it was committed to implementing all 27 recommendations in this report (62) which included the establishment of an Athletic Medicine Review Board to provide oversight of sports medicine, strength and conditioning, nutrition etc. The NCAA has published guidelines regarding independent medical care for college student-athletes (63). It was reported that both Durkin and Court had heavy influence, control or possibly a direct report over the football medical staff (64). Independent medical care may help prevent controversies that can occur with medical decisions. See *Class v. Towson University* (described in Chapter 3)—an ADA discrimination case brought by an athlete involving differing medical opinions with regard to his return to play after a heat injury.

Although the University of Maryland is commended for firing the wrongdoers and making important changes to help ensure the safety of their student-athletes, the University and the employees responsible for McNair's death may still face a lawsuit. In September 2018, the parents of Jordan McNair filed a notice of a possible lawsuit (65). They seek $30 million—$10 million each and another $10 million for Jordan's pain and suffering prior to his death. The document filed specifically listed head football coach DJ Durkin, Rick Court, and head athletic trainer Wes Robinson. The parents planned to make several claims including wrongful death, negligence, and gross negligence. The status of this possible lawsuit was unknown at the time this chapter was written.

High School Programs. In addition to addressing heat-related injuries in collegiate sports, they also need to be addressed in high school programs. Heat injury deaths are more prevalent in high school football programs than in collegiate football programs. Although best practices (e.g., position papers on heat injuries published by professional organizations on the prevention and treatment of athletic heat injuries) have been available for many years, it appears that many programs are still not following them. In June 2019, a high school football player in Florida died during conditioning drills in the heat (66). A law firm representing the family of the player sent a letter to the school requesting documents related to the workout. According to the school's superintendent, various failures occurred including incomplete paperwork and improper emergency procedures. The school employed an athletic trainer, but the trainer was not onsite when the player died. It was unknown at the time this chapter was written if the family filed a lawsuit. Although high school athletic programs have been encouraged to hire an athletic trainer at each school, trainers cannot be at every practice for all sports. They can, however, provide leadership to ensure that best practices are developed/implemented and that all coaching staff members are well-trained on how to properly carry them out. In addition, the Korey Stringer Institute provides state high school sports safety rankings to help incentivize high school programs to meet established policies related to best safety practices included in

the Inter-Association Task Force Document Preventing Sudden Death in Secondary School Athletics (67).

KEY POINT

Exertional Heat Injuries

Heat injuries and deaths are preventable according to many experts in the athletic field. Best practices regarding the prevention and treatment of heat injuries have been available (e.g., position papers published by professional organizations) for many years. However, too many strength and conditioning coaches and other athletic personnel are still not adhering to them or are not aware of them. Academic and certification preparation programs need to make a concerted effort to include knowledge and skills in this area. This was a recommendation from a study (68) that found collegiate strength and conditioning coaches lacked essential knowledge to prevent or recognize heat stroke (e.g., only 2.2% of the coaches surveyed scored 90% or higher on an assessment of heat stroke knowledge). The consequences of these injuries/deaths are not only devasting to the victims (athletes and their families) but also to academic institutions.

Exertional Rhabdomyolysis Cases

Many ER injuries have occurred due to intense training programs among student-athletes. Some of these that occurred between 2011 and 2019 include:

a) University of Iowa—13 football players, 2011 (69)
b) Ohio State University—6 women's lacrosse players, 2013 (70)
c) University of Oregon—3 football players, 2017 (71)
d) University of Nebraska—2 football players, 2018 (72)
e) University of Houston—12 women's soccer players, 2019 (73)

When serious, preventable injuries or deaths occur, there is often an investigation conducted by the university/college, as the University of Maryland conducted in the Jordan McNair case described above. These unfortunate events create a great deal of media attention and reflect negatively upon the athletic program and the institution. The investigations and policy changes that are made based on the investigative reports are costly. For example, the policy changes established at the University of Houston are expected to exceed $1 million (74). But the costs do not end there—costly litigation often follows as shown in the *Lee* case. One of the 13 football players at the University of Iowa and two of three players at the university of Oregon filed lawsuits.

Football player William Lowe at the University of Iowa filed a lawsuit that was eventually settled (75). He claimed he suffered acute renal failure and elevated creatine levels due to his ER diagnosis and continued to experience various mental and physical problems and mounting medical expenses. Interesting in this case were the findings in an internal, official report submitted to the Iowa state Board of Regents. It stated that the strength and conditioning coaches had no knowledge of ER (69). The report cleared all coaches, physicians, and trainers of any wrongdoing and provided recommendations including discontinuing the intense, high volume squat-lifting workout (69). Several questions arise regarding the knowledge/skills of the strength and conditioning coaches in this case. It is likely, in a Division I football program such as the University of Iowa, the strength and conditioning coaches possessed degrees and professional certifications in strength and conditioning. By 2011, they should all have known about ER and how to prevent it. At a minimum, they should have known about the signs and symptoms of overexertion through their educational and certification preparation programs. So why did they have the players perform another mandatory intense workout the day after the first intense workout? After the first workout, many players complained of substantial leg pain and stiffness and dark urine prior to the workout on the second day. Why did they not have the players seek medical care given their signs and symptoms?

University of Oregon football players, Doug Brenner and Sam Poutasi, filed lawsuits in 2019 (two years after their ER injuries) against the University, head coach Willie Taggart, and former strength coach Irele Oderinde seeking $11.5 million and $5 million in damages, respectively (71, 76). In his lawsuit, Brenner claimed the individual defendants imposed and carried out the workouts in a negligent manner and the institutional defendants were negligent in failing to regulate and supervise the individuals leading the workouts (71). In the Poutasi lawsuit, he claimed he suffered injuries in addition to ER such as muscle aches, kidney damage and the loss of use of his arms (76). These lawsuits were pending at the time this chapter was written.

NCAA Response to Help Prevent Exertional Rhabdomyolysis

In 2018, the NCAA Chief Medical Officer prepared an exertional rhabdomyolysis message that included five guiding principles regarding the prevention of ER (77). The fifth guiding principle specified that all strength and conditioning workouts should (a) "be documented in writing, (b) reflect the progression, technique, and intentional increases in volume, intensity, mode, and duration of the physical activity, and (c) be available for review by athletic departments" (77, p. 2).

Common Themes Among Exertional Heat and Rhabdomyolysis Injury Cases

In reviewing the negligence claims filed in the lawsuits, investigative reports compiled by the universities, statements made by the injured players, and the commentary of various experts, several common themes are evident as to what caused the heat-related and ER injuries to occur as follows:

a) *Strength and Conditioning Coaches Designing/Delivering Overly Aggressive Workouts,* e.g., Douglas Casa of the Korey Stringer Institute stated in reference to the Iowa case "they did a grossly inappropriate workout…really intense and novel on the first day these people were back" and he also stated that the injuries were 100% preventable (78).

b) *Student-Athletes Performing Grueling Workouts as Punishment,* e.g., Houston's soccer team had a "culture of extreme workouts and systematic physical punishments" (79) as one player stated "the physical punishment involved a grueling workout (80), and in Brenner's lawsuit (Oregon), it was alleged that the workouts were designed to be punishing (71).

c) *Failure to Properly Supervise Athletes Carefully While Workouts are Being Performed*

d) *Failure to Respond Properly When Athletes Report Signs/Symptoms of Overexertion*

e) *Lack of Oversight/Supervision from Head Coaches and Athletic/University Administrators*, e.g., based on the findings of investigative reports, it appeared that top officials were not aware of the inappropriate conduct of their employees in the athletic programs, and it wasn't until after the report was completed, the university made recommendations for changes. This is a prime example of being reactive versus proactive. As Douglas Casa stated, "there needs to be more oversight and people need to be more accountable" (78).

f) *Lack of Accountability Within the Strength and Conditioning Profession*, e.g., although some strength and conditioning coaches (and others involved) have been fired in these cases, the strength and conditioning profession needs to make a concerted effort to enhance the competence of its coaches and develop cultures that reflect safety and professionalism.

Strength and conditioning coaches and athletic administrators should keep abreast of information regarding the "well-being" of athletes prepared by the NCAA Sport Science Institute (SSI) available on the NCAA website (www.ncaa.org). For example, see a 24-page document titled: Preventing Catastrophic Injury and Death in Collegiate Athletes. They may also be interested in accessing various positions, editorials, etc. posted on The Drake Group's website (www.thedrakegroup.org). For example, a 34-page position paper titled: College Athlete Health and Protection from Physical and Psychological Harm is posted on the website. The Drake Group serves as a "watchdog" of sorts regarding a variety of issues facing collegiate sports. In addition, those who lead collegiate athletic programs may want to stay informed of H.R. 5528—a bill introduced in the House of Representatives in December 2019 to establish a Congressional Advisory Commission on Intercollegiate Athletics (available at: https://www.govtrack.us/congress/bills/116/hr5528). This Commission would investigate the relationship between institutions of higher education and intercollegiate athletic programs regarding various factors including policies on the health and safety of student athletes.

Clinical Exercise Programs

Research using legal databases did not find many negligence lawsuits involving cardiac and pulmonary rehabilitation programs. This may be due to the quality of instruction and close supervision provided to patients in these settings, or that these cases are settled out of court and, thus, not published. However, *Rannebarger v. Allina Health Systems* (81) is a good case to demonstrate the importance of providing proper instruction and supervision in these programs. In her first few sessions in Phase II cardiac rehabilitation, Edith Rannebarger exercised on a treadmill with side rails and received assistance getting on and off the treadmill. On the day of her injury, she was instructed to use a different treadmill with no side-rails, so she held on to the front handrail. In addition, no timer was set, as with the first treadmill, to count down the time bringing the treadmill to a stop. No one came to her assistance when she wished to get off the treadmill, even though she tried to get the staff's attention. She tried to stop the treadmill on her own but was unsuccessful. There was no safety magnet clipped to her clothing that she could pull to stop the treadmill although the treadmill comes equipped with one. In another attempt to stop the treadmill, she straddled the belt holding on to the front handrail. However, she caught her foot on the treadmill belt. To prevent a fall, she pulled herself with her left arm on the front handrail. As she did this, she heard a loud cracking noise in her shoulder and felt a burning sensation After informing a staff member about her shoulder, she was instructed to finish her exercise routine that did not use her arms. She was then told to go home and put ice on it. Her injury was not documented by any of the staff members. She was later diagnosed with a dislocated shoulder and torn rotator cuff that required surgical repair.

Rannebarger filed several negligence claims against the defendant hospital, followed by the defendant filing a motion for summary judgment. Because this was a **medical malpractice** (negligence of a health care provider) case, expert testimony was required. An expert witness for the plaintiff set forth six standards of care, allegedly owed to the plaintiff that that the defendant breached. These duties were breached when the defendant:

1. Did not use a timer on the treadmill that would count down the time bring the treadmill to a safe stop;

2. Failed to affix the safety magnet to Plaintiff's clothing…;

3. Did not instruct Plaintiff as to how to obtain the attention of the staff if and when she required any attention or assistance;

4. Failed to reasonably observe and monitor Plaintiff while she was on the exercise equipment at Mercy Hospital…;

5. Failed to assess Plaintiff's safety on a treadmill without the side rail safety feature in place;

6. Did not inquire further after Plaintiff complained of her left shoulder cracking nor assess her shoulder for injury nor provide initial treatment in the form of ice and stabilization of her shoulder (81, pp. 23-24).

The court denied the defendant's motion for summary judgment stating that the defendant's acts and omissions violated standards of care and that these violations caused the plaintiff's injury.

Another area of litigation that has occurred in these types of clinical exercise programs involves allegations for not meeting Medicare requirements. The Medicare statute defines a cardiac rehabilitation program as a physician-supervised program and contains several requirements including that patients receive an individualized written treatment plan that is established, reviewed, and signed every 30 days by a qualified physician (medical director). The statute also requires a qualified supervising physician to be immediately available and accessible for medical consultation and emergencies, which is presumed if the program is offered in a hospital. In *United States ex rel. Martinez v. KPC Healthcare Inc.* (82), Martinez, an employee of the hospital, claimed "that the hospital billed its services as cardiac rehabilitation services knowing that it did not actually comply with Medicare's requirements" (p. 3). She filed this case under the False Claims Act, a federal law. Martinez alleged that no physician was assigned to the cardiac rehabilitation and that nurses, who lacked experience with cardiac treatment, made the determinations

about a patient's treatment. For example, the nurses did not provide the patients with "individualized" exercise prescriptions putting them at an increased risk of injury. There is much more regarding this case and the court's analysis of the False Claims Act. It is briefly discussed here so that clinical exercise physiologists, who work in these programs, are aware of supervision requirements specified in the Medicare statute.

First Responder and Military Exercise Programs

The need to have highly-fit first responders and military personnel is obvious—it is required to safely and effectively perform their jobs. However, sometimes the high intensity and demanding training programs to prepare them for their jobs have resulted in serious injuries, death, and subsequent litigation. This section will describe two cases involving improper instruction and supervision—one involving a state police cadet and the other, a Marine recruit. Although government immunity was a successful defense in the Marine recruit case, it was not in the police cadet case. Efforts to increase the safety of these programs are needed to minimize costs due to loss duty time, medical treatment, extensive rehabilitation, and also to recognize the legal and moral duties regarding the health and safety for those who serve our country and communities.

In *Martin v. Moreau* (83), a state highway patrol cadet was seriously injured. While participating in the North Carolina State Highway Patrol Basic School, a 29-week para-military boot camp training program, Jennifer Martin suffered multiple minor injuries but was able to receive her Basic Law Enforcement Training Certificate. She was then assigned to remedial training and instruction in the required Active Confrontational Tactics and Survival Course. About halfway through this training program, under the supervision of Sargent Whaley, she fell injuring her left arm and hip which she self-treated. Officer Moreau, who instructed and supervised the early morning training the next day, along with Officer Gentieu, was informed of her fall. Officer Moreau instructed Martin to run 30 minutes on the treadmill at six miles per hour. After 15 minutes, she could not maintain the speed due to pain in her left hip. She reduced the speed and leaned on the rails of the treadmill. Officer Moreau became angry with Martin and ordered her to speed up the treadmill and to stop leaning on the rails. She complied but after a few seconds, she began experiencing excruciating pain and was visibly sobbing in pain. Despite informing Moreau of her severe hip pain, he again ordered her to speed up the treadmill and made various derogatory and demeaning comments toward her. He then reached over and increased the speed on the treadmill. Martin could no longer stand up and stopped the treadmill. Moreau then ordered her to do crunches and leg lifts on the floor. When she could not perform the leg lifts, Martin ordered her to get to the showers. He also ordered another female cadet, Velasquez, to not help her.

Martin managed to drag herself out of the weight room and out to the parking lot. Velasquez asked officer Gentieu to assist Martin, but like Moreau, he did not. After making derogatory comments toward Martin, Gentieu eventually instructed three cadets to put her in a wheelchair. When they did, Martin screamed in pain as she felt the bone in her left hip separate when the cadets lifted her. They wheeled her to her dorm room and was left in the dark crying in pain. Velasquez wheeled Martin to the school's medical office at 8:00 am when Dr. Griggs arrived. He could not get her out of the wheelchair to examine her and made an immediate appointment at the Duke Sports Medicine Clinic. About an hour later, Officer Moreau transported Martin to the Clinic, again making derogatory comments toward her during the 30 minute trip to the Clinic. At the Clinic, she was diagnosed with a completely displaced left femoral fracture. Martin had emergency surgery leaving her left leg permanently shorter than her right leg.

Martin filed a complaint against Officers Moreau and Gentieu alleging willful and wanton negligence. The defendants filed motions to dismiss based on sovereign immunity and public officer immunity. The trial court granted these motions to dismiss and Martin appealed. The appellate court reversed the trial court's ruling stating, "Plaintiff's complaint sufficiently alleged Defendants exceeded the scope of their duties in that Plaintiff alleged she suffered a severe and obvious injury, of which Defendants were aware, and yet Defendants ordered Plaintiff to continue exercising and then abandoned her without medical treatment for almost

an hour" (83, p. 9). These allegations were sufficient to refute the Officers' defenses of sovereign and public official immunity because their actions were corrupt or malicious and outside and beyond the scope of their duties. In his affidavit, Officer Dave Cloutier stated that Officer's Moreau's actions "clearly violated the standards and practices as outlined in the Specialized Physical Fitness and Subject Control/Arrest Techniques Instructor Training manuals" and that "the failure to act in accordance with those standards exhibited a callous, reckless and willful disregard for the safety of plaintiff Martin" (p. 16). Officer Cloutier said basically the same thing about Officer Gentieu. Additional proceedings occurred in this case, but the ruling of the appellate court remained.

The *Hajdusek v. United States* (84) case involved a serious injury suffered by a Marine Corps recruit during an intense workout. The plaintiff, Joseph Hajdusek, participated in a Marine Corps Delayed Entry Program to help him better prepare for basic training. He alleged that his superior ordered him to participate in an unreasonable program of physical activity, which resulted in a serious injury. On the day of the injury, Hajhusek claimed the workout was much longer and much more strenuous than previous workouts and that he was given only two, twenty-second water breaks over a two-hour period. He suffered several ailments including exertional rhabdomyolysis that resulted in his left arm being permanently disabled. He sued the United States under the Federal Tort Claims Act (FTCA). The FTCA serves as a limited waiver of sovereign immunity that allows federal courts to determine if the Government was liable for an injury or death caused by the wrongful act or omission of any employee of the Government. However, there is an exception to this provision removing from the district courts' jurisdiction any claim based on **discretionary function**. If the claim is based on discretionary function as in this case, the case must be dismissed for want of jurisdiction. Discretionary function refers to the discretion an official has based on a delegated responsibility.

The United States moved to dismiss Hajhusek's claim on the ground that it "stemmed from the performance of discretionary function and since the United States has not waived sovereign immunity for such claims, the district court lacked subject matter jurisdiction" (p. 149). The trial court agreed and dismissed the case. Hajdusek appealed this decision, but the appellate court affirmed the trial court's ruling. The appellate court stated that "Congress has decreed that the federal courts cannot use tort claims to second-guess the discretionary choices of federal agents who implement the government's policy choices. In this specific instance, Congress's command means that we cannot second-guess the decision of a Marine about how hard to work out a potential recruit..." (84, p. 153). Making decisions regarding working a recruit too much or too little is not what Congress intended for judges. These decisions reflect the discretionary function of those leading the training programs.

It is unlikely that military personnel injured in physical training programs will prevail in their negligent claims due to the sovereign immunity of the federal government. However, it is in the best interest of all parties to provide safe and effective training programs. For example, a focus on preventing injuries is needed as emphasized in the consensus statement by Bergeron et al. (10) briefly described earlier. The authors stated that some warfighters believe these these programs, such as ECPs, better prepare them for the battlefield. However, physicians and other health care providers have reported their concern with the increasing number of serious injuries including ER associated with these military programs. The authors provide several recommendations to improve the safety of ECPs such as progression, suitable rest periods, and having well-qualified and competent physical fitness trainers.

KEY POINT

Sovereign Immunity

Sovereign immunity may protect exercise professionals and their employers from their own negligent conduct in certain government-sponsored exercise programs. However, sovereign or government immunity may not apply if the conduct was reckless or willful as demonstrated in the Martin case. In the best interest of all parties, exercise programs for first responders and military personnel should be designed and delivered in a safe/effective manner despite government immunity or other immunities that might apply. An essential first step to help ensure these programs are safe/effective is to have them directed by credentialed and competent professionals.

Each branch of the military has its own training program and published guidelines addressing policies and procedures that need to be followed.

Serious injuries and deaths have also occurred while military personnel complete their fitness tests. These incidences have warranted changes in testing protocols. In 2019, for example, the Navy ordered more supervision during these tests after recent deaths of four sailors. The new guidelines, in part, call for certain precautions to be taken when unusual distress or fatigue is observed (85). In addition, the Army announced it was conducting a trial of modified tests for injured soldiers (86) and the Air Force was assessing some changes with its fitness tests (87).

DEVELOPMENT OF RISK MANAGEMENT STRATEGIES

| Assessment of Legal Liability Exposures | | Development of Risk Management Strategies | | Implementation of the Comprehensive Risk Management Plan | | Evaluation of the Comprehensive Risk Management Plan |

As demonstrated in the cases described within this chapter and other cases throughout this textbook, improper instruction and supervision (commission) or the failure to provide proper instruction and supervision (omission) resulted in negligence claims/lawsuits against exercise professionals and their employers. In order to minimize litigation in this area, fitness managers can develop and implement the following eight risk management strategies to help ensure participants are receiving safe instruction/supervision provided by the facility's employees. Many of the risk management strategies covered in previous and later chapters also relate to instruction and supervision such as:

- *Chapter 5*—Hiring only credentialed and competent employees; Providing formal education and practical training for all new employees.
- *Chapter 6*—Establishing policies and procedures regarding pre-activity screening/medical histories and fitness testing. Providing staff training covering such policies and procedures.
- *Chapter 7*—Establishing scope of practice policies and procedures; Providing scope of practice training for staff; Providing clinical/medical oversight.
- *Chapter 9*—Providing proper instruction and supervision regarding the use of exercise equipment
- *Chapter 10*—Providing proper instruction during a facility orientation; Providing on-going transitional supervision of the fitness floor and other areas within the facility
- *Chapter 11*—Providing proper instruction and training regarding the facility's emergency action plans.

1 **Risk Management Strategy #1:** Comply with Published Standards of Practice Addressing Safe Instruction and Supervision.

As stated previously, it is the responsibility of fitness managers and exercise professionals to obtain copies of these published standards of practice. This textbook only provides a brief description of some of them. Several published standards of practice related to instruction and supervision have been summarized in other chapters such as standards and guidelines related to (a) staff credentials, (b) exercise prescription for apparently healthy adults, clinical populations, and older adults, and (c) facility orientation.

The following are examples of additional standards, guidelines, and position papers related to safe instruction and supervision. For example, AFAA (88) recommends that group exercise leaders consider the following five questions to determine the effectiveness and potential risk for injury when teaching any exercise:

1. What is the purpose of the exercise?
2. Are you doing that effectively?
3. Does the exercise create any safety concerns?
4. Can you maintain proper alignment and form for the duration of the exercise?
5. For whom is the exercise appropriate or inappropriate? (88, p. 16).

These five questions are applicable to all exercise professionals such as personal fitness trainers and strength and conditioning coaches, not just group exercise leaders. If the exercise professionals, named as defendants in the negligence lawsuits described earlier, had considered these five questions when designing/delivering their exercise programs, many of the injuries and subsequent litigation may have been prevented. AFAA (88) also provides additional information regarding high quality (safe and effective) exercise instruction such as (a) incorporating factors related to class level (e.g., teaching at an intermediate level but explaining and demonstrating how to modify to lower and higher intensities), and (b) avoiding certain exercises that can increase the risk of injury. In addition, AFAA provides standards and guidelines regarding instruction and supervision in prenatal, senior, and youth fitness programs as well as programs for large-sized participants.

Class Size. Other than the NSCA, it does not appear that most professional organizations provide any specific standards or guidelines regarding the maximum number of participants in group exercise classes. One industry practice is to allocate 40-60 square feet per participant in a group exercise class (92). The NSCA (89) provides two standards requiring close supervision by well-qualified and trained personnel and attentive spotting for certain exercises. They also provide guidelines regarding professional-to-athlete ratios such as, 1:10 or lower for junior high, 1:15 or lower for high school, and 1:20 or lower for college with greater supervision recommended for youth, novices, and special populations (89).

Fitness managers and exercise professionals need to establish policies regarding the maximum number of participants allowed in each exercise class. It is essential that each instructor can always observe all participants to help ensure they are properly executing the exercises and are not experiencing any signs of overexertion. In fact, all group exercise leaders should be well-trained on how to move around the classroom as they are teaching so they can assist individual participants when needed. This is especially important for indoor cycling instructors given the difficulty to observe those in the back of a room that is often dark. The following should be considered to help determine these policies: "space available in the classroom, level of expertise and experience of the instructor, type of participants (e.g., novices, general population, special populations…), type of group exercise class, and building/fire codes" (1, p. 239). For fitness managers who choose to have large classes such as, more than 15-20 participants, it is recommended having a second instructor moving around the room to help provide adequate supervision and assistance to those who may need it. Overcrowding is also an important issue to consider. Plaintiffs may list overcrowding as a negligent claim as the aerobic dance participant did in *Contino v. Lucille Roberts Health Spa.* (90).

Youth Programs. Several of the published standards of practice were listed above under youth exercise programs. A few of these are briefly described here. For example, the YMCA (53) provides a variety of recommendations for youth programs including strength training and organized sports. The YMCA often refers to the published standards of practice of other professional organization (e.g., they refer to the American Academy of Pediatricians and NSCA for youth strength training guidelines). The NSCA (89) has three guidelines regarding youth strength training programs with the first guideline recommending that children under the age of seven should not participate in strength training activities. The second and third guidelines address children between the age of 7 and 14 and 14 years and older, respectively. The NSCA has published position statements regarding youth programs, such as Youth Resistance Training and Long-Term Athletic Development, available on the NSCA website (www.nsca.com).

The *ACSM's Guidelines for Exercise Testing and Prescription (ACSM's GETP)* describes recommendations for screening, testing, and exercise prescription for youth programs (91). The *ACSM's Health/Fitness Facility Standard and Guidelines* (92) contains four standards regarding youth programs and services (e.g., compliance with all applicable state and local laws and regulations that address supervision of youth programs, certain documents that need to be signed by parents/guardians whose children will be using the facility's child care services, and various policies such as staff supervision of children). The MFA (93) has five standards (requirements) and 20 guidelines (recommendations) for youth programs and services that address policies and procedures in the areas of screening, compliance with applicable laws/regulations, information to be provided to parents/guardians, risk management, and age-appropriate activities. IHRSA (94) has a standard that addresses appropriate supervision of youth programs that includes the qualifications of staff members who oversee youth programs.

Strength and Conditioning Programs. Several organizations have published standards of practices or best practices (e.g., position papers, consensus statements) that address numerous health and safety issues that strength and conditioning coaches should follow. Recommendations regarding injury prevention and proper emergency care are the major goals of many of these publications. Strength and conditioning coaches, along with athletic administrators and athletic trainers, need to establish written policies and procedures that reflect these safety practices and conduct staff training programs to help ensure they are carried out properly. The following represent a just few of these published standards of practice related to heat injuries and sickle cell trait.

1. Exertional Heat Illnesses (September 2015)—National Athletic Trainers' Association (NATA)
2. Sickle Cell Trait in the Athlete (September 2016)—College Strength and Conditioning Coaches Association (CSCCa)
3. Exertional Heat Illness during Training and Competition (March 2007)—ACSM

Many resources are available such as the *2014-15 NCAA Sports Medicine Handbook* (95) which is a 144 page document that includes a plethora of recommendations regarding the health and safety of athletes.

In addition to following published standards of practice to help ensure safety of athletes, athletic programs are also using **wearable technology** to help prevent heat and other injuries (96). However, data privacy and security issues need to be addressed with these technologies as described in Chapters 3 and 10.

First Responder/Military Programs. In addition to following standards of practice published by professional organizations regarding safe instruction and supervision, exercise professionals who lead exercise programs for first responders need to follow policies and procedures published in the instructor manuals such as the one described by Officer Cloutier in the *Marlin* case above for state police officers. Policies and procedures published by each branch of the military need to be followed when leading military fitness programs (e.g., Air Force Instruction 36-2905, available at: https://www.e-publishing.af.mil). These policies and procedures for each branch include the fitness requirements that need to be met by military personnel. These fitness requirements can be found at: https://www.military.com/military-fitness.

Risk Management Strategy #2: Establish Policies and Procedures Regarding High Intensity Exercise Programs.

Because of the increased popularity of high-intensity exercise programs, fitness managers and exercise professionals need to consider adopting policies and procedures to help ensure these programs are safely designed and delivered such as the following:

a) Do not offer ECPs or HIT programs—high intensity programs with little or no recovery intervals. These programs are risky for any population, even for elite athletes as demonstrated in the negligence cases described in this chapter. This policy reflects an exposure avoidance strategy as described in Chapter 2.

b) Exercise professionals need to follow the exercise intensity level as indicated on the medical clearance form by the participant's health care provider. See PASQ Medical Clearance Form in Chapter 6 appendix. If the health care provider indicated "moderate" as the highest level for his/her patient, then the exercise professional needs to follow that recommendation. When the exercise professional feels his/her participant is ready to move to the next intensity level, then medical clearance should again be completed at that time to be sure the health care provider approves. This is best accomplished by estab-

lishing two-way communication as described in Chapter 7.

c) HIIT programs: Although these types of high intensity exercise programs can create a greater risk for injury than a typical moderate-vigorous exercise program, important precautions to minimize any increased risks of injury can be developed into fitness facility policies and procedures. For example, before a participant can enroll in a HIIT program, a credentialed and competent exercise professional employed by the facility needs to be sure:

   i. The participant has approval for participation in high-intensity exercise from his/her health care provider (this applies to those whose health screening or medical history data warranted medical clearance).

   ii. For body weight/resistance HIIT programs, the participant can properly and safely perform the exercises. Certain body weight/resistance exercises require precise technique and/or considerable skill, balance, and strength for them to be safely executed.

   iii. For cardiovascular HIIT programs, the participant needs to demonstrate that he/she can safely perform continuous (e.g., 30 minutes) moderate-vigorous intensity exercise.

d) Have only credentialed and competent exercise professionals lead these programs who (a) fully understand the importance of adequate recovery periods, (b) can meet individual health/fitness needs if taught in a group setting, (c) provide proper instruction as well as supervision by closely observing participants for signs of overexertion.

e) In consultation with legal counsel, consider having participants sign a specialized assumption of risk document that describes the potential "increased" risks associated with these programs. See Exhibit 4-2 in Chapter 4 for an example of an express assumption of risk.

As demonstrated in the cases described in this chapter and other chapters, sometimes exercise professionals have pushed their participants to continue exercising despite their complaints of pain or extreme fatigue and requests to stop. Fitness managers may want to adopt the C.A.R.D. approach as a policy for exercise professionals to follow. Developed by Paul Fenaroli, JD, it provides the following steps to address participant complaints:

◗ **Communicate.** Let your client know breaks are available upon request. If in a group setting, make this announcement before class begins. Provide directions for what to do if anyone becomes extremely fatigued during exercise and wishes to take a take a break. Lower the intensity, but have them keep moving at a walking level (active recovery). Once recovered, individuals can sit or lay down. Provide water, although water should always be available before, during, and after workouts.

◗ **Assess.** If an injury or extreme fatigue/discomfort is reported, STOP the exercise and assess the severity of the situation. There is nothing wrong with taking a break. Remember, achieving health and wellness is a marathon, not a sprint. Your goal should be for every client to leave feeling BETTER than when they arrived. If an injury occurred, exercise should not continue and the facility's emergency action plan needs to be followed.

◗ **Respond.** After the client recovers from extreme fatigue/discomfort and wants to continue exercising, continue with LOW INTENSITY exercises. NEVER encourage your client to "push through pain" or continue to exercise despite discomfort. See Table 6-3 in Chapter 6: Soreness vs. Pain: How to Tell the Difference.

◗ **Document.** Especially if pain or discomfort causes training to end prematurely, take a moment to write down what happened. This does not have to be formal, but record what caused the complaint to arise, how you handled the situation and how the event resolved. This information can be recorded on the Lesson Plan Evaluation (see Exhibit 8-4 below).

Exercise professionals also need to be aware of signs and symptoms of overtraining. There are several articles published on this topic in the literature. However, for a short article that can be discussed in staff trainings, see "Overreaching/Overtraining: More Is Not Always Better" (97).

③ Risk Management Strategy #3: Offer Beginner-Level Exercise Classes for Novices, Low-Fit Participants, and Individuals with Clinical Conditions.

Given the popularity of certain programs such as indoor cycling and boot camp that are often taught at high-intensity or strenuous levels (though they can be taught at moderate-vigorous levels) as well as programs like yoga that often involve advanced or difficult poses, it is best to have novices, low fit participants, and individuals with clinical conditions to first participate in a beginner-level class. Offering these classes will help lower the risk of injuries and subsequent litigation. For example, as described above, first-time participants in indoor cycling classes have suffered serious injuries such as exertional rhabdomyolysis and musculoskeletal injuries, primarily because they were improperly instructed and supervised.

Offering well-taught beginner-level classes will help participants gain the knowledge and skills needed to safely perform the activity. As explained by van der Smissen (2), specific supervision (instruction) provides the participant an opportunity to gain knowledge of the activity, an understanding of one's own capabilities, and an appreciation of the potential injuries that can occur so that he/she can assume the inherent risks of the activity. An effective primary assumption of risk defense, as described in Chapter 4, requires the participant to possess a full understanding of the risks and voluntarily encounter those risks. Providing beginner classes with proper instruction and adequate experience can help beginners obtain a full understanding of the risks. Having documentation of class dates and the names of participants successfully completing the class can provide evidence to help prove that they did know, understand, and appreciate the risks and voluntarily chose to encounter those risks, if they later become injured and file a complaint. Documentation should include the knowledge and skills taught in the class (e.g., lesson plans) and the name of the instructor. As demonstrated in many of the negligence cases throughout this textbook, the primary assumption of risk defense is a common defense used by defendants, especially when the waiver defense is ineffective for various reasons. But for it to be an effective defense, it may help to have evidence to demonstrate that the participant received proper instruction and experience.

Some individuals may not be able to take a beginner-level class due to time conflicts. In addition, there may be some fitness facilities that cannot offer such classes and can only offer, for example, one boot camp class, one yoga class, and one indoor cycling class. In these situations, it is essential that instructors take special steps to instruct and supervise beginners or others who would benefit from a beginner-level class. Often, instructors will only tell a beginner something like "go at your own pace" or provide only partial instruction like the instructor in the *Scheck* spotlight case. A concerted effort to properly instruct a beginner (or others needing individualized instruction) is needed to minimize injury and subsequent litigation. For example, these individuals can be asked to come to the class 20-30 minutes ahead of time so the exercise leader can provide an orientation that includes basic instruction and explanation of safety issues such as how to keep the intensity low, etc. It is best for fitness managers and exercise professionals to develop a check-list of the content to be covered in this 20-30 minute orientation. Once completed, the instructor should sign and date the checklist and have the participants sign it verifying that they have received basic instruction. The checklist is evidence that instruction took place which may help strengthen the primary assumption of risk defense. These individuals should be placed in the front of the class so that the instructor can closely supervise them.

Most participants will appreciate having the opportunity to take beginner-level classes or having individual instruction prior to taking a new class. Offering these special instructional programs is also an excellent marketing strategy—helping maintain and increase the number of participants. Most individuals will enjoy a fitness facility that provides programs and services that focus on their safety. At the same time, these programs/services will help provide legal protection for the facility and its personnel. As described above by attorney

and Professor John Wolohan (46), having beginners take intermediate or advanced classes increases their risk of injury for which the defendants may be liable. He also stated that instructors, who fail to properly instruct beginners, will likely discover that courts will find them and their employers not only negligent, but potentially grossly negligent.

4 **Risk Management Strategy #4:** Have All Exercise Professionals Who Lead Exercise Programs Prepare Written Lesson Plans and Lesson Plan Evaluations.

Having written documentation such as lesson plans and lesson plan evaluations may help refute negligence claims/lawsuits made against defendants (instructors/trainers/coaches and their employers). These written documents can help provide evidence that proper instruction and supervision took place on the day of a participant's injury and that management took concerted efforts to help ensure that it did. Preparing lesson plans is an effective risk management strategy that can prevent injuries from occurring in the first place. For example, to reduce the number of exertional rhabdomyolysis injuries occurring in collegiate athletic programs, the NCAA Chief Medical Officer published five guiding principles for athletic personnel to follow. The fifth guiding principle specified that all strength and conditioning workouts should (a) "be documented in writing, (b) reflect the progression, technique, and intentional increases in volume, intensity, mode, and duration of the physical activity, and (c) be available for review by athletic departments" (80, p. 2).

Fitness managers and supervisors need to review and critique prepared written lesson plans and lesson plan evaluations of their employees who lead exercise programs. For newly hired exercise professionals, this needs to take place continually for several weeks during the employee's probationary period or when there is evidence that the instructional conduct of an employee needs to improve. Policies and procedures regarding this process need to be established (e.g., staff training on how to properly prepare these forms, procedures on how to submit them, timeframe for managers to review/critique them, lesson plan feedback that is shared with the employee prior to teaching the class/training session, and feedback on the lesson plan evaluations after teaching the class/training session). The major purpose of the review/critique and provision of feedback of the lesson plan is for the manager or supervisor to recommend any changes in the plan to help ensure participant safety. Managers/supervisors, obviously, need to possess proper credentials and competence to properly perform these tasks.

The lesson plan template in Exhibit 8-3 can be revised/adapted to reflect various types of exercise professionals and programs. For example, the lesson plan template can be designed differently for a group exercise leader, personal fitness trainer, and strength and conditioning coach. The lesson plan template reflects the basic components of an exercise training session (warm-up, etc.) as described in *ACSM's GETP* (91). Exercise professionals need to apply the FITT-VP principle (described in Chapter 7) when designing the exercise training session and describe how these factors will be individualized when leading a group training session. The template includes the objectives and safety principles to be taught or reviewed. It is important to realize that it is the responsibility of exercise professionals to teach their participants principles of safe exercise. It should never be assumed that they know and understand these important principles. Safety principles should be taught in a general orientation (see Chapter 10 for more information on facility orientations) and should also be taught/reviewed in structured exercise programs. This can easily be accomplished during the warm-up, cool-down, or stretching phases. Participants have responsibilities regarding their own safety such as applying safe principles of exercise and following the facility's safety policies, but they need to be well-informed of these responsibilities. In addition, this template includes listing certain participants (e.g., beginners, and the precautions the exercise leader plans to take to help ensure their safety). This documentation may serve as evidence that the duty to provide a reasonably safe program for participants was not breached.

The lesson plan evaluation template can be found in Exhibit 8-4. This template can be revised/adapted to reflect various types of exercise professionals and programs. The major purposes of lesson plan evaluations are to (a) provide a mechanism for the instructor/trainer/coach to reflect or self-evaluate each class/training session, and (b) to document situations that occurred during the class/training session. Completing this evaluation can help instructors/trainers/coaches improve their instruction and also provide documentation of any situations that occurred that may serve as a helpful defense if any future litigation occurs. For example, if a class participant complained about knee pain and the instructor recommended to seek medical evaluation, the date of that complaint/recommendation is recorded on the lesson plan evaluation. This documentation may provide a helpful defense if that participant later has a serious knee injury while working out in the facility and sues the facility. If certain situations occur such as a fight between two participants or a serious injury to a participant, they need to be documented on the lesson plan evaluation and also on the facility's Incident Report or Injury Report as described in Chapters 10 and 11, respectively.

 Risk Management Strategy #5: Conduct Performance Appraisals of All Exercise Professionals (1).

Conducting performance appraisals of exercise professionals who instruct and supervise exercise programs is an essential risk management responsibility of all fitness managers and supervisors. Performance appraisal, as defined by Mathis and Jackson (98), is "the process of evaluating how well employees perform their jobs when compared to a set of standards and then communicating that information to those employees" (p. 342). There are various administrative functions of performance appraisals (e.g., provide data to help make decisions regarding employee promotions or pay raises). There are developmental functions as well such as identifying strengths, areas of growth, and career planning (98). This discussion will focus on developmental functions.

The key to a fair and effective performance appraisal process is to have a written tool to evaluate an employee's job performance. A well-developed written tool provides the same criteria and performance standards to evaluate exercise professionals. Using the same

Exhibit 8-3: Lesson Plan Template

Name of Instructor/Trainer/Coach: _____   Date/Time of Class/Training Session: _____

Name of Class/Training Session or Client(s): _____

Major Objectives of this Class/Training Session:

Safety Principles to be Taught or Reviewed in this Class/Training Session:

Warm-Up Activities: (Estimated Time: ___ minutes)

Conditioning Activities:

> **Aerobic Activities:** (Estimated Time: ___ minutes)

> **Resistance Activities:** (Estimated Time: ____ minutes)

> **Neuromotor and/or Other Activities:** (Estimated Time: ____ minutes)

Cool-Down Activities: (Estimated Time: ___ minutes)

Stretching Activities: (Estimated Time: ___ minutes)

List the Names of Beginners, Low-Fit/Deconditioned Participants, and/or Individuals with Medical Conditions Participating in this Class/Training Session:

Describe Precautions for Each that will be Taken to Help Ensure Their Safety:

Exhibit 8-4: Lesson Plan Evaluation Template

Name of Instructor/Trainer/Coach: _____   Date/Time of Class/Training Session: _____

Name of Class/Training Session or Client(s): _____

Reflection/Self-Evaluation

1. Were the objectives of the lesson plan met? If not, explain.

2. Describe any changes made with the lesson plan and why.

3. How could the lesson plan be improved?

Situations that Occurred

_____ Check (√) here if no situations occurred.

1. Check (√) if any the following occurred?

_____ Participant behavior problem

_____ Participant complaint of pain or overexertion

_____ Concerning comment made by a participant

_____ Participant overexertion or injury

_____ Equipment problem

_____ Facility problem

_____ Other, explain _____

2. For each item checked above, describe the situation occurred and list names of the participant(s), if applicable. Also, describe how you responded to the situation.

NOTE: Facility Policy: Some of the items checked require completion of the certain Facility Forms such as an Incident Report or Injury Report. See the Manager on Duty for assistance. Also, inform your supervisor if you checked any of the above items that occurred.

criteria and performance standards helps to objectify the process and addresses one of the major criticisms of performance appraisals that they are unfair or biased. An example of a well-developed and pilot-tested Performance Appraisal Tool (PAT) for Group Exercise Leaders is provided in this chapter's appendix (99). Minor changes/updates have been made to the PAT since it was first introduced. Fitness managers and supervisors can adapt/revise this PAT for any type of exercise professional such as personal fitness trainers, strength and conditioning coaches, etc.

The PAT was developed based on the following factors as identified by Mathis and Jackson (98):

1. Type of performance criteria to be assessed—(a) behavior-based (behaviors required of the job), (b) trait-based (subjective characteristics), and (c) results-based (accomplishments)
2. Job criteria—the key responsibilities of the exercise professional's job
3. Performance Standards—levels of performance for each criterion are rated

There are three sections in the PAT: (a) In-Class Evaluation, (b) Out-of-Class Evaluation, and (c) Performance Appraisal Feedback. The In-Class section is completed during direct observation (e.g., a group exercise coordinator should observe an instructor in two-three different classes, a personal fitness trainer coordinator should observe a trainer training two-three different clients). The criteria under each of the nine "in-class evaluation" categories are all behavior-based and focus on instructional safety. The Out-of-Class section contains performance standards for all three areas—behavior-based, trait-based, and results-based. This section focuses on assessing the professionalism of the employee. The Performance Appraisal Feedback section documents that feedback was provided and identifies any action steps to be taken. Additional information regarding the development of the PAT is provided elsewhere (99).

One of the major goals of conducting performance appraisals is to help exercise professionals improve their job performance. Therefore, fitness managers and supervisors should communicate this process in a positive manner with their employees. Another major goal is to detect any issues related to participant safety before an injury occurs. It is likely that the injuries, due to

improper instruction and supervision described in the lawsuits throughout this textbook, would not have occurred if unsafe instruction/supervision had been detected during a performance appraisal and corrected. It is important that exercise instructors/trainers/coaches know and understand that improper instruction and supervision is a major legal liability exposure and that performance appraisals are conducted to help them minimize this exposure.

Although some managers/supervisors may believe the PAT is too lengthy, that was not the view of most of the managers//supervisors who participated in the PAT pilot-study (99). Comments from the pilot-test participants (program supervisors) included: "Once I was familiar with the form, it was very easy and quick to use" and "When giving feedback to the instructors, they really appreciated all the areas that were evaluated, and they were surprised by the detail." Managers/supervisors will experience many benefits when using a tool such as the PAT. Although it takes time to administer the PAT, much of a manager's or supervisor's time is saved by having employees properly performing their jobs, so managers/supervisors spend less time "putting out fires." Most importantly, it helps to minimize the great deal of time and stress associated with injuries and subsequent litigations.

Administrative Procedures

Often during a job interview, the candidate receives a job description that provides a general list of job functions. It is recommended to review and explain the PAT that will be used to evaluate the candidate's performance during the probation period and on a needed or annual basis thereafter. The PAT provides more detail than a job description and clearly communicates the many job expectations. Discussing the PAT during an interview informs the candidate how it relates to the facility's mission to provide a safety culture as described in Chapter 2.

The timeframes for conducting the performance appraisal are listed at the top of the PAT. It is recommended that this process be completed during the Introductory period (or probationary period) at least a couple of times or as needed. This early feedback "sets the stage" as to expectations and can prevent problems down the road. The Follow-Up period can be any time when a performance appraisal may be indicated (e.g., a manager observes inappropriate conduct during informal supervision, participant complaint, co-worker complaint, or when an action plan is established after an appraisal). The Regular Interval appraisal is generally completed on an annual basis. During each of these time periods, it is recommended to have the employee also complete the PAT (i.e., a self-appraisal). During the Performance Appraisal Feedback session, the employee and supervisor can compare the two appraisals which may be helpful if there are significant differences with any of the ratings. If needed, an action plan is established during the feedback session to help the employee improve his/her job performance. At the end of this confidential session, both parties sign the document with a copy given to the employee, and the original stored in the employee's personnel file.

6 **Risk Management Strategy #6:** Obtain Anonymous Feedback from Fitness Participants Regarding the Quality of Instruction Provided by Instructors/Trainers/Coaches.

Another method to help evaluate the quality of instruction and supervision provided by the facility's exercise professionals is to obtain anonymous feedback from participants. This feedback should be obtained two-three times during an employee's probationary period and then periodically, thereafter. It is best to use a written survey that is easy and quick for participants to complete. Examples of such surveys can be found on the Internet using search terms such as Participant Evaluation of Fitness Instructors. For example, Campus Recreation at the University of Maine has a well-designed Group Fitness Participant Evaluation that can be easily completed and submitted from its website (100). Once the data are analyzed, a summary should be shared with the exercise professional in a private setting and in a timely fashion, as well as discussed at the time of a performance appraisal. See Section 2 (Results-Based Performance) in the PAT provided in the appendix. This type of participant feedback is especially important for employees such as massage therapists. Given the private nature of massage, managers

and supervisors will not be able to directly or indirectly observe the conduct of massage therapists. Obviously, if there are any job performance concerns identified from the feedback of fitness facility participants, managers and supervisors need to take immediate action to address the concerns. Some facility managers and supervisors may also want to conduct peer evaluations if they can provide additional helpful information to evaluate an employee's job performance.

7 **Risk Management Strategy #7:** Provide an In-House Continuing Education Program that Focuses on Safe Instruction and Supervision.

Although fitness managers and supervisors need to be sure that employees are keeping their certifications current by meeting their continuing education (CE) requirements, they might not be aware of the content that employees receive in these programs. It may be that some certified individuals have worked many years in the exercise profession but have never earned CE credits/units that focused on safe instruction and supervision. This may be due to certifying organizations not requiring their certified professionals to obtain any "safety" continuing education credits/units. Therefore, providing an in-house CE program that focuses on safe instruction and supervision should be considered. Not only will the CE program continually reinforce the facility's mission to provide a safety culture but will remind employees how important it is to provide safe instruction and supervision. **Note:** Providing various employee in-service trainings has been addressed throughout this textbook (e.g., training upon hiring, training involving screening, testing, scope of practice, equipment/facility inspections, emergency procedures). The CE program proposed here is a special type of in-service training. Giving it a specific name, such as CE Safe Instruction program, will distinguish it from other in-service training programs and emphasize the importance of safe instruction and supervision.

There are a variety of resources that can be used in CE programs addressing safe instruction and supervision (e.g., published standard of practice (standards, guidelines, position papers), articles in professional journals, and presentations at professional conferences). A CE program that covers published standards of practice addressing safe instruction and supervision will provide excellent content to begin a CE program. These published standards of practice may have not been included in academic and certification preparation programs. Therefore, exercise professionals may not even be aware of them. Another CE program could involve having employees reading and discussing professional journal articles that address all types of topics on safe instruction and supervision. The *ACSM's Health & Fitness Journal* is an example of a professional journal that has published numerous articles focusing on safe instruction and supervision over the years. The following are a few of the many published in recent years:

1. *Targeted Resistance Training to Improve Independence and Reduce Falls in Older Adults*—September/October 2016
2. (a) *Exercise Strategies for Improving Quality of Life in Women with Stress Urinary Incontinence* and (b) *Exercise Considerations for Type 1 and Type 2 Diabetes*—January/February 2018
3. (a) *What is Functional/Neuromotor Fitness?* and (b) *Strategies for Implementing Safe and Effective Yoga Programs*— November/December 2018
4. (a) *Exercise Programming for Rheumatoid Arthritis* and (b) *The Lat Pulldown*—March/April 2019

These articles apply to all types of exercise professionals working in a variety of settings. Many other professional journals also publish articles that address safe instruction and supervision for professionals working with general and special populations.

Fitness managers or other employees who have attended sessions at professional conferences (or professional workshops or seminars) that have addressed instructional safety can also provide CE programs where they share what they learned with subordinates and/or co-workers. This may provide an opportunity for group exercise leaders and personal trainers who are not in management/supervisory positions to lead a CE program. In these cases, as well as all cases, the content of what is presented in a CE program needs to be reviewed so that it is accurate and appropriate. For example, content can be reviewed by the facility's clinical exercise physiologist or other exercise physiologists

who have degrees, professional certifications, and experience. CE programs can also be provided by experts in the community.

There are a variety of ways to administer the CE program and track CE credits/units earned. For example, fitness managers/supervisors could offer a certain number of CE programs (various safety topics related to instruction/supervision) each month and then require employees to attend, for example, at least one/month. Recognition for those employees who attend more than one (e.g., an accomplishment listed on the employee's annual performance appraisal, employee of the month, pay increase, etc.) would create incentives for high participation. Providing CE programs that focus on safe instruction and supervision is one of the best investments a fitness facility can make. It will help reduce injuries and costly litigation, increase participant satisfaction and retention, and enhance the reputation of the exercise profession.

⑧ Risk Management Strategy #8: Establish Policies and Procedures Regarding Proper Documentation Related to Instruction and Supervision (1).

Exercise professionals who provide safe instruction and supervision are less likely to cause harm to a participant and, thus, have a lower risk of facing negligent claims/lawsuits. However, if they are ever named as a defendant, it will be essential that they have kept documents to help prove they were not negligent such as screening and medical clearance forms, informed consents, etc. as described in previous chapters. Regarding the provision of safe instruction and supervision, they need to keep documents such as lesson plans and lesson plan evaluations. Facility managers may be able to have employees post their lesson plans and lesson plan evaluations on the facility's Intranet. However, each employee would need to have a secure site that only he/she and his/her supervisor would be able to access. This would make it easy and convenient for supervisors to review these employee documents. Fitness managers should establish policies and procedures that reflect all types of documents that their employees (instructors/trainers/coaches) need to keep as well as documents that supervisors need to retain. How long documents are retained will depend on the statute of limitations and the advice of legal counsel.

As described in Chapter 5, employers can be found vicariously liable for the negligent acts of their employees (e.g., instructors and trainers who failed to provide proper instruction and supervision) or directly liable for not properly hiring, training, and supervising their employees. Risk management strategies regarding proper hiring and initial training were covered in Chapter 5. The above risk management strategies that address on-going training and supervision of employees can be effective in preventing and defending both vicarious and direct liability claims. However, documentation that these strategies were implemented is necessary to help refute such claims. This documentation should include:

    a) Compliance with published standards of practice regarding safe instruction and supervision

    b) Policies and procedures related to high-intensity exercise programs

    c) Documentation of participants completing beginner-level classes, e.g., dates, instructors, and content covered as well as pre-class orientations, e.g., checklists completed by the instructor

    d) Lesson plans and lesson plan evaluations

    e) Performance appraisal tools

    f) Summaries of anonymous feedback from fitness participants

    g) Employee participation records in the facility's CE program

Some of the above items are documented in the Facility's Risk Management Policies and Procedures Manual such as the policies/procedures related to high-intensity exercise programs, but most of the items are kept by the employee and/or in the employee's personnel file. As with all personal information, policies and procedures need to be established so that the data are kept private, confidential, and secure.

RISK MANAGEMENT AUDIT
Instruction and Supervision

RISK MANAGEMENT (RM) STRATEGY*	YES ✔	NO ✔
1. Comply with Published Standards of Practice Addressing Safe Instruction and Supervision.		
2. Establish Policies and Procedures Regarding High Intensity Exercise Programs.		
3. Offer Beginner-Level Exercise Classes for Novices, Low-Fit Participants, and Individuals with Clinical Conditions.		
4. Have All Exercise Professionals Who Lead Exercise Programs Prepare Written Lesson Plans and Lesson Plan Evaluations.		
5. Conduct Formal Performance Appraisals of All Exercise Professionals.		
6. Obtain Anonymous Feedback from Fitness Participants Regarding the Quality of Instruction Provided by Instructors/Trainers/Coaches.		
7. Provide an In-House Continuing Education Program that Focuses on Safe Instruction and Supervision.		
8. Establish Policies and Procedures Regarding Proper Documentation Related to Instruction and Supervision.		

*See the section above—Development of Risk Management Strategies—for the recommendations associated with each risk management strategy and then, for each RM Strategy marked NO, create a list of action steps that need to be completed to meet the recommendations described in that RM strategy.

KEY TERMS

- Compartment Syndrome
- Developmentally Appropriate Programs
- Discretionary Function
- Exertional Rhabdomyolysis
- General Supervision
- High Intensity Training (HIT)
- High-Intensity Interval Training (HIIT)
- Medical Malpractice
- Non-Traditional Personal Fitness Training
- Professional Standard of Care
- Sovereign Immunity
- Specific Supervision
- Transitional Supervision
- Wearable Technology

STUDY QUESTIONS

The Study Questions for Chapter 8 can be found on the Fitness Law Academy website (www.fitnesslawacademy.com) under Textbook. They are provided in a fillable format for convenience.

APPENDIX

This chapter's appendix follows the References.

REFERENCES

1. Eickhoff-Shemek JM, Herbert DL, Connaughton, DP. *Risk Management for Health/Fitness Professionals: Legal Issues and Strategies.* Baltimore, MD: Lippincott Williams & Wilkins, 2009.

2. van der Smissen B. *Legal Liability and Risk Management for Public and Private Entities,* Volume Two. Cincinnati, OH: Anderson Publishing Company, 1990.

3. Voris HC, Rabinoff M. When is a Standard of Care Not a Standard of Care? *The Exercise Standards and Malpractice Reporter,* 25(2), 20-21, 2011.

4. Abbott AA. Injury Litigations. *ACSM's Health & Fitness Journal,* 17(3), 28-32, 2013.

5. Thompson PD, Franklin BA, Balady GJ, et al. Exercise and Acute Cardiovascular Events: Placing the Risks into Perspective. *Medicine & Science in Sports & Exercise,* 39(5), 886-897, 2007.

6. Franklin BA, Thompson PD, Al-Zaiti SS, et al. Exercise-Related Acute Cardiovascular Events and Potential Deleterious Adaptations Following Long-Term Exercise Training: Placing the Risks Into Perspective—An Update. *Circulation,* 141:e705-e736, 2020. Doi: 10.1161/CIR.0000000000000749. Available at: https://www.ahajournals.org/doi/10.1161/CIR.0000000000000749.

7. Ciccolella ME, Moore B, VanNess JM, Wyant. Exertional Rhabdomyolysis and the Law: A Brief Review. *Journal of Exercise Physiology Online,* 17(1), 19-27, February 2014.

8. Rider BC, Coughlin AM, Carlson C, et al. Exertional (Exercise-Induced) Rhabdomyolysis. *ACSM's Health & Fitness Journal,* 23(3), 16-20, 2019.

9. Glassman G. CrossFit Induced Rhabdo. *CrossFit Journal,* October 1, 2005. Available at: http://journal.crossfit.com/2005/10/crossfit-induced-rhabdo-by-gre.tpl. Accessed April 3, 2019.

10. Bergeron MF, Nindl BC, Deuster PA, et al. Consortium for Health and Military Performance and American College of Sports Medicine Consensus Paper on Extreme Conditioning Programs in Military Personnel. *Current Sports Medical Reports,* 10(6), 383-389, 2011.

11. Casa DJ, Anderson SA, Baker L, et al. The Inter-Association Task Force for Preventing Sudden Death in Collegiate Conditioning Sessions: Best Practice Recommendations. *Journal of Athletic Training,* 47(4), 477-480, 2012.

12. Springer BL, Clarkson PM. Two Cases of Exertional Rhabdomyolysis Precipitated by Personal Trainers. *Medicine & Science in Sports & Exercise,* 35(9), 1499-1502, 2003.

13. Hagerman P. Exertional Rhabdomyolysis. *Strength and Conditioning Journal,* 27(3), 73-74, 2005.

14. Thomas DQ, Carlson KA, Marzano A, et al. Exertional Rhabdomyolysis: What Is It and Why Should We Care? *Journal of Physical Education, Recreation & Dance,* 83(1), 4546-4549, 51, 2012.

15. Deyhle M, Kravitz K. Exertional Rhabdomyolysis: When Too Much Exercise Becomes Dangerous. *IDEA Fitness Journal,* 10(4) 16-18, 2013.

16. Bergeron M. Presentation at the 17th Annual ACSM Health & Fitness Summit March 12-15, 2013. Las Vegas, NV *Extreme Conditioning Programs—Are They Worth the Risk?* Available at: http://forms.acsm.org/Summit2013/pdfs/9%20Bergeron.pdf. Accessed April 3, 2019.

17. Diaz M. A Dozen UH Women Soccer Players Sidelined with Serious Medical Conditions Called Rhabdo. Available at: https://www.click2houston.com/news/a-dozen-uh-women-soccer-players-sidelined-with-serious-medical-condition-called-rhabdo. Accessed April 4, 2019.

18. Howley ET. ACSM's Top 10 Fitness Trends: What's Hot and What's Not: A Look Back. *ACSM's Health & Fitness Journal,* 22(6), 18-23, 2018.

19. Rynecki ND, Siracuse BL, Ippolito JA, et al. Injuries Sustained During High Intensity Interval Training: Are Modern Fitness Trends Contributing to Increased Injury Risks? *The Journal of Sports Medicine and Physical Fitness,* February 12, 2019. Available at: https://www.ncbi.nlm.nih.gov/pubmed/30758171. Accessed April 17, 2019.

20. Zuhl M, Kravitz L. HIIT vs. Continuous Endurance Training: Battle of the Aerobic Titans. IDEA Health & Fitness Association, January 26, 2012. Available at: https://www.ideafit.com/fitness-library/hiit-vs-continuous-endurance-training-battle-of-the-aerobic-titans. Accessed April 16, 2019.

21. Kilpatrick, MW, Jung ME, Little JP. High-Intensity Interval Training: A Review of Physiological and Psychological Responses. *ACSM's Health & Fitness Journal,* 18(5), 11-16, 2014.

22. Sabrena J. A Comparison of High-Intensity Interval Training in Different Populations. American Council on Exercise. Available at: https://ace-webcontent.azureedge.net/SAP-Reports/HIIT_SAP_Reports.pdf. Accessed April 16, 2019.

23. Physical Activity Guidelines for Americans, 2nd Ed., 2018. Available at: https://health.gov/paguidelines/secondedition/pdf/Physical_Activity_Guidelines_2nd_edition.pdf. Accessed March 27, 2019.

24. Campbell WW, Kraus WE, Powell KE, et al. High-Intensity Interval Training for Cardiometabolic Disease Prevention. *Medicine & Science in Sports & Exercise,* 51(6), 1220-1226, 2019.

25. Dalleck L. High-Intensity Interval Training for Clinical Populations. *ACE Certified News,* June 2012. Available at: https://www.acefitness.org/certifiednewsarticle/2589/high-intensity-interval-training-for-clinical. Accessed April 16, 2019.

26. van der Smissen B. Elements of Negligence. In: Cotten DJ, Wolohan JT, eds. *Law for Recreation and Sport Managers,* 4th Ed. Dubuque, IA: Kendall/Hunt Publishing Company, 2007.

27. Abbott A. Online Impersonal Training Risk Versus Benefit. *ACSM's Health & Fitness Journal,* 20(1), 34-38, 2016.

28. *Zehnder v. Dutton,* No. 1-16-2668. (Ill. App. Ct., 2017).

29. Caria MA, Tangianu F, Concu A, et al. Quantification of Spinning® Bike Performance During a Standard 50-Minute Class. *Journal of Sports Sciences,* 25(4), 421-429, 2007.

30. Battista R, Foster C, Andrew J, et al. Physiological Responses During Indoor Cycling. *Journal of Strength & Conditioning Research,* 22(4), 1236-1241, 2008.

31. Lopez-Minaro PA, Muyor Rodreguez JM. Heart Rate and Overall Perceived Exertion During Spinning® Cycle Indoor Session in Novice Adults. *Science & Sports,* 25(5), 238-244, 2010.

32. Muyor JM. Exercise Intensity and Validity of the Ratings of Perceived Exertion (Borg and OMNI Scales) in an Indoor Cycling Session. *Journal of Human Kinetics,* 39, 93-101, 2013.

33. Brogan M. Ledesma R, Coffino, et al. Freebie Rhabdomyolysis? A Public Health Concern. Spin Class-Induced Rhabdomyolysis. *The American Medical Journal,* 130(4), 484-487, 2016.

34. O'Connor A. As Workouts Intensify a Harmful Side Effect Grows More Common. *New York Times,* July 7, 2017. Available at: https://www.nytimes.com/2017/07/17/well/move/as-workouts-intensify-a-harmful-side-effect-grows-more-common.html. Accessed April 3, 2019.

35. *Wallis v. Brainerd Baptist Church,* 509 S.W.3d 886, 2016 WL 7407485 (Tenn., 2016).

References continued...

36. *Levine v. GBC, Inc.*, Case No. GJH-16-2455, 2016 WL 7388392 (S.D. Md., 2016).

37. *Horowitz v. Luxury Hotels International of Puerto Rico, Inc.*, 322 F. Supp. 3d 279 (D. P.R., 2018).

38. Swain TA, McGwin G. Yoga-Related Injuries in the United States From 2001 to 2014. *Orthopaedic Journal of Sports Medicine*, 4(11), 1-6, 2016.

38a. Sekendiz B. An Epidemiological Analysis of Yoga-Related Injury Presentations to Emergency Departments in Australia. *The Physician and Sportsmedicine.* January 2020. DOI: 10.1080/00913847.2020.1717395.

39. Quandt E, Porcari JP, Steffen J, et al. ACE Study Examines Effects of Bikram Yoga on Core Body Temps. *ACE Prosource*, pp. 1-5, May 2015. Available at: https://acewebcontent.azureedge.net/certifiednews/images/article/pdfs/ACE_BikramYogaStudy.pdf. Accessed August 2, 2019.

40. *Webster v. Claremont Yoga*, 26 Cal. App. 5th 284 (Cal. Ct. App., 2018).

41. Richardson TE. Expert Contributor, Angie's List. Beware of Boot Camp Classes. October 9, 2015. Available at: https://www.angieslist.com/articles/beware-boot-camp-fitness-classes.htm. Accessed August 2, 2019.

42. DeGregory P. Woman Sues Gym After 400-Pound Tire Crushes Ankle During Workout. *New York Post*, December 9, 2018. Available at: https://nypost.com/2018/12/09/woman-sues-gym-after-400-pound-tire-crushes-ankle-during-workout. Accessed August 2, 2019.

43. Inouye J, Nichols A, Maskarinec G, et al. A Survey of Musculoskeletal Injuries Associated with Zumba. *Hawaii Journal of Medicine & Public Health*, 72(12), 433-436, 2013.

44. *Marchese v. Gamble*, No. CV030827832, 2006 LEXIS 572 (Conn. Super. Ct., 2006).

45. *Honeycutt v. Meridian Sports Club*, 231 Cal. App. 4th 251 (Cal. Ct. App., 2014).

46. Wolohan JT. No Leg to Stand On. A Novice Kickboxing Student Claims Gross Negligence After Rupturing an ACL in Health Club's Class. *Athletic Business*, May 2015, pp. 18-19.

47. Donnelly FC, Mueller SS, Gallahue DL. *Developmental Physical Education for All Children: Theory into Practice*, 5th Ed. Champaign IL: Human Kinetics, 2017.

48. Rahl RL. *Physical Activity and Health Guidelines: Recommendations for Various Ages, Fitness Levels, and Conditions from 57 Authoritative Sources*. Champaign, IL: Human Kinetics, 2010.

49. Railey K. Child Care Centers at Gyms Not Always Regulated. *USA Today*, August 17, 2013. Available at: https://www.usatoday.com/story/news/nation/2013/08/17/unregulatedchildcare/2656615. Accessed August 6, 2019.

50. *Lyle v. 24 Hour Fitness*, Case No. A-14-CV-300 LY, 2016 WL 3200303 (W.D. Tex., 2016).

51. Bogage J. Youth Sports Still Struggling with Dropping Participation, High Costs and Bad Coaches, Study Finds. *The Washington Post*, October 16, 2018. Available at: https://www.washingtonpost.com/sports/2018/10/16/youth-sports-still-struggling-with-dropping-participation-high-costs-bad-coaches-study-finds/. Accessed August 6, 2019.

52. Friesen P, Saul B, Kearns L, et al. Overuse Injuries in Youth Sport: Legal and Social Responsibilities. *Journal of Legal Aspects of Sport*, 28, 151-169, 2018.

53. *Safeguarding Health and Well-Being, Medical Advisory Committee Recommendations: A Resource Guide for YMCAs*. Chicago, IL: YMCA of the USA, February 2011. Available at: http://safe-wise.com/downloads/MAC_2010a_Collection.pdf. Accessed November 5, 2018.

54. Kucera KL, Klossner D., Colgate B, et al. Annual Survey of Football Injury Research. February 15, 2019. National Center for Catastrophic Sport Injury Research. Available at: https://nccsir.unc.edu/files/2019/02/Annual-Football-2018-Fatalities-FINAL.pdf. Accessed June 13, 2019.

55. *Lee v. Louisiana Board of Trustees for State Colleges*, 280 So.3d 176, 2019 WL 1198551 (La. Ct. App., 2019).

56. Schoepfer-Bochicchio K. College Pays for Coach Who Used Exertion as Punishment. Legal Action. *Athletic Business*, June 2019, pp. 22-25.

57. An Independent Evaluation of Procedures and Protocols Related to the June 2018 Death of a University of Maryland Football Student-Athlete. Prepared by Walters Inc., September 21, 2018. Available at: https://www.usmd.edu/newsroom/Walters-Report to USM Board-of-Regents pdf. Accessed June 15, 2019.

58. Report to the University System of Maryland of an Independent Investigation of the University of Maryland Football Program. Prepared by Commissioners and Attorneys, October 23, 2018. Available at: https://www.usmd.edu/newsroom/Report-to-USM-Independent-Investigation-UMD-Footbal-10-23-2018.pdf. Accessed June 15, 2019.

59. When the Death of a Player Isn't Enough… In: *Sports Litigation Alert*, 15(21), Hackney H. (ed). Austin, TX: Hackney Publications, 2018.

60. Byrum T. Maryland's Strength and Conditioning Coach Risk Court Resigns After the Death of Jordan McNair, August 14, 2018. Available at: https://www.nbcsports.com/washington/maryland-terps/marylands-strength-and-conditioning-coach-rick-court-resigns-after-death-jordan. Accessed June 15, 2019.

61. Kirshner A. The Maryland Scandal Fallout Continues to Topple Powerful University Leaders. November 7, 2018. Available at: https://www.sbnation.com/college-football/2018/11/1/18051438/maryland-scandal-board-regents-firing. Accessed June 15, 2019.

62. University of Maryland Resources on Football Program External Review, April 4, 2019. Available at: https://umdrightnow.umd.edu/news/university-maryland-resources-football-program-external-review. Accessed June 16, 2019.

63. Athletics Health Care Administration Best Practices. Independent Medical Care for College Student-Athletes Guidelines. NCAA. Available at: http://www.ncaa.org/sport-science-institute/athletics-health-care-administration-best-practices-0. Accessed July 31, 2019.

64. Casmus B. The University of Maryland Tragedy: "Best Practices" Not Practiced. *From the Gym to the Jury*, 27(5), 1, 7, 2018.

65. Dinich H. Family of Jordan McNair Files Notice of Possible Lawsuit. September 11, 2018. Available at: https://www.espn.com/college-football/story/_/id/24648379/parents-late-maryland-terrapins-ol-jordan-mcnair-file-notice-possible-lawsuit. Accessed June 14, 2019.

66. Berg A. Lapse in Safety Prior to High School Player's Heat Death. *Athletic Business E-Newsletter*, July 2019. Available at: https://www.athleticbusiness.com/athlete-safety/lapse-in-safety-prior-to-high-school-player-s-heat-death.html. Accessed July 31, 2019.

67. Korey Stringer Institute. State High School Sports Safety Policies. University of Connecticut. Available at: https://ksi.uconn.edu/high-school-state-policies-2-2-2/. Accessed August 13, 2019.

68. Valdes AS, Hoffman JR, Clark MH, et al., National Collegiate Athletic Association Strength and Conditioning Coaches' Knowledge and Practices Regarding Prevention and Recognition of Exertional Heat Stroke. *Journal of Strength & Conditioning Research*, 28(11), 3013-3023, 2014.

69. Steinbach P. Overly Aggressive Workouts Put Athletes at Risk of Rhabdomyolysis. *Athletic Business E-Newsletter*, March 2011. Available at: https://www.athleticbusiness.com/Health-Fitness/overly-aggressive-workouts-put-athletes-at-risk-of-rhabdomyolysis.html. Accessed June 17, 2019.

References *continued...*

70. Jones T. Rhabdomyolysis Laid Low 6 Athletes. *The Columbus Dispatch,* March 9, 2013. https://www.dispatch.com/article/20130309/NEWS/303099822. Accessed June 18, 2019.

71. Scott J. Lawsuit Seeks $11.5M from Rhabdo-Causing Incident. *Athletic Business E-Newsletter,* January 2019. Available at: https://www.athletic-business.com/college/lawsuit-seeks-11-5m-from-rhabdo-causing-incident.html. Accessed June 18, 2019.

72. Berg A. Two Nebraska Football Players Hospitalized with Rhabdo. *Athletic Business E-Newsletter,* January 2018. Available at: https://www.athletic-business.com/safety-security/two-nebraska-football-players-hospitalized-with-rhabdo.html. Accessed June 18, 2019.

73. Steinbach P. U. of Houston Fires Strength Coach Over Rhabdo Cases. *Athletic Business E-Newsletter,* February 2019. Available at: https://www.athleticbusiness.com/athlete-safety/u-of-houston-fires-strength-coach-over-rhabdo-cases.html. Accessed June 18, 2019.

74. Steinbach P. U. of Houston Sets Policies in Wake of Rhabdo Cases. *Athletic Business E-Newsletter,* May 2019. Available at: https://www.athletic-business.com/athlete-safety/u-of-houston-sets-policies-in-wake-of-rhabdo-cases.html. Accessed June 18, 2019.

75. Iowa Rhabdo Lawsuit Settled. *Training & Conditioning.* Available at: http://training-conditioning.com/content/iowa-rhabdo-lawsuit-settled. Accessed June 17, 2019.

76. Scott J. Second Lawsuit Filed in Oregon Rhabdo Case. *Athletic Business E-Newsletter,* January 2019. Available at: https://www.athleticbusiness.com/athlete-safety/second-lawsuit-filed-in-oregon-rhabdo-case.html. Accessed June 18, 2019.

77. Sitzler B. NCAA Addresses Exertional Rhabdomyolysis, *NATA Now,* February 1, 2018. Available at: https://www.nata.org/blog/beth-sitzler/ncaa-addresses-exertional-rhabdomyolysis. Accessed June 19, 2019.

78. Jordan E. Former Hawkeye Sues Over 2011 Football Training Hospitalization. March 11, 2014. Available at: https://www.thegazette.com/2014/03/11/former-hawkeye-sues-state-over-2011-rhabdo-incident. Accessed June 17, 2011.

79. Berg A. Rhabdo Rampant at University of Houston. *Athletic Business E-Newsletter,* April 2019. Available at: https://www.athleticbusiness.com/safety-security/rhabdo-rampant-at-university-of-houston.html. Accessed June 18, 2019.

80. Berg A. UH Launches Internal Investigation into Rhabdo Cases. *Athletic Business E-Newsletter,* June 2019. Available at: https://www.athletic-business.com/athlete-safety/houston-launches-internal-investigation-into-rhabdo-cases.html. Accessed June 18, 2019.

81. *Rannebarger v. Allina Health System,* No. C0-04-7944, 2006 LEXIS 47 (D. Minn., 2006).

82. *United States ex. rel Martinez v. KPC Healthcare, Inc.,* No. 8:15-cv-01521-JLS-DFM, 2017 WL 10439030 (C.D. Cal., 2017).

83. *Martin v. Moreau,* 770 S.E.2d 390 (N.C. Ct. App., 2015).

84. *Hajdusek v. United States,* 895 F.3d 146 (1st Cir., 2018).

85. Berg A. Navy Orders More Supervision During Test After Deaths. *Athletic Business E-Newsletter,* May 2019. Available at: https://www.athleticbusiness.com/athlete-safety/navy-orders-more-supervision-during-test-after-deaths.html. Accessed August 9, 2019.

86. Berg A. Army Trialing Modified Fitness Test for Injured Soldiers. *Athletic Business E-Newsletter,* May 2019. Available at: https://www.athletic-business.com/military/army-trialing-modified-fitness-test-for-injured-soldiers.html. Accessed August 9, 2019.

87. Steinbach P. Is Running-Based Fitness Test Coming to the Air Force? *Athletic Business E-Newsletter,* March 2019. Available at: https://www.athleticbusiness.com/military/is-running-based-fitness-test-coming-to-air-force.html. Accessed August 9, 2019.

88. *Exercise Standards & Guidelines Reference Manual.* 5th Ed. Sherman Oaks, CA: Aerobics and Fitness Association of America, 2010.

89. NSCA Strength and Conditioning Professional Standards and Guidelines. *Strength and Conditioning Journal,* 39(6), 1-24, 2017. Available at: https://www.nsca.com/education/articles/nsca-strength-and-conditioning-professional-standards-and-guidelines/. Accessed November 5, 2018.

90. *Contino v. Lucille Roberts Health Spa,* 509 N.Y.S 2d 369 (N.Y. App. Div., 1986).

91. *ACSM's Guidelines for Exercise Testing and Prescription.* Riebe D. (ed). 10th Ed. Philadelphia, PA: Lippincott Williams & Wilkins, 2018.

92. *ACSM's Health/Fitness Facility Standards and Guidelines.* Sanders ME. (ed.) 5th Ed. Champaign, IL: Human Kinetics, 2019.

93. *Medical Fitness Association's Standards & Guidelines for Medical Fitness Center Facilities,* Roy B. (ed.). 2nd Ed. Monterey, CA: Healthy Learning, 2013.

94. IHRSA Club Membership Standards. In: *IHRSA's Guide to Club Membership & Conduct.* 3rd Ed. Boston, MA: International Health, Racquet & Sportsclub Association, 2005. Available at: http://download.ihrsa.org/pubs/club_membership_conduct.pdf. Accessed November 5, 2018.

95. *2014-15 NCAA Sports Medicine Handbook.* The National Collegiate Athletic Association. Indianapolis, IN, 2014. Available at: http://www.ncaapublications.com/productdownloads/MD15.pdf. Accessed August 13, 2019.

96. Antony A. What Wearable Technologies Can Prevent Sports Injuires? Prescouter, September, 2017. Available at: https://www.prescouter.com/2017/09/wearables-sports-injuries/. Accessed August 19, 2019.

97. Roy B. Overreaching/Overtraining: More Is Not Always Better. *ACSM's Health & Fitness Journal,* 19(2), 4-5, 2015.

98. Mathis RL, Jackson JH. *Human Resource Management* (10th ed.). Mason, OH: Thomson, 2003.

99. Eickhoff-Shemek JM, Selde S. Evaluating Group Exercise Leader Performance: An Easy and Helpful Tool. *ACSM's Health & Fitness Journal,* 10(1), 20-23, 2006.

100. Group Fitness Participation Evaluation. University of Maine Campus Recreation. Available at: https://umaine.edu/campusrecreation/program/fitness/group-fitness-participant-evaluation/. Accessed August 21, 2019.

The Performance Appraisal Tool (PAT) for Group Exercise Leaders appears on the following five pages. The three sections within the PAT are described under Risk Management Strategy #5 along with recommendations on how to properly carry out the performance appraisal process. This form can be adapted for personal fitness trainers and others who teach exercise programs.

NOTE: *The PAT is available on the Fitness Law Academy website (www.fitnesslawacademy.com) under Textbook Resources.*

PERFORMANCE APPRAISAL TOOL—GROUP EXERCISE LEADER (GEL)

Name of GEL_____ Name of Supervisor _____

Date of Class Observation _____ Name of Class _____

Number of participants attending _____ Date/Time of Class _____

Reason for Appraisal: _____ Introductory/Probationary _____ Follow-Up _____ Regular Interval

Rate the performance as I, M, E, or NA as follows:

I—Improvement is needed; performance standard is not met
M—Meets performance standard
E—Exceeds performance standard
NA—Not Applicable

> *Note:* **Explanation** sections are available to describe ratings.

SECTION 1: IN-CLASS EVALUATION

Behavior-Based Performance

	I	M	E	NA
Criterion #1—Pre-class Conduct				
1. Arrives prior to class time	——	——	——	——
2. Sets up equipment	——	——	——	——
3. Greets participants as they arrive	——	——	——	——

Explanation: _____

Criterion #2—Beginning of Class Conduct	I	M	E	NA
1. Starts class on time	——	——	——	——
2. Introduces self and class format	——	——	——	——
3. Welcomes everyone	——	——	——	——
4. Makes announcements, e.g., anything related to today's class	——	——	——	——
5. Encourages participants to exercise at own level	——	——	——	——

Explanation: _____

Criterion #3—Safe Instruction

Safe Instruction With Each Class Component

Warm-Up	I	M	E	NA
1. Teaches warm-up which is specifically appropriate for the class	——	——	——	——
2. Incorporates appropriate duration of warm-up	——	——	——	——
Conditioning				
3. Teaches appropriate intensity given fitness levels of participants	——	——	——	——
4. Incorporates proper progression of intensity	——	——	——	——
5. Incorporates proper progression of complexity	——	——	——	——
6. Monitors intensity by having participants take their heart rates	——	——	——	——
7. Monitors intensity by having participants rate their perceived exertion (RPE)	——	——	——	——

	I	M	E	NA
8. Observes each participant for signs of overexertion	—	—	—	—
9. Takes proper action if a participant appears to be overexerted	—	—	—	—
10. Incorporates appropriate duration of stimulus	—	—	—	—
11. Gradually decreases the intensity of exercises prior to cool-down	—	—	—	—

Cool-Down and Stretching

12. Incorporates appropriate duration and activities in the cool-down	—	—	—	—
13. Incorporates appropriate stretching activities	—	—	—	—

Safe Instruction Throughout Class

14. Teaches and demonstrates proper form and execution of exercises	—	—	—	—
15. Corrects improper form/execution of exercises	—	—	—	—
16. Demonstrates modifications given various levels of fitness	—	—	—	—
17. Teaches exercises in an appropriate sequence and progression	—	—	—	—
18. Avoids contraindicated exercises	—	—	—	—
19. Avoids patterns/combinations that can contribute to balance/coordination problems	—	—	—	—
20. Incorporates appropriate number of sets/reps when teaching muscle strength/endurance exercises	—	—	—	—
21. Incorporates exercises that utilize a variety of muscle groups	—	—	—	—
22. Incorporates exercises that focus on muscle balance/coordination	—	—	—	—
23. Incorporates exercises to address muscles that are commonly tight and/or weak	—	—	—	—
24. Incorporates safe transitions, e.g., standing to non-standing	—	—	—	—

Explanation: _____

Criterion #4—Effective Teaching Methods

1. Uses simple, command or cue words	—	—	—	—
2. Incorporates proper timing of command or cue words	—	—	—	—
3. Provides verbal encouragement/positive feedback	—	—	—	—
4. Utilizes appropriate voice quality including projections, volume, and enunciation	—	—	—	—
5. Utilizes appropriate nonverbal communication	—	—	—	—
6. Moves around the room while teaching	—	—	—	—
7. Uses appropriate music volume	—	—	—	—
8. Uses appropriate music tempo	—	—	—	—
9. Selects appropriate music	—	—	—	—
10. Teaches to the beat of the music; demonstrates proper rhythm	—	—	—	—
11. Utilizes room space effectively	—	—	—	—
12. Teaches/reviews exercise concepts and safety principles	—	—	—	—

Explanation: _____

Criterion #5—Class Management	I	M	E	NA
1. Comes to class prepared	—	—	—	—
2. Demonstrates control and command of the class	—	—	—	—
3. Uses class time effectively	—	—	—	—

Explanation: _____

Criterion #6—Professionalism				
1. Dresses appropriately	—	—	—	—
2. Demonstrates professional conduct and attitude	—	—	—	—
3. Supports and adheres to the facility's GEL policies and procedures	—	—	—	—
4. Handles equipment properly	—	—	—	—

Explanation: _____

Criterion #7—Interaction with Participants				
1. Uses an appropriate approach when correcting form/execution	—	—	—	—
2. Shows maturity when dealing with difficult participants	—	—	—	—
3. Encourages a noncompetitive atmosphere	—	—	—	—
4. Establishes a positive rapport	—	—	—	—
5. Incorporates humor appropriately	—	—	—	—
6. Demonstrates enthusiasm	—	—	—	—
7. Creates an enjoyable class	—	—	—	—
8. Welcomes late comers and encourages them to warm-up	—	—	—	—

Explanation: _____

Criterion #8—End of Class Conduct				
1. Ends class on time	—	—	—	—
2. Thanks participants	—	—	—	—
3. Gives positive feedback	—	—	—	—
4. Makes announcements, e.g., promotes other classes/upcoming events	—	—	—	—
5. Available to address participant questions/comments	—	—	—	—

Explanation: _____

Criterion #9—Post-class Conduct				
1. Puts away equipment	—	—	—	—
2. Leaves classroom on time	—	—	—	—
3. Follows procedures, e.g., turning off lights, locking door, etc.	—	—	—	—

Explanation: _____

SECTION 2: OUT-OF-CLASS EVALUATION

Behavior-Based Performance	I	M	E	NA

Criterion #1—Behavior outside the Classroom

	I	M	E	NA
1. Demonstrates dependability regarding teaching responsibilities	—	—	—	—
2. Makes prior arrangements for class when absent	—	—	—	—
3. Attends required in-service trainings, e.g., emergency plan, etc.	—	—	—	—
4. Supports and adheres to the facility's safety polices/procedures	—	—	—	—
5. Maintains current CPR/AED certification	—	—	—	—
6. Maintains current First-Aid certification	—	—	—	—
7. Maintains current GEL certification	—	—	—	—
8. Available to substitute classes for other instructors	—	—	—	—
9. Completes and maintains records/documents, e.g., lesson plans	—	—	—	—

Explanation: _____

Trait-Based Performance

Criterion #1—Communication Traits

	I	M	E	NA
1. Demonstrates appropriate interpersonal communication	—	—	—	—
2. Responds to constructive criticism appropriately	—	—	—	—
3. Responds to phone/email messages in a timely manner	—	—	—	—

Explanation: _____

Criterion #2—Professional/Personal Traits

	I	M	E	NA
1. Demonstrates a positive attitude	—	—	—	—
2. Demonstrates an unbiased attitude	—	—	—	—
3. Exhibits creativity	—	—	—	—
4. Shows a desire to learn	—	—	—	—
5. Takes responsibility for actions	—	—	—	—
6. Demonstrates self-motivation	—	—	—	—

Explanation: _____

Results-Based Performance

Criterion #1—Accomplishments Related to Participants

	I	M	E	NA
1. Obtained high attendance adherence in classes taught	—	—	—	—
2. Obtained positive participant evaluations	—	—	—	—

Explanation: _____

Criterion #2—Accomplishments Related to Program/Facility	Yes	No	In Progress
1. Created a new program or class	——	——	——
2. Improved an operational procedure(s)	——	——	——
3. Developed skills to teach another class or perform another job	——	——	——
4. Developed and/or taught "beginner-level" classes or orientations	——	——	——

Explanation: _____

Criterion #3—Professional Accomplishments			
1. Obtained additional degree or certification	——	——	——
2. Obtained an award or recognition	——	——	——
3. Attended conferences/workshops for continuing education	——	——	——

Explanation: _____

SECTION 3: PERFORMANCE APPRAISAL FEEDBACK

Discussion/Feedback Date _____ (Discussed self-performance appraisal, supervisor performance appraisal and developed an action plan).

Action Plan: (Steps to address performance standards rated "I" with a projected timeframe)

General/Positive Feedback:

GEL Signature _____ Date:_____

Supervisor Signature _____ Date: _____

Copy of written Performance Appraisal Tool given to GEL and original placed in GEL Personnel File on _____ (date).

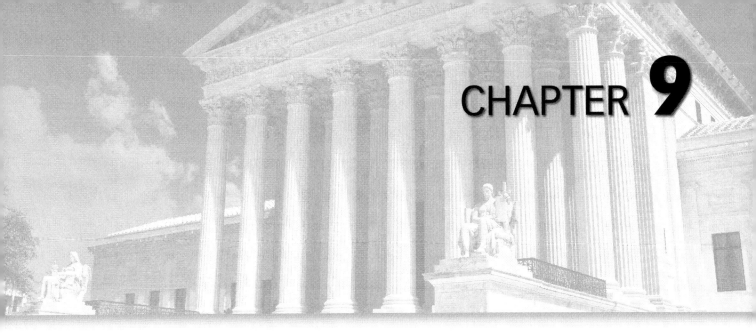

Exercise Equipment Safety

 LEARNING OBJECTIVES

After reading this chapter fitness managers and exercise professionals will be able to:

1. Realize that using exercise equipment is potentially hazardous creating risks of injuries and possible subsequent litigation.

2. Describe four major areas of legal liability exposures regarding exercise equipment.

3. Discuss and analyze negligence cases involving improper instruction and supervision of exercise equipment.

4. Describe five categories of strength training programs and three general types of injuries that can occur from participation in strength training activities.

5. Identify six major causes of strength training injuries and describe strategies that exercise professionals can implement to minimize or eliminate each.

6. Discuss why it is important to have individuals, who want to perform heavy resistance training, to first obtain medical clearance and read/sign a document that informs and warns them of the risks associated with heavy resistance training.

7. Describe why, from a legal perspective, it is essential that exercise professionals inform their participants of the warnings and instructional safety tips provided in the owner's manual provided by the equipment's manufacturer.

8. Describe how fitness facilities can comply with the Americans with Disabilities Act (ADA) by providing inclusive exercise equipment.

9. Using case law examples, summarize the many legal duties and responsibilities associated with exercise equipment that fitness managers/owners have for the facility such as: (a) purchasing/leasing equipment, (b) installing equipment properly, (c) keeping equipment clean/disinfected, (d) conducting equipment inspections and maintenance according to the manufacturer's specifications, and (e) removing equipment from use when in need of repair, after an injury, and after a manufacturer's recall (1).

10. Describe certain standards published by the American Society for Testing and Materials (ASTM International) regarding exercise equipment.

11. Compare and contrast exercise equipment standards of practice published by professional organizations and explain why the National Strength and Conditioning Association (NSCA) standards and guidelines are, perhaps, the most comprehensive from a legal liability perspective.

12. Using case law examples, discuss comparative fault systems that defendants can use when a participant's injury is due to his/her own fault.

13. Define manufacturing, design, and marketing defects as they relate to product liability.

14. Develop and implement 10 risk management strategies that will be effective in minimizing injuries and subsequent litigation involving exercise equipment (1).

INTRODUCTION

Many legal liability exposures (situations that create a risk of injury or reflect a violation of laws) exist involving exercise equipment. This chapter organizes these liability exposures into four major categories as shown in Figure 9-1. Of the four areas, the *negligence of exercise professionals*, such as the failure to properly instruct a participant on how to safely use exercise equipment, and the *negligence of fitness facility managers/owners*, such as the failure to properly maintain exercise equipment, appear to be the most common liability exposures. Four spotlight and several other cases are described to help fitness managers and exercise professionals gain an understanding and appreciation of these two major areas of legal liability exposures. Additional cases are described regarding the *negligence of participants* and the *fault of manufacturers*. Toward the end of this chapter, 10 risk management strategies are described that will help minimize legal liability associated with exercise equipment.

Figure 9-1: Legal Liability Exposures and Exercise Equipment Injuries

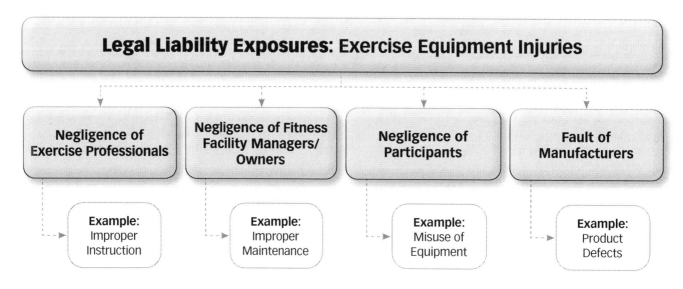

ASSESSMENT OF LEGAL LIABILITY EXPOSURES

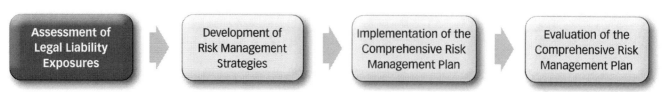

This section describes the four major areas of legal liability exposures associated with exercise equipment injuries: (a) negligence of exercise professionals, (b) negligence of fitness facility managers/owners, (c) negligence of participants, and (d) fault of the manufacturer.

Negligence of Exercise Professionals

As described in Chapter 8, improper instruction and supervision is a major allegation of negligence. Many injuries and subsequent lawsuits, described in Chapter 8 and other chapters in this textbook, have involved

Table 9-1	Exercise Equipment Negligence Lawsuits: Improper Instruction/Supervision	
SPOTLIGHT CASE (CHAPTER)	**EXERCISE EQUIPMENT**	**TYPE OF INJURY**
Corrigan v. MuscleMakers Inc. (4)	Treadmill	Fractured Ankle
Santana v. Women's Workout and Weight Loss Centers, Inc. (4)	Step Bench	Fractured Ankle
Stelluti v. Casapenn Enterprises, LLC, dba Powerhouse Gym (4)	Indoor Cycle	Back & Neck Injuries
Howard v. Missouri Bone and Joint Center (6)	Squat Lift	Back Injury
Layden v. Plante (7)	Smith Squat	Herniated discs
Levy v. Town Sports International, Inc. (7)	BOSU Ball	Fractured Wrist
Scheck v. Soul Cycle (8)	Indoor Cycle	Torn Quadriceps
Vaid v. Equinox (8)	Rower	Massive Stroke
ADDITIONAL CASES (CHAPTER)		
Parks v. Gilligan (4)	Bench Press	Crushed Finger
Makris v. Scandinavian Health Spa, Inc. (6)	Leg Press	Herniated discs
Moore v. Jackson Cardiology Associates (6)	Treadmill	Knee Injury
Mellon v. Crunch (7)	Step Bench	Both Wrists Fractured
Burgos v. Active Health and Fitness Club (8)	Heavy Tire	Crushed Ankle
Horowitz v. Luxury Hotels International of Puerto Rico, Inc. (8)	Indoor Cycle	Exertional Rhabdo
Martin v. Moreau (8)	Treadmill	Fractured Hip
Rannebarger v. Allina Health Systems (8)	Treadmill	Dislocated Shoulder

negligent instruction and supervision. Those related to exercise equipment are listed in Table 9-1. Several of these cases involved injuries that occurred on cardio equipment such as treadmills, indoor cycles, and rowers because the plaintiff (a) was not instructed on how to use the equipment properly (e.g. *Corrigan, Stelluti, Scheck*) or, (b) was instructed to begin at an inappropriate intensity level (e.g., *Vaid, Horowitz*).

Special Focus: Strength Training Equipment Injuries Due to Negligent Instruction and Supervision

A few of the negligence instruction and supervision cases listed in Table 9-1 involved various types of strength training equipment. However, due to the increased popularity of strength training programs (e.g., in 2020 (2), *training with free weights* was ranked fourth out of the top 20 fitness trends), a special focus on negligent instruction/supervision is needed. Additional reasons include:

- Negligence instruction and supervision cases in Chapter 8 focused on various types of exercise programs including personal fitness training, group exercise, youth, strength and conditioning, clinical exercise, and first responder/military—only one case involved strength training equipment.
- Almost all of the exercise professionals who lead the programs described in Chapter 8 have their participants perform exercises using strength training equipment such as machines, free weights, exercise balls, kettlebells, resistance bans, and BOSU® Balance Trainers.

This section begins with an overview of strength training injuries. Exercise professionals need to understand the types and causes of these injuries in order to develop instructional practices that can help prevent them. A description of several negligent instruction and supervision cases involving strength training equipment follows, including the spotlight case, *Butler v. Saville*.

Overview of Strength Training Injuries: Types and Causes

According to Lavellee and Tucker (3), strength training can be broken down into five categories:

a) Strength or resistance training—the goal is to increase muscle strength and endurance to improve health and fitness and includes using, for example, free weights (dumbbells and barbells), machines, bodyweight exercises, and resistance bands

b) Bodybuilding—the goal is less about strength but more on physique enhancement by increasing muscle size and muscular definition

c) Power lifting—the goal is to lift a maximal weight for one repetition in three lifts: the squat, the dead lift, and the bench press

d) Olympic weightlifting—the goal is to lift a maximal weight to achieve the highest total in two lifts: the clean and jerk and the snatch

e) Style-dependent strength sports, such as strongman competitions, Highland games, and field events

In their review of the literature regarding strength training injuries, Lavellee and Tucker (3) concluded that 60-75% of injuries were **acute non-emergent** (e.g., muscular strains, ligamentous sprains) and approximately 30% were **chronic-type injuries** (e.g., overuse injuries, tendonitis). **Acute emergent injuries** such as musculoskeletal (e.g., fractures, dislocations) and non-musculoskeletal (e.g., stroke, myocardial infarction), although rare, can occur. One of the many studies they cited was an epidemiology study authored by Kerr et al. (4) published in 2010 that analyzed weight training injuries using National Electronic Injury Surveillance System (NEISS) data between 1990 and 2007. These researchers found that (a) sprain/strains accounted for 46% of the injuries, (b) the most commonly injured body parts were the upper trunk (25%) and the lower trunk (20%), (c) the most common mechanism of injury was weights dropping on the person, and (d) free weights accounted for 90% of the injuries.

Weights dropping on individuals can be serious. In 2009, University of Southern California (USC) football player Stafon Johnson suffered a ruptured larynx when a bar fell onto his neck (5). Johnson claimed that an assistant strength coach was negligently and carelessly inattentive when placing a bench-press bar back into his hands after an exercise. After going through several emergency surgeries and recovery, he sued USC in 2011. The case was settled in 2012 with a confidential agreement (5).

Lavelle and Tucker (3) also describe injury sites among the different categories of strength training.

For example, shoulder injuries were more common among power lifters, elbow and knee injuries were more common among weightlifters, and power lifters and Olympic weightlifters experienced low-back muscular strains at a higher rate than bodybuilders. Recent epidemiology studies or systematic reviews of weight training injuries have shown similar results to Lavelle and Tucker (3) and Kerr et al. (4). For example, Keogh and Winwood (6) found that the shoulder, lower back, knee, elbow, and wrist/hand were the most common injury sites with strains, tendonitis, and sprains being the common types of injuries. Aasa et al. (7) found that the spine, shoulder, and knee were the most common injury sites in both Olympic weightlifters and power lifters. The authors of these studies concluded that there is need for more research regarding injury prevention.

Many strength training injuries can be prevented by addressing the underlying causes. Physician Herbert L. Fred (8) lists six common causes of injuries associated with weightlifting:

a) Poor conditioning or technique

b) Inadequate strength or endurance

c) Improperly selected resistance

d) Insufficient warm-up or stretching

e) Loss of balance

f) Fatigue

These causes of injuries were evident in the negligence cases involving strength training equipment listed in Table 9-1 and in the cases described below. Many of

KEY POINT

There are various categories of strength training programs with each having different goals. Injuries can occur with participation in all categories, but they can often be prevented. Exercise professionals need to first become aware of the common causes of strength training injures such as (a) poor conditioning or technique, (b) inadequate strength or endurance, (c) improperly selected resistance, (d) insufficient warm-up or stretching, (e) loss of balance, and (f) fatigue (8). To minimize injuries and subsequent litigation, exercise professionals need to obtain the necessary knowledge and skills (competence) to address these common causes of injury *before* they begin designing and delivering strength training programs.

the injuries could have been avoided if the instructors/trainers/coaches possessed the knowledge to fully understand these causes of injuries and the skills on how to address them when instructing and supervising strength training programs.

According to Fred (8), these causes of injuries exist among three classifications of weightlifting injuries (musculoskeletal, neurologic, and cardiovascular). He states that musculoskeletal injuries are frequently reported, but neurologic injuries, such as subarachnoid hemorrhage (SAH) and cardiovascular injuries such as aortic dissection, can also occur. For example, in an article published in *Cardiology* (9), the authors reported 31 patients who were diagnosed with aortic dissection that occurred predominantly during weightlifting involving extreme exertion. In a negligence lawsuit (Bursik case described below), the plaintiff documented 32 cases from NEISS data between 2002 and 2010 in which individuals suffered a stroke or subconjunctival hemorrhage (broken blood vessel in the eye) in conjunction with weightlifting (10). Fred (8) states that the chief culprit is vascular stress through an exceptionally elevated blood pressure. Therefore, he recommends individuals with certain medical conditions lift weights cautiously, if at all.

Resistance Training and the Valsalva Maneuver. The **Valsalva maneuver** occurs when individuals hold their breath against a closed glottis. It can occur with daily activities such as straining during defecating or lifting a heavy object. The question is: does the Valsalva maneuver, when performed with resistance training (RT), further increase risks over and beyond the risks associated with resistance training alone? The authors of a scientific statement published by the American Heart Association (AHA) state that "the Valsalva maneuver and high levels of muscle tension to lift...a heavy weight can result in somewhat dramatic changes to the physiological responses to RT" (11, p. 573). These physiological changes include a substantial rise in both systolic and diastolic blood pressure (BP) depending on the intensity and duration of the maneuver and the resistance. The authors of this AHA publication state that "although excessive BP elevations have been documented with high-intensity RT...such elevations are generally not a concern with low- to moderate-intensity RT performed with correct breathing technique and avoidance of the Valsalva maneuver" (11, p. 577). A

position paper of the NSCA published in 2019 included a similar statement: "Resistance exercise-induced elevations in blood pressure are dampened in low- to moderate-intensity resistance exercise performed with correct breathing technique (i.e., avoidance of the Valsalva maneuver) and training" (12, p. 2035). The AHA statement includes 10 absolute and six relative contraindications to resistance training (e.g., absolute contraindications include incontrollable hypertension and aortic dissection).

The Bursik Case. Debra Bursik claimed she suffered an intra-cerebral stroke when she engaged the Valsalva maneuver while lifting heavy weights during a personal training session (10). She referred to NEISS data to support her case regarding the prevalence of these injuries. The 32 NEISS documented cases in 100 hospitals were used to estimate the number of similar cases nationwide. This estimate was 1,287 cases during the same eight-year time period, 2002-2010. In her lawsuit, she claimed her personal fitness trainer was negligent (i.e., failed to supervise her to ensure she was breathing properly while lifting weights and failed to warn her of the dangers of the Valsalva maneuver during resistance training, a common risk she claimed based on the NEISS data). The case was settled out of court, but the testimony of the witnesses is relevant. An expert witness for the plaintiff stated that he would have been able to "provide a specific explanation of the Valsalva maneuver and the potential consequences if the warning is not adhered to, given the number of people that are experiencing this issue each year" (10, p. 12). Defense witnesses, exercise science professors and practitioners, believed there was no need to warn given that a stroke during weight training is rare. They did not know about the NEISS data. Another witness who had oversight of approximately 185 personal fitness trainers said he would not warn participants of such risks because it would scare them and keep them from exercising.

Note: *Not informing individuals of risks because it will scare them is not a legitimate legal defense.*

In an article titled "The Valsalva and Stroke: Time for Everyone to Take a Deep Breath," physician Jonathan M. Sullivan provides his views of the Bursik case (13). However, he first provides background information about the Valsalva maneuver and its effects on hemodynamics during each of its four phases, an overview of stroke, and case studies involving activities that preceded SAH. For example, one study that investigated 500 consecutive cases of SAH found no reliable documentation of Valsalva. "Lifting heavy loads and sporting/exercising preceded 2.4% and 3.8% of events, respectively, less than sex (6.4%), pooping (7.6%), standing up (5.4%) or sitting down (8.8%)" (13, p. 11). Sullivan also describes several studies and a systematic review that investigated resistance training and Valsalva (RT+V). The authors of these studies concluded that RT+V "increases blood pressure, but not as much as Valsalva alone" …and recommended "that the Valsalva should not be exaggerated under a load, but it should not be avoided, either, considering the moderating effect of Valsalva on TMP" (13, p. 9). TMP is an acronym for cerebral transmural pressure.

Note: *Intentionally engaging the Valsalva is often recommended while performing heavy weightlifting with the premise it might protect the lower back. However, Sullivan argues that Valsalva's protective effect is that it helps to generate less stress across the vascular wall than lifting weights without a Valsalva. In addition, he states Valsalva is an everyday occurrence and it is difficult to avoid with heavy lifting even when instructed not to do it.*

Sullivan (13) then presents his deep dive into the 32 NEISS cases cited by Bursik. He found that these cases did not document (a) that these individuals were lifting heavy, (b) which exercises they were doing, (c) the weight lifted, the medical histories, and (d) whether they were using barbells—nothing, except that they were lifting weights and then had a hemorrhage. In his review of these NEISS data, Sullivan indicated that a major problem with the 32 cases was that there was no documentation of Valsalva in any of them. Therefore, he concluded that using these data to make a causal connection between resistance training plus Valsalva increases the risk of stroke is quite weak. In fact, he states that nobody has ever demonstrated a cause-and-effect relationship between RT+V and intracranial hemorrhage. However, in a negligence lawsuit, the plaintiff does not have to prove a cause-and-effect relationship. Only the preponderance of the evidence is needed (i.e., was it more likely than not (over 50%)

that the defendant's breach of duty caused the plaintiff's injury).

Bursik's injury (stroke) could have happened to her by lifting "heavy" weights alone and not because of the combination of RT+V. As described in the above studies, lifting heavy weights can lead to neurologic and cardiovascular injuries due to extreme elevations of blood pressure. Perhaps the negligence of the trainer was having her lift heavy weights, which might have been contraindicated due to her medical history. Her medical history and whether the trainer had conducted proper medical screening were not provided in the case description (10). Sullivan (13) concludes that the dangers of Valsalva are imaginary. However, he does caution that some individuals with medical conditions should not lift, Valsalva or no Valsalva, until they are cleared by a physician. To minimize potential legal liability, Sullivan recommends that exercise professionals inform their participants of the risks and have them read/sign an explicit assumption of risk that includes risks of "cardiovascular, ocular, pulmonary and cerebrovascular complications from exercising under Valsalva" (13, p. 15). See Exhibit 9-1 for a summary regarding minimizing injury risks and legal liability in strength training programs.

Strength Training Cases: Negligent Instruction and Supervision

The following cases and the spotlight case (*Butler v. Saville et al.*) describe injuries due to the negligent instruction and supervision of exercise professionals involving strength training equipment. To learn more about strength training injuries and subsequent litigation, it is recommended that fitness managers and exercise professionals read an article by highly-experienced expert witness, Dr. Anthony Abbott, titled "Resistance Training and Litigation" (14). He describes several lawsuits involving free-weight exercises, fixed-weight exercises, and body-weight exercises, many of which involved improper instruction and supervision as well as improper equipment maintenance. Improper maintenance is described below under Negligence of Fitness Facility Managers/Owners.

Assaf Blecher v. 24 Hour Fitness Inc. and David Stevens (15). In this case, the plaintiff was awarded

---

Exhibit 9-1: Summary: Minimizing Injury Risks and Liability in Strength Training Programs

Exercise professionals should be aware of the following:

- Musculoskeletal injures are the most common but other injuries can occur such as neurologic (e.g., stroke) and cardiovascular (e.g. aortic dissection).
- All types of injuries (musculoskeletal, neurologic and cardiovascular) can be minimized if individuals are properly instructed and supervised including proper execution/technique and progression (i.e., obtain certain skill/strength before performing advanced lifting exercises) and avoiding fatigue (i.e., provide appropriate recovery periods between sets).
- Heavy resistance training (RT) causes significant increases in blood pressure. The Valsalva maneuver causes significant increases in blood pressure. RT combined with the Valsalva maneuver may cause further increases in blood pressure. However, it is difficult to avoid Valsalva with heavy RT.
- Heavy RT, with or without Valsalva, can increase the risk of neurologic and cardiovascular injuries (as well as musculoskeletal) especially in individuals with certain medical conditions.
- Individuals with certain medical conditions should not perform strength training activities or need to, first, obtain medical clearance. See AHA Scientific Statement (11) for absolute and relative contraindications.
- Elevations in blood pressure are, generally, not a concern with low- to moderate-intensity RT performed with correct breathing technique and avoidance of the Valsalva maneuver (11, 12).
- Prior to instructing heavy RT activities, exercise professionals should have participants obtain medical clearance and read/sign a document that informs and warns them of the risks. ***Note:*** Consultation with a competent lawyer is needed to prepare such a document.

$892,650 in damages ($142,650 for medical expenses and $750,000 for pain and suffering). On January 26, 2010, Blecher's personal fitness trainer, Stevens, dropped a 145-pound barbell on Blecher's face causing various facial injuries and emergency plastic surgery. Blecher claimed that Steven's conduct was grossly negligent for failing to (a) follow safety procedures such as properly gripping the bar, and (b) provide "spotting" responsibilities for a weight that was heavier than Blecher could handle. In addition, he claimed that 24 Hour Fitness was negligent for not properly educating its trainers on safety techniques. Although Blecher signed a waiver/release, it was unenforceable due to the gross negligence of Stevens.

The failure to provide spotting (omission) as well as improper spotting (commission) can lead to injuries and subsequent litigation as demonstrated in *Assaf Blecher* and other cases. See *Parks v. Gilligan* described in Chapter 4 in which a volunteer spotter and the facility were liable for the plaintiff's injury due to improper spotting. *Sicard v. University of Dayton* (16) is another case to demonstrate the importance of providing proper spotting. A basketball player was injured (pectoral muscle rupture) when a school-employed spotter and two volunteer spotters failed to contain 356 pounds of weight during a bench press. The basketball player sued the employee spotter and the University claiming that the spotter's actions/inactions constituted reckless and wanton misconduct. The appellate court found that the trial court erred when it granted summary judgment for the defendants and, therefore, reversed the trial court's ruling.

Note: *Some fitness facilities have opted to not provide free weights such as barbells because of the potential increased risk of injury and the added costs to employ competent exercise professionals to supervise the free-weight area and provide spotting of participants.*

Lemaster v. Grove City Christian Sch. (17). Hayden Lemaster, a 97-pound middle-school football player, was injured during an off-season workout after coach Swank instructed the young athletes to max out (i.e., attempt to lift their personal maximal weight one time). Student spotters and Coach Swank were available to assist Hayden, but when he attempted to squat 200 pounds without the assistance of spotters, he felt dizzy and experienced pain in his back and legs. He was later diagnosed with compression fractures in his spine. In their complaint, Hayden's parents claimed that Swank's conduct "showed a reckless disregard for the safety of others when he intentionally instructed members of the football team to max out on the squat lift…when he knew or had reason to know facts that would lead a reasonable person to realize that his conduct created an unreasonable risk of harm" (pp. 4-5). The parents also named the school as a defendant based on **respondeat superior.**

The trial court granted the motions for summary judgment for both defendants. At trial, Coach Swank claimed that he taught all the athletes proper weight training techniques and that Hayden injured himself due to poor positioning of the bar. The parents appealed and the appellate court reversed and remanded both summary judgments. To support their argument, Hayden's parents provided an affidavit from an expert strength and conditioning coach who stated that a strength and conditioning coach "who allows a sixth or seventh grader to max out is reckless and creates a substantial increase in harm to the kids" (17, pp. 9-10). Quoting previous case law, the court stated that "reckless conduct is characterized by the conscious disregard of or indifference to a known or obvious risk of harm to another that is unreasonable under the circumstances" (p. 7). The court also indicated that Hayden could not have assumed the risks because a 12 or 13-year-old "sixth grader is only halfway to full brain development… and cannot be expected to fully appreciate the danger his coach is asking him to experience" (17, p. 11).

Note: *To help ensure the safety of children participating in strength training programs, safety standards and guidelines such as those published by the NSCA (18) need to be followed.*

Gallant v. Hilton Hotels Corp. (19). The plaintiff in this case, Eric Gallant, claimed he was injured when he was struck in the back of his head by a kettlebell while taking a class taught by KettleBell Concepts, Inc. The class was held in a space that KettleBell Concepts Inc. rented from the Hilton Hotels Corp. Gallant sued Hilton Hotels Corp. and Hilton Worldwide, Inc. (Hilton) and KettleBell Concepts, Inc. and David Ganulin (KettleBell) claiming that he sustained the injuries when a kettlebell was swung by another participant in the class "who was negligently permitted, allowed and instructed to continue swinging kettlebells, despite people

moving about the room resulting from defendants' recklessness, negligent supervision, and negligent hiring." (p. 1). The defendants (Hilton and KettelBell) jointly filed a motion for summary judgment arguing that Gallant's action was barred based on the waiver/release he signed. However, Gallant claimed that the waiver/release was unenforceable because Hilton had a duty to protect its guests against the gross negligence by its lessee, KettleBell.

An expert witness for the plaintiff, a certified kettlebell trainer, stated that "during any type of break, when no instructors are maintaining the required vigilant supervision, no movement or swinging of kettlebells should occur" (19, p. 3). This expert also stated that the NSCA "recommends a six foot by four foot safety cushion, as a minimum, between kettlebell lifters at free weight stations. Such safety areas must be maintained whenever kettlebells are allowed to be lifted. Kettlebell lifters should be permitted to work only in designated lifting areas and…an area of at least five feet (side to side) and seven feet (front to back) should be maintained around all lifters when lifting is being performed…Moreover, for safe egress and ingress, there should be at least a 36 inch walkway maintained into the lifting area and a clear path provided to exits. No lifting should ever occur in this area, especially when student lifters are moving in or out of the facility" (p. 3).

In its analysis of the waiver/release, the court referred to New York's statute (GOL § 5-326) and stated that the defendants do not fall within the establishments listed within this statute. Based on this statute, waivers are against public policy and unenforceable in establishments such as health clubs and gymnasiums. Therefore, the waiver that Gallant signed could have been enforceable but it was ambiguous. It was also unenforceable because the court stated it is well settled that waivers for grossly negligent acts are void. The court granted the summary judgment for Hilton stating that their duty was to exercise reasonable care in maintaining their properties and there were no allegations that they breached that duty. However, summary judgment was denied for KettleBell and the court ordered that this plaintiff's action shall continue.

Jafri v. Equinox Holdings (20). In this case, the plaintiff, Saad Jafri, claimed he sustained permanent back injury while he was being trained by personal fitness trainer, Ryan Hopkins, an employee of Equinox. Jafri alleged that Hopkins instructed him to perform squats with a heavy load and then had him perform eccentric pulls which involved running away from Hopkins while Hopkins pulled back on a large rubber-band that was wrapped around his waist. At that point Jafri felt a pop in his lower back. He was unable to walk, and an ambulance transported him to the hospital. Jafri's complaint alleged that (a) Equinox had noticed that Hopkins used unsafe methods with members he trained, (b) Hopkins ignored warnings that Jafri had given him regarding his low back weakness, and (c) Hopkins failed to give him simple, beginner workouts. Hopkins moved to dismiss the complaint based on the waiver and primary assumption of risk defenses. He also argued that the complaint was totally frivolous.

The court ruled the waiver did not bar the plaintiff's claims based on its ambiguity and New York's statute (GOL § 5-326). For an effective primary assumption of risk defense, the plaintiff must possess a full understanding of the risks and voluntarily encounter those risks. The court stated that this doctrine "is not an absolute defense, but a measure of the defendant's duty of care" (20, p. 5) and that "awareness of risk is not to be determined in a vacuum…rather to be assessed against the background of the skill and experience of the particular plaintiff" (20, pp. 4-5). The court described several facts that needed to be determined during discovery regarding the background of Jafri such as his level of fitness, low back weakness, and experience with performing these exercises. Therefore, Hopkin's motion to dismiss, based on this doctrine, was denied.

Regarding the complaint being totally frivolous, the court referred to 22NYCRR 130-1.1(c) that permits courts to sanction attorneys for engaging in **frivolous conduct**. Conduct is frivolous if:

(1) it is completely without merit in law and cannot be supported by a reasonable argument for an extension, modification or reversal of existing law;

(2) it is undertaken primarily to delay or prolong the resolution of the litigation, or to harass or maliciously injure another; or

(3) it asserts material factual statements that are false (22NYCRR 130-1.1(c)).

Hopkins claimed that a Facebook posting made by the plaintiff was done for the sole intention of harassment. However, the court did not find that the plaintiff's conduct was frivolous based on the above definitions.

KEY POINT

To minimize injuries and subsequent legal liability, exercise professionals need to possess the necessary knowledge and skills to safely teach exercises using strength training equipment. Fitness managers/owners have a responsibility to properly hire, train, and supervise exercise professionals to avoid vicarious liability and direct liability (described in Chapter 5) as demonstrated in the negligence cases in this and other chapters.

Negligence of Fitness Facility Managers/Owners

Fitness facility managers have numerous responsibilities regarding exercise equipment safety. As described in previous chapters, fitness managers/owners are *the* risk management managers for the facility (see Figure 9-2) and have a vested interest, from a legal liability perspective, to take these responsibilities seriously. They have a duty to provide a reasonably safe environment, which means taking precautions to help prevent foreseeable injuries such as those presented in Table 9-1. As described in Chapter 5, employers can be vicariously liable (e.g., failure of an employee to provide safe instruction), and directly liable (e.g., failure to properly hire, train, and supervise employees). This section focuses on additional responsibilities of fitness managers/owners regarding equipment safety.

Figure 9-2: The Fitness Manager/Owner is *the* Risk Management Manager of the Facility

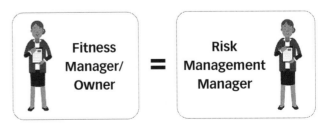

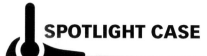

SPOTLIGHT CASE

Butler v. Saville et al.
No. CV116023310, 2014 WL 3805719 (Conn. Super Ct., 2014)

FACTS

Historical Facts:

In August 2009, Susan Butler, age 62, signed a contract with Planet Fitness Branford that included a release of liability that stated, in part, "from any responsibility or liability for an injury or damage to myself, including those caused by the negligent act or omission of Planet Fitness" (p. 1). In September of 2009 while participating in one of her first personal training sessions, trainer John Saville had Butler stand onto a BOSU ball (ball side down) and then he walked away leaving her unattended. Butler tried to maintain her balance but fell to the floor fracturing her wrist and hip resulting in subsequent surgeries (A). Note: The court uses "BOSU ball" to refer the BOSU® Balance Trainer.

Procedural Facts:

Butler, the plaintiff, filed a complaint against the defendants, Saville and several corporations collectively referred to as Planet Fitness. The defendants filed a Second Special Defense arguing that the contract Butler signed waived liability. Butler then filed a motion for summary judgment as to the defendant's Second Special Defense claiming that the release of liability violates public policy in Connecticut. The defendants then argued that Butler's injury was an activity with inherent risks and, thus, she assumed these risks.

ISSUE

Did the court grant Butler's motion for summary?

COURT'S RULING

Yes, the court granted Butler's motion for summary judgment – the release of liability (waiver) violated public policy and the primary assumption of risk defense was ineffective due to the negligence of the defendants.

COURT'S REASONING

The court stated that in Connecticut it is well established that, "the enforcement of a well drafted exculpatory agreement that releases a provider of a recreational activity from prospective liability for personal injuries sustained as a result of the provider's negligence may violate public policy if certain conditions are met" (p. 1). Factors regarding nonenforcement of the exculpatory clause applicable to this case include: "(1) Thousands, if not millions, of ordinary people go to gyms like Planet Fitness, and there is a societal expectation that such activities will be reasonably safe. (2) It would be illogical to relieve a professional gym like Planet Fitness, with superior expertise and information concerning the dangers of activities conducted on its premises, from the responsibility of reasonable care in conducting those activities. (3) The release at issue was a standardized adhesion contract, lacking equal bargaining power between the parties, and offered to Butler on a 'take it or leave it' basis" (p. 1).

Given the likely unenforceability of the release, the defendants then argue that the specific activity of BOSU ball that caused the injury was an activity with "inherent risks" and, therefore, Butler assumed those risks. To address this argument, the court stated that it is:

> common knowledge that some recreational activities are inherently more dangerous than others… Few people would go to a provider of sky-diving or bungee-cord jumping activities expecting such activities to be risk-free. But the societal expectation of gyms like Planet Fitness is entirely different. Ordinary people attend gyms like

Butler continued...

Planet Fitness hoping to achieve—what else? —fitness. They do not go to such establishments expecting physical risk. If the particular activity of BOSU ball is, as the defendants now claim, inherently risky, then the very act of directing an ordinary person to engage in that risky activity without proper supervision may itself be an act of negligence. A jury could, at a minimum, so find, and the defendants may not, consistently with public policy, shield themselves with the exculpatory clause in issue (p. 2).

Plaintiff Awarded Large Settlement—$750,000

After this court's ruling and during mediation, this case was settled for $750,000 (B). As analyzed by this court, the defenses (release of liability and primary assumption of risk) presented by the defendants were likely ineffective. If the case had gone to trial, the plaintiff's expert witness would have provided testimony supporting many of the negligent claims against Saville and Planet Fitness. There were 13 and seven negligent claims made against the trainer and Planet Fitness, respectively (B). These included the following against the trainer and Planet Fitness: Saville "failed to properly instruct the plaintiff on how to perform the physical exercise on the BOSU ball" and Planet Fitness "failed to provide properly trained and qualified fitness trainers" (B, p. 67).

Lessons Learned from *Butler*:

Legal

▸ Employers have a responsibility (duty) to properly hire, train, and supervise all their fitness staff members.

▸ The employer in this case was named as a defendant along with the trainer based on the legal principle of respondeat superior in which employers can be held liable for the negligent conduct of their employees.

▸ Releases of liability in some jurisdictions, such as Connecticut in this case, are not valid for personal injuries caused by negligent conduct because they violate public policy when certain factors are met (e.g., the release was an adhesion contract).

▸ The primary assumption of risk defense may not be effective, as in this case, when "risky" fitness activities are taught to ordinary persons because such instruction may itself be an act of negligence.

Risk Management/Injury Prevention

▸ Personal fitness trainers need to be well-trained on the importance of providing proper instruction and supervision (e.g., never leave a client unattended, provide safe instruction given the client's age, health status, and experience). Balance exercises on BOSU balls are considered advanced exercises (and "risky" as stated by this court) and should only be taught to those who have acquired adequate balance/coordination/skill to safely perform the exercise.

▸ Exercise professionals need to heed the BOSU warning "standing on the platform (flat part) is not recommended" as well as other safety guidelines. For more on the proper use of a BOSU ball, see an article titled: The BOSU Ball (C)

▸ Supervisors of personal fitness trainers should regularly observe and evaluate the job performance of their trainers. When it is observed that unsafe exercises are being taught, supervisors need to provide direct, constructive feedback immediately to the trainers on how to improve their instruction.

A. Herbert DL. Connecticut Case Against Planet Fitness Results in Ruling for Plaintiff and Large Settlement. *The Exercise, Sports and Sport Medicine Standards and Malpractice Reporter,* 4(4), 62, 2015.

B. Herbert DL. Case Against Personal Trainer in Connecticut Results in $750,000 Settlement. *The Exercise, Sports and Sport Medicine Standards and Malpractice Reporter*, 4(5), 65, 67-70, 2015.

C. Wing CH. The BOSU Ball. *ACSM's Health & Fitness Journal,* 18(4), 5-7, 2014.

Although risk management is, ultimately, the responsibility of fitness managers/owners, they will likely delegate many of the responsibilities regarding exercise equipment safety to other staff members in supervisory roles. Therefore, proper training of staff members who will have these responsibilities is important. The following are examples of issues that reflect legal liability exposures that fitness managers/owners/supervisors need to address to help ensure exercise equipment safety as well as compliance with various laws:

a) Following the ADA
b) Making informed decisions when purchasing/leasing equipment
c) Installing equipment properly such as spacing and signage
d) Keeping equipment clean and disinfected
e) Conducting equipment inspections and maintenance according to the manufacturer's specifications
f) Removing equipment from use when in need of repair, after an injury, and a manufacturer's recall
g) Following standards of practice published by professional and independent organizations
h) Providing proper storage for equipment such as dumbbells and exercise balls

Each of these issues are discussed in this section except for the last one, which is described in Chapter 10. The three spotlight and other cases described in this section help demonstrate the importance of addressing these safety-related issues in order to minimize negligence claims/lawsuits against fitness facility managers and owners.

Following the ADA

The ADA is described in Chapter 3. However, this discussion will briefly focus on exercise equipment issues relevant to the ADA. The American Society of Testing and Materials (ASTM International) Subcommittee on F08.30 on Fitness Products has 16 active standards regarding all types of commercial exercise equipment (21). Certain specifications included in two of these standards, F2115 and F1749, are described below (see Installing Equipment Properly). Most of these ASTM standards are designed for manufacturers. They focus on specifications related to the design and manufacturing of exercise equipment. However, fitness managers/owners should also be aware of some of these specifications and adhere to them.

One ASTM standard (F3021-17) is titled "Standard Specification for Universal Design of Fitness Equipment for Inclusive Use by Persons with Functional Limitations and Impairments" (22). This standard provides specifications that are not addressed in other ASTM commercial exercise equipment standards with a major goal to increase access and user independence by individuals with functional limitations or impairments. Additional goals of this standard are to (a) "promote proper design and manufacturing practices for fitness equipment intended for use by people with functional limitations or impairments" and (b) "assist designers and manufacturers in reducing the possibility of injury when the products are used in accordance with the operational instructions" (p. 1). This standard is quite lengthy with several sections. One section, Design and Construction Requirements, contains a subsection titled "General Requirements" and contains specifications under each of the following:

- Access and Set Up
- Seats, Sitting Surfaces, and Back Supports
- Adjustment Mechanisms
- Hand Grips
- Instructions for Use
- Labeling Requirements, e.g., see Figure 9-3 for an inclusive fitness symbol to be placed by the instructional panel on the equipment

Figure 9-3: Inclusive Fitness Symbol*

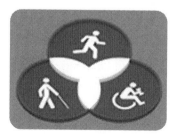

*Reprinted, with permission, from ASTM F3021-17 Standard Specification for Universal Design of Fitness Equipment for Inclusive Use by Persons with Functional Limitations and Impairments, copyright ASTM International, 100 Barr Harbor Drive, West Conshohocken, PA 19428.

The ADA does not require that fitness facilities provide special exercise equipment that is designed for persons with functional limitations or impairments. It does require fitness facilities to make reasonable accommodations for individuals with disabilities and to provide programs and services for them as described in Chapter 3. Fitness facilities that want to increase their membership numbers and participation rates may want to consider obtaining exercise equipment that meets the specifications of ASTM F3021-17. These participants will appreciate the equipment's easier access and user independence. Providing **inclusive exercise equipment,** along with well-educated and trained exercise professionals to work with individuals with limitations/impairments, is an effective way to increase physical activity among this population—a *Healthy People 2020* objective (23). This "inclusive" exercise equipment can be used by individuals with and without functional limitations or impairments. Therefore, when managers/owners are looking to purchase or replace exercise equipment, it may be wise to consider inclusive equipment.

Providing inclusive exercise equipment may help prevent ADA discrimination lawsuits. For example, in September 2019, a Clearwater, Florida man filed a lawsuit against the local YMCA for numerous violations to the ADA (24). Louis Jorgl is blind and uses a cane to get around. In his lawsuit, he claimed that the YMCA ignored his concerns more than a decade. He claimed that exercise machines were bunched too close together and that members blocked pathways with gym bags that caused him to trip and break his cane. According to his lawyer, Jorgl had asked for reasonable accommodations that were necessary considering his disability—not for any special favors. His lawyer also stated that Jorgl should not have "to use a fitness room at the risk of getting hit by other members because the machines are too close together, or tripping over obstructions that are left in the pathways of the fitness room in violation of YMCA policies..." (p. 3). Simple training of employees regarding the needs of disabled members would have solved much of the problem according to Jorgl's lawyer.

Note: *ASTM standard (F3021-17) includes specifications regarding access to and around the inclusive exercise equipment. It is essential that safety policies of the facility, such as no gym bags in the fitness area, are always enforced.*

Purchasing/Leasing Equipment

Only commercial-grade equipment should be considered for fitness facilities—not equipment designed for home use. Exercise equipment buying guides serve as a valuable resource for fitness manager/owners and are easily available. For example, Athletic Business has an online Buyers Guide (25) and IHRSA provides a "free" download of its Commercial Fitness Guide (26). Managers/owners need to consider and research a variety of factors when making equipment purchasing/leasing decisions such as (a) populations served, (b) spacing and storage issues, (c) costs, (d) quality of equipment (e.g., does it meet ASTM design and manufacturing specifications), (e) brand selection, (f) reputation and quality of services provided by the manufacturer/distributor, (g) safety and recall history, and (h) warranties. In addition, factors related to equipment safety need to be considered such as inspecting and cleaning procedures performed by staff members and maintenance service contracts with the manufacturer and/or distributor.

Whether purchasing or leasing exercise equipment, contract law will apply. See Chapter 1 for more information regarding the four required elements of a contract, the Uniform Commercial Code (e.g., Article 2 addresses the sale and/or purchase/lease of goods), and the Statute of Frauds that requires contracts be in writing for the sale of goods over $500. It may be wise for fitness managers/owners to first have a competent lawyer review the terms of exercise equipment purchasing/leasing contracts.

Used Equipment. Additional factors need to be considered when purchasing used exercise equipment such as the designation of the equipment. For example, one company (27) provides three designations: (a) as is, (b) refurbished, and (c) certified remanufactured. The criteria that the equipment needs to meet for each designation is different, with the certified remanufactured designation meeting the most stringent criteria.

Note: *Some fitness facilities such as community, non-profit facilities may receive offers to have used commercial exercise equipment donated to them. It is best to turn down these offers unless the equipment can first be refurbished/remanufactured by a reputable company.*

Technology. Various technologies should also be considered. Some manufacturers offer a digital platform where individuals can track their workouts while using exercise equipment and more. For example, Technogym developed Mywellness®—the first cloud-based open platform in the industry (28). Features of Mywellness® include enabling (a) personal fitness trainers to manage their client's program, and (b) users to easily track both indoor and outdoor training. Prior to accessing Mywellness®, individuals have an option to not have their personal data tracked. Technogym, a global company, established the opt-out mechanism to be compliant with the General Data Protection Regulation (GDPR). The GDPR was adopted by the European Union (EU) in 2018 and contains many privacy rules and hefty penalties for violations (29). In addition, **predictive asset management technologies** exist that can track exercise equipment usage as well as an alert system to notify facility operators when the equipment needs maintenance. The statistics obtained are useful for decision-making and record-keeping. For more information on predictive asset management technology, see an article published on the IHRSA's website (30).

Installing Equipment

Safety factors need to be considered regarding the installation of exercise equipment such as spacing, signage, and electrical issues. The equipment owner's (or user's) manual contains these specifications. See appendix 9 for an excerpt from Technogym's User's Manual of the Technogym Skillmill Treadmill. This manual states that "the installation, maintenance and setting operations must be carried out by qualified Technogym staff or persons authorized by Technogym" (p. 5). Reputable equipment manufacturers/distributors have their own designated, trained, and certified employees who properly install the equipment including assembling, inspecting, and testing the equipment according to the specifications in the owner's manual. Prior to purchasing/leasing exercise equipment, fitness managers/owners should review the specifications in the manuals, in consultation with the manufacturer's representatives, to be sure the facility can comply with them. It is wise to have at least one designated employee (e.g., a professional in a supervisory role assigned to oversee the exercise equipment including inspections and maintenance). This employee can serve as the liaison with the manufacturer's certified technician and even complete the training and certification offered by the manufacturer.

Spacing of Equipment

A major installation issue is equipment spacing. Too often, exercise equipment is spaced too close together which can lead to injuries. For example, the spotlight case, *Jimenez v. 24 Hour Fitness*, demonstrates the importance of (a) providing adequate spacing behind treadmills to prevent serious injuries and, (b) following published spacing specifications to minimize legal liability. Spacing specifications are included in the treadmill's owner's manual as shown in appendix 9 and in ASTM Standard F2115-18 (31). This ASTM standard specifies minimum clearances needed behind (2 meters or 79.2 inches) and between (0.5 meter or 19.5 inches) treadmills (see Figure 9-4). Spacing specifications for all exercise equipment should be followed as stated in the owner's manual as well as other specifications such as certain equipment being properly bolted to the floor (see *Barnhard vs. Cybex International, Inc.* under Fault of the Manufacturer) or in some cases, to the wall or ceiling, such as TRX Suspension equipment.

Figure 9-4: Minimum Clearance Specifications Behind and Between Treadmills*

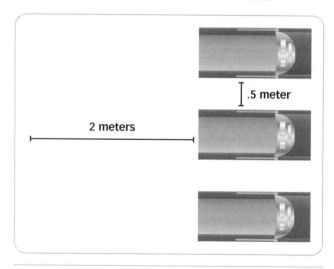

.5 meter

2 meters

*Based on ASTM F2115-18 Standard Specification for Motorized Treadmills

Treadmill Falls. Providing proper spacing of treadmills may help prevent serious injuries such as the plaintiff, Etelvina Jimenez, experienced in the spotlight case. Falls off treadmills are quite common. After the death of SurveyMonkey's CEO, David Goldberg, who suffered severe head trauma after slipping from a treadmill, *USA Today* published an article titled "Treadmill Injuries Send Thousands to the ER Every Year" in 2015 (32a). Based on NEISS data, there were 24,400 treadmill-related injuries in 2014 that were treated in hospital emergency rooms and 30 deaths between 2003-2012 (32a). Given these statistics, fitness managers and exercise professionals need to take precautions, such as providing proper instruction and supervision, to help ensure participants are safely exercising on the treadmills. They may also want to consider not providing treadmills as an exposure avoidance strategy. Alternatives include providing a walking/jogging track as well as other cardio equipment where falls are less likely.

SPOTLIGHT CASE

Jimenez v. 24 Hour Fitness
188 Cal. Rptr. 3d. 228 (Cal. Ct. App., 2015)

FACTS

Historical Facts:

While exercising at 24 Hour Fitness, Etelvina Jimenez fell backwards off a moving treadmill and sustained severe head injuries when her head hit the exposed steel foot of a leg exercise machine that was placed approximately three feet 10 inches behind the treadmill. About two years prior, Jimenez joined 24 Hour Fitness. Justin Wilbourn, the membership manager, required her to sign a membership agreement that included a liability release provision. He knew that Etelvina could not read or speak English and he did not ask a Spanish-speaking employee to assist in the administration of the waiver. "Instead, he pointed to his computer screen to a figure, $24.99, indicating the membership fee, and made pumping motions with his arms like he was exercising. Etelvina understood the numbers, which are identical in Spanish, and she understood Wilbourn's physical gestures to mean that if she paid that amount, she could use the facility. She could not read anything else" (p. 231). Without making any other indications about the release and what it meant, he pointed to the signature lines where Etelvina needed to sign. She believed she was signing to only to pay the monthly fee of $24.99.

Procedural Facts:

The plaintiffs, Etelvina and Pedro Jimenez, filed a negligence lawsuit claiming that 24 Hour Fitness was grossly negligent because they did not set up the treadmill as specified in the manufacturer's safety instructions and that the release signed by Etelvina was obtained by fraud and misrepresentation. The defendant, 24 Hour Fitness, moved for summary judgment contending that it was not liable because of the liability release signed by Etelvina.

The trial court agreed with the defendants and granted summary judgment. In their ruling, regarding gross negligence, the court stated, "a space of three to four feet as opposed to the recommended six-foot safety zone cannot constitute gross negligence...at most, ordinary negligence" (p. 234). Regarding the release was obtained by fraud and misrepresentation, the court stated that although Etelvina signed the agreement without understanding all its terms, that was not the fault of 24 Hour Fitness. The plaintiffs appealed claiming the trial court erred in granting 24 Hour Fitness summary judgment because "(1) the liability release is not enforceable against plaintiffs' claim of gross negligence; (2) the release was obtained by fraud and misrepresentation..." (p. 230).

Jimenez continued...

ISSUE

Was the basis provided by the trial court to grant summary judgment to 24 Hour Fitness regarding the issues of gross negligence and fraud and misrepresentation in error?

COURT'S RULING

Yes, the appellate court ruled that trial court erred on both issues and reversed the trial court's decision.

COURT'S REASONING

Regarding gross negligence and citing various previous case law decisions, the appellate court stated: "A release cannot absolve a party from liability for gross negligence...Gross negligence long has been defined in California and other jurisdictions as either a 'want of even scant care' or 'an extreme departure from the ordinary standard of conduct'" (pp. 235-236). The defendant claimed that no industry standard existed regarding a treadmill safety zone. However, the plaintiffs presented three pieces of such evidence: "(1) the treadmill manufacturer's owner's manual instructed in its Treadmill Safety Features section that 'the *minimum space* requirement *needed* for user safety and proper maintenance is three feet wide by six feet deep'...; (2) the manufacturer's assembly guide for the treadmill also instructs that the treadmill requires a minimum six-foot-deep clearance behind it '*for user safety* and proper maintenance'...; and (3) plaintiffs' expert, Waldon, declared that 'for the safety of the users and in order to minimize injury, it is important that a safety zone behind the treadmill be kept clear of other machines and obstacles...'" (p. 237).

The court concluded that because 24 Hour Fitness did not provide a six-foot safety zone, a standard practice in the industry, their "failure to provide the *minimum* safety zone was an extreme departure from the ordinary standard of conduct..." (p. 237). The court stated "24 Hour knew it was violating the manufacturer's express safety directions when it deliberately arranged the gym equipment without providing a six-foot safety zone for the treadmills. It can be inferred that 24 Hour did so for the purpose of placing more machines into its facility to accommodate more members to make more money..." (p. 238).

Regarding the issue of fraud and misrepresentation and relying on previous case law, the court stated: "Generally, a person who signs an instrument may not avoid the impact of its terms on the ground that she failed to read it before signing... However, a release is invalid when it is procured by misrepresentation, overreaching, deception or fraud" (p. 243). Etelvina contended that Wilbourn's nonverbal gestures indicated that what she was signing related only to the price on the computer screen. The court stated: "It is undisputed that Etelvina did not speak or read English and Wilbourn did not speak Spanish. Further, Wilbourn knew Etelvina did not speak or read English. And he knew that Etelvina did not read the contract, including the terms setting forth the release, even though, as the membership manager, he must have known that the release says 'By signing below, you acknowledge and agree that you have read the foregoing...' provisions of the release...Under these circumstances, already ripe for misrepresentation and overreaching, Wilbourn's gestures and pointing may very well have misrepresented the nature of the document Etelvina signed" (p. 245).

Lessons Learned from *Jimenez:*

Legal

- A release is unenforceable when a defendant's conduct is considered grossly negligent (e.g. a defendant knows of a violation of specific safety specifications but chooses not to correct it).

- Courts may allow evidence such as specifications published in an equipment manufacturer's owner's manual to help determine the duty owed to the plaintiff.

- Improper administration of a release may result in claims of fraud/misrepresentation making the release (contract) illegal and unenforceable (e.g., have a staff member who speaks the language of the participant explain the release and/or provide the release in the language of the participant).

Jimenez continued...

Risk Management/Injury Prevention

▶ Treadmills, as well as other pieces of exercise equipment, need to be installed following the spacing requirements established in the owner's manual and other published industry standards.

▶ Participants, especially first-time users of treadmills, need to be instructed on how to properly use the machine to help prevent falls.

▶ Proper warning labels need to be posted on treadmills as well as on other exercise equipment. Have instructional placards posted on or near each piece of exercise equipment.

Warning Labels and Signage

Providing warning labels and proper signage is essential when installing exercise equipment. Along with instructional placards posted on or close to the equipment, warning labels need to be placed on the equipment. Exercise equipment warning labels are provided by the manufacturer and are placed on the equipment in a location easily visible to the user. The location of the warning label for each piece of equipment is included in the owner's manual. For example, see page 18 in the Technogym's manual provided in the appendix. ASTM F1749-15 (32) provides specifications for warning labels including the signal icon (triangle) and signal word (Warning) appearing at the top of the warning label. This ASTM standard also provides hazard classifications that are noted by signal words according to the relative seriousness of the potential hazards as follows:

▶ **DANGER**—Indicates an imminently hazardous situation which, if not avoided, will result in death or serious injury...

▶ **WARNING***—Indicates a potentially hazardous situation, which, if not avoided, could result in death or serious injury.

▶ **CAUTION**—Indicates a potentially hazardous situation, which, if not avoided, may result in minor or moderate injury... (32, p. 2).

*Exercise equipment requires "warning" labels because it is potentially hazardous. Using exercise equipment can result in serious injury as demonstrated in the exercise equipment injuries and lawsuits described in this textbook.

It is difficult to place a warning label on certain equipment such as dumbbells, barbells, kettlebells, exercise balls, resistance bands, etc. Fitness managers/owners should consider posting a sign that describes the

warnings as specified in the owner's manual in the area where this equipment is stored. The warning signal icon and signal word could be included at the top of the sign. In addition, exercise professionals who use this type of equipment need to inform their participants of these warnings specified in the owner's manual.

In addition to warning labels, ASTM F1749-15 (32) provides a Fitness Facility Safety Sign that is to be posted in the facility (see Figure 9-5). The manufacturer is to provide one facility safety sign with each equipment order along with instructions on proper locations for posting the sign. For large facilities with multiple areas where exercise equipment is used, it is a good idea to post the facility safety sign in each equipment

Figure 9-5: Fitness Facility Safety Sign*

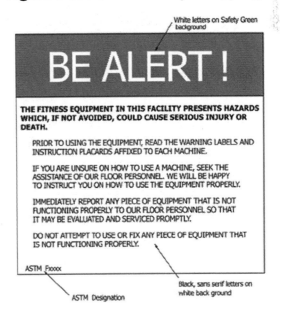

*Reprinted, with permission, from ASTM F1749-15. Standard Specification for Fitness Equipment and Fitness Facility Safety Signage and Labels, copyright ASTM International, 100 Barr Harbor Drive, West Conshohocken, PA 19428.

area (e.g., cardio, selectorized strength, free weight). As with all important signs, it needs to be large enough to be noticeable and easily read. According to this standard, other general safety signs are to "use signal words such as *safety first* and *be careful and think*" (p. 2). Warning labels and signs should be inspected periodically in case they are no longer readable and need to be replaced.

KEY POINT

The failure to warn participants of injury risks is a common allegation of negligence. Because using exercise equipment is potentially hazardous, it is essential that participants are warned of such risks. One way to inform them of these risks is through warning labels placed on the equipment (provided by the manufacturer) and warning signage posted near equipment storage racks such as exercise balls, kettlebells, etc.

Keeping Equipment Clean/Disinfected

A study conducted by FITRATED in 2017 involved gathering bacteria samples from 27 different pieces of exercise equipment (treadmills, exercise bikes, free weights) at three gyms affiliated with national chains (33). EMLab P&K performed all the laboratory testing to determine the bacteria levels based on colony-forming units (CFUs)—the number of viable bacterial cells. The results are summarized in Table 9-2. To put these numbers into perspective, the bacteria levels found on the exercise equipment were compared with the number of germs found on everyday items. For example, exercise bikes had 39 times more bacteria than a plastic reusable cafeteria tray, free weights had 362 times more bacteria than a toilet seat, and treadmills had 74 times more bacteria than a water faucet.

Another study (34) also investigated the prevalence of bacteria on exercise equipment and other surfaces in four membership-based fitness centers in Memphis, Tennessee. Many categories of microbes were found, which was likely due to poor personal hygiene of facility users and inadequate cleanliness of fitness centers. The authors concluded that "it is critical to underscore the need of proper hygienic practices in fitness centers and gyms for minimizing the spread of disease-causing organisms" (p. 12555).

Questions arise given the prevalence of bacteria on exercise equipment. What is the likelihood of gym users getting sick with a bacterial infection and what are the liability risks of the facility if an individual claims his/her infection came from the use of the equipment? According to one expert, microbiologist and author Jason Tetro, it is unlikely you'll become sick as long as you don't (a) lick the equipment, (b) wipe your face with your hands instead of towel, or (c) wipe your face with a towel that's been all over the equipment (35). The Centers for Disease Control and Prevention (CDC) (36) offers the following tips for preventing bacterial infections for fitness facility users:

- Use barriers, like a towel or clothing, between your skin and the surface.
- Shower immediately after activities where you have direct skin contact with people or shared surfaces or equipment…
- Clean your hands regularly with soap and water or an alcohol-based sanitizer.
- Keep cuts and scrapes clean and covered with bandages or dressing until healed.

Table 9-2	Bacteria Levels on Gym Equipment*	
TYPE OF BACTERIA	**DESCRIPTION**	**PERCENTAGE**
Gram-positive cocci	Most common cause of skin infections and a frequent cause of pneumonia and septicemia.	41%
Gram-negative rods	90-95% are harmful to humans and can be resistant to antibiotics.	31%
Gram-positive rods	Tend to not be harmful to humans, although there are a few exceptions.	14%
Bacillus	Found throughout nature, most notably in soil, with strains that are both harmful and helpful to humans.	14%

*From: Examining Gym Cleanliness. FITRATED. Available at: https://www.fitrated.com/resources/examining-gym-cleanliness. Accessed May 20, 2020.

The New York State Department of Health (37) also provides several suggestions to help prevent skin infections under each of the following questions:

- What is the most important way to prevent the spread of skin infections?
- As an athlete, what can I do to prevent getting or spreading skin infections?
- What should coaches, trainers, or other authorized persons do to reduce the spread of skin infections in athletes?
- What should schools and clubs do to prevent the spread of skin infections?

Following these preventive tips, as well as providing disinfectant wipes for participants to wipe down the exercise equipment before and after use, will help minimize the risk of skin infection injuries and possible subsequent litigation. However, if such a negligence lawsuit against a facility does occur, it may be difficult for plaintiffs to prove that their infection was caused from using the equipment/facility, given that bacteria are essentially everywhere. See three cases described in Chapter 10 involving bacterial infections. Facility cleanliness is discussed in Chapter 10. According to one legal source, LegalMatch (38), certain factors may help prove the fitness facility was liable for skin infection injuries such as:

- If several members are all experiencing the same symptoms…
- If the gym has failed to provide sanitation measures such as soaps or disinfectants…
- If the conditions of the gym are visibly unsanitary…
- If gym personnel had been informed of the unsanitary…conditions, but failed to take actions to remedy it… (38)

Regardless of the likelihood of skin infections occurring and the potential difficulty in proving negligence, it is essential that fitness and sport managers/owners take steps to keep the exercise equipment clean and disinfected to meet their legal duty to provide a reasonably safe environment for their participants. Cleaning specifications described in the equipment's owner's manual need to be followed (e.g., see page 26 in the Technogym's manual provided in the appendix). Additional resources are available to guide decisions on cleaning and disinfecting exercise equipment.

A CDC website (39) describes several guidelines for athletic facilities regarding cleaning and disinfecting procedures. The Environmental Protection Agency (EPA) provides a list of approved disinfectants effective against Methicillin-resistant Staphylococcus aureus (MRSA) and approved disinfectants against viruses such as COVID-19.

- **MRSA:** https://www.epa.gov/pesticide-registration/list-h-epas-registered-products-effective-against-methicillin-resistant
- **COVID-19:** https://www.epa.gov/pesticide-registration/list-n-disinfectants-use-against-sars-cov-2#filter_col1 This list includes the "contact" time for each product such as 5-10 minutes that the disinfectant must be present on a surface before it effectively kills the virus—an important factor to consider when establishing disinfecting procedures.

Regarding products, the CDC recommends reading the label before using them. Such labels will include:

- How the cleaner or disinfectant should be applied
- If you need to clean the surface first before applying the disinfectant (e.g., precleaned surfaces)
- If it is safe for the surface. Some cleaners and disinfectants, including household chlorine bleach, might damage some surfaces (e.g., metals, some plastics).
- How long you need to leave it on the surface to be effective (i.e., contact time)
- If you need to rinse the surface with water after using the cleaner or disinfectant (39)

Conducting Equipment Inspections/Maintenance

The failure to conduct proper exercise equipment inspections and maintenance is a common allegation of negligence. Often, courts will refer to the maintenance specifications in the owner's manual to help determine if the defendant facility was negligent, as demonstrated in cases previously described in this textbook and in the two following spotlight cases—*Chavez v. 24 Hour Fitness* and *Grebing v. 24 Hour Fitness*. For an example, see pages 26-27 in the appendix (routine maintenance) provided in the Technogym's manual. In the

Chavez case, the facility was liable for gross negligence for not following the maintenance specifications in the owner's manual, whereas in the *Grebing* case, the facility was not liable because it had evidence that regular inspections and preventative maintenance were conducted by a trained technician. The *Grebing* case demonstrates the legal protection that documentation can provide. Following the spotlight cases, additional cases are briefly described involving claims of improper inspections and maintenance.

Note: *In the* Grebing *case and in the* Balinton *case (described under Fault of Manufacturer), the courts used the term "products liability" versus "product liability"—the term used in this textbook.*

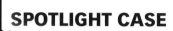

SPOTLIGHT CASE

Chavez v. 24 Hour Fitness
189 Cal. Rptr. 3d. 449 (Cal. Ct. App., 2016)

FACTS

Historical Facts:

While exercising at 24 Hour Fitness on February 11, 2011, Stacey Chavez was injured when the back panel of a FreeMotion cable crossover machine (cross-trainer) struck her in the head. She suffered a traumatic brain injury and experiences many signs and symptoms including lapses in consciousness, severe headaches, dizziness, decreased appetite, and personality changes that have interfered with her work, marriage, and other relationships. She had just recently joined 24 Hour Fitness on January 2, 2011 and on that date, signed a membership agreement that included a release of liability.

Procedural Facts:

The plaintiffs, Stacey Chavez and her husband Ruben (who sought recovery for loss of consortium), filed a complaint against 24 Hour Fitness alleging claims of ordinary and gross negligence on November 30, 2012. The plaintiffs claim that 24 Hour Fitness did not properly maintain the cross-trainer in accordance to the specifications set forth in the owner's manual and that 24-Hour Fitness knew or should have known that proper maintenance was not performed. The defendant, 24 Hour Fitness, moved for summary judgment on October 25, 2013 contending that the written release of liability was a complete defense to the plaintiffs' claims.

The trial court agreed with the defendant and granted summary judgment. The court ruled that the claim of ordinary negligence was barred by the release of liability in the membership agreement. Regarding gross negligence, "the court concluded 24 Hour met its burden to show it was not grossly negligent by establishing 'it had a system of preventative and responsive maintenance of its equipment in place at its locations at the time Plaintiff was injured'" (p. 455). The court also stated, "to maintain the machines according to some industry standard or as recommended in the owner's manual ... is a common enough occurrence that no reasonable juror could find it to be such an 'extreme departure from the ordinary standard of conduct' as to constitute gross negligence" (p. 455). The plaintiffs appealed.

ISSUE

Did the trial court error when it granted summary judgement in favor of the defendant?

COURT'S RULING

Yes, the appellate court ruled that 24 Hour Fitness was grossly negligent and reversed the trial court's decision to grant summary judgment.

Chavez continued...

COURT'S REASONING

Several individuals provided testimony that was reviewed by the appellate court. 24 Hour Fitness submitted the testimony of John Reb, area manager of facilities overseeing equipment maintenance, and Gabriel Galan, the service manager at the facility where Chavez was injured. "Reb declared that 24 Hour employs a facilities technician at each club who is responsible for maintenance, inspection, and repair of exercise equipment. The facilities technician is tasked with performing monthly preventative maintenance on each piece of exercise equipment. In doing so, the facilities technician is to 'follow and complete' the preventative maintenance chart provided...Reb further declared that the facilities technician is also responsible for repairing equipment as needed. A maintenance log of such repairs is stored in the computer program..." (pp. 452-453).

Galan stated, "facilities technicians are required to complete a Preventative Maintenance Chart, documenting the preventative maintenance performed on the equipment" (p. 453). He also stated that the chart showed the cross-trainer underwent preventative maintenance on February 7, 2001, four days prior to the plaintiff's injury.

The plaintiffs submitted the testimony of (a) John Manning, a mechanical engineer specializing in the design of exercise equipment, (b) Ronald Labrum, a consultant and supplier of exercise equipment, (c) two members who witnessed the injury to Chavez, and (d) the depositions of both Reb and Galan. Manning stated, "the back panel should be held in place by four metal brackets and magnetic strips" and at the time of his inspection, "the upper right bracket and upper left magnetic strips were missing. Three remaining brackets were bent or worn and beginning to separate from the machine" (p. 453). Labrum testified that "it is custom and practice in the fitness industry to perform preventative maintenance on all machinery in compliance with the applicable owner's manual" and "that the cross-trainer's owner's manual required that the rear access panel be removed weekly for maintenance" (p. 453).

The members, who witnessed the injury, indicated that problems often existed with machines and they had reported such issues. One had observed cables break on the machines while in use and the weights come slamming down but never a panel fall off a machine. Their testimony also implied that regular preventive maintenance on the machines was not performed.

The testimony of both Galan and Reb provided evidence of gross negligence. Galan testified that he "did not know whether facilities technicians were required to be familiar with the owner's manual for each piece of equipment or whether the 24 Hour facilities keep such manuals on hand" (p. 454). Galan and Reb both testified that:

> ...the club facilities technician—Mark Idio—should have performed preventative maintenance on each piece of equipment each month. They agreed that the February 2011 preventative maintenance chart for the...facility indicated preventative maintenance should have been performed on the cross-trainer during the week of February 7, 2011. Reb testified that the February 2011 preventative maintenance chart was blank, such that he could not say whether the called-for maintenance had been performed. Galan likewise did not know whether the preventative maintenance listed on the February 2011 preventative maintenance chart was completed (p. 457). (See "note" below regarding Mark Idio).

The court concluded "that notations should have been made on the preventative maintenance chart to indicate the completion of each task. The absence of such notations supports the influence that no preventative maintenance was performed in February 2011" (p. 457). Because of this evidence, the court stated that 24 Hour Fitness failed to exercise even scant care and that the failure of 24 Hour Fitness to comply with preventative maintenance specified in the owner's manual would constitute an extreme departure from the ordinary standard of conduct.

Note: An additional issue in this case is worth discussing. Two weeks after 24 Hour Fitness moved for summary judgment (November 8, 2013), the plaintiffs subpoenaed Idio to appear at a deposition on December 23, 2013. Idio indicated he was just informed of the subpoena on Dec. 21, 2013 in an e-mail correspondence with one of the plaintiff's attorneys and in the e-mail, he invited the attorney to call him on his cell phone. The attorney stated that she contacted Idio at least three times to set up his deposition but he had not returned her calls. 24 Hour Fitness indicated it would produce Idio but by this time he was no longer an employee. The plaintiffs requested a continuance of the case so that Idio's deposition could be obtained. The trial court denied this request, but the appellate court reversed this decision and granted their request for continuance.

Chavez continued...

Lessons Learned from *Chavez*:

Legal

▸ Facilities need to have a system in place to carry out maintenance procedures of a facility's exercise equipment. However, this is not enough – the maintenance procedures must be carried out properly. The failure to have maintenance procedures would be negligent omission, whereas, not properly carrying them out would be negligent commission (both are ordinary negligence).

▸ The release of liability did not protect against gross negligence in this case. Gross negligence occurred in this case when the defendant knew (or should have known) that maintenance procedures were not being properly carried out. Gross negligence, defined by this court, reflects the failure to exercise even scant care.

▸ Expert witnesses educate the court as to the duty or standard of care owed to the plaintiff. Courts, as the one in this case, generally allow expert witnesses to include specifications published in the equipment owner's manual (e.g., proper maintenance procedures) as admissible evidence in negligence cases. Fact witnesses, such as the members who testified in this case, can also provide evidence.

▸ A facility's documentation/records can be used as evidence to help determine if the facility was negligent or grossly negligent.

▸ It is important to adhere to a subpoena (a court order) to prevent any potential legal consequences.

Risk Management/Injury Prevention

▸ Facilities need to have an exercise equipment maintenance system in place that reflects the procedures set forth in owner's manual (as well as other published standards) for each piece of exercise equipment.

▸ Facilities need to have well-trained employees (and/or contractors) that know how to properly carry out the equipment maintenance procedures and keep documentation of such maintenance.

▸ Facility managers need to supervise maintenance procedures and check documentation records on a regular basis to be sure they are completed properly and make corrections when needed (e.g., retrain staff members).

SPOTLIGHT CASE

Grebing v. 24 Hour Fitness
184 Cal. Rptr. 3d. 155 (Cal. Ct. App., 2015)

FACTS

Historical Facts:

Timothy Grebing was injured while using a low row machine at 24 Hour Fitness. As he was pulling the handlebar, the clip that connects the handlebar to the cable failed causing the handlebar to break free from the cable striking him in the forehead. He suffered injuries to his head, back, and neck. He was a frequent user of the low row machine and acknowledged he had read the warning label on the machine: PRIOR TO USE, BE SURE THE 'SAFTEY CLIP' IS IN PROPER WORKING CONDITION AND SHOWS NO SIGNS OF WEAR!

When joining 24 Hour Fitness, Grebing signed a membership agreement including a release of liability. In part, it stated "24 Hour...will not be liable for any injury...resulting from any negligence of 24 Hour or anyone on 24 Hour's behalf...You understand that 24 Hour is providing recreational services and may not be held liable for defective products" (pp. 160-161).

Grebing continued...

Procedural Facts:

Grebing, the plaintiff, filed a complaint asserting the following causes of action against 24 Hour Fitness: (a) negligence (they failed to properly assemble or maintain the low row machine), and (b) strict products liability. The defendant, 24 Hour Fitness, moved for summary judgment claiming the release signed by Grebing was a complete defense for any negligence on its part. 24 Hour Fitness also argued that it could not be liable for strict products liability because it provided services only and was not in the business of designing, manufacturing, distributing, or selling exercise equipment.

Opposing the motion, Grebing claimed that the defendant was grossly negligent and, therefore, the release could not absolve 24 Hour Fitness of liability for gross negligence. However, the trial court granted summary judgment in favor of the defendant. Grebing appealed the judgment of the trial court.

ISSUE

Did the trial court err when it grant summary judgment in favor of 24 Hour Fitness?

COURT'S RULING

No, the appellate court affirmed the ruling of the trial court.

COURT'S REASONING

In providing an explanation of summary judgment, the court stated "A defendant moving for summary judgment must show that one or more elements of the plaintiff's cause of action cannot be established or that there is a complete defense. If the defendant meets this burden, the burden shifts to the plaintiff to present evidence creating a triable issue of material fact" (p. 160).

Regarding the issue of negligence, the court stated that the release encompassed the type of injury sustained by Grebing whether or not his injury was due to poor maintenance or improper assembly of the equipment. The Court stated, "when a release expressly releases a defendant from any liability, it is not necessary that the plaintiff have specific knowledge of the particular risk that ultimately caused the injury" (p. 161). Citing *Tunkl v. Regents of University* (1963) and other case law, the court indicated:

> An exculpatory contract releasing a party from liability for future ordinary negligence is valid unless it is prohibited by statute or impairs the public interest...A valid release precludes liability for risks of injury within the scope of the release...A release of liability for future gross negligence, in contrast, generally is unenforceable as a matter of public policy...Ordinary negligence consists of a failure to exercise reasonable care to protect others from harm, while gross negligence consists of a 'want of even scant care' or 'an extreme departure from the ordinary standard of conduct' (p.160).

Grebing argued that the testimony of a club member, Lozoya, provided the evidence required to demonstrate gross negligence, i.e., the "want of even scant care or an extreme departure of from the ordinary standard of conduct" (p. 161). However, the court stated that Grebing was mistaken because Lozoya testified that the clips were not broken and that the only problem was that they are often missing because members steal them from different machines.

The court also indicated that 24 Hour Fitness took several measures to maintain their facility and equipment. They hired a technician who conducted daily inspections and performed preventative maintenance and if the technician was unavailable, other staff members performed these tasks. Given these measures, and even Grebing's evidence that may have raised inferences regarding the measures' effectiveness, the court concluded that 24 Hour Fitness was not grossly negligent.

Regarding products liability, the court citing previous case law indicated that "unlike claims for ordinary negligence, products liability claims cannot be waived...However, a defendant cannot be liable based on products liability if the dominant purpose of the defendant's transaction with the plaintiff was providing services rather than supplying a product" (p. 162). The court

Grebing continued...

ruled that 24 Hour Fitness could not be liable based on a claim for products liability because it established "that it did not manufacture the exercise machine on which Grebing was injured, and that it purchased or leased exercise equipment for use by its members...As such, it cannot be liable based on a claim for products liability" (p. 163). In addition, as stated in 24 Hour Fitness membership agreement, their dominant purpose was to provide services rather than supply products.

Lessons Learned from *Grebing*:

Legal

▶ Based on this court, the release of liability covered the type of injury sustained by the plaintiff. It was not necessary that the plaintiff have specific knowledge of the particular risk that caused the injury.

▶ This court ruled that a release of liability will not protect a defendant from gross negligence.

▶ Strict products liability claims (i.e., injuries caused by a product defect), cannot be waived (via a release of liability) and need to be made against the manufacturer of the equipment, not the fitness facility that provides services only.

Risk Management/Injury Prevention

▶ Fitness facilities need to have an exercise equipment maintenance system in place (e.g., the court in this case indicated that 24 Hour Fitness took several measures to maintain their equipment such as hiring a technician who conducted daily inspections and performed preventive maintenance).

▶ Though not an issue raised in this case as in the Jimenez case, those assigned to carry out the inspections and maintenance of the exercise equipment need to be well-trained (and supervised) to help ensure they are properly performing these tasks and documenting such.

Additional Negligence Cases: Improper Inspections/Preventive Maintenance

In an article by Dr. Anthony Abbott titled "Facility Layout and Maintenance Concerns" (40), he describes several cases involving issues of improper layout and maintenance of exercise equipment. He describes one case in which the plaintiff was seriously injured while sitting on a bench doing bicep curls. There were no records of any inspections of the 15-year old bench and its pull-pin mechanism used to adjust height. Dr. Abbott emphasized the importance of conducting inspections and keeping proper records as well as having designated, trained employees and/or contract maintenance companies to conduct inspections and preventive maintenance of all exercise equipment.

In *Rampadarath v. Crunch Holdings* (41), Rosealin Rampadarath was injured when a pedal on an indoor cycling bike broke off causing injuries to her left knee and elbow, shoulders, and cervical and thoracic spine. She alleged that the pedal was not property attached, fastened, and/or tightened which allowed the pedal to remain loose. Rampadarath's negligent claims against the defendant included failing to inspect, maintain, or repair the defective pedal and that the defendant had actual or constructive notice of the hazardous condition that should have been recognized and remedied. The defendant moved for summary judgment stating that there was no admissible evidence to establish that Crunch created the condition or had actual or constructive notice that there was a defective pedal.

Relying on previous case law decisions, the court stated that a defendant owner "who is responsible for maintaining premises who moves for summary judgment in a case involving a defective condition on the property has the initial burden to make a prima facie showing that it neither created the hazardous condition nor had actual or constructive notice of its existence for a length of time to discover and remedy" (pp. 8-9). The court agreed with the plaintiff's attorney who argued that the defendant was unable to meet this burden given the testimony of Carl Hall (Rampadarath's instructor) who stated he did not know if regular inspections and maintenance were done on the bikes and if maintenance records were kept. The defendant failed to submit inspection or maintenance records for the bike which allegedly caused the injuries to the plaintiff. Therefore, the court denied the defendant's motion for summary judgment stating that when a there is a failure of a defendant to make reasonable inspections, it constitutes negligence and may make the owner liable for the injures caused by the condition.

In *Geczi v. Lifetime Fitness* (42), Jodi Geczi was injured while exercising on a treadmill. She claimed the treadmill began jerking violently. To steady herself, she grabbed the side rails with both hands at which time she suffered a severe pull on her left arm. She, allegedly, reported the incident to a Lifetime employee who told her that he knew the treadmill was broken. She also alleged that later that evening, a manager informed her that he had known the night prior that the treadmill was malfunctioning. In her negligence lawsuit, Geczi claimed that Lifetime failed to maintain the treadmill, warn her that the machine was not working properly, and that her injuries resulted from willful and wanton misconduct of the defendant. The trial court ruled that the exculpatory provisions in two documents that she signed upon joining Lifetime Fitness barred her negligent claims but not the claim for the willful/wanton conduct. The court stated that genuine issues of fact exist as to whether Lifetime acted willfully/wantonly. The court stated, "that it was unclear whether Lifetime had taken any action before the incident to decommission the treadmill either by placing an out-of-order sign on it, unplugging it, or in some other way making it unavailable or inoperable to patrons" (pp. 803-804). However, "Geczi's willful and wanton claim was tried to a jury which returned a verdict for Lifetime" (p. 804).

Geczi appealed claiming the trial court erred when it concluded that the language in the release she signed protected the defendant from its willful/wanton conduct (i.e., Lifetime knew the treadmill was defective and could cause injury). The appellate court stated that the exculpatory language "extended to liability for *any* injury resulting from Lifetime's negligence...in maintaining equipment, negligence in leaving defective equipment available to users, and negligence in failing to warn patrons of defective equipment" (42, p. 809). The appellate court also stated that if the defendant's conduct rose to the level of willful/wanton conduct, the release signed by Geczi would not have protected the defendant from liability.

Note: *Generally, if a defendant has actual or constructive notice of a defective condition and then chooses to not correct it or warn of the defective condition, it would be considered gross negligence, willful/wanton, or reckless conduct. In this case, the appellate court ruled that leaving defective equipment available to users and failing to warn of defective equipment reflected "ordinary" negligence (not willful/wanton conduct) and, thus, the waiver protected the defendant.*

KEY POINT

Conducting inspections and preventive maintenance of "all" exercise equipment is an essential risk management strategy. Fitness managers/owners need to follow the manufacturer's specifications in the owner's manuals and document that such inspections and preventive maintenance procedures were properly completed. Courts allow expert witnesses to introduce these specifications as evidence of the duty the defendant owed to the plaintiff.

Removing Equipment from Use

In several situations, fitness managers/owners need to remove exercise equipment from use including (a) when it needs repair, (b) after an injury, and (c) after a recall from the manufacturer. It is best to remove the equipment from the facility. If equipment removal is not feasible, Dr. Anthony Abbott (40) states that "then professional-looking signage such as 'out-of-order' must be placed where easily observed from all angles" (p. 39). However, he also warns that some participants may ignore such signage and try to use the potentially dangerous equipment so it would be best to seal off the area with yellow tape like that used in hazardous scenes.

Remove from Use—Need of Repair

Regarding removing exercise equipment in need of repair, fitness managers/owners should consider adopting policies and procedures reflected in the following NSCA (18) standard:

> *Exercise devices, machines, equipment, and free weights that are in need of repair...must be immediately removed from use until serviced and repaired and be re-inspected and tested to ensure that they are working properly before being returned to service... (p. 11).*

Inspections and preventive maintenance of all exercise equipment (including equipment such as exercise balls, resistance bands, dumbbells, benches) need to be completed properly in accordance with the manufacturer's specifications. Records of the inspections and maintenance should be stored in a secure location. This documentation can be very effective to help refute negligence claims as demonstrated in the *Grebing* case above. Of course, if a piece of exercise equipment is found, while completing inspections and maintenance, to not be working properly, is worn, or defective in any way, it should be immediately removed from use as described above.

If a participant or employee reports a problem with a piece of equipment, it should be properly document (e.g., completion of an **Incident Report** by an authorized employee such as the manager on duty). Manager on duty is discussed in more detail in Chapters 10 and 11 and an example of an Incident Report can be found in Chapter 10. For example, in *Beglin v. Hartwick Coll.* (43), a college student was injured when the metal weight plates of a weight machine jammed causing a serious injury to his hand. The main issue in this case was if the fitness center had actual or constructive notice of a dangerous condition with the weight machine. The defendant provided testimony from an athletic trainer at the facility and the center supervisor. Both denied any knowledge of any problems with the machine prior to the plaintiffs' injury. The plaintiff provided testimony from the fitness center's custodian who was responsible for cleaning and servicing the exercise equipment. He testified that the metal plates on the weight machine could easily become jammed and that this was a recurring problem. He also testified that he had notified the athletic trainer at the facility of the problem. After reviewing the totality of the evidence,

the appellate court upheld the trial court's ruling to deny the defendant's motion for summary judgment to dismiss the complaint.

Note: *It appears in this case, there was no formal reporting system (i.e., there was no completion of an Incident Report). If such a procedure had been in place along with proper follow-up to remove the weight machine from use, the injury to the plaintiff would, likely, not have occurred.*

Once exercise equipment is removed from use because of needed repair, fitness managers/owners should quickly have the equipment repaired or replaced for safety reasons and to provide quality customer service and maintain high retention rates. One article (44) listed 'broken equipment not getting fixed in time' as the #1 reason individuals should look for a new gym. Obviously, it is essential that the equipment is repaired properly by a trained technician. In one case, a cable on a leg extension machine that had snapped or broke was repaired with duct tape by the defendant YWCA (45). After the repair is made, the equipment needs to be inspected and tested to be sure it is working properly—again, following such specifications in the owner's manual.

Remove from Use—After an Injury

If a participant is injured while using a piece of equipment or at the time when such a report is made, it is essential to remove that piece of equipment from use. Fitness managers/owners need to realize that litigation may follow. Therefore, they need to not only remove the equipment from use but still retain it. Such policies and procedures should be developed in consultation with the facility's legal counsel and included in the facility's Risk Management and Policies Procedures Manual. Legal counsel can provide advice regarding **spoliation of evidence**, which can occur "when evidence is hid, withheld, changed, or destroyed during or before litigation or a similar legal proceeding" (46, p. 1). Certain jurisdictions have statutes against spoliation of evidence in which a defendant can face fines and prison time; other jurisdictions may rely on case law (46). The following two cases, *Malouf* and *Keevil* address the issue of spoliation of evidence.

In the first case involving a treadmill injury, *Malouf v. Equinox Holdings, Inc.* (47), the treadmill was not preserved by the defendant club. The defendant club argued that the treadmill was functioning properly at the time of the injury. However, because it was missing, the defendant was unable to provide the treadmill for inspection to demonstrate that it was operating properly. In addition, all paperwork involving the treadmill was missing. The plaintiff "established that defendant's failure to take affirmative steps to preserve the treadmill constituted spoliation of evidence by demonstrating that defendant was on notice that the treadmill might be needed for future litigation" (p. 422). The evidence showed that the plaintiff had reported the injury immediately and that a defendant's employee prepared a claims defense form that was submitted to its legal department. Therefore, the trial court denied the defendant's opportunity to show that the treadmill was functioning properly, and the appellate court upheld the trial court's ruling. Retaining the equipment and records such as injury reports and equipment inspections/ maintenance is essential to help defend negligence claims made by plaintiffs.

In the second case, *Keevil v. Life Time Fitness, Inc.* (48), Kevin Keevil was injured in the defendant's swimming pool while using a Spri exertube that he had anchored to the pool's ladder posts. When the exertube broke, the recoil of the band snapped it into his face injuring his right eye. He put the two pieces of the exertube on the deck beside the pool, got out of the pool, and sat down on a nearby bench. He informed a couple lifeguards what happened and that he could not see out of his right eye. He was hospitalized for two days and, then, underwent several operative procedures over the next month. His vision remained impaired and was informed by his specialists that his eyesight would not improve. In his complaint, Keevil made several negligent claims against the defendant Life Time Fitness including the failure to warn and instruct patrons of the dangerous nature of exertubes and that the defendant supplied him with a defective and unreasonably dangerous exertube when it knew or should have known it was defective and dangerous. He also alleged spoliation of evidence for the defendant's failure to preserve the exertube given that the band was material to a potential civil action.

The head of the aquatics department at Life Time Fitness testified that the exertubes were used by some of the aqua group fitness instructors and by members on their own in the pool but never in the manner that Keevil used the exertube. She also testified that she had warned Keevil to not perform the exercises with the exertube anchored to the ladder's railing because the tubing can snap and hurt you. However, Keevil did not heed her warning and continued using the exertube in the same manner. The aquatics director also testified that she did not recall seeing the broken exertube after Keevil's injury and did not know what happened to it. The court ruled that under Illinois law, the waiver/release that Keevil signed barred his negligence claims as well as his derivative spoliation claim. Regarding spoliation of evidence, the court stated that "it is not an independent tort, but a derivative action that arises out of other causes of action" (p. 35).

Serious eye injuries have occurred in other cases as well when exercise resistance bands have broken. See *Oden v. YMCA* (49) in which a YMCA member suffered severe and permanent injuries to his face and eye and *Evans v. Thobe* (50) in which a university student suffered serious injuries to her eye requiring surgery and resulting in permanent vision impairment. Fitness managers/owners need to realize that serious injuries can occur using exercise resistance bands, but can be prevented by instructing participants on how to properly use them and to be sure participants use them only as intended. In the *Keevil* case, there was a question as to whether (a) the exertubes were intended to be used in swimming pools, and (b) Keevil's misuse of the exertube caused his injury. In addition, they need to be inspected in accordance with the manufacturer's specifications and removed from use if worn or damaged. It is also best to warn participants of the risks of injury associated with using such bands if they are not used as intended. Once a participant has been informed of his/her improper use and/or warned of the risks associated with misuse of any exercise equipment, it is important to document the instruction/warning provided by completing an Incident Report. See Chapter 10 for an example of such a form.

Remove from Use—After a Recall from Manufacturer

On November 27, 2009, James McDonald was using a Valeo exercise ball when it suddenly burst causing him to forcefully fall to the ground and sustain severe injuries. He made several negligence claims against the defendant, Health Fitness Corporation, including that it failed to remove the Valeo balls from use after the manufacturer of the balls (EB Brands) issued a recall several months prior to his injury (51). In fact, the U.S. Consumer Product Safety Commission (CPSC) along with the EB Brands (a subsidiary of E&B) issued a report titled: 3 Million Fitness Balls Recalled after Users Report Injuries (52) on April 16, 2009. This report indicated 47 cases of the balls unexpectedly bursting when they were overinflated. Federal law requires manufacturers to report to the CPSC when they know they have a product that contains a defect that could create an unreasonable risk of serious injury or death. Interestingly, E&B failed to make such a report to the USPC when it knew of 25 incidents related to defective balls as early as 2007 (53). This reporting mistake cost E&B $550,000 in civil penalties (53). Although the McDonald case occurred several years ago, it demonstrates the importance of fitness managers/owners to follow recalls from manufacturers to help ensure participant safety and, to avoid possible negligent claims/lawsuits for failing to adhere to such recalls.

Dr. Betul Sekendiz (54) summarized 11 CPSC treadmill recall cases between 1998 and 2008 affecting more than 168,000 treadmills involving various types of defects. These defects created hazards such as an electrical short in the motor, overheating of circuitry, and malfunctioning of the electric control unit. As described below under Fault of Manufacturer, manufacturers can be liable for various types of product defects and, thus, it is essential for them to recall defective products to help minimize injuries and liability. The following are examples of additional recalls of various exercise equipment:

- Fall Injuries Prompt TRX Suspension Trainer Recall—Recall on October 2, 2012 (55): Hazard was with early models (sold before 2009) having a defective strap- adjustment buckle that could break; 82 reports of falls and 13 reports of injuries to the head, shoulder, face, and hip.
- Cybex Recalls Weight-Lifting Equipment Due to Serious Injury Hazards—Recall on August 29, 2018 (56): Smith Press Model 5340; Hazard was the weight bar that could fall; 27 reports of

injuries including serious injures of paralysis and spinal fracture.
- Core Health & Fitness Recalls Stairmaster Stepmill Exercise Equipment Due to Fall Hazard—Recall on August 30, 2018 (57): Hazard was the steps quickly accelerating without input from users posing a fall injury; 52 incidents resulting in 12 minor injuries.
- Fit for Life Recalls SPRI Ultra Heavy Resistance Bands Due to Injury Hazard—Recall on October 4, 2019 (58): Hazard was the rubber resistance bands can separate from the handle and strike consumers, posing an injury hazard; 10 reports of incidents including contusions, abrasions and lacerations.

Following Published Standards of Practice

As demonstrated in the negligence cases above, adherence to specifications published by the independent organizations such as the ASTM International and equipment manufacturers is essential for safety and legal liability reasons. Professional organizations have also published standards and guidelines related to exercise equipment. It is important for fitness managers/owners to adhere to these as well. A description of the standards and guidelines published by seven different professional organizations was provided in Chapter 4. The following briefly describes the equipment standards and guidelines published by four of these professional organizations. Fitness managers/owners need to obtain these publications to review the standards and guidelines in their entirety.

- ACSM (59): Two standards related to adequate spacing of all types of continuous-motion exercise equipment and proper signage (e.g., warning labels) in accordance to ASTM F1749 (ASTM F1749 is described above); Five guidelines that address issues such as equipment safety (e.g., preventive maintenance program in accordance with manufacturer's specifications, a system for removing broken or damaged equipment) and accessibility for individuals with physical limitations.
- NSCA (18): Four standards and three guidelines; Standards, in part, require (a) proper assembly

based on manufacturer's instructions with accompanying safety signage, instruction placards, and warnings posted based on ASTM standards, (b) inspection and testing of all exercise devices, machines, free weights by strength and conditioning professionals prior to use, (c) inspection and maintenance in accordance to the specifications of the manufacturer, and (d) removal from use of equipment in need of repair, and in case of an injury, consult with legal advisors prior to service/repair; Guidelines address issues such as preserving user manuals and warranties provided by the manufacturer and cleaning/disinfecting equipment in accordance to the manufacturer's specifications and/or OSHA.

- IHRSA (60): One standard that requires exercise equipment to be maintained in working order, malfunctioning equipment to be repaired/replaced in a timely fashion, and signs to be posted on or near equipment that is malfunctioning to inform patrons of risk of injury.

- MFA (61): Under Facility Operations, there are three guidelines that address (a) exercise equipment spacing recommended by the manufacturer, (b) preventive maintenance program based on the manufacturer's guidelines and record keeping of maintenance inspections, and (c) provision of inclusive exercise equipment for those with disabilities and other special populations. Under Risk Management and Emergency Response, there is one standard and two guidelines regarding appropriate signage on equipment (e.g. warnings, instructional) as well as areas throughout the facility. In the free-weight area, MFA recommends having a spotter.

Negligence of Participants

As described in Chapter 1, when a participant's injury is due to his/her own fault or negligence, the defendant may have an effective defense based on contributory or comparative negligence. Each state employs certain systems for allocating fault and damages such as (a) pure contributory negligence, (b) pure comparative fault, and (c) modified comparative fault (62). Each of these were described in Chapter 1. Most states have adopted one of the comparative fault systems. For example, in the *Baldi-Perry v. Kaifas and 360 Fitness Center* case (63, 64), described in Chapter 2, the jury returned a verdict of $1.4 million. However, the verdict was reduced to $980,000 due to the jury's finding that the plaintiff was 30% at fault. This case occurred in New York which has pure comparative fault system (62). In *Vaid v. Equinox* (65), spotlight case described in Chapter 8, the jury returned a verdict of $14,500,000. However, it was reduced to $10,875,000 based on a finding that Dr. Vaid was 25% at fault. This case occurred in Connecticut which has a modified comparative fault system (62). Another spotlight case described in Chapter 10, *Thomas v. Sport City* (66), occurred in Louisiana which has a pure comparative fault system (62). The trial court awarded the plaintiff $45,000 and $13,703.35 in general and special damages, respectively. Comparative fault assigned to the plaintiff was 30% and 35% each to the two defendants (the facility and manufacturer). However, the appellate court reversed this decision finding no fault of either defendant. Therefore, the plaintiff's injury was 100% his own fault and instead of receiving 70% of the monetary damages, the plaintiff received no damages.

To help show that a plaintiff's injury was due to his/her own fault (in part or all), fitness managers/owners need to have a system in place to provide such evidence. For example, when a participant is (a) misusing the exercise equipment, (b) not following warning or other signage posted on/near the equipment, or (c) not following safety policies related to equipment use, a facility staff member needs to correct and/or inform the participant. Obviously, staff members need to be well-trained on how to communicate properly and professionally with participants when these situation arise. At that time, an Incident Report needs to be completed, submitted, and securely stored following the policies and procedures of the facility. A sample of an Incident Report is provided in Chapter 10. If a future injury occurs and subsequent litigation, this form will provide evidence that might be helpful in showing the plaintiff's actions/inactions contributed to his/her own injury. If the participant continues with the same unsafe behaviors, this should also be documented. For more information on how to address inappropriate behaviors of participants, see Chapter 10.

Fault of Manufacturer

As described in Chapter 1, **product liability** is a form of strict liability. Product liability not only applies to manufacturers but can also apply to distributors and sellers of exercise equipment even though they had nothing to do with the making of the product. It is also important to realize that product liability law is based on state law (67). For example, some states have innocent seller statutes that can protect distributors and sellers from a plaintiff's product liability claims. In addition, defendants (e.g., manufacturers) have available defenses to help refute such claims such as the plaintiff misused the equipment, assumed the risks, and/or was a sophisticated user of the equipment (67), which are like some of the defenses used by defendants (e.g., fitness managers/owners) in negligence claims/lawsuits.

Liability only arises if the product is defective. As presented in the *Restatement Third of Torts* (68), there are three types of defects: (a) **manufacturing defect**, (b) **design defect**, (c) **marketing defect**. See Exhibit 9-2 for definitions of each. It is important to realize that fitness managers/owners are not liable for exercise equipment defects as demonstrated in *Grebing v. 24 Hour Fitness* (69), spotlight case described earlier. As stated by this

appellate court, fitness facilities are not in the business of designing, manufacturing, distributing, or selling exercise equipment and, therefore, are not subject to strict product liability. The following cases describe various product liability claims/lawsuits involving exercise equipment. As demonstrated in these cases, the plaintiff needs to prove that the exercise equipment was defective and that the defect was the cause of his/her injury.

In *Thomas v. Sport* City (66), a spotlight case presented in Chapter 10, the trial court found the manufacturer of the hack squat machine (Capps Welding) liable for a design defect. However, the appellate court reversed the trial court's ruling. To determine if there was a design defect, the appellate court required Thomas (the plaintiff) to prove that there was an alternate design that would meet the purpose of the hack squat machine—a machine that would allow for a full squat and capable of preventing his injury. Expert witnesses for the defendant Capps Welding, who were experts in the design of exercise equipment, testified that the design of their hack squat machine was similar in design to other manufacturers' hack squat machines. Thomas was unable to establish an alternate design and the court concluded that the Capps Welding hack squat machine did not have a design defect and that "the trial court committed manifest error in finding the hack squat machine to be unreasonably dangerous" (p. 1157).

Design and marketing defects were addressed in *Barnhard v. Cybex International* (70). While working

---

Exhibit 9-2: Types of Product Defects*

A product is defective when it:

(a) contains a manufacturing defect when the product departs from its intended design even though all possible care was exercised in the preparation and marketing of the product;

(b) is defective in design when the foreseeable risks of harm posed by the product could have been reduced or avoided by the adoption of a reasonable alternative design by the seller or other distributor, or a predecessor in the commercial chain of distribution, and the omission of the alternative design renders the product not reasonably safe;

(c) is defective because of inadequate instructions or warnings when the foreseeable risks of harm posed by the product could have been reduced or avoided by the provision of reasonable instructions or warnings by the seller or other distributor, or a predecessor in the commercial chain of distribution, and the omission of the instructions or warnings renders the product not reasonably safe.

with a patient, Natalie Barnhard, a physical therapy assistant employed by Amherst Orthopedic Physical Therapy, stood next to the weight-stack side of a Cybex leg extension machine and pulled on it to stretch her arms and shoulder. The machine, weighing more than 600 pounds, was not secured to the floor. It tipped over onto Barnard fracturing her neck rendering her a quadriplegic. Barnhard claimed Cybex was negligent (the machine had design and marketing defects) as well as her employer. The trial court (jury) awarded her damages of $66 million and assigned comparative fault as follows: (a) Cybex 75% or $49.5 million, (b) Amherst 20%, and (c) Barnhard 5% (71, 72).

The appellate court concluded "that a fair interpretation of the evidence supports the jury's verdict that Cybex was negligent and that its negligence was a substantial factor in causing the plaintiff's injuries" (70, p. 1555). Cybex claimed that Barnhard was injured as a result of her misuse of the machine. However, the court stated that although the plaintiff was not using the machine for its intended purpose, the use of the machine for stretching was common and, thus, foreseeable. The court also stated that the machine was defectively designed based on the testimony of a plaintiff's expert that it could have been made safer and that the design defect was a substantial factor causing the plaintiff's injury. In addition, the court ruled that Cybex did not provide adequate warnings (a marketing defect) when it failed to warn purchasers and users of the machine's potential tipping hazard, which was also a substantial factor in causing the plaintiffs' injuries. The appellate court did, however, reduce Cybex's damages to $44 million. Regarding Amherst, the court stated that the evidence supported the jury's verdict finding (20% fault) that it was negligent, and its negligence was also a substantial factor in causing the plaintiff's injury. This ruling occurred on November 18, 2011 but two parties, Barnhard and Cybex, agreed to a settlement of $19.5 million (72) in February 2012. This case demonstrates the need for some exercise equipment to be bolted to the floor and the importance of providing warnings.

As indicated in this case, misuse of exercise equipment may be an available defense to product defect claims/lawsuits. However, if an individual is misusing exercise equipment (i.e., not using the equipment as intended) but is performing an exercise that is commonly done with the machine, the misuse defense may not be an effective defense. This could also apply to misuse defenses used by defendant fitness facilities. Therefore, it is important for fitness facilities to have staff members well trained on how to provide proper instruction to participants, not only when they are misusing exercise equipment in a way that does not reflect its intended purpose, but also when using the equipment in a manner that is commonly performed that can increase a risk of injury. Documentation of such instruction (e.g., completion of an Incident Report) is important to provide evidence that proper instruction took place. In addition, this case demonstrates the importance of equipment manufacturers having adequate product liability insurance. It was reported that Cybex only had $4 million in available insurance to cover the incident (71).

In *Balinton v. 24 Hour Fitness* (73), Egnacio Balinton exercised frequently at several 24 Hour facilities in the San Francisco area between 2003 and 2011. On August 6, 2011, he was using a hack squat machine at 24 Hour's North Beach facility that did not have a safety brake (safety catch) that prevents the "weight apparatus from descending all the way to the bottom of the frame in the event that the user is unable to return the weight apparatus to its starting position" (p. 1). While performing a set of exercises on the hack squat machine, Balinton's legs became fatigued and he was unable to return the weight to its starting position causing the weight to descend too low into a crunch position and injuring him. Balinton filed products liability claims and negligence claims against 24 Hour Fitness. He appealed the trial court's rulings that his products liability claims failed as a matter of law because 24 Hour was a provider of services and not of products, and that his negligence claims were barred by the primary assumption of risk doctrine.

The appellate court upheld the trial court's rulings. Regarding the products liability claims, the California court stated that the strict products liability doctrine has expanded to reach nonmanufacturing parties outside the vertical chain of distribution, but it does not apply to transactions whose primary objective is obtaining services, and that the dominant purpose of 24 Hour was the provision of services. Regarding his negligence claims, Balinton argued that 24 Hour increased the inherent risks when he used the hack squat machine at the North Beach location because it provided hack squat machines with the safety brake feature at other locations. He claimed that the North Beach location "set a trap" for him to injure himself by expecting a safety brake on its hack squat machine. However, when considering the primary assumption of risk defense, the court stated that the "plaintiff's subjective awareness or expectation is not relevant" (p. 4), and that 24

Hour did not violate its duty not to increase the inherent risks in weightlifting. Citing previous case law, the court stated that "the doctrine of primary assumption of the risk bars claims for personal injury where the plaintiff is injured by a risk inherent in a sport or activity itself, but recognizes the duty of defendants not to act so as to *increase* the risk of injury over that inherent in the activity" (p. 8).

DEVELOPMENT OF RISK MANAGEMENT STRATEGIES

| Assessment of Legal Liability Exposures | Development of Risk Management Strategies | Implementation of the Comprehensive Risk Management Plan | Evaluation of the Comprehensive Risk Management Plan |

As demonstrated in the negligence cases described above, injuries involving exercise equipment are very common. Many of these negligence cases were due to improper instruction/supervision, maintenance, spacing, and provision of warning signage. As described in Chapter 8, improper instruction and supervision is considered *the* most common allegation of negligence. In addition to improper instruction/supervision, expert witnesses, Voris and Rabinoff (74), with more than 30 years each as expert witnesses, listed the following as common allegations of negligence related to exercise equipment:

- Failure to maintain or inspect the equipment
- Failure to warn
- Failure to properly label equipment... (74)

The following risk management strategies regarding exercise equipment safety focus on minimizing injuries and subsequent claims/lawsuits related to the (a) negligence of exercise professionals and, (b) negligence of fitness managers/owners. Several of these strategies emphasize the importance of complying with published standards of practice such as those from independent organizations (e.g., owner's manuals provided by equipment manufacturers). As described in Chapter 4 (see Table 4-1), expert witnesses often refer to these in their testimony to help educate the court as to the standard of care (duty) owed to the plaintiff as demonstrated in the *Jimenez* and *Chavez* spotlight cases presented earlier. It is important to develop policies and

procedures to be included in the facility's Risk Management Policy and Procedures Manual (RMPPM) that reflect these risk management strategies. Facility staff members need to be well-trained on these policies/procedures to help ensure they are properly carried out.

 Risk Management Strategy #1: Comply with the Americans with Disabilities Act (ADA) Regarding Exercise Equipment.

The ADA is described in Chapter 3. However, one requirement of the ADA is that fitness facilities provide services for individuals with disabilities such as functional limitations or impairments. This includes providing exercise equipment that can be used by these individuals. However, it does not, necessarily, mean that the facility must provide inclusive equipment as specified in the ASTM Standard F3021-17 (22), previously described. However, to better serve this population, fitness managers/owners should consider purchasing or leasing inclusive exercise equipment. Providing inclusive exercise equipment may help reduce ADA discrimination claims/lawsuits such as the Louis Jorgl case described earlier. Jorgl claimed that exercise machines were bunched too close together and they were difficult to access. The ASTM standard (F3021-17) includes specifications regarding access to and around the inclusive exercise equipment. Fitness facilities who opt not to provide designated inclusive equipment still need to comply with the ADA by providing exercise equipment that can be used by those with disabilities and provide proper spacing to access the equipment. Inclusive equipment is available from reputable manufactures and is equipment that can be used by individuals with and without functional limitations or impairments. Therefore, it is a good investment from a variety of perspectives.

2 **Risk Management Strategy #2:** Provide Proper Instruction and Supervision by Competent Exercise Professionals on the Safe Use of All Exercise Equipment (1).

As demonstrated in many of the cases described in this chapter including the *Butler v. Saville et al.* (75) spotlight case and other cases presented throughout this textbook (see Table 9-1), exercise equipment injuries are often due to improper instruction and supervision. It is essential that personal fitness trainers, group exercise leaders, and strength and conditioning coaches are well-trained on how to properly use exercise equipment themselves *before* instructing their participants. Training needs to focus on practical skills such as *teaching* proper positioning/execution and progression for all the equipment exercise professionals will have their participants use. Many injuries are due to improper execution and progression, such as poor technique or lifting too much weight. Follow-up, practical assessments are needed to determine if they have acquired the necessary skills to teach safely. More information regarding training of exercise professionals, including assessment of teaching skills, is described in Chapters 5 and 8.

Proper instruction includes informing participants of the information/risks found on the warning labels placed on the equipment or on the warning signage posted near equipment (see Risk Management Strategy #3). Exercise professionals should carefully review the specifications in the equipment manufacturer's owner's/user's manual regarding safe instruction, potential risks, and warnings so they can inform their participants of these important safety features and include/document these safety features in their lesson plans. The personal fitness trainer in *Butler* did not appear to know how to teach safe exercises using a BOSU ball,

especially for a 62-year old novice, nor did he appear to be aware of safety tips provided in the manufacturer's owner's manual. For example, in the BOSU Elite owner's manual (76), there are 18 safety tips. Tip #11 states, in part, the following: "STANDING ON THE PLATFORM SIDE OF THE BOSU® ELITE IS NOT RECOMMENDED. IT IS AN ADVANCED EXERCISE AND INCREASES YOUR RISK OF FALLING WHICH COULD CAUSE SERIOUS INJURY..." (p. 5). This owner's manual also provides three warning labels and the location for their placement on the BOSU ball. Safety tips in the Technogym's user's manual are described on pages 16-17 in the appendix.

In addition, proper instruction includes informing and warning participants of injury risks associated with a particular risky or advanced activity such as standing on the platform side of a BOSU ball and heavy RT. As described earlier, heavy RT causes a significant rise in blood pressure compared to low-to moderate-intensity RT and, thus, may lead to a risk of cardiovascular and neurologic injuries, especially in individuals with certain medical conditions. In addition to obtaining medical clearance, fitness managers and exercise professionals should consider having participants read and sign a document that describes these risks. As with all such documents, they need to be prepared by a competent lawyer. Once participants are informed of the risks, they may decide to opt out.

Injuries involving strength training equipment were a special focus in this chapter. Several negligence cases were described involving improper instruction and supervision. Exercise professionals need to be aware of various strategies to minimize injuries such as those summarized in Exhibit 9-1 as well as common causes of weightlifting injuries (8). It is essential that instructors/trainers/coaches be well-educated and trained on how to prevent these injuries when designing and delivering strength training activities. In addition to the case law examples and resources described in this chapter, there are many educational resources available to be used in staff training programs to help address the importance of safe instruction and supervision. A couple published in 2019 are: (a) Resistance Training for Older Adults: Position Statement From the National Strength and Conditioning Association (12), and (b) Developing a Lifelong Resistance

Training Program (77). Textbooks, such as *Essentials of Strength Training and Conditioning*, 4th ed. published by Human Kinetics and *ACSM's Foundations of Strength Training and Conditioning* published by Lippincott Williams & Wilkins, are also available.

Developing and implementing risk management strategies that focus on safe instruction and supervision may also help reduce injuries caused by a participant's own negligence. For example, participants who are properly instructed and supervised will be less likely to misuse exercise equipment. One of the major goals of risk management is to reduce injuries from happening in the first place, including those caused by a participant's own negligence.

③ Risk Management Strategy #3: Make Informed Decisions When Purchasing and/or Leasing Commercial-Grade Exercise Equipment.

Fitness managers/owners should only consider purchasing/leasing commercial-grade equipment from a reputable manufacturer. Equipment designed for home use should not be considered. As described earlier, there are a variety of factors fitness managers/owners need to consider when purchasing/leasing commercial-grade exercise equipment such as (a) populations served, (b) spacing/storage issues, (c) costs, (d) quality of equipment, e.g., does it meet ASTM design and manufacturing specifications, (e) brand selection, (f) reputation and quality of services provided by the manufacturer/distributor, (g) safety and recall history, and (h) warranties. Investing time to investigate these factors is essential so that cost-effective decisions are made as well as decisions related to equipment safety.

Fitness managers/owners should consider consulting with a competent lawyer to review the terms of exercise equipment purchasing/leasing contracts. It will be important to comply with Article 2 of the Uniform Commercial Code that addresses the sale and/or purchase/lease of goods. Legal review may also be helpful for exercise equipment purchases subject to the Statute of Frauds that requires contracts be in writing for the sale of goods over $500. As described earlier, there are several factors to consider when purchasing used exercise equipment (e.g., how the equipment is designated such as refurbished or certified remanufactured). Managers of non-profit

facilities, who receive offers to have used commercial exercise equipment donated to them, should turn down these offers unless the equipment can first be refurbished or remanufactured by a reputable company.

Risk Management Strategy #4: Install All Exercise Equipment in Accordance with the Manufacturer's Specifications (1).

As described above, reputable equipment manufacturers/distributors have their own designated, trained, and certified employees who properly install the equipment. This includes assembling, inspecting, and testing the equipment according to the specifications in the owner's manual. Fitness managers/owners should review the specifications in the manuals in consultation with the manufacturer's representatives at the time of making purchasing/leasing decisions, to be sure the facility can comply with them. Fitness managers/owners should designate at least one employee, a professional in a supervisory role, to oversee the exercise equipment including inspections and maintenance. This employee can serve as the liaison with the manufacturer's certified technician and even complete the training and certification offered by the manufacturer.

Proper installation includes providing proper spacing of exercise equipment and securing equipment so it does not tip over. These are important legal liability issues as demonstrated in the *Jimenez* and *Barnhard* cases described. In addition to specifications in the owner's manuals, fitness managers/owners should refer to ASTM Standard F2115-18 (31) regarding minimum clearances on the sides and back of treadmills (see Figure 9-4). Given the thousands of falls off treadmills that occur each year, complying with these specifications is essential to help prevent catastrophic injuries. Proper installation includes posting warning labels and signage as explained next in Risk Management Strategy #5. In addition, instructional signage needs to be placed on the equipment or near the equipment. Posting the ASTM Fitness Facility Safety Sign (32) will also help inform participants to seek the help of staff members when needing instruction on how to safely use the exercise equipment (see Figure 9-5). This sign is to be provided by the manufacturer and for large facilities with multiple exercise areas, one sign should be posted in each area.

⑤ Risk Management Strategy #5: Post Warning Labels On or Warning Signage Near All Exercise Equipment.

Exercise equipment requires "warning" labels because it is potentially hazardous. According to ASTM Standard F1749-15 (32), warning "indicates a potentially hazardous situation, which, if not avoided, could result in death or serious injury" (p. 2). As evident from cases described in this and other chapters, the failure to warn is a major legal liability exposure. It is often listed by plaintiffs as a negligent claim. In addition to directly informing participants of warnings associated with using exercise equipment, warning labels and signage need to be posted on or near the exercise equipment.

When exercise equipment is installed by a manufacturer's technician, the technician places the warning labels on the machines in the location indicated in the owner's manual. It will be important for fitness manager/owners to check this was done properly. However, certain exercise equipment (e.g., exercise balls, dumbbells, resistance bands, kettlebells) is often ordered directly from the manufacturer or distributor. It may be difficult to place warning labels on this type of equipment. However, participants still need to be warned of the risks involved in using the equipment. Fitness managers/owners should post a sign in the area where this equipment is stored that describes the warnings as specified in the owner's manual for each type of equipment. The ASTM warning signal icon and signal word, used in warning labels (see page 18 in the appendix), could be included at the top with the name of the equipment (e.g., Kettlebells—warnings would then be listed below). As with all signage, it needs to be readable and in large font so it is noticeable to users.

⑥ Risk Management Strategy #6: Keep All Exercise Equipment Clean and Disinfected in Accordance with the Manufacturer's Specifications and the Centers for Disease Control and Prevention (CDC) Recommendations (1).

It is essential that fitness managers/owners take steps to keep the exercise equipment clean and disinfected to meet their legal duty to provide a reasonably safe environment for their participants. The studies described above (33, 34) demonstrate the prevalence of all types of bacteria found on exercise equipment. Although it may be difficult for plaintiffs to prove their infection was caused from using the exercise equipment, certain factors such as those listed previously (38) may help them prove a breach of duty.

Participants should have access to disinfectant wipes they can use before and after using the equipment. However, they also need to be encouraged to use the wipes by their trainers/instructors/coaches and during the facility orientation (described in Chapter 10) for new participants. In addition, using the disinfectant wipes provided should be included as one of the safety policies posted in the facility. Fitness managers/owners and exercise professionals may want to provide participants additional tips from the CDC (36) on how they can prevent bacterial infections when using the exercise equipment.

Cleaning specifications described in the equipment's owner's or user's manual need to be followed. For example, see appendix for proper cleaning procedures of the TechnoGym Skillrun Treadmill. The CDC (39) also provides several guidelines regarding cleaning and disinfecting procedures. The EPA provides a list of approved disinfectant products effective against MRSA and viruses such as COVID-19. Regarding cleaning and disinfectant products, the CDC (39) recommends reading the label before using them.

⑦ Risk Management Strategy #7: Conduct Inspections and Maintenance of All Exercise Equipment in Accordance with the Manufacturer's Specifications (1).

As demonstrated in the spotlight cases (*Chavez* and *Grebing*) and other cases, fitness facilities can be found liable for their failure to conduct proper exercise equipment inspections and maintenance. To minimize injuries and subsequent litigation, fitness managers/owners need to follow the inspection and maintenance specifications in the owner's manual of each piece of exercise equipment. For example, see the appendix that describes inspection and maintenance procedures for the Technogym Skillrun Treadmill. Providing evidence of proper inspections and maintenance procedures is an important risk management strategy that can be quite effective in refuting negligence claims as demonstrated in *Grebing*.

Even though equipment owner manuals may not address daily inspections of the exercise equipment to determine if it is functioning properly, damaged, or worn, it is recommended "all" equipment be inspected at least once per day. As described in Chapter 10, participants of fitness facilities are classified as invitees. One of the duties owed toward invitees is to inspect the facility and equipment. Because exercise equipment can become unsafe for use at any time, daily inspections are needed to help meet this duty. During the inspection of the equipment, the warning labels and signage also need to be inspected to be sure they have remained on or near the equipment and are readable. If not, they need to be replaced immediately.

Fitness managers/owners should not become over-reliant on predictive asset management technologies that can notify them when equipment needs maintenance. Although this technology may be useful, it is not a substitute for following the maintenance specifications in the owner's manuals and conducting daily inspections. In addition, this technology may not be applicable to all types of exercise equipment.

 Risk Management Strategy #8: Remove Exercise Equipment From Use When Needing Repair, After an Injury, and After a Manufacturer's Recall (1).

As demonstrated in the case law examples above, removing exercise equipment is essential (a) when it needs repair, (b) after an injury, and (c) if recalled by the manufacturer. If the equipment cannot be physically removed from the facility, proper professional-looking "out of order" signage is needed or other methods to help ensure it will not be used by participants (e.g., gym equipment covers, sealed off using hazard-warning tape). Once equipment is repaired by a qualified technician, it needs to be inspected and tested before it is returned to service. Repairing (or replacing damaged equipment) in a timely fashion is important from a safety perspective and a customer service perspective. It is often a complaint of participants and a major reason they look for another facility (44).

In addition to needing repair, exercise equipment needs to be removed from use when a participant is injured from using the equipment or at the time when such a report is made. Because negligence claims or a lawsuit may follow, it is not only important to remove such equipment, but still retain it. As described above, fitness managers/owners should seek the advice of legal counsel to develop and implement policies and procedures, given state laws vary regarding the spoliation of evidence. As described in Chapter 11, the name, manufacturer, and serial number of the piece of equipment should be recorded. In addition, photos of the equipment and the area around the equipment (instructional and warning signage, etc.,) should be taken right after the injury. The evidence gathered may help determine the cause of the injury (e.g., participant misuse, product defect) which may be useful to refute negligence claims against the facility alleged by plaintiffs.

Exercise equipment also needs to be removed from use immediately when a recall from the manufacturer and/or the CPSC is issued. Recalls are issued based on reports of injuries with the use of the equipment usually caused by some type of product defect (e.g., design, manufacturing, and/or marketing). Federal law requires manufacturers to report to the CPSC when they know they have a product that contains a defect that could create an unreasonable risk of serious injury or death. Although the manufacturer can be found liable for product defects, fitness facilities can be found liable for failing to remove the equipment from use after receiving the recall. Defective exercise equipment further increases the risk of injuries and must be removed from use.

 Risk Management Strategy #9: Comply with Published Standards of Practice Addressing Exercise Equipment Safety.

Both independent and professional organizations have published standards and guidelines related to exercise equipment. Independent organizations include ASTM International and equipment manufacturers. The ASTM Subcommittee on F08.30 on Fitness Products has 16 active standards regarding all types of commercial exercise equipment (21). Three of these have been described—F2115, F1749, and F3021. Although these standards are primarily for manufacturers of commercial exercise equipment, fitness managers/owners should also be aware of them and follow certain specifications published in the standards. In addition, fitness managers/owners need to follow the specifications in the owner's (or user's) manuals for each piece of equipment. These manuals contain numerous specifications regarding various safety factors such as proper installation, warnings, cleaning/disinfecting, etc. See the appendix for an example of the typical content covered in a user's manual. As demonstrated in the *Jimenez* and *Chavez* spotlight cases described in this chapter and other cases in this textbook, adherence to these specifications is essential from a legal liability perspective

Professional organizations have also published standards and guidelines regarding exercise equipment. Some of these refer to certain ASTM standards. Those published by four organizations—ACSM, NSCA, IHRSA, and MFA—were previously briefly described. Of the four organizations, the NSCA standards (requirements) and guidelines (recommendations) are the most comprehensive. It is recommended that fitness managers/owners, at a minimum, follow the four NSCA standards that are reflected above in Risk Management Strategies #4, #5, #7, and #8. These four NSCA standards reflect common legal liability exposures involving exercise equipment as demonstrated in the negligence cases described in this and other chapters. Other professional organizations should consider adopting these four NSCA standards in their own future publications.

As stated in previous chapters, standards of practice published by professional organizations do not always reflect major legal liability exposures. Fitness managers/owners may believe that if they follow all the standards in these publications, they have taken steps to address major legal liability exposures. However, that may not be the case if important safety practices (e.g., inspecting and maintaining exercise equipment) are missing or not categorized as standards. When making decisions to determine what should be considered a standard, the editors/authors of these publications should consider reviewing common allegations of negligence that fitness facilities have faced.

 Risk Management Strategy #10: Establish Policies and Procedures Regarding Proper Documentation Related to Exercise Equipment Safety (1).

As described throughout this textbook, having documentation (evidence) to demonstrate that legal duties were carried out properly can be a very effective defense for defendants when faced with negligence claims/lawsuits. For example, the defendant in the *Chavez* spotlight case was found grossly negligent—there was no evidence that the defendant had maintained the exercise machine according to the specifications in the owner's manual. In the *Grebing* spotlight case, the defendant was not liable for gross negligence because of evidence that a technician conducted daily inspections and performed preventative maintenance of the exercise equipment. The following are examples of records that should be kept as documentation regarding exercise equipment:

- Records of instructional programs provided for fitness staff members on how to properly use the equipment as well as how to teach safe use
- Equipment installation records in accordance with the manufacturer's specifications such as inspection, testing, spacing, warning labels, and signage
- Inspections (daily) and preventive maintenance records according to the equipment manufacturer's specifications
- Records involving the removal from use when equipment needs repair, after an injury, and after a manufacturer's recall
- Records of service and/or repair
- Records of cleaning and disinfecting the equipment
- Records demonstrating compliance with standards of practice published by independent and professional organizations

As with all records, they need to be kept in a private, confidential, and secure location.

Note: *Records involving situations such as a participant's misuse of exercise equipment (e.g., an Incident Report) are described in Chapter 10.*

RISK MANAGEMENT AUDIT
Exercise Equipment Safety

RISK MANAGEMENT (RM) STRATEGY*	YES ✔	NO ✔
1. Comply with the Americans with Disabilities Act (ADA) Regarding Exercise Equipment.		
2. Provide Proper Instruction and Supervision by Competent Exercise Professionals on the Safe Use of All Exercise Equipment.		
3. Make Informed Decisions When Purchasing and/or Leasing Commercial-Grade Exercise Equipment.		
4. Install All Exercise Equipment in Accordance with the Manufacturer's Specifications.		
5. Post Warning Labels On or Warning Signage Near All Exercise Equipment.		
6. Keep All Exercise Equipment Clean and Disinfected in Accordance with the Manufacturer's Specifications and the Centers for Disease Control and Prevention (CDC) Recommendations.		
7. Conduct Inspections and Maintenance of All Exercise Equipment in Accordance with the Manufacturer's Specifications.		
8. Remove Exercise Equipment From Use When Needing Repair, After an Injury, and After a Manufacturer's Recall.		
9. Comply with Published Standards of Practice Addressing Exercise Equipment Safety.		
10. Establish Policies and Procedures Regarding Proper Documentation Related to Exercise Equipment Safety.		

*See the section above—Development of Risk Management Strategies—for the recommendations associated with each risk management strategy and then, for each RM Strategy marked NO, create a list of action steps that need to be completed to meet the recommendations described in that RM strategy.

KEY TERMS

- Acute Emergent Injuries
- Acute Non-Emergent Injuries
- Chronic-Type Injuries
- Design Defect
- Frivolous Conduct
- Incident Report
- Inclusive Exercise Equipment

- Manufacturing Defect
- Marketing Defect
- Predictive Asset Management Technologies
- Product Liability
- Respondeat Superior
- Spoliation of Evidence
- Valsalva Maneuver

STUDY QUESTIONS

The Study Questions for Chapter 9 can be found on the Fitness Law Academy website (www.fitnesslawacademy.com) under Textbook. They are provided in a fillable format for convenience.

APPENDIX

This chapter's appendix follows the References.

REFERENCES

1. Eickhoff-Shemek JM, Herbert DL, Connaughton, DP. *Risk Management for Health/Fitness Professionals: Legal Issues and Strategies.* Baltimore, MD: Lippincott Williams & Wilkins, 2009.

2. Thompson WR. Worldwide Survey of Fitness Trends for 2020. *ACSM's Health & Fitness Journal,* 23(6), 10-18, 2019.

3. Lavellee ME, Tucker B. An Overview of Strength Training Injuries: Acute and Chronic. *Current Sports Medicine Reports,* 9(5), 307-313, 2010.

4. Kerr ZY, Collins CL, Comstock RD, et al. Epidemiology of Weight-Training-Related Injuries Presenting to United States Emergency Departments, 1990 to 2007. *The American Journal of Sports Medicine,* 20(10), 1-7, 2010.

5. Moura P. USC and Stafon Johnson Settle Lawsuit. ESPN. Available at: https://www.espn.com/los-angeles/ncf/story/_/id/7477966/usc-trojans-settle-ex-player-stafon-johnson-negligence-lawsuit. Accessed August 29, 2019.

6. Keogh KW, Winwood PW, The Epidemiology of Injuries Across the Weight-Training Sports. *Sports Medicine,* 47(3) 479-501, 2017.

7. Aasa U, Svartholm, Anderson F, et al. Injuries Among Weightlifters and Powerlifters: A Systematic Review. *British Journal of Sports Medicine,* 51(4), 211-219, 2017.

8. Fred HL. More on Weightlifting Injuries. *Texas Heart Institute Journal,* 41(4), 453-454, 2014.

9. Hatzaras I, Tranquill M, Coady M, et al. Weight Lifting and Aortic Dissection: More Evidence for a Connection. *Cardiology,* 107(2), 103-106, 2007.

10. Bursik D, Conway G. Warning Clients of Possible Effects of Valsalva With Resistance Exercise - Implications to the Standard of Care for Fitness Professionals? *The Exercise, Sports and Sports Medicine Standards and Malpractice Reporter,* 2(1), 11-12, 2013.

11. Williams MA, Haskell WL, Ades PA, et al. Resistance Exercise in Individuals With and Without Cardiovascular Disease: 2007 Update. *Circulation,* 116, 572-584, 2007.

12. Fragala MS, Cadore EL, Dorgo S, et al. Resistance Training for Older Adults: Position Statement From the National Strength and Conditioning Association. *The Journal of Strength and Conditioning Research,* 33(8), 2019-2052, 2019.

13. Sullivan JM. The Valsalva and Stroke: Time for Everyone to Take a Deep Breath. Starting Strength. Available at: https://startingstrength.com/articles/valsalva_stroke_sullivan.pdf. Accessed September 2, 2019.

14. Abbott A. Resistance Training and Litigation. *ACSM's Health & Fitness Journal,* 20 (5), 61-65, 2016.

15. *Assaf Blecher v. 24 Hour Fitness Inc. and David Stevens,* No. BC43630 (Los Angeles Superior Court). In: Man Receives Large Jury Verdict After Personal Trainer Drops Weight on His Face. http://calbraininjury.com/personal-injury/man-receives-large-jury-verdict-after-personal-trainer-drops-weight-on-his-face/. Accessed September 4, 2019.

16. *Sicard v. University of Dayton,* 104 Ohio App.3d 27 (Ohio Ct. App., 1995).

17. *Lemaster v. Grove City Christian Sch.,* No. 16AP-587, 2017 LEXIS 4858 (Ohio Ct., App., 2017).

18. NSCA Strength and Conditioning Professional Standards and Guidelines. *Strength and Conditioning Journal,* 39(6), 1-24, 2017. Available at: https://www.nsca.com/education/articles/nsca-strength-and-conditioning-professional-standards-and-guidelines/. Accessed November 5, 2018.

19. *Gallant v. Hilton Hotels Corp.,* 988 N.Y.S.2d 522, 2014 LEXIS 853 (N.Y. Misc., 2014).

20. *Jafri v. Equinox Holdings, Inc.,* N.Y. Slip Op 33186(U), 2014 LEXIS 5330 (N.Y. Misc., 2014).

21. ASTM International. Subcommittee on F08.30 on Fitness Products. Available at: https://www.astm.org/COMMIT/SUBCOMMIT/F0830.htm. Accessed September 19, 2019.

22. ASTM International. ASTM F3021-17. Standard Specification for Universal Design of Fitness Equipment for Inclusive Use by Persons with Functional Limitations and Impairments. ASTM International: West Conshohocken, PA, 2017.

23. *Healthy People 2020.* Physical Activity. Available at: https://www.healthypeople.gov/2020/data-search/Search-the-Data#objid=5069. Accessed September 18, 2019.

24. Rosales I. Clearwater YMCA Sued for Large Number of Violations Against the Americans with Disabilities Act. Pinellas County News, September 3, 2019. Available at: https://www.abcactionnews.com/news/region-pinellas/clearwater-ymca-hit-with-federal-lawsuit-for-astonishing-number-of-violations-against-the-americans-with-disabilities-act. Accessed September 18, 2019.

25. Welcome to the Athletic Business Online Buyers Guide. Athletic Business Buyers Guide 2019. Available at: https://www.athleticbusiness.com/buyers_guide/. Accessed September 19, 2019.

26. F.I.T. 2019: IHRSA's Commercial Fitness Guide. Available at: https://www.ihrsa.org/publications/fit-2019-ihrsas-commercial-fitness-guide. Accessed September 19, 2019.

27. Refurbished Vs. Certified Remanufactured. Usedfitnesssales.com. Available at: https://www.usedfitnesssales.com/refurbished-vs-remanufactured/. Accessed September 19, 2019.

28. Mywellness®. Technogym. Available at: https://www.technogym.com/int/business-solution/mywellness-2/. Accessed September 19, 2019.

29. Waters CR. The Global Fitness Industry Prepares for GDPR, May 16, 2018. Available at:https://www.ihrsa.org/improve-your-club/the-global-fitness-industry-prepares-for-gdpr/. Accessed September 24, 2019.

30. Feld J. How Technology Can Help You Get the Most Out of Your Equipment, October 10, 2018. Available at: https://www.ihrsa.org/improve-your-club/how-technology-can-help-you-get-the-most-out-of-your-equipment. Accessed September 19, 2019.

31. ASTM International. ASTM F2115-18. Standard Specification for Motorized Treadmills. West Conshohocken, PA: ASTM International, 2017.

32. ASTM International. ASTM F1749-15. Standard Specification for Fitness Equipment and Fitness Facility Safety Signage and Labels. West Conshohocken, PA: ASTM International, 2015.

32a. Madhami A. Treadmill Injuries Send Thousands to the ER Every Year. *USA Today,* May 5, 2015. Available at: https://www.usatoday.com/story/news/2015/05/04/treadmill-emergency-room-injuries-exercise-equipment/26898487/. Accessed August 28, 2019.

33. Examining Gym Cleanliness. FITRATED, 2017. Available at: https://www.fitrated.com/resources/examining-gym-cleanliness. Accessed September 19, 2019.

34. Mukherjee N, Dowd SE, Wise A, et al. Diversity of Bacterial Communities of Fitness Center Surfaces in U.S. Metropolitan Area. *International Journal of Environmental Research and Public Health,* 11, 12544-12561, 2014.

35. Polish J. Germs On Your Workout Equipment Aren't As Big Of A Deal As You Think, An Expert Says. Bustle, July 18, 2019. Available at: https://

References *continued...*

www.bustle.com/p/germs-on-your-workout-equipment-arent-as-big-of-a-deal-as-you-think-expert-says-18170589. Accessed September 19, 2019.

36. Methicillin-resistant Staphylococcus aureus (MRSA). Cleaning and Disinfecting. Centers for Disease Control and Prevention. Available at: https://www.cdc.gov/mrsa/community/environment/index.html. Accessed September 24, 2019.

37. Preventing Skin Infections. New York State Health Department. Available at: https://www.health.ny.gov/diseases/communicable/athletic_skin_infections/hand_washing.htm. Accessed September 24, 2019.

38. What If I Have Developed a Skin Infection Due to Unsanitary Gym Conditions? LegalMatch. Available at: https://www.legalmatch.com/law-library/article/gym-liability-for-skin-infection-injuries.html. Accessed September 19, 2019.

39. Methicillin-resistant Staphylococcus aureus (MRSA). Athletic Facilities Cleaning and Disinfecting. Centers for Disease Control and Prevention, January 24, 2019. Available at: https://www.cdc.gov/mrsa/community/environment/athletic-facilities.html. Accessed September 19, 2019.

40. Abbott AA. Facility Layout and Maintenance Concerns. *ACSM's Health & Fitness Journal*, 22 (1), 37-41, 2018.

41. *Rampadarath v. Crunch Holdings*, 39 Misc. 3d 1205(A), 2013 LEXIS 1312 (N.Y. Misc., 2013).

42. *Geczi v. Lifetime Fitness*, 973 N.E.2d 801 (Ohio Ct. App., 2012).

43. *Beglin v. Hartwick Coll.*, 67 A.D.3d 1172 (N.Y. App. Div., 2009).

44. Giblin C. 10 Reasons to Dump Your Gym. *Mens' Journal*, Health & Fitness, n.d. Available at: https://www.mensjournal.com/health-fitness/10-reasons-to-dump-your-gym. Accessed September 30, 2019.

45. Herbert DL. Ohio Jury Awards Large Verdict in Weight Machine Case. *The Sports, Parks & Recreation Law Reporter*, 21(1), 65, 68-70.

46. Laws.com. Spoliation of Evidence. Available at: https://court.laws.com/spoliation-of-evidence. Accessed September 27, 2019.

47. *Malouf v. Equinox Holdings, Inc.*, 113 A.D.3d 422 (N.Y. App. Div., 2014).

48. *Keevil v. Life Time Fitness Inc.*, No. 1-15-1551, 2016 LEXIS 647 (Ill. App. Ct., 2016).

49. *Odom v. YMCA*, No. 2-15-1274, 2016 LEXIS 1790 (Ill. App. Ct., 2016).

50. *Evans v. Thone*, 958 N.E.2d 616, 2011 LEXIS 2969 (Ohio Ct. App., 2011).

51. Herbert DL. New Lawsuit Filed Against Fitness Facility in Wisconsin. *The Exercise Standards and Malpractice Reporter*, 25(4), 53-54, 2011.

52. 3 Million Fitness Balls Recalled after Users Report Injuries. *Consumer Reports News*, April 16, 2009. Available at: https://www.consumerreports.org/cro/news/2009/04/3-million-fitness-balls-recalled-after-users-report-injuries/index.htm. Accessed September 30, 2019.

53. E&B Giftware Agrees to $550,000 Civil Penalty for Failing to Report Defective Fitness Balls. *NEWS from USPC*, December 11, 2011. Available at: https://www.cpsc.gov/Newsroom/News-Releases/2012/EB-Giftware-Agrees-to-550000-Civil-Penalty-for-Failing-to-Report-Defective-Fitness-Balls/. Accessed September 30, 20019.

54. Sekendiz B. Risks of Treadmills in Health/Fitness Facilities. *ACSM's Health & Fitness Journal*, 20(4), 10-14, 2016.

55. Fall Injuries Prompt TRX Suspension Trainer Recall, October 2, 2012. The Schmidt Firm, PLLC. Available at: https://www.schmidtlaw.com/fall-injuries-prompt-trx-suspension-trainer-recall. Accessed October 1, 2019.

56. Cybex Recalls Weight-Lifting Equipment Due to Serious Injury Hazards, August 29, 2018. U.S. Consumer Product Safety Commission. Available at: https://www.cpsc.gov/Recalls/2018/cybex-recalls-weightlifting-equipment-due-to-serious-injury-hazards. Accessed October 1, 2019.

57. Core Health & Fitness Recalls Stairmaster Stepmill Exercise Equipment Due to Fall Hazard (Recall Alert), August 30, 2018. U.S. Consumer Product Safety Commission. Available at: https://www.cpsc.gov/Recalls/2018/Core-Health—Fitness-Recalls-Stairmaster-Stepmill-Exercise-Equipment-Due-to-Fall-Hazard-Recall-Alert. Accessed October 1, 2019.

58. Fit for Life Recalls SPRI Ultra Heavy Resistance Bands Due to Injury Hazard, October 4, 2019. Available at: https://www.cpsc.gov/Recalls/2019/fit-for-life-recalls-spri-ultra-heavy-resistance-bands-due-to-injury-hazard. Accessed October 10, 2019.

59. *ACSM's Health/Fitness Facility Standards and Guidelines*. Sanders ME. (ed). 5th Ed. Champaign, IL: Human Kinetics, 2019.

60. IHRSA Club Membership Standards. In: *IHRSA's Guide to Club Membership & Conduct*. 3rd Ed. Boston, MA: International Health, Racquet & Sportsclub Association, 2005. Available at: http://download.ihrsa.org/pubs/club_membership_conduct.pdf. Accessed November 5, 2018.

61. *Medical Fitness Association's Standards & Guidelines for Medical Fitness Center Facilities*, Roy B. (ed.). 2nd Ed. Monterey, CA: Healthy Learning, 2013.

62. Contributory Negligence/Comparative Fault in All 50 States. Matthiesen, Wickert & Lehrer, S.C., February 19, 2018. Available at: https://www.mwl-law.com/wp-content/uploads/2018/02/COMPARATIVE-FAULT-SYSTEMS-CHART.pdf. Accessed October 10, 2010.

63. *Baldi-Perry v. Kaifas and 360 Fitness Center, Inc.* Complaint. Index No. 2010-1927, Supreme Court, Erie County, New York. February 19, 2010.

64. Herbert DL. Recent Verdict Against Personal Trainer – Lessons to be Learned. CPH & Associates. Available at: https://www.cphins.com/recent-verdict-against-personal-trainer-lessons-to-be-learned/. Accessed August 3, 2018.

65. *Vaid v. Equinox*, No. CV136019426, 2016 LEXIS 828 (Conn. Super. Ct., 2016).

66. *Thomas v. Sport City, Inc.*, 738 So. 2d 1153 (La. Ct. App., 2 Cir., 1999).

67. Product Liability in All 50 States. Matthiesen, Wickert & Lehrer, S.C., April 25, 2019. Available at: https://www.mwl-law.com/resources/product-liability-laws-50-states/. Accessed October 11, 2019.

68. *A Concise Restatement of TORTS Third Edition*. Compiled by: Bublick EM, Rogers JE. St. Paul, MN: American Law Institute, 2013.

69. *Grebing v. 24 Hour Fitness*, 184 Cal. Rptr. 3d 155 (Cal. Ct. App., 2015).

70. *Barnhard v. Cybex International, Inc.*, 89 A.D.3d 1554, 2011 LEXIS 8278 (N.Y. App. Div., 2011).

71. Friedman J, O'Neill PS. Exercising Caution After The Big Verdict In *Barnhard v. Cybex International, Inc.*, January 3, 2012. Available at: https://www.sfia.org/press/397_Exercising-Caution-After-The-Big-Verdict-in. Accessed October 15, 2019.

72. Cohen A. Products Liability in IHRSA's Cybex Agenda. *Athletic Business E-Newsletter*. February 22, 2012. Available at: https://www.athleticbusiness.com/corporate/products-liability-on-ihrsa-s-cybex-s-agenda.html. Accessed October 15, 2019.

73. *Balinton v. 24 Hour Fitness USA, Inc.*, No. A140576, 2017 WL 541914 (Cal. Ct. App., 2017).

74. Voris HC, Rabinoff M. When is a Standard of Care Not a Standard of Care? *The Exercise Standards and Malpractice Reporter*, 25(2), 20-21, 2011.

75. *Butler v. Saville et al.*, No. CV116023310, 2014 WL 3805719 (Conn. Super Ct., 2014).

76. BOSU Elite by WeckMethod Owner's Manual. Available at: https://cdn.shopify.com/s/files/1/0250/2533/files/BOSU_Elite_Owner_s_Manual_8.16.17.01.pdf?7767772137240965716. Accessed March 24, 2020.

77. Kravitz LR. Developing a Lifelong Resistance Training Program. *ACSM's Health & Fitness Journal*, 23 (1), 9-15, 2019.

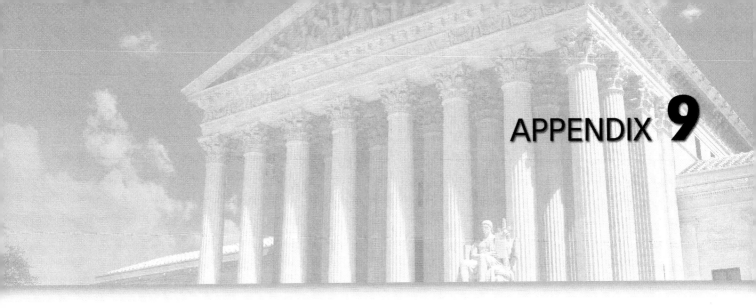

The following information has been reprinted from the User's Manual of the TechnoGym Skillrun Treadmill. The Manual Contents, items covered in this Manual, are listed below. The following pages are excerpts from the Manual including:

Page 5: Personal Safety

Pages 16–18: Safety Devices and Warnings

Page 19: Place of Usage

Pages 26–27: Routine Maintenance

NOTE: *Reprinted with permission from TECHNOGYM USA CORP., Copyright, 2017. 700 US Highway 46 East, Fairfield, NJ 07004*

CONTENTS

PERSONAL SAFETY

Use of the product is subject to a medical examination to assess your suitability to the type of workout exercise you intend to perform, and in compliance with the conditions for use laid down by Technogym.

Persons suffering from certain physical conditions may only use the product under the strict supervision of a doctor with specific qualifications.

If, during exercise, the message "HIGH HEART RATE" appears, your heart rate is too high and you should slow down the exercise.

Before starting any workout, make sure your position on the product is correct, paying attention to any components that may obstruct use.

Plan the workout according to your physical characteristics and state of health, beginning with less demanding workloads.

Do not overexert yourself or work to exhaustion. Incorrect or excessive exercise may cause physical harm or sudden death. If you feel any pain or abnormal symptoms, stop your workout immediately and consult your physician.

Wear proper workout clothing and shoes during training; do not wear garments that block perspiration; do not wear loose clothing. Tie long hair back. Keep garments or towels away from moving parts.

When using the product, other people must remain at a safe distance.

Do not use the product when children or pets are present.

The person in charge of the gym must explain proper and improper use of the equipment to users.

Fully assemble the product before using it. Check the product before each use. Do not continue to use the product if it is not working properly.

Assemble and use the product only on a solid and flat surface.

Keep all the components (such as the power cable and the on/off switch) away from liquid substances, to avoid all risk of electric shock.

Keep the product in good working condition. If you see signs of wear, contact Technogym's technical support service.

Do not attempt any maintenance work on the product other than the operations described in the user manual.

The installation, maintenance and setting operations must be carried out by qualified Technogym staff or persons authorised by Technogym.

The electrical system must conform to the standards and legal requirements in the country of use.

SKILLRUN

5

SAFETY DEVICES AND WARNINGS

STOP button (A). This button can be used to stop the exercise without having to use the normal controls.

Emergency switch (B). This switch stops the exercise immediately. It is equipped with a cord with a peg to clip on to the user's clothing as shown in the illustration. Check that the peg grips onto clothing sufficiently well to operate the emergency switch. The user triggers the emergency switch if he/she moves too far away from the control panel, that is if the cord becomes taught.

To restore all the functions of the equipment after an emergency stop, reset the switch as shown in the illustration.

After finishing the exercise, replace the emergency switch peg back into its slot, as shown in the illustration.

If the emergency switch is activated while the product is in use at any gradient, the treadmill belt runs freely, and no form of braking is applied. Under such conditions, the user's weight and gravity may cause an unintended acceleration. Hold onto the side supports.

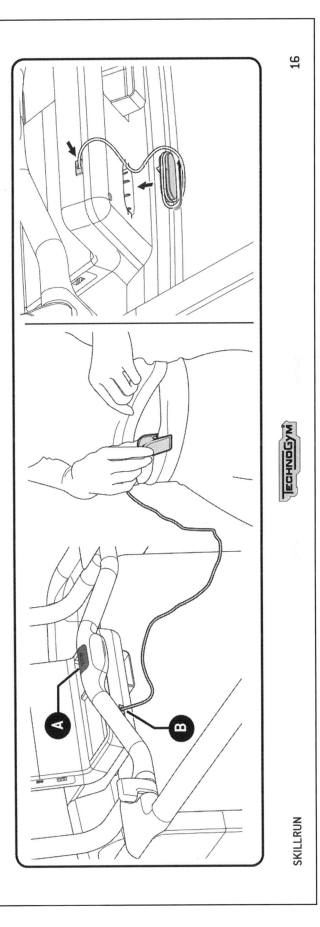

16

TECHNOGYM

SKILLRUN

SAFETY DEVICES AND WARNINGS

Main switch (C). Turns the power to the product on and off.

Circuit breaker (D). Protects the electrical components of the product. When a power surge occurs, the protection device opens, thus preventing damage to the electronics inside.

To access to the main switch and circuit breaker, open the panel (E).

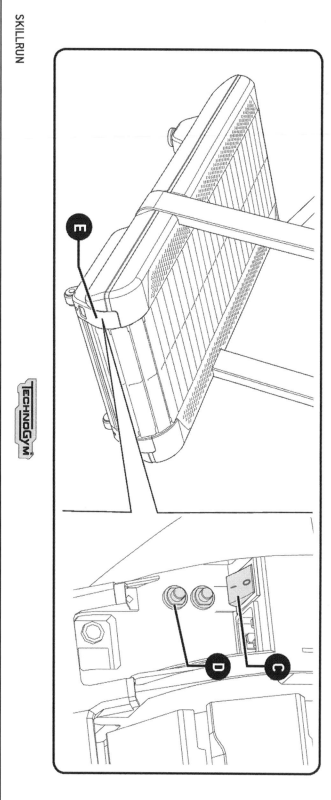

SKILLRUN

17

SAFETY DEVICES AND WARNINGS

⚠ WARNING

Please read the adhesive labels on the equipment, which provide information about possible risks and hazards.

Before using the product, read all the warnings on the label applied to the right-hand column.

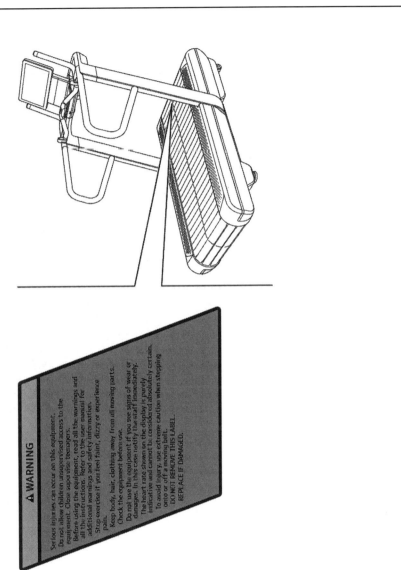

⚠ WARNING

Serious injuries can occur on this equipment.
Do not allow children unsupervised access to the equipment. Close supervise teenagers.
Before using the equipment, read all the warnings and all the instructions. Refer to the user manual for additional warnings and safety information.
Stop exercise if you feel faint, dizzy or experience pain.
Keep body, hair, clothing away from all moving parts.
Check the equipment before use.
Do not use the equipment if you see signs of wear or damages. In this case notify the staff immediately.
The heart rate shown on the display is purely indicative and cannot be considered absolutely certain.
To avoid injury, use extreme caution when stepping onto or off a moving belt.
DO NOT REMOVE THIS LABEL.
REPLACE IF DAMAGED.

SKILLRUN

18

PLACE OF USAGE

To ensure that exercising with the equipment is easy, safe and effective, the place where it is used should comply with certain specific requirements; in particular, before choosing where to install the equipment we recommend that you check that the following conditions are present.

- The temperature is between +10°C and +25°C;

- Enough air is circulating to keep humidity during exercise to between 20% and 90%;

- The lighting is good enough to make the area a safe and relaxing place to exercise in;

- There is plenty of free space all around each item of equipment and a safety perimeter of 2x1 m, as shown in the illustration;

- The floor is flat, stable and vibration-free, and strong enough to bear the weight of the equipment plus user.

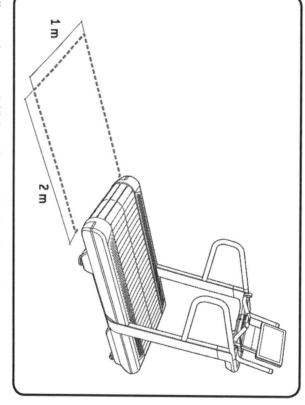

The place in which the equipment is installed must comply with all the suitability requirements laid down in current legislation on this matter.

In order to guarantee the performance indicated by the manufacturer, you are advised against using the equipment in areas where there are high short-wave or similar emissions.

Do not expose the equipment to direct sunlight.

Do not use outdoors. Do not leave the equipment outdoors, exposed to the elements (rain, sun, wind, etc.) Do not expose the equipment to water jets.

Do not operate the equipment where aerosol (spray) products are being used or where oxygen is being handled.

Do not install the equipment in areas with high humidity levels, for example close to swimming pools, whirlpools or saunas.

SKILLRUN

19

ROUTINE MAINTENANCE

As the equipment is used in a sports centre by more than one person, it should always be kept clean and free of dust, in accordance with normal hygiene and sanitary rules.

To clean the control panel, proceed as follows:

- turn the equipment off by moving the switch to the OFF (0) position;
- unplug the equipment power cable from the wall socket;
- clean the control panel with a damp, but not wet, cloth.

Every week, clean the equipment completely:

- turn the equipment off by moving the switch to the OFF (0) position;
- unplug the equipment power cable from the wall socket;
- clean the external parts with a damp sponge;
- move the equipment to one side so that you can vacuum underneath it.

Do not use chemical products or solvents.

 WARNINGS

Do not rub too hard on the control panel and diagrams, or on the written instructions on the labels.

The safety of the equipment is assured only on the condition that it is carefully inspected every two weeks for any signs of damage and/or wear.

Danger of falling. If the product is not connected to the power supply, the belt will turn freely. You must hold onto the side supports when getting on and off the product

For maintenance operations not described in this manual, contact the Technogym Technical Support Service.

SKILLRUN

26

ROUTINE MAINTENANCE

WARNINGS

Routine maintenance, adjustment and lubrication jobs must be performed by the Technogym Technical Support Service.

Before starting any job, turn the equipment off by switching the switch to the OFF (0) position and unplugging the power cable from the wall socket

Every two weeks, check:

- that the individual elements of the treadmill belt and the belt itself are not damaged;

- that the plastic protective devices are undamaged.

Emergency switch

Check the condition of the emergency switch each month.

- ensure that the cord and the spring are present and in good condition.

- check that the emergency switch is undamaged.

- with the treadmill belt in motion at 5 km/h, pull the cord with the spring to trigger the emergency switch and ensure that the belt stops.

- with the treadmill belt in motion at 5 km/h, press the emergency push button to ensure that the belt stops.

If the emergency switch does not work properly, place the product out of service and contact the Technogym Technical Support Service.
To replace defective or damaged components, contact the Technogym Technical Support Service.

SKILLRUN

27

CHAPTER 10

Managing Facility Risks

LEARNING OBJECTIVES

After reading this chapter, fitness managers and exercise professionals will be able to:

1. Identify major risks that exist in the daily operations of a fitness facility and describe how they can be properly managed.

2. Realize the importance of complying with OSHA standards such as noise exposure levels and ADA standards regarding accessible design (1).

3. Describe state consumer protection laws involving membership contracts and deceptive practices.

4. Using case law examples, discuss how courts determine legal duties owed to invitees (1).

5. Describe the legal importance of conducting and documenting daily inspections of the facility.

6. Develop and implement an educational facility orientation for new fitness participants.

7. List and describe the types of signage that are needed in the facility and explain the legal protection that signage can provide.

8. Using case law examples, describe the importance of keeping the facility well-maintained, clean, and disinfected.

9. In consultation with legal and data security experts, develop and implement policies and procedures that reflect data privacy and security laws.

10. Help ensure live streaming/ on-demand digital fitness classes and workouts are safely taught by credentialed and competent instructors.

11. Develop and implement policies and procedures to help protect the safety and physical security of facility participants.

12. Comply with standards of practice published by independent and professional organizations related to facility operations (1).

13. Appreciate the legal significance of completing and maintaining proper documentation regarding facility operations.

14. Provide proper supervision of the facility and develop and implement strategies that may provide some legal protection in unsupervised or partially-supervised facilities.

15. In consultation with legal and insurance experts, obtain the necessary insurance to protect the facility including events that are organized or sponsored by the facility.

16. Develop and implement 10 risk management strategies that will be effective in minimizing legal liability exposures related to facility risks.

INTRODUCTION

Managing facility risks is a complex and essential task of fitness managers and exercise professionals. Numerous risks exist that can lead to injury and subsequent litigation. This chapter focuses on facility risks that are common to most fitness facilities and, therefore, does not include all facility risks. For example, many risks and/or issues related to fitness facility construction and design are not addressed as well as legal liability and risk management issues associated with swimming pools. It is recommended that fitness managers/owners refer to a comprehensive resource titled *Facility Planning and Design for Health, Physical Activity, Recreation, and Sport* (2), published in 2019. This book contains 33 chapters. Three of these are:

- Chapter 5—Electrical, Mechanical, and Energy Management
- Chapter 13—Aquatic Facilities
- Chapter 32—Facility Maintenance

As an example of the content included in this book, the chapter on Aquatic Facilities covers a variety of topics such as construction and design, applicable laws, emergency management, supervision issues, and pool operations. References to a variety of organizations that have published standards/guidelines (e.g., National Swimming Pool Foundation—NSPF, YMCA, American Red Cross) as well as those that offer a certification in pool and spa operations such as NSPF's Certified Pool and Spa Operator®, are also included.

In addition, it is recommended that fitness managers/owners refer to standards and guidelines regarding facility construction and design published by independent organizations such as ASTM International, American National Standards Institute (ANSI), and Consumer Products and Safety Commission (CPSC) as well as professional organizations such as ACSM. For example, ACSM (3) has three standards and 15 guidelines addressing design/construction issues such as the ADA, building codes, spacing, storage, illumination, HVAC, and floor surfaces. The NSCA (4), MFA (5) and AACVPR (6) have similar standards and/or guidelines.

This chapter begins with identifying and describing several categories of common legal liability exposures involving facility risks. Three spotlight cases are described along with other legal cases to help gain an understanding and appreciation of these common legal liability exposures. Toward the end of the chapter, 10 risk management strategies are provided that describe how fitness managers and exercise professionals can minimize these risks.

ASSESSMENT OF LEGAL LIABILITY EXPOSURES

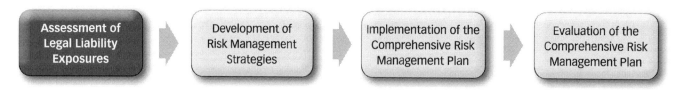

The legal liability exposures described in this section have been categorized into eight areas. These include:

1) Federal, State, and Local Laws
2) Legal Duties Toward Invitees
3) Facility Maintenance and Cleaning
4) Supervision of Facilities
5) Technology and Data Privacy/Security
6) Facility Security
7) Inappropriate Behaviors of Fitness Participants
8) Event Organizer and Sponsor

Specific legal liability issues associated with commercial lease agreements and facility rental agreements are not addressed in this section. Fitness facilities need to use such agreements when they lease and/or rent space (e.g., leasing space for an onsite physical therapy clinic, leasing/renting space to exercise programs such as Silver Sneakers™ and Rock Steady Boxing, and renting space for events such as birthday parties). Several examples of these types of agreements are available on the Internet. However, it is essential to have a competent lawyer prepare such contracts and address legal liability and insurance issues. A few cases in this textbook address lease and rental agreements, such as *Hoffner v. Lanctoe* described later in this chapter (lease agreement) and *Gallant v. Hilton Hotels Corp.* described in Chapter 9 (rental agreement).

Federal, State, and Local Laws

The failure to comply with federal, state, and local laws can lead to costly fines. This section describes some of these laws related to the management of the facility. Described are federal laws such as OSHA's signage and noise exposure regulations and the ADA's 2010 Standards for Accessible Design regarding service animals. State and local laws involving health club membership contracts and deceptive practices are also described.

Federal Laws

Certain OSHA requirements were previously described in Chapter 3 such as General Duty Clause and the Hazard Communication Standard. Chapter 11 covers the OSHA General Industry Standard and Bloodborne Pathogens Standard. To enhance compliance with OSHA requirements, employers and employees can take a "general industry" online training course offered by OSHA that offers 10-hour and 30-hour options (7). OSHA also provides many free publications including a booklet titled All About OSHA (8) that summarizes many of OSHA's requirements.

Employers need to comply with OSHA's specifications for accident prevention signs and tags (9). These specifications apply to the design, application, and use of signs or symbols that indicate and, insofar as possible, define specific hazards that could harm workers or the public, or both, as well as property damage. OSHA provides free signage (e.g., a free OSHA Job Safety and Health poster (10) plus other free posters). OSHA compliant signage can also be purchased from various commercial providers as well as signage indicating the location of first-aid kits and automatic external defibrillators (AEDs). Another standard involves noise exposure limits which is a safety issue that fitness managers/owners need to address.

OSHA Standard: Noise Exposure Limits

OSHA has established legal limits on noise exposure based on a worker's time weighted over an average 8-hour day (11). OSHA's permissible exposure limit (PEL) for noise is 90 decibels (or 90 dBA) for all workers for an 8 hour day (12). The National Institute for Occupational Safety and Health (NIOSH) recommends these exposure limits to 85 decibels (or 85 dBA) over an 8-hour average (11). The noise dose is based on both the sound exposure level and how long it lasts (duration) as shown in Table 10-1. Fitness managers/owners not only should comply with this standard for their employees but for their participants as well.

Table 10-1	OSHA Standard: Occupational Noise Exposure*	
TIME TO REACH 100% NOISE DOSE	**EXPOSURE LEVEL PER OSHA PEL****
8 hours	90 dBA
4 hours	95 dBA
2 hours	100 dBA
1 hour	105 dBA
30 minutes	110 dBA
15 minutes	115 dBA

*Adapted from: https://www.cdc.gov/niosh/topics/noise/reducenoiseexposure/regsguidance.html. (Accessed December 12, 2019).
**PEL—permissible exposure limit

Several articles have been published regarding the noise levels in fitness facilities, especially in exercise classes like indoor cycling and Zumba. For example, author Lisa Packer (13) summarized a study conducted by researchers at George Mason University. The researchers found that noise levels were 100-110 decibels and over 90 decibels in indoor cycling and Zumba classes, respectively. In addition, the sound levels associated with banging of weights, dropping heavy objects, and flipping tires in CrossFit programs were equivalent to intense shock waves, similar to explosions. Given that fitness classes are 45-60 minutes in duration, these high decibel levels may exceed the noise exposure levels as specified in Table 10-1. Instructors, especially those who teach more than one class/day, may experience hearing damage or loss due to these noise exposures. However, participants can also experience hearing damage, as demonstrated in *Levine v. GBG, Inc.*

In *Levine v. GBG, Inc.* (14), the plaintiff claimed the instructor, in his indoor spin class, played the stereo at an unreasonably high and dangerous volume causing acoustic trauma to his inner ear and associated nervous system. In his negligence lawsuit against the instructor and GBG, he alleged that the instructor was required to be familiar with the Gold's Gym Group Fitness Instructor Manual, which specified that the music volume be played at a safe level at all times. Due to jurisdiction issues, the case was remanded to a Circuit Court in Maryland. Although the outcome of this case was unknown at the time this chapter was written, it demonstrates the importance of following OSHA's standard on noise exposure levels to minimize hearing injuries and subsequent litigation.

In a study published in the *Archives of Environmental & Occupational Health* (15), the authors indicated that 85% of instructors who teach high-intensity exercise classes (e.g., indoor cycling) found loud music motivating, whereas, about one-fifth of participants found it stressful. They also found that music volume was higher in high-intensity classes than in low-intensity classes. However, the low-intensity classes still averaged above 85 decibels. They concluded that the noise exposure, particularly in high-intensity classes, poses a potential risk to hearing. Comments from readers of a *New York Times* article (16) regarding indoor cycling injuries included the following related to noise levels:

- I wouldn't go to a spinning class just because of the music. It's really loud, brain-dead music, with an instructor shouting on top of it. No thanks.
- I've never understood the spin class. When they run it, the instructor has the lights off, so it's dark, the music jacked up SO loud it's painful anywhere CLOSE to that gym, and she's shouting amplified instructions at volumes louder than the music…How does damaging hearing in the dark improve health?

For more information on noise levels in fitness classes and facilities see IDEA Opinion Statement titled "Recommendations for Music Volume in Fitness Settings" (17), and an IHRSA article titled "Bad Vibrations: Why You Need to Protect Your Gym from Excessive Noise" (18).

The Federal Trade Commission Act (FTCA) and the ADA were covered in Chapter 3. As described in Chapter 3, regulations of the FTCA include (a) unfair and/or deceptive acts or practices, (b) consumer data privacy and security, and (c) advertising and social media posts. Chapter 3 provided a description of the requirements in Titles I and III of the ADA and examples of discrimination cases. Chapters 6 and 7 addressed the ADA as it relates to pre-activity health screening/fitness testing and exercise prescription, respectively. Chapter 7 briefly described standards of practice published by professional organizations (e.g., ACSM, NSCA, IHRSA, and MFA) that require or recommend the provision of programs/services for people with disabilities. The importance of fitness facilities providing inclusive exercise equipment was presented in Chapter 9. The following presents some additional topics regarding ADA requirements.

ADA: Standards for Accessible Design and Service Animals

Chapter 3 briefly described the 2010 ADA Standards for Accessible Design. Effective on March 15, 2012, compliance with the 2010 standards was required for new construction and alterations under Titles II and III (19). This law is lengthy and quite complex. It will be important for fitness managers/owners to consult with legal counsel to help ensure compliance with this law and its many requirements such as spacing and signage specifications. Some helpful resources regarding the 2010 ADA Standards are:

- ADA Checklist for Existing Facilities: https://www.adachecklist.org/doc/fullchecklist/ada-checklist.pdf. (Accessed December 23, 2019).
- Quick Reference Guide to ADA Signage: https://www.accentsignage.com/wp-content/uploads/ADA-Quick-Reference.pdf. (Accessed December 23, 2019).

As described in Chapter 3, studies have shown that fitness facilities had a high degree of inaccessibility in several different areas such as customer-service desks, restrooms, locker rooms, drinking fountains, and areas around the exercise equipment. As listed in Table 3-2 in Chapter 3, there are a variety of resources to help fitness managers and exercise professionals improve in these areas. For example, the National Center on Health, Physical Activity and Disability (NCHPAD) has many resources including a video (How to Choose a Fitness Facility) that highlights these common areas of inaccessibility (20). This video could be shown to employees in an ADA training program to increase awareness of issues facing individuals who use wheelchairs. ADA staff training programs should include the importance of using disability-friendly language that places the person first, such as (a) person with a disability (versus disabled or handicapped), (b) person who uses a wheelchair (versus wheel-chaired-bound), and (c) person with epilepsy (versus epileptic).

Fitness facilities may want to obtain the Universal Global Design (UGD) certification. A YMCA in Michigan was the first in the world to receive this prestigious recognition (21). The certification involves standards such as the facility design process and facility management policies that consider "an aging population, individuals with disabilities, those recovering from medical procedures and those with temporary injuries, musculoskeletal disease, and hearing and sight challenges" (21, para. 4). Some facilities may want to consider another certification—the WELL Building Standard. In 2019, a YMCA in San Francisco (22) was the first fitness facility to receive this certification. It requires meeting criteria such as air quality (e.g., air filtration, proper ventilation, low-chemical cleaning standards) and comfort (e.g., noise levels).

The ADA has requirements addressing **service animals** as part of the 2010 Standards for Accessible Design (23). Service animals are dogs and miniature horses that have been trained to do work or perform tasks for people with disabilities. Several rules apply such as staff members having limited inquiries. They can only ask two questions—is the service animal required because of a disability and what work or task has the service animal been trained to perform. **Emotional support animals** are not considered service animals under the ADA (24). They are often used as part of a medical treatment plan to help individuals improve their physical, social, emotional, and/or cognitive functioning.

Fitness facilities need to be sure their website is accessible to comply with ADA, Title III (places of public accommodation). According to Helen Durkin (25), IHRSA's executive vice president of public policy, the number of website accessibility lawsuits are growing dramatically with plaintiffs' attorneys suing businesses including health clubs. For strategies to help protect from such lawsuits, see IHRSA's article titled "Technology Can Grow Your Fitness Business—But Know the Risks" (25).

State Laws

Fitness manager/owners need to be aware of state laws involving **membership contracts** and other consumer protection statutes applicable to fitness facilities. For example, the Massachusetts Health Club Membership Contracts Law (26) contains the following provisions, in part:

- prohibits the sale of lifetime membership contracts or contracts for more than three years;
- regulates financing arrangements by prohibiting contracts from requiring payments for more than one month beyond the expiration of the contract, and requiring that installments be in substantially equal amounts and due at substantially equal intervals, not more frequently than once a month;
- requires health clubs to post on the premises all of its courses and membership prices, discounts, sales or offers;
- makes many kinds of misrepresentations by health clubs a violation of the Consumer Protection Act, including misrepresentations of the club's facilities, services, programs, training methods, or pricing structure, or of the number, qualifications or experience of its personnel, or of the consumer's cancellation rights (26, para. 2).

Massachusetts also has a law covering cancellation rights that requires the membership contract to include the following notice in ten point bold font:

CONSUMER'S RIGHT TO CANCELLATION. YOU MAY CANCEL THIS CONTRACT WITHOUT ANY PENALTY OR FURTHER OBLIGATION BY CAUSING A WRITTEN NOTICE OF YOUR CANCELLATION TO BE DELIVERED IN PERSON OR POSTMARKED BY CERTIFIED OR REGISTERED UNITED STATES MAIL WITHIN THREE (3) BUSINESS DAYS OF THE DATE OF THIS CONTRACT OR THE DATE OF YOUR RECEIPT TO THE ADDRESS SPECIFIED IN THIS CONTRACT (27, para. 1).

Fitness facility members have made claims against facilities alleging their facility violated provisions within these types of statutes (28). Other claims made by members related to membership contract violations have involved laws such as the Telephone Consumer Protection Act (29) and the Electronic Funds Transfer Act (30).

States have laws similar to the FTCA described in Chapter 3 that prohibit, among other things, unfair and/or deceptive acts or practices For example, New York's statute—Deceptive Trade Practices by Health Clubs; Seller's Misrepresentation (31)—states the following, in part: It is an unfair and deceptive trade practice and unlawful for a seller to:

- misrepresent directly or indirectly in its advertising, promotional materials, or in any manner the size, location, facilities, or equipment of its studio or place of business or the number or qualifications of its personnel.
- use or refer to fictional organization divisions or position titles or make any representation which has the tendency or capacity to mislead or deceive consumers as to the size or importance of the business, its divisions, or personnel or in any other material respect.
- misrepresent directly or indirectly the size, importance, location, facilities, or equipment of the business through the use of photographs, illustrations, or any other depictions in catalogs, advertisements, or other promotional materials.
- misrepresent the nature of its courses, training devices, methods, or equipment or the number, qualifications, training, or experience of its personnel whether by means of endorsements or otherwise (31, para. 1).

For an example of a case in which the fitness facility violated the Connecticut Unfair Trade Practices Act (CUTPA) because of deceptive advertising regarding the qualifications and experience of their personal fitness trainers, see *D'Amico v. LA Fitness,* spotlight case in Chapter 5.

Washington D.C. also has consumer protection laws, such as the Consumer Protection Procedures Act (CPPA). On January 8, 2019, Attorney General Karl A. Racine announced that his office filed a lawsuit against Town Sports International (TSI) for violating this law (32). Racine alleged that:

"TSI is misleading consumers into signing up for memberships, failing to disclose all sign-up fees, refusing to provide written membership contracts, failing to inform consumers that memberships auto-renew, misleading consumers about cancellation policies, and continuing to charge consumers even after they cancel their memberships" (32, para. 7).

Interestingly, TSI had an agreement with the attorney general's office in 2016 to comply with the CPPA and promised to not mislead members. However, since 2016, Racine's office received approximately 50 complaints about TSI's violations of the CPPA.

Local Laws

Fitness managers/owners need to be aware of local laws. For example, the city of Philadelphia has an ordinance that requires businesses, including health clubs, to accept cash for their goods and services (33). It was reported that a number of gyms and fitness centers in Philadelphia, including 13 Planet Fitness locations, were in violation of this city's cashless ban. These health clubs require people to have a bank account in order to become a member of the facility as well as to purchase a bottle of water. A fine of up to $2,000 per transgression is included in the regulation. The goal of this law was to prohibit discrimination against people with lower incomes who, likely, do not have a bank account.

KEY POINT

To comply with many federal laws and regulations such as those promulgated by OSHA, ADA, and FTCA, fitness managers/owners should consult with their legal counsel to establish policies and procedures to comply with these laws as well as state and local laws. State laws address a variety of consumer protection laws that cover membership contracts and unfair or deceptive practices. Similar local laws may also be applicable to fitness facilities. To avoid violations and costly fines, daily operations need to reflect compliance with these laws.

Legal Duties Toward Invitees (Fitness Participants)

As described in Chapter 4, a special relationship is formed between a person(s) on land (e.g., a participant of a fitness facility) and a land owner/occupier (e.g., an owner/manager of a fitness facility). The law classifies persons who enter a fitness facility (or any business) as trespassers, licensees, or invitees. Each of these classifications were discussed in *Duncan v. World Wide Health Studios* (34), described in Chapter 4, including the legal duties that fitness managers and exercise professionals have toward persons in each classification. To determine whether the defendant health club was negligent, the court in *Duncan* first examined the relationship between the plaintiff and the health club. The court determined that the plaintiff was an invitee defined as follows:

An invitee is a person who goes on the premises with the express or implied invitation of the occupant...for their mutual advantage; and to him, the duty owed is that of reasonable and ordinary care, which includes the prior discovery of reasonably discoverable conditions of the premises that may be unreasonably dangerous, and correction thereof or a warning to the invitee of the danger (34, p. 837).

Because this discussion focuses on invitees, it is important to remember that invitees can be all types of fitness participants such as members, program participants, or guests who participate in the programs/services offered by a fitness facility. Invitees are owed a different standard of care (duty) than a trespasser or a licensee because a mutual benefit exists between an invitee and the land owner/occupier. For example, an owner of a fitness facility receives a monetary benefit from the fees that a member pays, and the member receives all the benefits that the membership provides. The *Duncan* court stated that the defendant health club had a duty of reasonable and ordinary care toward invitees. This duty includes reasonable inspection of the property for dangers and correction or warning of dangers. In the following spotlight case, *Crossing-Lyons v. Town Sports International, Inc.*, the fitness facility failed to meet these duties. Following the *Crossing-Lyons* case are eight additional cases involving duties toward invitees.

SPOTLIGHT CASE

Crossing-Lyons v. Town Sports International, Inc. (d/b/a New York Sports Club)
No. L-2024-14, 2017 WL 2953388 (N.J. Super. Ct. App. Div., 2017)

FACTS

Historical Facts:

When Janet Crossing-Lyons became a member of New York Sports Club, she was required to sign a waiver and release which included, in part:

This waiver and release of liability includes, without limitation, all injuries which may occur as a result of ... (a) your use of all amenities and equipment in the facility; (b) your participation in any activity, including, but not limited to, classes, programs, personal training sessions or instruction; and (c) the sudden and unforeseen malfunctioning of any equipment (p. 1).

On the day of her accident, Crossing-Lyons was on her way to meet her trainer when she tripped over a weight belt that was left on the floor by another member, which resulted in substantial injuries requiring hip surgery. She claimed the trainer knew of the existence of the weight belt and failed to remove it, despite the fitness center's policy to pick up items left on the floor.

Crossing-Lyons continued...

Procedural Facts:

The plaintiff, Crossing-Lyons, filed a complaint against the New York Sports Club charging the club with negligence due to failing to pick up the weight belt off the floor. The club filed a motion of summary judgment, which was granted by the trial court. In dismissing the case, the trial court judge relied on *Stelluti v. Casapenn Enterprises L.L.C*, 203 N.J. 286 (N.J. Lexis 750, 2010) in which the waiver protected the defendants for an injury due to negligent instruction.

Crossing-Lyons appealed this decision arguing that the trial court judge misapplied the *Stelluti* decision. She contended that the exculpatory clause was unenforceable and requested the order to grant summary judgment be reversed.

ISSUE

Did the waiver and release of liability, signed by the plaintiff, absolve the New York Sports Club of liability for its negligence to properly carry out its common law duty owed to invitees?

COURT'S RULING

No, the waiver/release did not absolve the club from liability for the injury incurred to the plaintiff. The trial court erred and its decision to grant summary judgment was reversed by the appellate court.

COURT'S REASONING

The appellate court stated that a business owner "has a duty to guard against any dangerous conditions that the owner knows about or should have discovered; and to conduct reasonable inspections to discover latent dangerous conditions. Any attempt to limit these conditions by directing patrons to sign exculpatory agreements requires careful attention by our courts" (p. 1) especially given that historically, exculpatory clauses are disfavored in law. The exculpatory agreement, signed by Crossing-Lyons, was unenforceable because it violated a common law duty of care that the fitness center owed to its invitees. "It adversely affects the public interest by transferring the redress of civil wrongs from the responsible tortfeasor to either an innocent injured party or society-at-large" (p. 2).

In making its decision, the appellate court relied on *Walters v. YMCA*, 437 N.J. Super. 111 (App. Div. 2014). In this case, the plaintiff's injury, like the injury incurred by Crossing-Lyons, occurred while on the premises (in *Walters*, the plaintiff slipped on a step leading to the indoor pool) versus from participation in physical activity or using the exercise equipment. The injuries suffered by Crossing-Lyons and Walters could have occurred in any business setting. A waiver/release to protect from these types of injuries is not enforceable because it adversely affects the public interest. If the plaintiff's injury was due to negligent instruction as in *Stelluti,* the waiver might have protected the defendant.

Lessons Learned from *Crossing-Lyons*

Legal

- Duties owed to invitees (e.g., inspections, correct/remove or warn of dangers) need to be properly carried out by staff members.

- According to this court, the waiver/release signed by the plaintiff violated the public interest based on "common law" duties owed to invitees.

- The court stated that a waiver/release would be enforceable for negligent instruction as it was in another New Jersey case *(Stelluti)* but not for failing to carry out duties toward invitees.

Risk Management/Injury Prevention

- Facility staff members need to be well-trained to follow the facility's policy to pick up (and properly store) equipment laying around on the floor and to remind those participants who fail to follow this policy of its importance.

- Participants need to be informed of this facility's policy upon joining and list this policy in the Facility's Safety Policies posted in the facility.

Legal Cases: Duties to Invitees

Unlike the court's ruling in *Crossing-Lyons,* courts, generally, have ruled that if the waiver/release is enforceable, it will protect defendants from **premise liability** claims involving injuries to invitees, as demonstrated in several of the following eight cases. Premise liability is a legal concept that typically applies when an injury was caused by some type of unsafe or defective condition on one's property (35). To prevail with a premise liability claim, the injured party needs to prove that the property owner/occupier knew or should have known that the premises were in an unsafe/defective condition and failed to take proper action to correct the condition. Of the eight cases (descriptions to follow), the court rulings varied with six ruling *for* the defendant and only two *for* the plaintiff as follows:

▶ **Court Rulings for the Defendants**

Grijalvla: Waiver/release was enforceable—protected defendant against the plaintiff's premise liability and negligence claims.

Toro: Waiver/release was enforceable; however, it may have not been if the plaintiff could have proven that the defendant created or had actual notice of the dangerous condition and did not take steps to correct the condition.

Anderson: Waiver/release was enforceable; however, it may have not been if the plaintiff could have proven that the defendant was grossly negligent (e.g., conduct that substantially or unreasonably increases the inherent risk of an activity or actively concealed a known risk).

Anast: Waiver/exculpatory agreement was enforceable—it explicitly stated negligent failure to warn or remove a hazardous, unsafe, dangerous, or defective condition.

Hoffner: No duty owed to an invitee when a defect (ice patch on the sidewalk) is open and obvious.

Gibson: Waiver/release was enforceable—it was unambiguous and covered any and all injuries due to negligence.

▶ **Court Rulings for the Plaintiff**

Roer—waiver/release unenforceable—it did not contain any exculpatory language; however, even if it did, it would likely have been unenforceable due to a New York statute (waivers/releases are void).

Lik—defendant was unable to provide any evidence that daily walkthroughs of the gym were conducted to inspect for defective conditions.

Several of these cases involved trip and falls and slip and falls. As described in Chapter 2, injuries due to falls in fitness facilities have resulted in a high number of liability claims. Therefore, to minimize these types of injuries, it is best to take steps to prevent them from occurring which includes carrying out the duties owed to invitees.

Fitness Floor Injuries: Improper Storage of Equipment

In *Roer v. 150 West End Owners Corp.* (36), the plaintiff fell off a treadmill when an exercise ball got sucked under the belt of the TM. This caused the rear of the TM to be lifted a couple of inches which propelled the machine forward several feet where it hit the wall causing the fall. The facility had video surveillance of the incident. The plaintiff claimed that the facility failed to take reasonable measures to ensure that the exercise ball would be secured. The court agreed stating that the defendant's "failure to provide storage racks…to prevent free movement of the balls…was a proximate cause of the Plaintiff's injuries." The waiver/release did not protect the defendant from its own negligence. First, it did not contain any exculpatory language to absolve the defendant from its own negligence and second, if it had, it would likely have been unenforceable under New York's General Obligations Law in which waivers are unenforceable. See Chapter 4 for more detail on this law.

In *Grijalva v. Bally Total Fitness* (37), the plaintiff, Ruben Grijalva, was injured while he was lifting fifty-five pound dumbbells. When he lowered the weights to the floor his right middle finger was caught between his own weights and a set of eighty-pound dumbbells left on the floor by another member. Ruben claimed he would not be able to return to work as a carpenter because his finger remained disfigured and not fully functional, even after reconstructive surgery. He filed several claims against Bally including premise liability and negligence. Regarding his premise liability claim, Ruben asserted that Bally breached its duty to maintain safe premises for invitees by failing to return the weights to their racks. He claimed that Bally's failure to assign employees to monitor the premises and remove weights and dumbbells from the floor constituted negligence. The appellate court upheld the trial court's ruling granting summary judgment in favor of Bally. The waiver/release that Ruben signed protected Bally regarding Ruben's premises liability and negligence claims.

Injuries From Falls: Locker/Shower Areas

In *Toro v. Fitness International* (38), the plaintiff claimed, as a member and business invitee, that his serious injuries from a slip and fall in the men's locker room were caused by a dangerous and hazardous condition (i.e., wet and slippery floor). In addition, he claimed that the defendant should be held liable because it knew or should have known about the dangerous and hazardous condition. The appellate court upheld the trial court's ruling that the waiver/release signed by the plaintiff was enforceable. It would be unenforceable if the plaintiff, a business invitee, could prove that the property owner "either created or had actual or constructive notice of the dangerous condition" (p. 977). When a defendant has actual knowledge of a dangerous condition and then does not take steps to correct that condition, it could constitute gross negligence. Although the plaintiff argued that the defendant did not keep accurate logs of its inspections and they failed to place mats on the locker room floor, the court ruled this was insufficient evidence. The plaintiff offered no evidence that the floor tended to be wet on a regular basis or that the defendant had actual knowledge of the wet floor.

In *Anderson v. Fitness International* (39), Kirk Anderson fell in the shower causing his humerus (long bone in the arm) to snap in two. He underwent surgery to repair his humerus requiring a plate and screws. In his gross negligence lawsuit against Fitness Intl., he alleged that the defendant knew or should have known of the dangerous condition in the shower area (i.e., tile floor layered with soapy residue with no handrails,

shower mats, or friction strips). He claimed he had fallen twice in the men's locker room and had informed employees at the front desk, but they seemed marginally interested in his complaints and requests. He also claimed that he had observed numerous other patrons fall in the shower area. The appellate court upheld the trial court's ruling granting summary judgment in favor of the defendant based on the waiver that Anderson signed and the fact he was unable to provide evidence of gross negligence. The trial court stated that "you don't know whether those complaints came under the nose of someone with authority to give you something about them and that person tossed them in the air with reckless abandonment, or whether a secretary accidentally threw away all of the complaints so they never came to the attention of anybody who was in a position to do anything about it. Until you have those facts, you're just pleading a conclusion of gross negligence" (p. 796). However, the court also stated that "conduct that substantially or unreasonably increases the inherent risk of an activity or actively concealed a known risk could amount to gross negligence which would not be barred by a release agreement" (p. 881). The court also concluded that the failure to guard against or warn of a dangerous condition typically does not constitute gross negligence.

Injuries from Falls: Basketball Courts

In *Lik v. LA Fitness, Inc.* (40), the plaintiff, while playing basketball, alleged that he suffered a knee injury after jumping up and landing on a defective floor board. After filing a claim involving an allegedly negligent condition against the defendant, the defendant claimed the plaintiff's injury was not due to negligence because he assumed the inherent risks of playing basketball. Relying on previous case law, the court stated owners of a sporting venue "owe a duty to exercise care to make conditions as safe as they appear to be. If the risks of the activity are fully comprehended or perfectly obvious, the plaintiff has consented to them" (p. 4). The court also stated that the standard for applying the assumption of risk depends on whether the conditions caused by the defendant's negligence created a dangerous condition over and above the usual dangers that are inherent in the sport. The court ruled that doctrine of primary assumption of risk was not applicable in this case because defective floorboards are not part of the usual dangers inherent in the sport of basketball. The plaintiff also alleged that his injury was due to the defendant's failure to provide actual and constructive notice of the defective condition. The facility's operation manager testified that general daily walkthroughs of the gym were conducted but was unable to provide evidence that records of inspections were kept. The manager offered no testimony regarding the last time an employee checked the basketball court prior to the plaintiffs' injury. Therefore, the court denied the defendant's motion for summary judgment.

In *Anast v. LTF Club* (41), the plaintiff, while playing basketball, saw an employee who appeared to be sweeping or mopping the floor but did not see exactly what he was doing. While chasing a loose ball, he slipped and fell fracturing his ankle. After the fall, he noticed the water standing on the floor where he had slipped. Anast sued LTF and LTF moved for summary judgment. Referring to previous court rulings in Illinois, the court stated that the "operator of a business owes its customers a duty to exercise reasonable care to maintain the premises in a reasonably safe condition for their use" and "when a business invitee like Anast is injured in a fall, the business owner is liable if the condition that caused the fall was placed there by the operator's agents or if the operator or its agents had actual notice of the condition or it was there long enough that it should have been discovered with ordinary care" (p. 1). LTF argued that the exculpatory language in the agreement that Anast signed barred his claim that his injury resulted from an employee's failure to remove or warn of a hazardous condition (e.g., rope off the dangerous area while cleaning the floors). The court agreed with LTF stating that the exculpatory agreement specifically mentions "negligent failure to warn or remove a hazardous, unsafe, dangerous or defective condition" (p. 5). Therefore, the court granted the motion for summary judgment in favor of the defendants.

Injuries From Falls: Exterior Areas

In *Hoffner v. Lanctoe* (42), Charlotte Hoffner was a member of Fitness Xpress located in a commercial building in Michigan. There is only one entrance into the facility, which is serviced by a sidewalk that runs the length of the building and connects the building with the parking lot. Under the lease agreement, the building, sidewalk, and parking lot are owned and maintained by the tenants, Richard and Lori Lanctoe. On the day of Hoffner's injury, the Lanctoes had earlier cleared and salted the icy parking lot and sidewalk. However, by the time the plaintiff arrived, the sidewalk was icy at the facility's entrance. She said she could see the ice but thought she could make it inside the building being it was only a few steps. Unfortunately, she fell on the ice injuring her back. Hoffner brought a premises liability lawsuit against the Lanctoes and Fitness Xpress. Both defendants moved for summary judgment. The trial court denied these motions.

The appellate court reversed the trial court's ruling concluding that Fitness Xpress was entitled to summary judgment because they did not own or control the sidewalk. However, the appellate court affirmed the trial court's denial to grant the Lanctoes summary judgment. Although the Lanctoes claimed they were not liable based on the **open and obvious doctrine,** the appellate court disagreed. The Lanctoes then appealed to the Michigan Supreme Court.

After an analysis of Michigan premises liability law and the open and obvious doctrine, the Supreme Court stated that the "duty owed to an invitee considers whether a defect is open and obvious. The possessor of land owes no duty to protect or warn of dangers that are open and obvious because such dangers, by their nature, apprise an invitee of the potential hazard, which the invitee may then take reasonable measures to avoid" (p. 460-461). An exception to this general rule exists when *special aspects* of a condition make even an open and obvious risk unreasonable. This exception permits recovery only in certain circumstances (e.g., a condition that presents a high likelihood of harm notwithstanding a hazard's obvious nature). The Court concluded that the "ice patch on the sidewalk that plaintiff chose to confront was open and obvious, and plaintiff has not provided evidence of special aspects of the condition to justify imposing liability on defendants despite the open and obvious nature of the danger" (pp. 481-482). Therefore, the Court reversed the appellate court's ruling and granted summary judgment in favor of the Lanctoes.

In *Gibson v. YMCA* (43), the plaintiff fell and sustained injuries when she tripped on an allegedly, uneven or cracked sidewalk approximately twenty feet from the entrance to the YMCA. She sued the YMCA claiming the YMCA was negligent for not properly maintaining its premises. The YMCA moved for summary judgment based on the release that the plaintiff had signed. The trial court denied this motion because the language in the release did not include that the plaintiff assumed the risk of an injury from a defectively constructed or maintained sidewalk. There was a question as to whether the YMCA intended that the release contemplated a trip and fall on a cracked sidewalk or area of disrepair. Upon appeal, the appellate court reversed the trial court's ruling and granted summary judgment to the YMCA. The release signed by the plaintiff absolved the YMCA "for any and all injuries…even if such damage or injury results from a negligent act or omission" (p. 6). Whether or not the plaintiff contemplated that exact injury was immaterial because the language in the release was unambiguous.

Fitness Facility Orientation: Educating Invitees of Their Safety Responsibilities

Professional organizations have published standards of practice regarding fitness facility orientations. For example, ACSM has a standard that states, in part, "facility operators shall…offer the new member or prospective user a general orientation to the facility"

(3, p. 29). The Medical Fitness Association (MFA) has a guideline that states, "all facility users should be offered an initial orientation to the facility, the facility's equipment, basic program concepts, and emergency/safety guidelines" (5, p. 25). These standards/guidelines do not provide much guidance on *what* topics to cover in the facility orientation and do not address *why* a facility orientation is important from safety and legal liability perspectives, and how to develop and implement a facility orientation program. The what, why, and how are described below—see Topics #1 through #6.

As presented in Chapter 2, one essential feature of creating a safety culture is to inform participants of their safety responsibilities. Fitness managers/owners cannot assume that fitness participants will be aware of safety practices such as following the facility's safety policies, using the exercise equipment properly, and applying principles of safe exercise. Regarding proper instruction on how to use the equipment, the court in the spotlight case, *Thomas v. Sport City*, stated:

> "members of health clubs are owed a duty of reasonable care to protect them from injury while on the premises… [This duty] necessarily includes a general responsibility to ensure that their members know how to properly use gym equipment" (p. 1157).

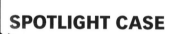

SPOTLIGHT CASE

Thomas v. Sport City, Inc.
738 So. 2d 1153 (La. Ct. App., 2 Cir. 1999)

FACTS

Historical Facts:

Thomas, a weight lifter and member of Sport City health club for several years, was an experienced user of the club's hack squat machine. One day, after completing a set of 180 pounds of weights that was on the carriage of the machine, he thought he had properly engaged the hook to secure the weights. However, he did not secure the hook and the rack of weights fell, fracturing his ankle and crushing his foot.

Procedural Facts:

The plaintiff, Thomas, filed a negligence lawsuit against Sports City, Inc., its insurer, Scottsdale Insurance Company, claiming that the health club failed to warn, supervise and instruct him on the proper use of the hack squat machine. He also

Thomas continued...

filed a products liability claim against Capps Welding, manufacturer of the hack squat machine, claiming the machine had a design defect. The trial court ruled in favor of the plaintiff awarding him general damages of $45,000 and special damages of $13,703.35. Comparative fault was assigned as follows: 30% to the plaintiff, 35% to Sports City, and 35% to Capps Welding. The defendants (Sport City and Capps Welding) appealed the decisions of the trial court.

ISSUES

1) Was Sport City negligent because they did not meet the duty of reasonable care owed to the plaintiff?

2) Was Capps Welding liable for products liability because their hack squat machine had a design defect and, thus, was unreasonably dangerous?

COURT'S RULING

1. No, the appellate court ruled that Sport City was not negligent because the injury to Thomas was not caused by a breach of duty.

2. No, the appellate court ruled that Capps Welding was not liable for products liability because the design of the hack squat machine was not defective or unreasonably dangerous.

COURT'S REASONING

Regarding the negligence lawsuit and citing previous case law, the court stated that "members of health clubs are owed a duty of reasonable care to protect them from injury while on the premises...and this duty necessarily includes a general responsibility to ensure that their members know how to properly use gym equipment" (p. 1157). The court stated if Sport City had not instructed or supervised the plaintiff on the proper use of the machine it would normally be a breach of duty because the machine could easily cause injury. However, the plaintiff testified, he knew how to use the machine and did not feel it was necessary for him to be shown how to use the hack squat machine. The plaintiff acknowledged he had been a user of the machine for years and if he had properly latched the hooking mechanism, the weight would have not fallen. Therefore, the court found that Sport City's failure to warn or instruct the plaintiff was not the cause of the plaintiff's injury and that the trial court erred in finding Sport City at fault.

Regarding the products liability claim, the court describes three elements that the plaintiff must prove to show a defect by design under La. Rev. Stat. § 9:2800.56:

> First, he must prove that another way to design the product existed at the time it was placed on the market. Next he must show that the alternative design was significantly less likely to cause the accident, or that the alternative design would have significantly reduced the damage. Thirdly, the claimant must prove that, at the time the product left the manufacturer's control, the likelihood that the product as designed would cause the claimant's damage and the gravity of that damage outweighed the burden on the manufacturer of adopting the alternative design identified by claimant and the adverse effect, if any, this different design would have on the product's utility (pp. 1154-1155).

To determine if there was a design defect, the appellate court required Thomas to prove that there was an alternate design that would meet the purpose of the hack squat machine—a machine that would allow for a full squat and capable of preventing his injury. Two weightlifting experts for the plaintiff were not, according to the court, qualified to testify about the design of the hack squat machine but both stated that the weightlifter is responsible for his own safety. Two additional experts for the defendant Capps Welding, who were experts in the design of exercise equipment, testified that the design of hack squat machine was similar in design to other manufacturer's hack squat machines. Therefore, Thomas was not able to establish an alternate design and the court concluded that the Capps Welding hack squat machine did not have a design defect and that "the trial court committed manifest error in finding the hack squat machine to be unreasonably dangerous" (p. 1157).

Thomas continued...

Lessons Learned from *Thomas:*

Legal

▶ Fitness facility staff members have a duty to instruct participants on how to properly use exercise equipment.

▶ To prove negligence, the plaintiff must show that a breach of duty (e.g., failure to instruct) was the "cause" of the injury. Negligent instruction was not the cause of the injury in this case given the plaintiff was an experienced user of the hack squat machine.

▶ Monetary damages can be awarded based on the percentage of fault of each party as the trial court assigned in this case. However, the appellate court found that the defendants (Sport City and Capps Welding) were not liable for the injury.

▶ Plaintiffs making a products liability claim against a manufacturer need to prove there was a manufacturing, design, or marketing defect.

▶ Courts may rely on expert testimony and state statutes, as in this case, to determine if certain elements have been met to prove there was a design defect.

Risk Management/Injury Prevention

▶ Fitness facility staff members need to carry out their duty to instruct participants on how to properly use the exercise equipment, which can be done by:

- Providing instruction/demonstration in the facility orientation.
- Referencing "instructional" signage posted in the facility and on (or next to) each piece of equipment in the facility orientation.
- Encouraging new participants to ask a staff member to show them how to use the equipment.
- Training staff members, who supervise the fitness floor, on how to properly communicate with and instruct participants who are not using the equipment properly or misusing the equipment

Topic #1: Purpose of the Facility Orientation

Explain that management is committed to safety and has taken many steps (e.g., developed/implemented safety standards/guidelines published by professional organizations) to create a safety culture to help ensure the safety of all participants. However, participants also have safety responsibilities and the main purpose of the orientation is to describe these responsibilities.

Topic #2: Facility Safety Policies

Review the sign posted in the facility that lists the facility's safety policies. For an example of safety polices to include on this sign, see Exhibit 10-1. Explain each of these along with the reason for each. Emphasize that all participants need follow these for their own safety and the safety of others. For large facilities, it may be necessary to post this sign in several areas. It may also be

wise to provide the list of these policies in the membership agreement (with a signature line where they sign and agree to follow them), on the facility's website, and a written copy to distribute in the orientation. These steps will underscore the importance of the safety policies and may serve as evidence in refuting future negligence claims/lawsuits (e.g., an injury caused by not following safety policies).

Topic #3: Instruction on the Proper Use of the Exercise Equipment

It is not feasible to provide instruction on every piece of equipment in a facility orientation. However, it may be wise to demonstrate the proper use on one piece of cardio equipment (e.g., a treadmill) and on one weight training machine. During the instruction on proper form and execution, point out the warning labels and instructional placards posted on the machines. It will also be important to review the warning

---

Exhibit 10-1: Example: Fitness Facility Safety Policies to be Posted in the Facility

- Return equipment such as dumbbells and exercise balls back to their storage racks after use.
- No personal equipment is allowed anywhere in the facility, e.g., gym bags, purses, exercise equipment, etc. Lockers are available to store personal belongings.
- Proper workout attire is required. Shirts must be worn at all times. Closed toe athletic shoes must be worn in the Fitness Facility.
- Please wipe down equipment after use. Disinfectant wipes are provided throughout the facility.
- No one under the age of 16 is permitted in the Fitness Facility without parent/guardian supervision. No one 13 or younger is allowed to use the Fitness Facility unless enrolled in one of our youth programs.
- No tobacco use of any kind including vaping, food or chewing gum is permitted in the Fitness Facility. Spill-proof water bottles are allowed.
- Please be courteous of others using the Fitness Facility and display appropriate behavior at all times.
- Cell phones must be turned off or put on vibrate. Do not use a cell phone while performing any exercises.
- **No photos or video recordings are allowed anywhere in the facility without the permission of management.**
- Follow all signage that is posted on the equipment and throughout the Facility.

---

signage and any instructional placards posted near equipment such as free weights, kettlebells, and exercise balls. Related to instruction, it is best to also go over the items listed in the posted Facility Safety Sign (see Figure 9-5 in Chapter 9) such as "if you are unsure on how to use a machine, seek the assistance of our floor personnel…". In addition, it is recommended to emphasize the importance of seeking instruction on treadmills and free weights, given the high number of injuries with these types of equipment as described in previous chapters.

Topic #4: Facility Safety Signage

In addition to the safety polices posted in Exhibit 10-1, it is important to point out and explain other safety and/or policy signage posted throughout the facility during the orientation such as:

a) Warning and/or caution signage posted in swimming pools, saunas/steam rooms, hot tubs/spas, and shower areas.

b) Policy and usage guidelines in group exercise studios, locker/shower areas, indoor tracks, and other areas.

c) Emergencies—signage regarding the location of first-aid kits and AEDs as well as medical emergency plans, evacuation plans, and emergency phones

d) Outdoor exercise precautions—signage addressing weather and safety precautions. For an example, see Exhibit 10-2.

e) Exit and restroom signage

Note: *Regarding the last item in Exhibit 10-2 (for more information, ask one of our professional staff members), exercise professionals can refer participants to reliable information from various reputable websites as well as information provided by ACSM and other organizations for consumers. For example, see a short article entitled "Exercising in Hot and Cold Environments" (available in the ACSM's Resource Library).*

Fitness facilities need to be sure that certain signage within the facility meets OSHA and ADA specifications. Signage should also meet specifications published by the American Society of Testing and Materials (ASTM) as described in Chapter 9. In addition, fitness managers/owners should review signage standards and guidelines published by professional organizations. For example, ACSM (3) has five standards and two guidelines, MFA (5) has three standards and several guidelines, and IHRSA (44) has one standard.

Note: *Signage in languages other than English may be needed given the facility's clientele.*

Exhibit 10-2: EXERCISER'S ALERT*

Warning! Off-Premises Activities

Fitness activities carried out "off-premises" such as walking and jogging should be carefully considered. Not only should exercisers undergo pre-activity health screening, proper warm-up, and professional prescription for activity, special care should be given to environmental conditions and safety issues.

Environmental Conditions

Exercise in high temperatures (above 80° Fahrenheit) or at high humidity should be undertaken only in moderation. Prolonged activity in sustained heat, humidity, and/or sun should be avoided. If you choose to exercise during these conditions, such activity should be undertaken before 11:00 a.m. or after 3:00 p.m. Fluid should be taken liberally during exercise, particularly at high temperatures and before thirst is indicated.

Exercising during severe cold weather, snow, sleet, severe rain, hail, high winds, storms, or similar conditions should also be avoided.

Activity at high altitude should be undertaken gradually and progressively by beginning slowly and increasing over several days until normal activity can be undertaken. Fluid intake also should be increased during high altitude exercise.

Safety Issues

In addition to environmental conditions, special caution regarding the area to be used for exercise activity must be considered. Answer the following questions before beginning activity:

    a) Is this a high crime area? If so, avoid it. If you don't know, avoid until you find out. The police department is your best source of information for this purpose. If you cannot find out, don't use the area.

    b) Is the area properly illuminated at night? If not, avoid it.

    c) Is the ground surface in good condition? If not, avoid it.

    d) Is the area in a remote location or interspersed with hiding places for assailants? If so, avoid it.

Helpful Hints

- Do not wear headphones
- Exercise in pairs
- Carry and be prepared to use a whistle, if needed, to obtain attention.
- Carry mace or keys in fist to use if attacked.
- Carry mobile phone to call 911 in case of an emergency
- Exercise during daylight hours if possible
- For more information, ask one of our professional staff members

---

*Reproduced and adapted with permission from: Herbert DL. *Jogger's Attack in High Crime Area Leads to Suit*. *The Exercise Standards and Malpractice Reporter*. 5(2), 30, 1991. Copyright 2019 by PRC Publications, Inc. Canton, Ohio. All other rights reserved.

Topic #5: Principles of Safe Exercise

During the orientation, it is essential to describe basic principles of safe exercise such as warm-up, cool-down, progression, signs/symptoms of overexertion, and potential risks of exercise and how to minimize those risks. This is best accomplished by providing a handout with this information such as the 32-page booklet briefly described in Exhibit 10-3. The instructor can verbally highlight some of these principles in the booklet and encourage individuals to read through it sometime after the orientation. This information could also be available on the facility's website.

Having evidence that the facility provided instruction of safe principles of exercise may be helpful to defend any future litigation involving negligent instruction. For example, in an article by Dr. Anthony Abbott (45), he describes several negligent lawsuits in which the plaintiff's cardiac arrest was likely due to the failure of the fitness staff to carry out their legal duty to orient/educate the plaintiff on the importance of proper cool-down and the concept of blood pooling. In addition, as presented in this textbook, there are many injury cases involving exercise intensity being too high or the exercises too advanced, given the individual's health/fitness status.

Topic #6: Programs/Services Offered and Credentials of Exercise Professionals

As described in Chapter 8, it is essential for fitness facilities to offer "beginner level" programs such as beginner indoor cycling, yoga, and boot camp classes. In the orientation, these programs can be promoted, as well as other types of classes and personal fitness training, for both general and special populations as shown in Figure 7-2 in Chapter 7. Special population programs can include those for youth, women who are pregnant or postpartum, older adults, individuals with disabilities and/or chronic diseases. It will be important to describe the credentials of the exercise professionals who provide these programs/services. Be sure this information is accurate and honest to help prevent any violations of statutes involving unfair and deceptive practices as described earlier. For example, do not make statements like "our clinical exercise programs are taught by clinical exercise physiologists" unless they truly are (e.g., they possess the credentials commensurate with ACSM's certified clinical exercise physiologist).

Facility Maintenance and Cleaning

Serious injuries have occurred from failing to properly maintain and clean fitness and athletic facilities such as saunas, steam rooms, hot tubs, whirlpools, and locker/shower areas. Certain laws are applicable regarding the maintenance/cleaning of these types of facilities as well as standards and/or guidelines published by professional organizations such as the ACSM (3) and the YMCA (46). This section includes a spotlight case (*Miller v. The YMCA of Central Massachusetts et al.*) in which there were numerous failures to properly maintain the steam room that led to a death. Following

---

Exhibit 10-3: Benefits of Providing a Written Handout on Safe Principles of Exercise

For fitness participants:

- They learn about safety principles and why they are important.
- The information can be presented in a user-friendly format—easy, quick to read and understand such as in the Physical Fitness booklet.*
- Provides a "free" resource for them to review and demonstrates management's commitment to their safety.

For fitness managers and exercise professionals:

- Provides important information to review with new participants during Facility Orientations—a unique benefit to the facility.
- When unsafe principles are observed, participants can be reminded of this information provided to them in the Facility Orientation.
- Helps minimize legal liability by carrying out the legal duty to provide proper instruction—the written resource can serve as evidence in negligence claims/lawsuits.

Physical Fitness: Guidelines for Safe and Effective Exercise. Available at: www.fitnesslawacademy.com (32-page booklet)

---

the spotlight case, three legal cases are described involving bacterial infections that the plaintiffs claimed were caused by the failure of the defendants to properly clean and disinfect their facilities.

Legal Cases: Improper Cleaning and Disinfecting Procedures

Serious injuries that can occur, such as severe burns from using a steam room, were evident in the *Miller* spotlight case. Other injuries such as bacterial skin infections can also occur, especially in warm environments such as steam rooms/saunas and hot tubs/whirlpools. In an article by Dr. Anthony Abbott (47) entitled "A Hot Topic," he described several of these bacterial infections and how they can thrive in these environments. He also described other injury risks related to

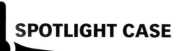

SPOTLIGHT CASE

Miller v. The YMCA of Central Massachusetts et al.
33 Mass. L. Rep. 562, 2016 LEXIS 323 (Mass. Super. Ct., 2016)

FACTS

Historical Facts:

Mr. Thomas Miller, a member of the Silver Sneakers program, attended his local YMCA to exercise. Prior to joining, Mr. Miller signed a release absolving the Silver Sneakers program of any negligence liability which stated: "I hereby release, waive, discharge and covenant not to sue…from any and all demands, liabilities, losses and demands (including death), *caused…by the negligence of any of the foregoing people or entities"* (p. 7). Mr. Miller checked in at the YMCA's front desk around 5:55 am and at some point, went to use the steam room. At about 7:00 am another member noticed Mr. Miller lying unconscious on the floor of the steam room with hot steam blasting upon his body. After he could not enter the steam room because it was locked, he activated the emergency call button outside of the steam room, which alerted the front desk and a call to 911 was placed.

In the meantime, two YMCA employees went to the steam room to try to gain entry to the control room to shut off the steam vent but were unable to because they did not have access to a master key. Another employee who had a master key refused to unlock the door because he was not authorized to use it. Only YMCA employee Kenneth McArthur was authorized to open the door. However, it wasn't until after McArthur watched EMS for five minutes, trying to gain access to the steam room, that he used his key so they could access the steam room. The YMCA disputes some of these facts claiming that (a) one of its employees did obtain a key and was able to unlock the door to the steam room and shut off the steam vent, (b) another employee tried to use a defibrillator but it did not work because of the moisture on Mr. Miller's body and lack of extra defibrillator pads. Mr. Miller was taken by ambulance to the hospital where he was diagnosed with second degree burns covering 12-15% of his body that required multiple surgeries. Mr. Miller died three weeks after the incident.

Procedural Facts:

Mr. Miller's estate filed a lawsuit alleging "a violation of the wrongful death statute on behalf of Mr. Miller's beneficiaries (count I), conscious pain and suffering (count II), and gross negligence (count III)" (p. 2). Counts I and II allege negligence. The lawsuit claims the YMCA officials had:

1. no steam room safety policy;
2. no "walk through locker room logs";
3. no regular staff inspections of the steam room;
4. no risk management classes for its employees;
5. no discussion of members' health risks in using the steam room;
6. no discussions about "having any doctors or other medical professionals present or on-call" if an older member's health became emergent;
7. no official member clearance was required of Silver Sneakers members; and
8. no written logs of inspections of the steam room (pp. 3-4).

"Perhaps more importantly, the estate claims that when the EMT personnel responded to the scene, they still were unable to gain access to the control room shut off valve in the steam room where Mr. Miller's body still lay, with his flesh burning, unconscious on the floor" (p. 4).

In their defense, all of the defendants (the YMCA and its two officers President Kathryn Hunter and Vice President Ken Mierzykowski), claimed they were protected because Miller had signed a release of liability and because there was a

Miller continued...

danger sign posted outside the steam room cautioning people, among other things, to not use the steam room alone. All the defendants filed motions for summary judgment.

ISSUE
Did the court grant the motions for summary in favor of the defendants?

COURT'S RULING
No. The court denied all motions of summary judgment.

COURT'S REASONING
Regarding the release, the court stated the very existence of the release concedes that the YMCA was aware of its duty to provide a safe environment for its members. The court also stated that "there can be little question that one who pays for admission to a facility of a commercial establishment has the right to expect to be reasonably safe while on the its premises" (p. 5). The release that Mr. Miller signed absolved the Silvers Sneakers program of all negligence liability but nowhere in the release is the YMCA mentioned. Even if it had included the YMCA, the release would not apply to count I (where the decedent could have released his own claims but not those of his beneficiaries) as well as count III, gross negligence.

The court did not address the danger sign posted outside the steam room but did address a section within the YMCA published safety recommendations, *Safeguarding Health and Well-Being,* titled: The Use of Saunas, Steam Rooms and Whirlpool/Hot Tubs in the YMCA. This document recommended that steam rooms have easily-accessible emergency shut-off systems. However, the defendants claimed that this document should not be applied because it was the February 2012 edition and Mr. Miller's accident occurred on January 2, 2012. The court's response to this was that "Nevertheless, the last page of this Guide shows that there were six iterations of this guide in the previous 20 years...The court has no idea which, if any, of these previous editions contained recommendations that would have applied to the horrible incident involving Mr. Miller's..." (p. 7). The court added that these published guidelines present genuine issues of material fact in this case, in addition to the eight issues raised by Mr. Miller's estate.

Note: This YMCA document (46) that has been cited in this textbook is the 2011 edition and was likely current at the time of this incident. It includes three pages of recommendations for these types of facilities including "Controls to shut off the equipment in the event of an emergency should be easily accessible by users" (p. 127). The court also indicated that the YMCA had no working defibrillator (AED) on its premises which was in violation of G.L. c. 93, section 78A, a Massachusetts statute that requires health clubs to have an AED.

Lessons Learned from *Miller*

Legal
- For a release to be an effective defense, it must be written very carefully to include all potential defendants. The YMCA was not mentioned in the "Silver Sneakers" release in this case.

- As demonstrated in this case, waivers/releases can be an effective defense for ordinary negligence but not for gross negligence.

- A waiver/release, in states where they are enforceable, releases the negligent claims made by the individual who signed it, but perhaps not for the claims made by his/her beneficiaries as demonstrated in this case.

- Facilities that allow non-members to use the facility (e.g., third parties that rent/lease space for programs/services) need to address potential legal liability issues that can arise.

- The YMCA, in this case, did not even follow the YMCA recommendations established by the Medical Advisory Committee of the YMCA of the USA. Published standards of practice help courts determine duty and breach of duty as they did in this case.

- Fitness facilities need to comply with state AED laws that require fitness facilities to have an AED as well as other related requirements (e.g., having two sets of pads which the YMCA did not have in this case).

Miller continued...

Risk Management/Injury Prevention

▶ Managers of fitness facilities have many risk management responsibilities. It was evident in this case that YMCA managers were not aware of these important responsibilities based on their testimony:

- The YMCA Director of Operations testified he was responsible for the day-to-day training and supervision of employees in steam room safety and developing any safety protocol for the steam room at this YMCA branch and three others.
- The YMCA President testified that she was the strategic leader of the facility whose duties included personally supervising staff responsible for safety programs and that she never participated in the drafting of any safety plan.

▶ Fitness facilities that provide facilities like steam rooms, saunas, whirlpools/hot tubs need to follow safety standards of practice published by professional organizations such as the YMCA and ACSM but also those published by independent organizations (manufacturers).

▶ Risk management strategies regarding steam rooms, saunas, whirlpools/hot tubs include:

- Having a well-written safety plan
- Providing employee training regarding the safety plan for new employees and on a regular basis for all employees, e.g., four times/year
- Having employees supervise the facilities
- Conducting regular inspections and completing logs of inspections
- Having immediate access by employees
- Having an emergency alarm button inside and outside the facility
- Informing participants of potential risks
- Providing facility policy and safety signage

▶ Regarding AEDs, fitness facilities need to comply with state statutes, if applicable, as well as perform regular inspections of the AED based on the manufacturer's specifications. See Chapter 11 for more on this topic.

using these types of facilities and offered several risk management strategies to help prevent these risks. The following three cases involve bacterial infections. The first two, *Manerchia* and *Pecora*, involve infections the plaintiffs claimed came from exposure to the fitness facility's hot tub and sauna, respectively. The third case, *Tynes v. Buccaneers Limited Partnership*, involves a bacterial infection suffered by a professional football player.

In *Manerchia v. Kirkwood Fitness & Racquetball Clubs* (48), Jack Manerchia claimed his diagnosis of cellulitis (bacterial skin infection) came from his use of the Kirkwood Club's hot tub. In his lawsuit, he alleged that the Club's negligence caused his injury. An expert witness, the plaintiff's physician, testified that his cellulitis could have come from the Club's hot tub but it was also likely that it came from somewhere else. The trial court ruled that the Club was entitled to summary judgment

but gave Manerchia 30 days to find new counsel and submit expert opinions to support the cause of his illness and the cleanliness of the Club's hot tub. He submitted another expert opinion, Dr. Charles Hesdorffer. Dr. Hesdorffer stated, "with reasonable degree of medical certainty...and following a careful evaluation of Manerchia's medical records...the cellulitis that he developed was a direct result of his immersion in the hot tub..." (pp. 3-4). Despite this testimony, the trial court granted summary judgment in favor of the Club stating that Mancheria could not prove that the Club was negligent and that its negligence caused his illness.

Upon appeal, Mancheria claimed that the Club failed to comply with the state's regulatory requirements for the maintenance of hot tubs and that such a violation is negligence per se. However, the Delaware Supreme Court stated that he offered no proof of that failure other than the hot tub looked dirty on the day he used it and that it was closed off with caution tape on his next visit to the Club. The Court ruled those facts do not establish the Club's failure to properly maintain the hot tub. Although the Club had discarded its records showing compliance with the State's requirements, it did not violate any regulations by discarding such records because they only needed to be kept for one year. The Court did not address the negligence per se issue. Regarding Dr. Hesdorffer's testimony, the Court stated that he merely confirmed Mancheria's condition, but failed to provide any proof that the injury was caused by the use of a hot tub, let alone the Club's hot tub. Therefore, the Supreme Court affirmed the trial court's ruling.

In *Pecora v. Fitness Intl., LLC* (49), the plaintiff claimed that he contracted Methicillin-resistant *Staphylococcus aureus* (MRSA) after his use of the health club's sauna. The defendants argued that the plaintiff did not have any evidence to support his claim that the bacteria existed at the health club or the sauna prior to his infection. The defendants submitted an Affidavit from a physician with a subspecialty in infectious disease who stated "it is well recognized in the field of infectious diseases that MRSA can be transmitted in a variety of common everyday interactions…MRSA can also be transmitted from one person to another by merely being in close proximity to a person who is colonized by MRSA who is coughing or sneezing. It is common for individuals who are 'colonized', to be unaware of that fact, making it virtually impossible to trace whether physical contact or other methods of transferring MRSA…there is no evidentiary foundation or scientific methodology, which is generally accepted in the infectious disease medical community to attribute the cause of the plaintiff's MRSA infection to his use of the sauna in question" (pp. 2-3).

The court stated that a landowner may be liable for an injured plaintiff but "it must be established that a defective condition existed and that the landowner affirmatively created the condition or had actual or constructive notice of its existence" (p. 5). However, the plaintiff did not put forth any facts to support his allegations that the defendants knew or should have known about MRSA bacteria being present in the health club. The plaintiff only offered speculation regarding health code violations related to record keeping. The court granted the defendants' motion for summary judgment

concluding that "mere speculation as to the cause of an accident, when there could have been many possible causes, is fatal to a cause of action" (p. 6).

As demonstrated in *Manerchia* and *Pecora*, it may be difficult for plaintiffs to prove that their skin bacterial infections resulted from the use of the fitness facilities. However, as described in Chapter 9, if certain factors are present, plaintiffs may be able to make a good case (50). Of major concern is the incidence of MRSA in athletic facilities. Based on a study published in *Medicine & Science in Sports & Exercise* (51), community-associated MRSA (CA-MRSA) infection incidence has increased among high-school and collegiate athletes (e.g., 15.5 per 10,000 athletes in 2012-2013 to 20.3 per 10,000 athletes in 2016-2017). This study also found that the week preceding the infection, the CA-MRSA-infected, student athletes came into contact with locker rooms, playing surfaces, weight rooms, athletic training facilities, weight room weights, locker room showers, athletic training facility tables, and athletic training facility whirlpools. The authors concluded that despite practitioner (i.e., athletic trainers) knowledge of CA-MRSA treatment options and preventative recommendations, such as those published by the CDC and the National Athletic Trainers' Association (NATA), it has not curtailed the incidence of CA-MRSA. Organizational and institutional policies and resources are needed to ensure preventive and management protocols are implemented and updated.

As described in *Tynes v. Buccaneers Limited Partnership* (52), NFL veteran place kicker, Lawrence Tynes, joined the Buccaneers Limited Partnership in July 2013. As he did in each of his nine prior seasons in the NFL, Tynes voluntarily visited a podiatrist for a minor procedure on the toe-nail on the big toe of his kicking foot on July 30, 2013. Each visit to these podiatrists was without incident. The Buccaneers Limited Partnership (Buccaneers) was aware of this procedure. As part of his treatment, Tynes needed to soak his toe in hot and cold tubs, which he did at the defendant's facility—One Bucs Place. This state-of-the-art facility provides locker rooms, showers, training room, and soaking tubs used by the football players, coaching staff, and others including members of the public. After using the facilities, Tynes developed a MRSA infection resulting in permanent damage which ended his professional career.

In 2015, Tynes filed a $20 million lawsuit in the Thirteenth Judicial Circuit in Hillsborough County (located in Tampa, Florida) against the defendant Buccaneers claiming that unsanitary conditions at the facility lead to him contracting a MRSA infection (53). He alleged two Florida premises liability claims (Count I) and negligent misrepresentation (Count II). The two premises liability claims arise from the duties landowners owe to invitees (a) duty to use reasonable care to maintain the premises in a reasonably safe condition, and (b) duty to provide invitees notice of latent and concealed perils known to the premise owner or should have been known. In his negligent misrepresentation claim, Tynes alleged that the defendant "supplied him with false information regarding the precautions and procedures designed to prevent the spread of infection" (52, p. 1356) in order to convince him to undergo his treatment regimen at the Buc's facility. A negligent misrepresentation claim involves a common law duty to exercise reasonable care or competence in supplying information. There are four elements: "(1) there was a misrepresentation of material fact; (2) the representer either knew of the misrepresentation, made the misrepresentation without knowledge of its truth or falsity, or should have known the representation was false; (3) the representer intended to induce another to act on the misrepresentation; and (4) injury resulted to a party acting in justifiable reliance upon the misrepresentation" (52, p. 1356).

The defendant removed this case to federal court (U.S. District Court) arguing that Tynes' claims are intertwined with the NFL's collective bargaining agreement (CBA) because they dealt with medical treatment he received in rehabilitating his football-related injury. However, Tynes then moved to remand the case to the Hillsborough County court claiming that his claims have nothing to do with the CBA and that his complaint focused entirely on the defendants' mismanagement of its facility's conditions. The U.S. District Court (52) agreed with Tynes stating his claims do not arise from any provisions in the CBA. The CBA does not address duties owed to invitees and issues related to negligent misrepresentation claims. The court held that the "duty underlying negligent misrepresentation is a duty owed by any professional to any person acting in justifiable reliance on that professional…" (p. 1357).

The court added that the defendant's representations were untrue and misleading stating the following:

> Defendant failed to 'institute rigorous sanitation/cleanliness protocols' to prevent the spread of MRSA infection inside the Facility. For instance, Defendant failed to ensure that 'sterile techniques' were used, such that equipment, devices, and surfaces used by multiple people throughout the Facility were properly cleaned and disinfected. Moreover, Defendant failed to warn Tynes that several other people using the Facility at the same time—including a coach, a trainer, and several players—were suffering from bacterial infections. These people 'used the same hot and cold tubs, soak buckets, and other therapy devices, equipment, and surfaces' as Tynes, and Defendant 'failed to properly and reasonably … sterilize, disinfect and/or clean' them (p. 1354).

Although the U.S. District court remanded the case to the Hillsborough County court, Tynes reached a settlement with the Buccaneers (53) on February 10, 2017. The terms of the settlement were not disclosed. See Risk Management Strategy #4 for recommendations on keeping facilities well-maintained, clean, and disinfected.

In addition to skin infections, legal cases involving Legionnaires' disease have also occurred. Legionnaires' disease is a severe type of pneumonia. The bacteria thrive in warm water such as in hot tubs and spas. In one of the Legionnaires' disease cases (54), the plaintiff claimed she was sickened with the disease after using the facility's amenities. She claimed the facility failed to properly inspect the showers, water fountains, spas, pools, and water fixtures to determine if the bacteria, Legionella, was present.

Supervision of Fitness Facilities

Legal scholar, Betty van der Smissen stated that the "lack of or inadequate supervision is the most common allegation of negligence" (55, p. 163). Many of the injuries in the cases described in this chapter, as well as other chapters throughout this textbook, could have been prevented if there had been proper supervision of the facility. The failure to provide proper supervision can lead to terrible consequences as demonstrated in the *Miller* spotlight case earlier. As in *Miller*, the lack of proper supervision of a steam room resulted in another death. A woman was found dead inside the steam room at a 24 Hour Fitness Club in Littleton, Colorado (56). She had entered the club after 1:00 pm and was found dead at 7:45 am the next day. The manager of the facility told investigators that the closing employee did not make sure everyone had exited the club that evening. The coroner determined that she had been dead for at least 12 hours and died from renal failure due to dehydration. If proper staff supervision had been provided (e.g., on-going, routine supervision of the facility and carrying out proper closing procedures), it is unlikely that this death would have occurred.

Several professional organizations have published standards and guidelines regarding supervision of various programs and services. Many of these have been previously described (e.g., see Risk Management Strategy #1 in Chapter 8). Regarding general supervision of the facility, ACSM (3) has one guideline that recommends having a **manager on duty (MOD)** or supervisor on duty (SOD) who has the responsibility to oversee the facility's operations during all open hours and another guideline that recommends regular walk-throughs of the facility. Given that the lack of or improper supervision is a common allegation of negligence, it is recommended that fitness managers and exercise professionals consider implementing these guidelines (recommendations) as standards (or requirements) to minimize liability.

Proper supervision of facilities and/or activities such as trampoline parks, climbing walls, and obstacle courses (e.g., Ninja Warrior gyms) is also essential. Injuries from participation in these facilities/activities also appear to be quite prevalent as evident in just conducting a simple Internet search. These injuries have resulted in negligence claims/lawsuits. It is beyond the scope of this chapter to address these types of claims/lawsuits. However, as these types of facilities/activities continue to increase in popularity, it is likely that the number of injuries and litigations will also increase. Managers/owners who provide these types of facilities/activities, need to consider certain legal liability exposures, such as the increased risk of injuries, that exist due to the "risky" nature of these types of activities.

Consultation with a competent lawyer is needed to address these liability exposures. In addition, professional instruction (e.g., proper progression) and close supervision are essential to help minimize injury risks.

Unsupervised Fitness Facilities

Many fitness facilities are open 24/7 in which staff supervision is limited (i.e., only available during certain hours of operation). Other facilities such as those in hotels and apartment complexes do not provide any staff supervision. These types of facilities allow "key access" so individuals can enter the facility any time (24/7) or during limited hours (e.g., 6:00 am to 10:00 pm). Although unstaffed or limited-staffed facilities face many legal liability exposures, the most concerning is when there is a serious injury, such as a cardiac arrest, and there is no one available to provide the proper first aid or to call Emergency Medical Services (EMS). Additional risks include property damage or theft and the possibility of an assault (57).

Fitness managers/owners need to make an informed decision, in consultation with legal counsel, to weigh the benefits of having an unstaffed or limited-supervised facility (e.g., personnel cost savings) in light of the liability risks (e.g., participant injuries that may go unattended and subsequent litigation). Managers/owners should consider their moral duties to provide safe and effective programs and facilities. However, moral duties are not often considered and only a "business decision" is considered that maximizes profits and minimizes legal liability risks through the use of a waiver/release and having adequate insurance.

Regarding a waiver/release, these types of facilities should have individuals sign a specially-written document upon joining or using the facility that absolves the facility for its own negligence (including the failure to provide supervision) and informs them that the facility has limited (or no) staff supervision and that they use the facility at their own risk. For the type of specific language to include in these waivers/releases, see an article entitled "Unsupervised Facility May Require Specialized Waivers" (58). Waivers/releases can be effective in protecting these types of facilities, but as described in Chapter 4, they are not enforceable in all states. And, of course, they do nothing to prevent injuries and/or deaths—only the development and implementation of sound risk management strategies can help prevent injuries and deaths as described throughout this textbook. Adequate insurance needs to be obtained in consultation with competent insurance experts to help purchase the insurance coverage needed for situations that may occur in unsupervised facilities.

Regarding facilities that are unstaffed during certain times of operation or not staffed at all, the ACSM (3) recommends providing signage to inform users of the risks of using the facility when there is no supervision and steps they can take if they observe an emergency situation. However, the following risk management strategies should be considered, in consultation with legal and insurance experts:

1) For facilities that provide limited staff supervision, individuals should read and sign a specially-written waiver/release upon joining the facility that is properly administered by a well-trained staff member.

2) For facilities that provide no staff supervision, individuals should read and sign a specially-written waiver/release that, perhaps, can be completed electronically. It also may be a good idea to have the waiver/release prominently displayed at the facility's entrance.

3) For facilities that provide limited supervision, professional staff members need to first have participants complete pre-activity screening procedures and participate in the facility orientation prior to using the facility.

4) Post signage (e.g., warnings, exercise at your own risk—no supervision provided).

5) Provide video surveillance (e.g., closed-circuit television (CCTV) that monitors all areas in the facility, including entry and exit points but excludes locker/shower areas and restrooms). It should have the capacity to be monitored by a third party who has authority to alert emergency services (59).

6) Install panic buttons/emergency phones such as panic alarms that are fixed and mobile (on lanyards) and are easily accessible and prominently displayed. The panic alarm system to be monitored by the same third party with access to the CCTV footage (59).

7) Follow any applicable laws (e.g., those described above and throughout this textbook) and best practices (published standards/guidelines) such as daily inspections of the facility/equipment, maintenance, and cleaning/disinfecting of the facility.

8) Encourage individuals to not use the facility alone.

9) Avoid providing exercise equipment that poses a potential increased risk of injury without supervision such as treadmills and free weights.

10) Avoid providing facilities such as saunas/steam rooms and hot tubs/whirlpools or close them during unsupervised hours.

As described in Chapter 4, unstaffed fitness facilities will likely be held to the reasonable person standard of care. In other words, the courts will weigh two factors—the magnitude (severity and probability) of the risks and the burden of taking precautions. If the magnitude is high (e.g., high probability of a serious injury) and the defendant's burden to take precautions is low (e.g., implementing low-cost strategies such as those listed above), the defendant could be liable for a plaintiff's injury if the precautions were not implemented.

Unsupervised Outdoor Fitness Facilities

To provide access to various exercise equipment and activities, outdoor fitness parks are being built throughout the U.S. For example, the American Association of Retired Persons (AARP) and nonprofit FitLot™ have built such parks and plan to provide these parks in all 50 states as well as Washington D.C., Puerto Rico, and the U.S. Virgin Islands (60). The first of these AARP-branded parks, located in or near existing parks, opened in St. Petersburg, Florida on April 24, 2019. AARP plans to invest three years of programming to include 45-60 minutes of instructor-led demonstrations of the equipment that will engage people of all ages in the community. No information was provided by AARP on how they (or the city/county park departments) will address various legal liability exposures that exist with such outdoor fitness parks.

Fitness facilities, such as campus recreation facilities, are also providing outdoor fitness spaces and equipment. For example, the University of Oregon provides 6,000 square feet of open-air fitness space which is half asphalt and half natural turf (61). According to the assistant director for facilities, the area complements their CrossFit programming and includes equipment such as plyometric boxes, oversized tires, sleds, and parallel bars. The assistant director indicated that the equipment is designed for outdoor use. For example, it will hold up to elements such as rain and UV light. The turf area is used for exercise classes such as yoga and tai chi. The outside area is open any time the building is open for drop in use. However, even when the building is closed, someone could still use the space when there is no staff supervision. Heavy signage is the main way the university manages the risk of providing no staff supervision of the area. Although the assistant director and others would like to add more of these outdoor spaces, the university has not done so due to the risks of fitness equipment in uncontrolled spaces. This is often the major reason why other facilities have opted to not provide outdoor fitness areas.

Those planning such facilities need to consider a variety of factors such as the weather and the risk management strategies listed above for unsupervised facilities. In addition, equipment should be purchased from manufacturers that have implemented the specifications in ASTM F3101—ASTM Standard Specification for Unsupervised Public Use Outdoor Fitness Equipment (62). This ASTM specification includes parameters for the design and manufacture of outdoor fitness equipment and its installation with the intent to minimize the likelihood of serious injuries.

Technology and Data Privacy/Security

Over recent years, a variety of technology applications have been used in fitness facilities and programs. Many of these have advanced the profession and have changed common practices in the design and delivery of exercise programs and daily operations of a fitness facility. Technology applications will continue to be a "hot topic" in the years ahead. Previous chapters have included content regarding technology and data privacy such as the following:

- **Chapter 3**—Federal privacy laws (FTCA, HIPAA), state privacy laws, wearable technology,

wellness products/devices including mobile apps, authorization for release of protected health information (PHI)
- **Chapter 6**—Keeping pre-activity health-screening data, fitness testing data, and related forms (e.g., informed consents, medical clearance forms, medical releases) private, confidential, and secure
- **Chapter 7**—Keeping exercise prescription data private, confidential, and secure
- **Chapter 8**—Internet training using live platforms; Wearable technology to prevent heat and other injuries
- **Chapter 9**—Cloud-based platforms, General Data Protection Regulation (GDPR), and predictive asset management technologies regarding exercise equipment

In addition, many published articles and conference program presentations have provided a plethora of information regarding the many issues related to technology applications in the field. A nonprofit organization, Fitness Industry Technology Council (http://www.fittechcouncil.org) was formed in 2016 and provides a variety of educational programs/services and technology updates for its members. Keeping on top of ever changing technology is an on-going challenge for fitness managers and exercise professionals. However, it is essential, especially, from a legal liability perspective regarding data privacy/security as discussed next. But first, because of its popularity, a brief description of some of the safety/legal liability issues regarding live streaming/on-demand fitness programs is presented.

On-Demand Fitness Classes and Workouts

Various fitness facilities and organizations are offering on-demand fitness classes and workouts for their members and participants that are provided by various vendors. For example, HealthPartners, a company that offers health insurance and health care, announced in October 2019 that they were expanding their well-being program to include on-demand virtual fitness classes that will be provided by a vendor (Wellbeats) (63). Fitness managers, when contracting with vendors who provide these types of fitness classes and workouts, need to consider a variety of safety and legal liability issues such as:

a) Review the vendor providing the fitness classes/workouts carefully—see Chapter 5 for factors to consider (e.g., litigation history, compliance with laws including data privacy and security laws, liability/insurance issues).

b) Review the credentials and competency of the fitness instructors who teach the classes/workouts.

c) Review the fitness classes/workouts provided to determine if they are taught in a safe and effective manner.

d) Are the fitness classes/workouts available for beginner, intermediate, and advanced levels and are they categorized accordingly?

e) Does the provider (vendor) of the fitness classes/workouts include a statement specifying the "terms of agreement" to which the user agrees prior to accessing the fitness classes/workouts as well as a statement describing the vendor's privacy policy? For examples of a "terms" agreement and "privacy" policy, see the SaveTrainer website (https://savetrainer.com). SaveTrainer is a program that includes a variety of on-demand exercise videos offered by the Save Institute. Prior to accessing the videos, an individual must first "agree" to the terms by agreeing to a document that includes several sections such as a medical disclaimer, limitation of liability, and indemnification.

f) Consult with the facility's legal counsel to, perhaps, add a description of these types of classes/workouts in the facility's waiver/release of liability document and check the facility's liability insurance to be sure it covers these programs.

As with all contracts, these agreements with vendors who provide these types of fitness classes/workouts need to be reviewed by competent legal counsel. Fitness facilities that have their own employees design and deliver on-demand classes and workouts that facility members and participants (or perhaps others) can access should discuss legal liability issues related to these types of programs with their legal counsel. Some of these issues were described in Chapter 8—see Individualized Legal Consultation: A Must for Virtual and Other Non-Traditional Exercise Programs.

Individual Data Privacy: PII and BIPA

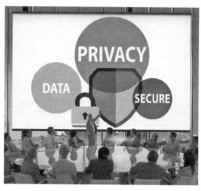

A helpful resource to stay abreast of the many data privacy issues associated with technology is IHRSA. This organization provides updated articles on this topic on a regular basis on their website (www.ihrsa.org). A couple of these articles are briefly described:

a) *Your Fitness Business Suffered a Data Breach. Now What?* September 2019 (64)

Author Jeff Perkins discusses how each state has a data breach law that defines **personally identifiable information (PII)** differently. However, generally these data include medical, biometric, and financial information as well as an individual's name, social security number or driver's license number. These state laws include a data breach notification requirement that also varies by state. Perkins states that a data breach can be very costly: "if your club has 2,000 members and half become victims of a data breach, it could cost your business up to $148,000" (p. 6).

b) *Tapping into the Biometric Revolution in a Shifting Landscape,* May 2019 (65)

In this article, author Jeff Perkins discusses biometrics including sensitive information such as fingerprint scans, body composition scans, VO2 max testing, and iris scans/facial recognition. He states that lawmakers are concerned about the erosion of privacy given the increasing interest in collection and use of **biometric data**. He mentions that some states already have laws regulating the collection and use of biometric data (e.g., Illinois has a **Biometric Information Privacy Act (BIPA)** and several other states are considering such proposals). In reviewing these laws, he described five principles (notice, consent, retention, security, and purpose) that will help fitness facilities comply with them.

Biometric Data—Recovery Facilities/Equipment. In addition to the biometric data obtained from scans described above, some fitness facilities are collecting other types of biometric data. For example, a health club in California has a Recovery Zone for its members with the goal to help its members recover from intense workouts (66). The amenities and equipment in the Recovery Zone feature products that produce a pulsed electromagnetic field and sound to target sore muscles as well as infrared light to stimulate mitochondria. Additional high-tech recovery facilities include infrared saunas, cryotherapy chambers, and compression equipment to enhance and improve blood flow. According to the manager of the Recovery Zone, the equipment is more effective than spending 16 or 18 weeks in physical therapy. In addition to biometric data privacy and security, other issues need to be considered before fitness facilities offer a recovery zone with these types of facilities and equipment. For example, what are the risks associated with the use of these facilities/equipment? Are special credentials and training required before exercise professionals have their participants use such equipment? Do these types of services cross over into the practice of physical therapy or other licensed professions?

Biometric Data—Student-Athletes. As described in Chapter 8, wearable technology is being used by athletic programs to help prevent heat and other injuries. In an op-ed in *Forbes* (67), Karen Weaver described a contract ($170 million deal) that University of Michigan signed with Jumpman, Nike's Michael Jordan branded apparel division. This contract allows Nike to harvest personal data from Michigan athletes through the use of wearable technology, such as biological or physical performance data, during practices and games. Numerous data privacy questions arise with these types of technologies. For example, has the athlete read and signed an informed consent that explains how these data will be used? Can the athlete choose to opt out? How will third-party contractors use the data? As an example, Weaver mentions Fusionetics and describes how they claim to have over 500 college and university teams using their program.

In addition to biometric data, colleges and universities are using technology, such as SpotterEdu, allowing coaches to track the locations of their student-athletes at all times. As a former coach and athletic administrator, Weaver states that "our students' personal data is not ours, especially their 'biometric' data about physical performance" (67, para. 11). She is concerned that athletic programs are trading off player's personal data to obtain lucrative contracts with third-party technology

providers. Athletic directors, coaches, and strength and conditioning coaches need to be cognizant of the legal implications that will likely arise with the use of this technology. They need to stay on top of state laws such as Biometric Information Privacy Acts, as described above, as well as review the Family Educational Rights and Privacy Act (FERPA), a federal law that protects the privacy of student records. In addition, if student data are being used for research purposes by the college/university and/or a third party, the research project first needs approval from the institution's Institutional Review Board as described in Chapter 6.

KEY POINT

Numerous technological applications that gather an individual's private information are widely used in fitness/athletic programs and facilities. It is essential that fitness and athletic managers have procedures in place that reflect compliance with various privacy and security laws that protect an individual's data. It is also important that they stay abreast of new privacy and security laws as technologies in this area continue to expand and grow. For example, some states already have Biometric Information Privacy Acts and several other states are considering such proposals.

Facility Security: Protecting Participant Safety

Several legal liability exposures exist regarding the security of the facility. Monitoring access to the facility is essential so that only authorized individuals can enter the facility. The ACSM (3) and MFA (5) have standards that require having an operational system in place to effectively monitor access to the facility. Historically, this has been accomplished through a membership card with a photo ID that can be shown to a staff member upon entrance. For unsupervised facilities, members are often provided key fobs that can be scanned to enter the front entrance to the facility. However, in recent years some facilities have used biometric technology such as a hand or fingerprint scan (68). This technology can be effective in terms of monitoring facility access as well as controlling personnel costs and hassles associated with individuals who forget their card. Issues such as the costs to set up and maintain the technology and data privacy should be considered. Facilities that use biometric data as a means to control access to the facility need to review data privacy laws and implement important strategies such as notice (e.g., informing individuals that their biometric data is being collected) and consent, such as obtaining consent from individuals to collect and use the data (65). Some fitness facilities are using other scanning methods to allow access such as smartphone apps as well as other digital platforms to free up front desk space and improve productivity (69).

The failure to monitor access to a fitness facility has been an issue in various negligence cases. For example, in *Lister v. Fitness International, LLC, d/b/a LA Fitness* (70), the plaintiff claimed that an employee who was working at the front desk allowed non-members to enter the club. One of these non-members was one of four men who attacked the plaintiff while playing basketball. In the defendant's motion for summary judgment, LA Fitness claimed that the exculpatory clause that the plaintiff signed protected against any liability. The plaintiff argued that the exculpatory clause was unenforceable because it cannot apply to reckless conduct stating:

> In this case, the defendant recklessly disregarded its own policies limiting guest access to its club, requiring photo identification to be produced by all guests, and prohibiting guests from playing on the basketball court…The club knew that a high volume of people entered the club but failed to provide adequate staffing at its front desk to obtain identification from all guests (p. 3).

Referring to the definition of recklessness from the Restatement (Second) of Torts and previous case law, the court noted that "recklessness, in contrast to negligence, requires conscious action rather than mere inadvertence" and is "an extreme departure from ordinary care, a wanton or heedless indifference to consequences" (p. 4). The court granted the defendant's motion for summary judgment because the plaintiff was

unable to present any evidence of reckless conduct on part of the defendant.

Note: *The outcome of this case might have been different, if the plaintiff could have proved that the defendant "knew" or had prior knowledge of non-members entering the facility who had harmed members in the past, and thus, creating a foreseeable risk or danger.*

Protecting the safety of fitness participants also involves protecting their physical privacy. In addition to cameras on smart phones, individuals can easily obtain mini cameras that can be used for spying and video-taping at a low cost. This can create a challenge for fitness facilities even those with stringent policies such as "no photos or video recordings are allowed anywhere in the facility without the permission of management". The following are examples of articles published in the *Athletic Business E-Newsletter* in 2019:

- Man Arrested for Taking Photos of Child at Gym—July 2019 (71)
- Camera in Soap Dispenser Recorded Women's Teams—October 2019 (72)
- Missouri Man Caught Filming Woman at Fitness Club—November 2019 (73)

In addition to federal and state privacy laws, fitness managers/owners need to be familiar with specific state laws regarding privacy in locker rooms such as the Wisconsin law described in Chapter 3. In consultation with legal counsel, it may wise to post a sign in locker rooms that informs participants of facility's photo/video-recording policy and relevant privacy laws. The consequences of violating policies and/or laws can be included in the signage. This may help deter any unlawful conduct and protect the privacy of participants.

In addition to physical fights like the one that occurred in the *Lister* case described above and invasion of privacy (e.g., illegal video-recording), other unlawful conduct can occur while fitness participants are in the facility. One common unlawful act is theft. Providing lockers for participants to safely store their property while using the facility is an effective strategy to help prevent theft. However, individuals can break into lockers and steal one's property such as described in the following articles published in the *Athletic Business E-Newsletter* in 2019:

♦ Thieves Strike at Campus Rec Fitness Center—October 2019 (74)

♦ Thieves Target Fitness Clubs in Chicago Suburbs—November 2019 (75)

♦ Duo Nabbed for Cross-County Fitness Club Thefts– December 2019 (76)

The best approach to help minimize any potential liability associated with personal property is to include language such as "not responsible for lost, stolen, or damaged personal property" in the facility's waiver/release of liability and post signage that states the same. Although waivers/releases are unenforceable for personal injury in some states, as described in Chapter 4, they are generally enforceable for personal property losses.

To prevent the facility's property being stolen/damaged or any other criminal acts, it is best to provide staff supervision during all operating hours and inform participants (e.g., in the membership contract, facility website, and signage) of the consequences (e.g., revoking of membership, contacting law enforcement) of such conduct. For example, one hospital fitness center listed 11 behaviors on its website that could lead to loss of membership privilege that included unlawful conduct such as destruction/theft of property, fighting on the premises, possession of illegal drugs (77). To help deter criminal conduct, it is also recommended to have video

KEY POINT

Protecting the safety of participants is a major responsibility of fitness managers/owners. Responsibilities include monitoring access to the facility and having policies and procedures that (a) reflect privacy laws that help protect the physical privacy of participants (e.g., no photos, videotaping) and, (b) minimize theft of personal property or other criminal acts. The failure to take such steps can lead to legal liability, especially after an incident has occurred. There is a common law rule that fitness facility managers/owners do not have a legal duty to prevent harm caused by the actions of third parties. However, if a manager/owner knew (or should have known) of harmful actions of third parties, such as criminal acts, and took no action to help prevent such foreseeable dangers, plaintiffs may be able to prevail in their negligence lawsuits.

surveillance, where feasible, and to have adequate lighting inside and outside the facility.

Inappropriate Behavior of Fitness Participants

In addition to unlawful conduct committed by facility participants, inappropriate behaviors can occur. When such behaviors happen, facility managers/owners need to have a response plan that is legally sound. Such a plan needs to be developed in consultation with legal counsel. Often, management's reaction when such conduct is first reported is to suspend or revoke the individual's membership and/or access to the facility. However, this type of initial reaction can lead to discrimination claims and other legal problems.

One of the first steps to develop a plan is to inform fitness participants of the facility's expected behaviors of all participants and, perhaps, describe the potential consequences of not following the specified behaviors. These behavior expectations, such as following the facility's safety and other policies, can be included in the membership contract, listed on the facility's website, and posted in the facility.

The next step is to have a plan to investigate the situation. Whether it is first reported by a staff member or a participant, a responsible, well-trained staff member (e.g., the manager on duty) must properly gather as specific information as possible and document what occurred. See Exhibit 10-4 for an example of an Incident Report that can be used to document all types of incidences. In addition to documenting inappropriate behaviors of participants or employees, an Incident Report can also document other situations that arise that need to be documented such as those listed in Exhibit 10-4. The documentation of the incident involving a participant's behavior can be shared with the facility's legal counsel if needed (e.g., before a decision to revoke a membership is made). In addition, documentation provides effective evidence to help refute and defend negligence and other claims such as discrimination.

Helen Durkin, IHRSA's executive vice president of public policy, describes such a discrimination case in her article entitled "6 Ways to Manage Difficult Situations at Your Health Club" (78). An African American member was conducting his own personal training business at the club. He was warned, repeatedly, to stop but he did not. The club terminated his membership for not following this club's policy. He alleged that the club discriminated against him because of his race. However, the club managers had documented all the warning incidents and the case was dismissed. As demonstrated in this case, a consequence of revoking a membership is a possible discrimination lawsuit. However, if the fitness facility has documentation to show repeated violations of the facility's policies and that all members are treated exactly the same, it will be difficult for the removed member to prove that the club's decision was discriminatory. Some fitness facilities have a three-strikes-and-you're-out policy. For example, after three documented incidents of not following the policies/expected behaviors, the membership is revoked. It is always best to review such policies with legal counsel before they are implemented.

KEY POINT

When faced with negligence claims/lawsuits, documentation (e.g., evidence to help demonstrate that duties were not breached) can provide a powerful defense for fitness facilities. The same is true when facilities are faced with claims for violating laws such as discrimination laws. Given the rise in discrimination cases as described in Chapters 2 and 3, such documentation is essential. For example, when revoking an individual's membership for not following the facility's policies, the individual may file a discrimination lawsuit against the facility. Having documentation of the individual's repeated inappropriate behavior, along with showing that all members were treated the same, can help refute such discrimination claims.

Event Organizer and Sponsor

Often, fitness facilities will organize and/or sponsor events such as marathons, triathlons, obstacle course racing (OCR), and walk/run races to support local non-profits such as the American Heart Association or Alzheimer's Association. Before fitness facilities consider organizing or sponsoring such events, fitness managers/owners need to become aware of various legal liability issues as well as follow safety guidelines published by organizations such as Road Runners Club of America (www.rrca.org), Running USA (www.runningusa.org) and Team USA (www.teamusa.org/USA-Triathlon).

Serious injuries and deaths have occurred in marathons and triathlons (79, 80). Many of these injuries/deaths (e.g., cardiac arrest, drowning) are due to the health/fitness status of individuals (e.g., coronary risk factors, inadequate training)—not to the negligence of organizers or sponsors. However, negligence lawsuits against event organizers and/or sponsors have occurred. For example, in *Angelo v. USA Triathlon* (81), Richard Angelo died while participating in the swim portion of a triathlon. His wife brought claims for wrongful death, conscious pain and suffering, punitive damages, and negligent infliction of emotional distress against USA Triathlon (sponsor of the event) and the United States of America, United States Coast Guard, and United States Coast Guard Auxiliary (collectively, U.S. Defendants).

The court granted USA Triathlon's motion for summary judgment based on the agreement Mr. Angelo signed prior to the event in which he "agreed to indemnify USA Triathlon for any losses arising from his participation in the triathlon, including losses associated with lawsuits arising from his participation, even if brought by his estate" (81, p. 1). The U.S. defendants argued that their motion for summary judgment should also be granted based on the release and indemnity provisions that applied to USA Triathlon. However, the court ruled that they did not have counterclaim for indemnification. The court stated that the plaintiff "has demonstrated that additional discovery is likely to uncover facts that may influence the outcome of the pending motion. Discovery would allow for a more detailed inquiry into the preparations leading up to the triathlon as well as the facts and circumstances of the attempted rescue" (p. 3). The court questioned the actions of Coast Guard personnel who spotted Mr. Angelo swimming outside the designated swim area and later found him face down in the water. They attempted to resuscitate him but were unsuccessful.

Serious injuries and deaths have also occurred in OCR events, such as paralysis and death from drowning as described in the following cases, *Sa* and *Sengupta*, respectively. Other injuries have included environmental illnesses (e.g., heat illness, hypothermia) and bacterial infections (e.g., norovirus, MRSA) from going through

---

Exhibit 10-4: Example: Incident Report*

Instructions: The Manager on Duty (MOD) has the responsibility of completing and submitting this form to management immediately following an incident. All parties involved in the incident need to be reminded to keep all aspects of the incident private, confidential, and secure.

Date of Incident: _____   MOD Completing this Form: _____

Check (√) the type of incident:

_____ Participant/Member behavior

_____ Participant/Member complaint

_____ Employee behavior

_____ Employee complaint

_____ Equipment issue, e.g. malfunctioning, broken, damaged, warning label missing

_____ Facility issue, e.g., security, flooring, electrical, HVAC, locker/shower area, cleaning

_____ Signage issue, e.g., missing, destroyed, unreadable

_____ Other, _____

Description of Incident (be specific):

_____

_____

_____

Incident Follow-Up (to be completed by management):

_____

_____

_____

Incident Report Filed and Securely Stored: _____ (Date)

*An incident is a situation that occurred during any hours of operation. If a personal injury occurred, an Injury Report must be completed. If an evacuation occurred, an Evacuation Report must be completed. This form is not a substitute for "daily" inspections of the equipment and facility—that is a separate form.

---

communal water and mud (82). For more on these types of infections, see an article titled "Infection from Outdoor Sporting Events—More Risk than We Think?" (83). Negligence lawsuits against the event organizers and sponsors have occurred as a result of these injuries. In *Sa v. Red Frog Events, LLC* (84), the plaintiff participated in a two-day Warrior Dash event in Michigan. He was injured as a result of diving head first into the mud pit leaving him paralyzed from the chest down. The plaintiff and others were encouraged to dive head first into the mud pit by an emcee. The plaintiff filed a three count claim against the defendant, Red Frog Events: Count I (negligence), Count II (gross negligence), and Count III (willful and wanton misconduct).

The court ruled that the waiver/release barred the plaintiff's negligence claim but not the other two claims. The court defined gross negligence as "conduct so reckless as to demonstrate a substantial lack of concern for whether injury results" (84 p. 778). Because the defendant was aware of the dangers presented by diving head first into a mud pit, the court stated that it was plausible that the act of encouraging participants to do so was gross negligence. The Michigan Supreme Court has distinguished gross negligence (high degree of carelessness or recklessness) and willful and wanton misconduct (in the same class as intentional wrongdoing). The court stated that a reasonable jury might conclude that the defendant's conduct could meet the willful and wanton misconduct standard.

In addition to potential legal liability of the event organizers (e.g., race directors), those who sponsor these events need to be aware of their potential legal liability. All types of sponsors need to realize that the plaintiff's attorney will try to name any party as a defendant that has a relationship with the event and/or have an impact on the event (85). Sponsors include:

- Minimal sponsors who give cash or goods such as financial sponsors
- Controlling sponsors who provide tactical support and/or assistance to help with the race
- Hosting sponsors who allow the event to be held on their property (85)

Sengupta v. Tough Mudder, LLC (86) is a good case to demonstrate the types of sponsors that can be named as defendants in negligence cases. Avishek Sengupta drowned while participating in the Tough Mudder walk-the-plank obstacle. In her complaint, the mother of Mr. Sengupta claimed the defendants failed to follow safety precautions and made false and misleading statements regarding the event's safety. The organizers of the event, Tough Mudder Mid-Atlantic and Peacemaker National Training Center, were named as defendants. Amphibious Medicus was also named as a defendant. Tough Mudder had retained Amphibious Medicus to provide personnel to help ensure the safety of participants while participating in the walk-the-plank obstacle such as water safety and emergency protocols. In addition, General Mills, Tough Mudder's corporate partner, was named as a defendant. The climbing wall for the walk-the-plank obstacle prominently displayed the General Mill's Wheaties® logo.

To help minimize legal liability associated with event sponsorship, sponsors should require a written contract that identifies its role and limits its liability such as a contract that includes an indemnity clause that transfers liability to the appropriate parties (85). In addition, sponsors should consider purchasing sponsorship insurance. Sponsors might assume they have no liability for merely sponsoring an event, but this may not be the case and need to take steps to minimize their potential liability.

Race organizers have numerous responsibilities and duties such as (a) warning participants of dangers and risks, (b) inspecting and ensuring a safe course and/or obstacle design, (c) providing an emergency action plan, and (d) providing well-trained staff and volunteer supervisors (85). They also need to realize the importance of having participants read and sign a well-written waiver/release and purchasing adequate insurance. The *Johnson v. Capitol Specialty Ins. Corp.* (87) case demonstrates the need to carefully review insurance policies for any exclusions they may include. The main issue is this case was to determine if a Capitol general commercial liability insurance policy, purchased by the event organizer, covered potential damages resulting from the death of an obstacle race participant or if exclusions in the policy barred recovery.

The race, known as the Extreme Rampage, was organized by Chris Johnson, the owner of Rampage, LLC. He paid for and signed the Capitol liability insurance policy. He received a copy of the policy that contained two exclusions:

a) A sponsor exclusion that stated, "With respect to any operations shown in the Schedule, this insurance does not apply to bodily injury to any person while practicing for or participating in any sports or athletic contest or exhibition that you sponsor" (87, p. 3).

b) A participant exclusion that stated, "This insurance does not apply to bodily injury, property damage, personal or advertising injury or medical expense arising out of any preparation for or participation in any of the activities or operations shown in the schedule above" (87, pp. 3-4).

After the death of the participant, Johnson submitted a claim but Capitol denied the claim "asserting it had no duty to defend or indemnify Johnson because the policy expressly excluded coverage for event participants" (87, p. 4). The trial court granted Capitol's motion for summary judgment ruling that the policy did not provide the coverage the organizer needed. Johnsen appealed. He claimed that he was never informed that participants would be excluded from coverage. However, the appellate court ruled that Johnson cannot plead ignorance regarding the content of the contract stating that "all persons are presumed to know the law and the mere lack of knowledge of the contents of a written contract for insurance cannot serve as a legal basis for avoiding its provisions" (87, pp. 9-10). Johnson also argued how the term "sponsor" in the sponsor exclusion was interpreted, given he was the race organizer, not a sponsor. However, the appellate court also upheld this trial court's ruling that the organizer was a sponsor as defined by the policy.

Regarding OCRs, race organizers and sponsors need to stay abreast of a new standard titled New Practice for Standard Practice for Obstacle Course Events (ASTM WK54714) being developed by the American Society for Testing Materials. This new standard will provide guidelines for design, construction, operation, inspection, safety, and maintenance of land-based pedestrian obstacle courses (88).

DEVELOPMENT OF RISK MANAGEMENT STRATEGIES

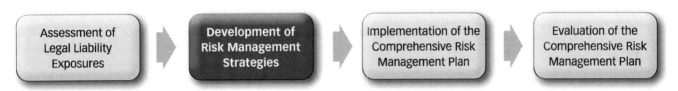

Given the many legal liability exposures involving facility risks, it is essential that fitness managers and exercise professionals develop effective risk management strategies to reduce these risks. By developing and implementing the following risk management strategies, injuries and subsequent negligent lawsuits, such as those described in this chapter, can be minimized. Once policies and procedures are developed that reflect these risk management strategies, they should be included in the facility's Risk Management Policies and Procedures Manual (RMPPM). As described throughout this textbook, staff members need to be well-trained on these policies/procedures to help ensure they are properly carried out.

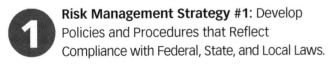

Risk Management Strategy #1: Develop Policies and Procedures that Reflect Compliance with Federal, State, and Local Laws.

To avoid substantial fines, it is essential that fitness managers/owners comply with federal, state, and local laws and regulations. Consulting with a knowledgeable lawyer is required to meet these obligations. It is unlikely that academic and certification programs adequately cover statutory and administrative laws applicable to fitness facilities and how to comply with them.

However, fitness managers/owners and other supervisory staff members can attend and complete online trainings, such as those offered by OSHA, to help obtain a certain level of knowledge and skills. In addition to OSHA online trainings described above, fitness managers can also contact their local OSHA office to inquire about having an OSHA-authorized outreach trainer provide employee training. OSHA standards covered in this textbook, such as signage specifications and noise exposure limits described in this chapter, and those described in Chapters 3 and 11, reflect only a few of the many OSHA standards that may be applicable to fitness facilities.

The ADA has been addressed in previous chapters. This chapter briefly described some of the standards in the 2010 ADA Standards for Accessible Design (i.e., signage and service dogs). Various resources are available to help fitness facilities develop polices/procedures to comply with these standards such as the ADA Checklist and Guide to ADA Signage (listed previously). Numerous resources from the National Center on Health, Physical Activity and Disability (NCHPAD) can also be helpful. For example, see their website (www.nchpad.org) to access videos such as "How to Choose a Fitness Facility" and resources such as Get the Facts (18-page booklet) and Discover Accessible

Fitness (52-page booklet). Although these NCHPAD resources are geared toward individuals with disabilities, they are also excellent resources for fitness facility managers and exercise professionals. The following are examples of additional resources available that may be helpful when developing policies/procedures and staff training programs that reflect ADA requirements as well as to help better serve individuals with disabilities:

a) Fact Sheet—Accessibility of Fitness Centers and Healthcare Facilities for People With Limb Loss (89), published by the Amputee Coalition

b) Removing Barriers to Health Clubs and Fitness Facilities (90), published by North Carolina Office on Disability and Health

Facility managers and exercise professionals need to comply with the FTCA as well as any similar consumer protection state and local laws regarding (a) unfair and/or deceptive acts or practices, (b) consumer data privacy and security, and (c) advertising and social media posts. Several states have statutes that regulate health club membership contracts as described earlier.

Once the policies and procedures are developed reflecting these laws, it will be important to provide staff training to help ensure that employees follow them. For example, if the facility has a policy that the noise exposure levels should be no higher than 90 decibels in group exercise classes, those teaching classes need to be informed of this policy and why it is important to follow such as: (a) OSHA standards help prevent injuries and subsequent litigation (*Levine v. GBG, Inc.* as a case example), and (b) reduction in complaints from participants about music being too loud. OSHA resources, as well as those published by IDEA (17) and IHRSA (18), can be used to help develop the content of the training program.

 Risk Management Strategy #2: Conduct Daily Inspections of the Facility to Meet the Legal Duties Owed to Invitees (1).

To meet the legal duties owed to invitees (individuals using the facility and equipment), fitness managers/owners have two basic responsibilities: (a) regularly inspect the facilities property and equipment to determine if there is any condition(s) that might be considered dangerous, and (b) if a condition could be considered "dangerous" by an invitee, it is necessary to correct the condition (e.g.,

repair or remove the dangerous condition) or warn the invitee of the possible danger (e.g., post proper warning signage that invitees will see and understand). The facility's property includes the indoor premises as well as outdoor premises such as sidewalks and parking lots if owned and/or leased by the fitness facility.

As demonstrated in the above cases involving injuries from falls, courts will analyze whether or not defendants met their legal duty owed to invitees. In most of these cases, the waiver/release protected the defendants, but not in all of the cases such as *Crossing-Lyons* and *Roer*. If the waiver/release is unenforceable for whatever reason, the facility's Commercial General Liability (CGL) policy should cover injuries due to falls and other injuries that might occur on the premises. Another important issue addressed in these cases was having documentation to show that the facility fulfilled its legal duty owed to invitees such as written records of inspections and posting of warnings. For example, if the manager in the *Lik* case had produced evidence (e.g., written records of inspections kept), the court might have granted the defendant's motion for summary judgment. Another risk management strategy is to have an Incident Report (see Exhibit 10-4) completed when fitness participants or employees report a possible danger. Quickly addressing the potential danger may help prevent future injuries and litigation.

Fitness managers/owners need to develop a written inspection checklist that can be completed by a well-trained staff member on a daily basis. This checklist can serve as documentation that the inspections occurred. The items on the checklist can include the exercise equipment, facilities such as locker/shower areas and saunas/hot tubs, flooring, signage, etc. as well as outdoor premises, if applicable. If dangers are identified, appropriate steps need to be immediately taken (remove/repair or warn) and described and dated on the inspection checklist. If dangers are identified at any other time by fitness floor/facility supervisors or others, the same steps need to be taken.

Risk Management Strategy #3: Develop and Implement an Educational Facility Orientation Program.

As stated by the court in spotlight case, *Thomas v. Sport City*, "members of health clubs are owed a duty of reasonable care to protect them from injury while on the premises… [This duty] necessarily includes a general responsibility to ensure that their members know how to properly use gym equipment" (p. 1157). In addition to instructions regarding proper use of exercise equipment, the facility orientation should include several other topics for safety and legal liability reasons as described previously.

Various methods on how to deliver the Facility Orientation can be considered such as personal orientations (e.g., an individual or small group) or electronic orientations (e.g., the facility's website or other electronic media such as smartphone applications). The personal option is best for obvious reasons. It also provides an excellent way to establish positive relationships with new participants. No matter which option, the six topics described earlier should be included.

First, it will be important that the front desk staff members are well-informed about the Facility Orientation (i.e., its purpose and importance and well-trained on how to promote it to new participants). Next, to help ensure that the staff members who lead the Facility Orientation provide quality education, it will be necessary to:

⭑ Develop a written lesson plan for them to follow that covers the six topics (e.g., a checklist with each topic listed and an outline of what to describe with each topic).

⭑ Provide staff training including having the staff members conduct a mock Facility Orientation where their teaching performance can be evaluated and documented.

At the end of each Facility Orientation, the staff member who provided the orientation should complete the following documents and keep them stored in a secure place. These documents can serve as future evidence to help refute negligence claims/lawsuits.

⭑ Lesson plan (checklist of topics)—Completed, signed, and dated by instructor

⭑ List of participants—Names of those who attended

⭑ Acknowledgement—Document signed by participants affirming their attendance and agreement to follow the instructions provided in the orientation

Refusal to Participate in the Facility Orientation

Some participants may not want to attend a Facility Orientation. For these individuals, it would be wise to

have them read and sign a Refusal Form such as the one in Exhibit 10-5. This form will verify their refusal and may be helpful in defending any future claims/lawsuits.

Note: *As with all such forms that contain exculpatory language, it must be reviewed by competent legal counsel before it is implemented. Once signed, this document needs to be stored in a secure place.*

 Risk Management Strategy #4: Develop and Implement Policies and Procedures Regarding Proper Maintenance and Cleaning of the Facility (1).

Providing proper maintenance of the facility includes numerous responsibilities of fitness managers/owners. They have a legal duty to provide reasonably safe facilities which means taking precautions to prevent foreseeable injuries. For example, if a danger or hazard is uncovered during daily inspections, actions must be taken to fulfill legal duties owed to invitees. Appropriate actions need to be taken any time a situation arises which could lead to an injury or harm. For example, if an Incident Report (see Exhibit 10-4) indicates a flooring problem that needs repair such as the floor defect in the *Lik* case, it needs to be repaired in a timely fashion. If it will take time to complete the repair, warning signage is needed. All types of problems can arise in fitness facilities (e.g., electrical, HVAC, lighting, etc.) that need to be addressed in a timely fashion for safety and legal liability reasons.

Keeping the facility clean and disinfected is also essential. The importance of keeping exercise equipment clean and disinfected was presented in Chapter 9. As described in Chapter 9, disease-causing bacteria can be found virtually everywhere. Because of this, it is difficult for individuals to prove that their skin infections were due to the facility's failure to keep it clean/disinfected as demonstrated in the *Manerchia* and *Pecora* cases described. However, NFL football player, Lawrence Tynes, was able to prove that his bacterial infection (MRSA) was caused by the failure of the facility's management at One Buccaneers Place to keep it clean/disinfected. The court stated "defendant failed to 'institute rigorous sanitation/cleanliness protocols' to

Exhibit 10-5: Refusal to Participate in the Fitness Facility Orientation*

To help ensure safe participation in fitness activities, several major professional fitness organizations have published standards and/or guidelines that require or recommend that fitness facilities provide all new members and participants an orientation to the facility that includes proper use of the exercise equipment. Therefore, to comply with these national standards and guidelines, _____ (name of fitness facility) ("Facility") has established a policy that requires all new members and participants to participate in the Facility's Orientation. However, though not recommended, participants may refuse to participate in this process by reading and signing the following:

I _____ (name of participant) understand that Facility requires all participants to complete a Facility Orientation that includes instruction/information regarding: (a) proper use of the exercise equipment and facility, (b) awareness of safety policies and procedures, (c) principles of safe/effective exercise such as warm-up, progression, and monitoring of sign/symptoms of overexertion, and (d) programs/services offered by the Facility to meet individual needs and interests

However, I have chosen not to participate in the Facility Orientation.

Risks associated with refusal to participate in the Facility Orientation

I understand and appreciate that there exists the possibility of adverse effects occurring during exercise testing and exercise. The purpose of my participation in a facility orientation is to familiarize myself with the facility and its equipment, in the proper use of the facility and that equipment, in the proper methods of my participation in the activities carried on within the facility and in the policies and procedures for use of the facility and the equipment, amenities and activities carried out in the facility. If I do not participate in the orientation, I acknowledge and agree that I may not fully understand and appreciate how equipment and amenities in the facility are to be operated and used and in accordance with applicable policies and procedures and that the risks of harm to me and others may be increased. I have been informed that the risks of activity, though remote, include abnormal blood pressure, fainting, disorders of heart rhythm, stroke, and very rare instances of heart attack or even death. In addition, I understand that I may experience musculoskeletal conditions or injuries such as fractured bones, muscle strains, muscle sprains, muscular fatigue, contusions, muscle soreness, joint injuries, torn muscles, heat-related illnesses, and back injuries. I understand that other risks not listed here, both minor and major, can also occur. By my refusal to participate in the Facility Orientation, the chances of the occurrence of one or more of these or other risks may be increased. Moreover, I recognize that I may hurt myself or others by not fully understanding how to use the equipment or amenities in the facility or as to how to use the facility itself or in my participation in activities in the facility due to my failure to participate in the orientation or to identify the policies and procedures applicable thereto.

Benefits of participating in the Facility Orientation

I understand that the benefits of participating in the Facility Orientation are to enhance my safety and to possibly minimize some of the risks stated above. I assert that my refusal to participate in the Facility Orientation is voluntary and that I knowingly assume all such risks.

Waiver/Release

My signature below indicates that I have been fully informed of, understand, and appreciate the benefits of participating in the Facility Orientation as well as the potential risks of not participating in the Facility Orientation. In addition, my signature also indicates that I have executed a release and waiver document with the Facility which, among other things, contractually binds me and my estate not to bring any type of legal claim and/or lawsuit against the Facility and/or its staff members for among other things, the failure of the Facility and/or its staff to conduct a Facility Orientation. I also understand that this release/waiver gives up and relinquishes my right to institute a claim or lawsuit against the Facility and/or its staff members for a number of other acts and/or omissions, including those which could be classified as ordinary negligence. I hereby reaffirm my understanding and agreement to that release and waiver documents and to this statement.

Exhibit 10-5 continued...

This Agreement shall be interpreted according to the laws of the State of _____. If any part of this agreement should ever be determined by a court of final jurisdiction to be invalid, the remaining portions shall be deemed to be valid and enforceable.

_____   _____
Signature of Participant   Date

_____   _____
Signature of Staff Member   Date

prevent the spread of MRSA infection inside the Facility…" (52, p. 1354).

For facilities such as saunas/steam rooms and hot tubs/whirlpools, it will be important to follow the cleaning procedures specified in the owner's manual. There may be state regulatory requirements that require proper cleaning (and record-keeping to demonstrate proper cleaning) of such facilities as addressed by the plaintiffs in *Manerchia* and *Pecora*. Other areas within the facility such as locker/shower areas also need to be properly cleaned, perhaps several times throughout the day such as after peak usage times. See an article by Paul Steinbach (91) that addresses maintenance and cleaning of locker areas. As described in Risk Management Strategy #6 in Chapter 9, fitness facility managers/owners should follow the CDCs recommendations for cleaning and disinfecting the facility (92). The CDC also provides recommendations regarding laundry procedures (93). In addition, the Environmental Protection Agency (EPA) provides a list of approved disinfectants effective against MRSA and viruses such as COVID-19:

- MRSA: https://www.epa.gov/pesticide-registration/list-h-epas-registered-products-effective-against-methicillin-resistant
- COVID-19: https://www.epa.gov/pesticide-registration/list-n-disinfectants-use-against-sars-cov-2#filter_coll

Response After A Pandemic

Unlike most bacterial infections, viral infections can lead to pandemics because they can spread quickly through human contact. The pandemic in 2009 (H1N1) did not lead to the government's mandate to close fitness facilities. However, in March of 2020, fitness facilities were required to close due to the COVID-19 pandemic. Many facilities began to re-open in May and June of 2020 depending on continuing guidance from state and local governments. All types of safety and legal issues became apparent in the re-opening phase. To enhance safety and minimize legal liability in the re-opening phase, fitness managers/owners can:

- Follow guidance provided by the federal, state, and local governments
- Refer to government websites such as the CDC, Health and Human Services (HHS), EPA, OSHA, and the Equal Employment Opportunity Commission (EEOC) for information to help ensure compliance with laws/regulations and guidance provided
- Develop policies and procedures that reflect government guidance and laws/regulations
- Train staff members and inform participants of the policies and procedures
- Check HVAC systems to help ensure they are meeting the standards/guidelines of the American Society of Heating, Refrigeration, and Air-Conditioning Engineers (ASHRAE—www.ashrae.org/technical-resources/standards-and-guidelines)
- Consult with legal counsel to address injuries/illnesses related to the virus (e.g., covered in the facility's waiver/release and liability insurance policies)
- Keep evidence (documentation) such as laws/regulations followed, implementation of staff

training programs, and information provided to participants regarding policies/procedures

⑤ Risk Management Strategy #5: Develop and Implement Policies and Procedures that Address Data Privacy/Security and Physical Safety/Security.

Many technological applications are used in the fitness field that gather an individual's personal data. This chapter and other chapters have described some of these technologies as well as federal and state laws regarding the protection of an individual's personal data. It is evident that these types of technologies will continue to be developed and new privacy and security laws will be enacted to help protect an individual's personal data such as Biometric Information Privacy Acts. Some risk management strategies to help increase compliance with these Acts were described earlier in this chapter such as notice and consent (65).

Compliance with state breach notification laws is important. Given the prevalence of data breaches and the costly penalties that employers can face for such violations, fitness managers/owners should consider having a data security analyst on their staff or hired as a consultant who has the expertise to help ensure that the facility is keeping individual data (fitness participants and employees) private and secure. They also need to consult with a lawyer, such as a cybersecurity and privacy lawyer, to stay on top of new data privacy and security laws. It may be wise to purchase cyber security insurance—briefly discussed under Risk Management Strategy #9.

The importance of protecting the physical safety and security of participants was described such as (a) allowing only authorized individuals to access the facility, (b) having participants fully informed of the facility's safety policies and behavior expectations and consequences for not following the policies/behavior expectations, and (c) reporting an incident that may lead to an increased risk of injury and correcting the incident in a timely fashion.

Note: *When completing an Incident Report (see Exhibit 10-4) that involves inappropriate behavior of a fitness participant or employee, it is essential that the procedures to complete the report follow the facility's investigation plan (approved by legal counsel) to help provide a legally defensible case if future litigation occurs such as a discrimination lawsuit.*

Risk management strategies include having safety policies/behavior expectations in the membership contract and posting them in the facility (see Exhibit 10-1). Special signage in areas such as locker/shower rooms regarding photos and video-recording policies should also be considered. For laws, such as the Wisconsin law regarding locker room privacy (described in Chapter 3), it might be wise to post a sign that summarizes the law and the consequences for violations. Having proper lighting throughout the facility (and exterior areas) and video surveillance can help protect the physical security of participants and employees.

⑥ Risk Management Strategy #6: Provide Proper Staff Supervision of the Facility.

Many injuries and subsequent litigation can be prevented by providing proper supervision of the facility by well-trained staff members of the facility. This includes having a designated manager on duty (MOD) who has the responsibility to oversee the facility's operations during all open hours. The MOD should be a professional staff member with credentials such as a degree in the field and professional certification. In addition to having a job description for MODs, they need to be well-trained on their many responsibilities and well-informed of how to properly carryout the fitness facility's policies and procedures including opening/closing procedures and completing Incident Reports (see Exhibit 10-4) and Injury Reports (see Chapter 11).

It is best for fitness facilities to have at least one "fitness floor supervisor" at all times in the main area where the exercise equipment is located. For large facilities, more than one fitness floor supervisor may be needed. In addition, there needs to be a facility supervisor(s) that roams all areas of the facility, such as locker/shower areas, saunas/steam rooms, hot tubs/whirlpools, gymnasiums, and racquetball courts. These fitness floor and facility supervisors should have, at a minimum, the credentials equivalent to those recommended by ACSM (3) for personal fitness trainers and group exercise leaders (e.g., two years of college education in fitness/exercise science, accredited certification, and AED/CPR certification). A job description for floor and facility supervisors is needed. They need to be well-trained regarding their many responsibilities such as:

- Provide general, specific, and transitional supervision as described in Chapter 8
- Enforce safety and other polices of the facility (e.g., replacing equipment to its proper storage racks, addressing inappropriate participant behaviors)
- Serve as first responder in case of a medical emergency/follow the facility's emergency action plan
- Develop professional relationships with participants
- Exhibit professional communication with participants at all times

Lesson plans for the educational trainings of fitness floor and facility supervisors should be developed and the training sessions need to be properly documented.

Regarding unsupervised facilities or partially-supervised facilities, see the 10 risk management strategies listed and described earlier under Unsupervised Fitness Facilities. It will be essential to share these strategies with legal counsel and insurance providers before they are implemented. Fitness facilities that offer activities outside, such as outdoor fitness facilities and classes, need to develop/implement some of these same strategies when these outdoor programs/services are provided with no supervision.

Risk Management Strategy #7: Post and Maintain Signage Throughout the Facility (1).

Having proper signage throughout the facility is an essential risk management strategy. Signage can help defend against negligent claims such as the failure to warn of risks, failure to provide instruction, and failure to inform of the facility's safety policies. As described in Chapter 9, proper warning labels or signage and instructional placards are needed for all exercise equipment as well as the ASTM Facility Sign (see Figure 9-6 in Chapter 9). In this chapter, signage

required by the OSHA and ADA and signage as shown in Exhibits 10-1 and 10-2 were described. Other types of signage were also listed and described (see Topic #4: Facility Safety Signage under Fitness Facility Orientation). In order for signage to be effective, it needs to be clearly visible and readable. It is best to have a checklist of all facility signs that can be completed during daily inspections to help ensure signage has not been removed or damaged. Signage may need to be provided in languages other than English, given the facility's clientele.

Risk Management Strategy #8: Comply with Published Standards of Practice.

As described throughout this text, it is important for fitness facility managers/owners to comply with standards of practice published by independent and professional organizations. The ASTM standard regarding outdoor fitness equipment and their pending standard on obstacle course events were described. Regarding professional organizations, the following standards of practice were briefly summarized previously: (a) design/construction—ACSM, NSCA, MFA, and AACVPR, (b) facility orientation—ACSM and MFA (c) signage—ACSM, MFA and IHRSA, (d) maintenance and cleaning—ACSM and YMCA, (e) facility access—ACSM and MFA, and (f) supervision—ACSM. Many more standards and guidelines exist regarding facility risks such as:

- IHRSA (44) has several standards regarding membership contracts
- YMCA (46) has many recommendations that address issues such as children in locker rooms, MRSA, and noise levels
- MFA (5) provides, in its appendices, many sample forms that reflect usage policies and guidelines for various areas within the facility and monthly safety inspection forms
- ACSM (3) provides many supplemental materials and forms related to facility risks.

As recommended in Chapter 4 (see Special Notice Regarding Published Standards of Practice), fitness managers and exercise professionals need to obtain these publications to review the standards and guidelines in their entirety.

Risk Management Strategy #9: Obtain Adequate Insurance to Protect the Facility and Facility Activities.

The importance of having both general liability insurance (i.e., a commercial general liability policy) and professional liability insurance was described in Chapter 5. Fitness manager/owners need to consider other types of insurance in consultation with legal and insurance experts. Given the many insurance companies that provide various insurance policies for fitness facilities, it is essential to investigate the reputation of the company before purchasing any policy. The following, although not an exhaustive list, briefly describes additional types of insurance to consider:

a) Property insurance—covers the building and contents damaged from natural disasters (e.g., floods, tornadoes), theft, and vandalism
b) Loss of business income—replaces lost revenue when the facility is closed due to major repair or reconstruction.
c) Employment practices insurance—covers the facility from lawsuits brought by employees such as discrimination, sexual harassment, and wrongful termination
d) Cyber security insurance—covers cyber-related incidents such as data breaches
e) Event cancellation insurance—for facilities organizing/sponsoring events, it covers loss of business income due to weather, venue unavailability, etc.
f) Workers' compensation insurance—covers injuries to employees while on the job; mandated by state law (state laws vary). See Chapter 1 for more on workers compensation, a form of strict liability.
g) Umbrella insurance—adds additional coverage to the limits stated in existing policies

Fitness managers/owners also need to investigate the need of a new insurance policy or an endorsement (addendum to a current policy) anytime they are considering adding new facilities/equipment and/or programs (e.g., climbing walls, Ninja Warrior obstacle courses) or planning to organize or sponsor an event, such as a community walk/run, to help ensure they have adequate liability insurance coverage. In addition, a careful review of all insurance policies is needed to be fully aware of the terms and exact coverages and any exclusions in the policy as demonstrated in the *Johnson* case. It is important to check if the policy covers the cost of the legal defense. Business owners and those who organize/sponsor events may need to consider additional endorsements to protect against mass violence and disruptions such as acts of terrorism and active shooter (94). Pandemic insurance may also need to be considered.

Risk Management Strategy #10: Properly Document and Securely Store Written Records Regarding Facility Operations (1).

Having documentation (evidence) to help demonstrate that legal duties were properly carried out can be a very effective defense for defendants when faced with negligence claims/lawsuits. Having documentation that federal laws/regulations and any state laws were properly followed can prevent hefty fines for violations of such laws. In this chapter, these included OSHA and ADA standards, the FTCA and state statutes such as consumer protection laws (e.g., membership contracts, deceptive practices), data privacy and security, and regulatory requirements for the maintenance/cleaning of facilities such as hot tubs and steam rooms. The following are examples of records related to facility risks that need to be properly completed and then kept in a private and secure location:

a) Compliance with federal and state laws
b) Compliance with published standards of practice
c) Daily inspections of the facility
d) Incident reports and follow-up, e.g., see Exhibit 10-4
e) Maintenance and cleaning schedules and reports
f) Opening and closing procedures
g) Records of warning signage and facility/equipment repairs
h) Facility orientations, e.g., attendance, lesson plan checklist, and related refusal forms
i) Lesson plans and dates of staff trainings, e.g., MODs, floor supervisors, and facility supervisors
j) Records of re-opening procedures as a result of pandemic or similar event

RISK MANAGEMENT AUDIT Managing Facility Risks		
RISK MANAGEMENT (RM) STRATEGY*	**YES ✔**	**NO ✔**
1. Develop Policies and Procedures that Reflect Compliance with Federal, State, and Local Laws.		
2. Conduct Daily Inspections of the Facility to Meet the Legal Duties Owed to Invitees.		
3. Develop and Implement an Educational Facility Orientation Program.		
4. Develop and Implement Policies and Procedures Regarding Proper Maintenance and Cleaning of the Facility.		
5. Develop and Implement Policies and Procedures that Address Data Privacy/Security and Physical Safety/Security.		
6. Provide Proper Staff Supervision of the Facility.		
7. Post and Maintain Signage Throughout the Facility.		
8. Comply with Published Standards of Practice.		
9. Obtain Adequate Insurance to Protect the Facility and Facility Activities.		
10. Properly Document and Securely Store Written Records Regarding Facility Operations.		

*See the section above—Development of Risk Management Strategies—for the recommendations associated with each risk management strategy and then, for each RM Strategy marked NO, create a list of action steps that need to be completed to meet the recommendations described in that RM strategy.

KEY TERMS

- Biometric Data
- Biometric Information Privacy Act (BIPA)
- Emotional Support Animals
- Invitee
- Licensee
- Manager on Duty (MOD)

- Membership Contracts
- Open and Obvious Doctrine
- Personally Identifiable Information (PII)
- Premise Liability
- Service Animals
- Trespasser

STUDY QUESTIONS

The Study Questions for Chapter 10 can be found on the Fitness Law Academy website (www.fitnesslawacademy.com) under Textbook. They are provided in a fillable format for convenience.

REFERENCES

1. Eickhoff-Shemek JM, Herbert DL, Connaughton, DP. *Risk Management for Health/Fitness Professionals: Legal Issues and Strategies.* Baltimore, MD: Lippincott Williams & Wilkins, 2009.

2. Facility Planning and Design for Health, Physical Activity, Recreation, and Sport. Sawyer TH, (ed.). 14th Ed. Urbana, IL: Sagamore Publishing LLC, 2019.

3. ACSM's Health/Fitness Facility Standards and Guidelines. *Sanders ME. (ed). 5th Ed. Champaign, IL: Human Kinetics, 2019.*

4. NSCA Strength and Conditioning Professional Standards and Guidelines. *Strength and Conditioning Journal,* 39(6), 1-24, 2017. Available at: https://www.nsca.com/education/articles/nsca-strength-and-conditioning-professional-standards-and-guidelines/. Accessed November 5, 2018.

5. *Medical Fitness Association's Standards & Guidelines for Medical Fitness Center Facilities,* Roy B. (ed.). 2nd Ed. Monterey, CA: Healthy Learning, 2013.

6. American Association for Cardiovascular and Pulmonary Rehabilitation (AACVPR). Guidelines for Cardiac Rehabilitation and Secondary Prevention Programs. Williams MA, Roitman JL (eds). 5th Ed. Champaign, IL: Human Kinetics, 2013.

7. OSHA-Authorized Outreach Training Online. OSHA Education Center. Available at: https://www.oshaeducationcenter.com/. Accessed December 12, 2019.

8. All About OSHA. Available at: https://www.osha.gov/pls/publications/publication.html. Accessed December 20, 2019.

9. Specifications for Accident Prevention Signs and Tags. Standard 1910.145. Occupational Health and Safety Administration. Available at: https://www.osha.gov/laws-regs/regulations/standardnumber/1910/1910.145. Accessed December 12, 2019.

10. Acquiring 'Free' OSHA Publications and Posters. Available at: https://www.osha.gov/Publications/workplace_poster_page.html. Accessed December 20, 2019.

11. Occupational Noise Exposure. Standard 1910.95. Occupational Health and Safety Administration. Available at: https://www.osha.gov/laws-regs/regulations/standardnumber/1910/1910.95. Accessed December 12, 2019.

12. Noise and Hearing Loss Prevention. Guidance and Regulations. The National Institute for Occupational Safety and Health. Available at: https://www.cdc.gov/niosh/topics/noise/reducenoiseexposure/regsguidance.html. Accessed December 12, 2019.

13. Packer L. Dangerous Decibels and Exercise Classes. March 30, 2015. Articles by Lisa Packer. Muck Rack. Available at: https://muckrack.com/lisa-packer/articles. Accessed December 12, 2019.

14. *Levine v. GBG, Inc.,* No. GJH-16-2455, 2016 WL 7388392 (S.D. Md., 2016).

15. Beach EF, Nie V. Noise Levels in Fitness Classes Are Still Too High: Evidence form 1997-1998 and 2009-2011. *Archives of Environmental & Occupational Health,* 69(4), 223-230, 2014.

16. O'Connor A. As Workouts Intensify, a Harmful Side Effect Grows More Common. *New York Times.* July 17, 2017. Available at: https://www.nytimes.com/2017/07/17/well/move/as-workouts-intensify-a-harmful-side-effect-grows-more-common.html. Accessed December 12, 2019.

17. IDEA Opinion Statement: Recommendations for Music Volume in Fitness Settings. IDEA Health & Fitness Association. September 1,

2001. Available at: https://www.ideafit.com/group-fitness/idea-opinion-statement-recommendations-music-volume-fitness-settings/. Accessed December 12, 2019.

18. Schmaltz J. Bad Vibrations: Why You Need to Protect Your Gym from Excessive Noise. December 6, 2017. Available at: https://www.ihrsa.org/improve-your-club/bad-vibrations-why-you-need-to-protect-your-gym-from-excessive-noise. Accessed December 12, 2019.

19. 2010 ADA Standards for Accessible Design. Available at: https://www.ada.gov/regs2010/2010ADAStandards/2010ADAstandards.htm. Accessed December 13, 2019.

20. How to Choose a Fitness Center. National Center on Health, Physical Activity and Disability. Available at: https://www.nchpad.org/1672/6768/How~to~Choose~a~Fitness~Center. Accessed December 13, 2019.

21. Godlewski L. Inside the First Universal Design-Certified Facility. *Athletic Business E-Newsletter.* May 2016. Available at: https://www.athleticbusiness.com/rec-center/behind-the-scenes-of-the-first-universal-design-certified-facility.html. Accessed December 13, 2019.

22. Scott J. First Fitness Facility Certified Under WELL Building Standard. *Athletic Business E-Newsletter.* September 2019. Available at: https://www.athleticbusiness.com/rec-center/first-fitness-facility-certified-under-well-building-standard.html. Accessed January 17, 2020.

23. ADA Requirements. Service Animals. Available at: https://www.ada.gov/service_animals_2010.htm. Accessed December 13, 2019.

24. Service Animals and Emotional Support Animals. ADA National Network. Available at: https://adata.org/guide/service-animals-and-emotional-support-animals. Accessed December 15, 2019.

25. Gluck E. Technology Can Grow Your Fitness Business—But Know the Risks. February 19, 2019. Available at: https://www.ihrsa.org/improve-your-club/industry-news/technology-can-grow-your-fitness-business-but-know-the-risks. Accessed January 6, 2020.

26. Health Club Contracts—Generally. 36A Mass. Prac., Consumer Law § 30:34 (3d.ed.), September 2019.

27. Health Club Contracts—Cancellation Rights. 36A Mass. Prac., Consumer Law § 30:36 (3d.ed.), September 2019.

28. Buckman DF. Construction and Applicability of State Statutes Governing Health Club Membership Contracts or Fees. *American Law Reports.* 48 A.L.R.6th 223. Westlaw, Thomson Reuters, 2009.

29. *Powell v. YouFit Health Clubs, LLC,* No. 17-cv-62328-BLOOM/Valle, 2019 WL 926131 (S.D. Fla., 2019).

30. *Lopez v. Blink Fitness Linden,* No. 17-6399 (JMV)(MF), 2018 WL 6191944 (D. N.J., 2018).

31. Deceptive Trade Practices by Health Clubs; Seller's Misrepresentation. 21 N.Y. Jur.2d Consumer and Borrower Protection § 419, November 2019.

32. Dominic A. Town Sports International Sued by Washington, DC, Attorney General. *Club Industry News.* January 10, 2019. Available at: https://www.clubindustry.com/news/town-sports-international-sued-washington-dc-attorney-general. Accessed December 20, 2019.

33. Scott J. Are Gyms Violating Ban on Cashless Businesses? *Athletic Business E-Newsletter.* November 2019. Available at: https://

References continued...

www.athleticbusiness.com/fitness-training/are-gyms-violating-ban-on-cashless-businesses.html. Accessed January 7, 2020.

34. *Duncan v. World Wide Health Studios*, 232 S.2d 835 (La. Ct. App., 1970).

35. What is Premises Liability? Available at: https://www.nolo.com/legal-encyclopedia/what-premises-liability.html. Accessed May 26, 2020.

36. *Roer v. 150 W. End Ave. Owners Corp.*, No. 112198/06, 2010 LEXIS 6214 (N.Y. Misc. 2010).

37. *Grijalva v. Bally Total Fitness,* No. 01-14-00217-CV, 2015 LEXIS 3277 (Tex. App., 2015).

38. *Toro v. Fitness International,* 150 A.3d 968 (Pa. Super. Ct., 2016).

39. *Anderson v. Fitness International*, 208 Cal. Rptr. 3d 792 (Cal. Ct. App., 2016).

40. *Lik v. LA Fitness, Inc.*, 41 N.Y.S.3d 452, 2016 LEXIS 1761 (N.Y. Misc., 2016).

41. *Anast v. LTF Club,* No. 16 C 8763, 2017 LEXIS 191751 (D. Ill., 2017).

42. *Hoffner v. Lanctoe,* 492 Mich. 450 (Mich., 2012).

43. *Gibson v. YMCA*, No. M2015-01466-COA-R9-CV, 2016 LEXIS 337(Tenn. Ct. App., 2016).

44. IHRSA Club Membership Standards. In: *IHRSA's Guide to Club Membership & Conduct.* 3rd Ed. Boston, MA: International Health, Racquet & Sportsclub Association, 2005. Available at: http://download.ihrsa.org/pubs/club_membership_conduct.pdf. Accessed November 5, 2018.

45. Abbott A. Cardiac Arrest Litigations. *ACSM's Health & Fitness Journal*, 17(1), 31-34, 2013.

46. Safeguarding Health and Well-Being, Medical Advisory Committee Recommendations: A Resource Guide for YMCAs. Chicago, IL: YMCA of the USA, February 2011. Available at: http://safe-wise.com/downloads/MAC_2010a_Collection.pdf. Accessed November 5, 2018.

47. Abbott AA. A Hot Topic. *ACSM's Health & Fitness Journal*, 19(1), 35-38, 2015.

48. *Manerchia v. Kirkwood Fitness & Racquetball Clubs*, 992 A.2d 1237, 2010 LEXIS 136 (Del., 2010).

49. *Pecora v. Fitness Intl., LLC*, NY Slip Op 32259(U), 2019 LEXIS 4196 (N.Y. Misc., 2019).

50. What If I Have Developed a Skin Infection Due to Unsanitary Gym Conditions? LegalMatch. Available at: https://www.legalmatch.com/law-library/article/gym-liability-for-skin-infection-injuries.html. Accessed September 19, 2019.

51. Braun T, Kahonov L. Community-associated Methicillin-Resistant Staphylococcus aureus Infection Rates and Management among Student-Athletes. *Medicine & Science in Sports & Exercise,* 50(9), 1802-1809, 2018.

52. *Tynes v. Buccaneers Limited Partnership*, 134 F.Supp.3d 1351 (M.D. Fla., 2015).

53. Buccaneers, Former Kicker Lawrence Tynes Reach Settlement in MRSA Lawsuit. ESPN.com new services. February 22, 2017. Available at: https://www.espn.com/nfl/story/_/id/18738780/buccaneers-former-kicker-lawrence-tynes-reach-settlement-mrsa-lawsuit. Accessed December 26, 2019.

54. Lawsuit Filed Against Orlando LA Fitness. Legionnaires' Disease News. Siegel Brill PA Attorneys at Law. April 18, 2018. Available at: https://www.legionnairesdiseasenews.com/2018/04/lawsuit-filed-orlando-la-fitness/. Accessed January 17, 2020.

55. van der Smissen B. *Legal Liability and Risk Management for Public and Private Entities*, Volume Two. Cincinnati, OH: Anderson Publishing Company, 1990.

56. Kufahl P. Woman's Undiscovered Death in Steam Room Shows How Routines Should Never Become Routine. *Club Industry News.* July 14, 2015. Available at: https://www.clubindustry.com/blog/womans-undiscovered-death-steam-room-shows-how-routines-should-never-become-routine. Accessed December 31, 2019.

57. 24 Hour Fitness Centers, Culture of Safety. Available at: https://cultureofsafety.thesilverlining.com/safety-tips/24-hour-fitness-centers. Accessed January 3, 2020.

58. Herbert DL. Unsupervised Facility May Require Specialized Waivers. Sport Waiver. January 25, 2010. Available at: https://www.sport-waiver.com/unsupervised-facility-may-require-specialized-waivers. Accessed January 3, 2020.

59. Recommendations for Unsupervised Fitness Facilities. Fitness Australia. August 15, 2018. Available at: https://fitness.org.au/articles/policies-guidelines/recommendations-for-unsupervised-fitness-facilities/4/1365/20. Accessed January 3, 2020.

60. AARP Donating Outdoor Fitness Parks for All Ages. By Media Relations, May 13, 2019. Available at: https://blog.aarp.org/aarp-media-relations/aarp-donating-fitness-parks-for-all-ages. Accessed January 3, 2020.

61. Cameron C. Designated Spaces Bring Fitness Programming Outdoors. *Athletic Business E-Newsletter.* August 2018. Available at: https://www.athleticbusiness.com/rec-center/designated-spaces-bring-fitness-programming-outdoors.html. Accessed January 3, 2020.

62. ASTM International. ASTM F3101-15. Standard Specification for Unsupervised Public Use Outdoor Fitness Equipment. West Conshohocken, PA: ASTM International, 2015.

63. HealthPartners Expands Well-Being Program to Include On-Demand Digital Fitness, Gym Membership Discounts. October 30, 2019. Available at: https://www.healthpartners.com/hp/about/press-releases/healthpartners-expands-well-being-program.html. Accessed January 7, 2020.

64. Perkins J. Your Fitness Business Suffered a Data Breach. Now What? September 19, 2019. Available at: https://www.ihrsa.org/improve-your-club/your-fitness-business-suffered-a-data-breach-now-what/. Accessed January 7, 2020.

65. Perkins J. Tapping into the Biometric Revolution in a Shifting Landscape. May 14, 2019. Available at: https://www.ihrsa.org/improve-your-club/tapping-into-the-biometric-revolution-in-a-shifting-landscape/. Accessed January 7, 2020.

66. Scott J. Incorporating Recovery Equipment, Services in Your Health Club. *Athletic Business E-Newsletter.* January 2020. Available at: https://www.athleticbusiness.com/fitness-training/incorporating-recovery-equipment-services-in-your-health-club.html. Accessed July 23, 2020.

67. Weaver K. Names, Images, Likenesses…And Data: Another Issue for NCAA Athletes to Take Seriously. *Forbes.* January 1, 2020. Available at: https://www.forbes.com/sites/karenweaver/2020/01/01/names-images-likenessesand-data/#6df2dccc21cc. Accessed January 8, 2020.

68. Biometrics Gaining Steam in College Rec Centers. *Athletic Business E-Newsletter.* April 2015. Available at: https://www.athleticbusiness.com/rec-center/biometrics-gaining-steam-in-college-rec.html. Accessed January 8, 2020.

References continued...

69. Springs S. Emerging Rec Center Technology: What Should Be On Your Radar? *Athletic Business E-Newsletter.* July 2019. Available at: https://www.athleticbusiness.com/rec-center/emerging-rec-center-technology-what-should-be-on-your-radar.html. Accessed January 8, 2020.

70. *Lister v. Fitness International, LLC, d/b/a LA Fitness,* No. 13-3013, 2014 WL 1327590 (E.D. Pa., 2014).

71. Berg A. Man Arrested for Taking Photos of Child at Gym. *Athletic Business E-Newsletter.* July 2019. Available at: https://www.athleticbusiness.com/civil-actions/man-arrested-for-taking-photos-of-child-at-gym.html. Accessed January 9, 2020.

72. Steinbach P. Camera in Soap Dispenser Recorded Women's Teams. *Athletic Business E-Newsletter.* October 2019. Available at: https://www.athleticbusiness.com/facility-security/camera-in-locker-room-soap-dispenser-recorded-women.html. Accessed January 9, 2020.

73. Berg A. Missouri Man Caught Filming Woman at Fitness Club. *Athletic Business E-Newsletter.* October 2019. Available at: https://www.athleticbusiness.com/civil-actions/missouri-man-caught-filming-woman-at-fitness-club.html. Accessed January 9, 2020.

74. Berg A. Thieves Strike at Campus Rec Fitness Center. *Athletic Business E-Newsletter.* October 2019. Available at: https://www.athleticbusiness.com/locker-room/thieves-strike-at-campus-fitness-center.html. Accessed January 9, 2020.

75. Berg A. Thieves Target Fitness Clubs in Chicago Suburbs. *Athletic Business E-Newsletter.* November 2019. Available at: https://www.athleticbusiness.com/fitness-training/thieves-target-fitness-clubs-in-chicago-suburbs.html. Accessed January 9, 2020.

76. Berg A. Duo Nabbed for Cross-Country Fitness Club Thefts. *Athletic Business E-Newsletter.* December 2019. Available at: https://www.athleticbusiness.com/facility-security/duo-charged-with-fitness-club-thefts-across-the-country.html. Accessed January 9, 2020.

77. Membership Benefits at the Fitness Center at UH Avon Health Center. Available at: https://www.uhhospitals.org/locations/uh-avon-health-center/fitness-center/features-and-benefits. Accessed January 9, 2020.

78. Durkin H. 6 Ways to Manage Difficult Situations at Your Health Club. May 2, 2018. Available at: https://www.ihrsa.org/improve-your-club/6-ways-to-manage-difficult-members-at-your-health-club/. Accessed January 9, 2020.

79. Sankoff J. Athlete Deaths in Triathlon and How to Prevent Them. TrainingPeaks Coach Blog. August 27, 2019. Available at: https://www.trainingpeaks.com/coach-blog/athlete-deaths-in-triathlon-and-how-to-prevent-them/. Accessed January 14, 2020.

80. Dayer MJ, Grenn I. Mortality During Marathons: A Narrative Review of the Literature. *BMJ Open Sport & Exercise Medicine,* 2019. Available at: https://bmjopensem.bmj.com/content/bmjosem/5/1/e000555.full.pdf. Accesses January 14, 2020.

81. *Angelo v. USA Triathlon,* Nos. 13-cv-12177-ADB, 14-cv-14260, 2016 WL 126248 (D. Mass., 2016).

82. Young S, Keiper M, Fried G, et al. A Muddied Industry: Growth, Injuries & Legal Issues Associated with Mud Runs (Part I). *ACSM's Health & Fitness Journal,* 18(3), 31-34, 2014.

83. DeNizio JE, Hewitt DA. Infection from Outdoor Sporting Events—More Risk than We Think? *Sports Medicine—Open,* August 14, 2019. Available at: https://www.ncbi.nlm.nih.gov/pmc/articles/PMC6694362/. Accessed January 14, 2020.

84. *Sa v. Red Frog Events, LLC.,* 979 F. Supp. 2d 767 (E.D. Mich., 2013).

85. Seidler T, Fried G, Young S, et al. A Muddied Industry: Essential Risk Management Strategies for Mud Run Participants, Race Organizers, and Sponsors (Part II). *ACSM's Health & Fitness Journal,* 18(5), 42-45, 2014.

86. *Sengupta v. Tough Mudder, LLC,* Analyzed In: Herbert DL. Tough Mudder Sued in West Virginia Wrongful Death Case. *The Exercise, Sports and Sports Medicine Standards & Malpractice Reporter,* 3(6), 81, 83-90. 2014.

87. *Johnson v. Capitol Specialty Ins. Corp.* Nos. 2017-CA-000171-MR, 2017-CA-000172-MR, 2018 WL 3090603 (Ky. Ct. App., 2018).

88. ASTM WK54714. New Practice for Standard Practice for Obstacle Course Events. Available at: https://www.astm.org/DATABASE.CART/WORKITEMS/WK54714.htm. Accessed January 14, 2020.

89. Fact Sheet. Accessibility of Fitness Centers and Healthcare Facilities for People With Limb Loss. May 2015. Amputee Coalition. Available at: https://www.amputee-coalition.org/resources/accessibility-of-fitness-centers-and-healthcare-facilities-for-people-with-limb-differences/. Accessed January 20, 2020.

90. Removing Barriers to Health Clubs and Fitness Facilities: A Guide for Accommodating All Members, Including People with Disabilities and Older Adults. 2008. North Carolina Office on Disability and Health. Available at: https://fpg.unc.edu/sites/fpg.unc.edu/files/resources/other-resources/NCODH_RemovingBarriersToHealthClubs.pdf. Accessed January 15, 2020.

91. Steinbach P. Keeping Locker Room Areas Dry, Inviting and Safe. *Athletic Business.* January/February 2020, pp. 44-46, 48.

92. Methicillin-resistant Staphylococcus aureus (MRSA). Athletic Facilities Cleaning and Disinfecting. Centers for Disease Control and Prevention, January 24, 2019. Available at: https://www.cdc.gov/mrsa/community/environment/athletic-facilities.html. Accessed September 19, 2019.

93. Laundry. Effective Laundry Procedures. Centers for Disease Control and Prevention. January 28, 2019. Available at: https://www.cdc.gov/mrsa/community/environment/laundry.html. Accessed January 17, 2020.

94. Saddler JM. Weighing the Need for Sports/Event Insurance for Terrorism, Active Shooter and Civil Unrest. *Sport Law Facilities,* 3(1), 5-7, 2018.

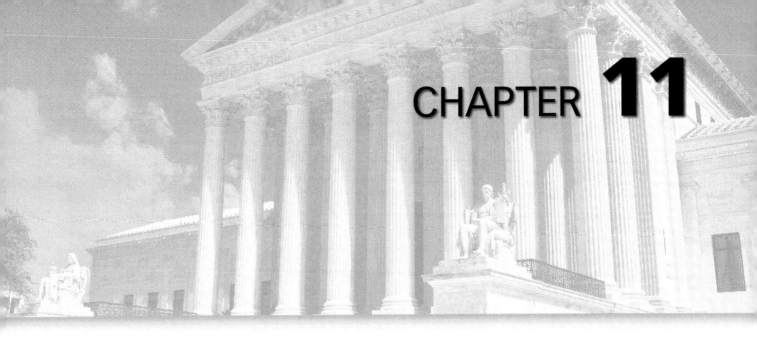

Emergency Planning and Response

 LEARNING OBJECTIVES

After reading this chapter, fitness managers and exercise professionals will be able to:

1. Realize the importance of taking a proactive approach to emergency planning and response.

2. Appreciate the importance of complying with federal laws applicable to emergency planning and response, such as the OSHA General Industry and Bloodborne Pathogen standards.

3. Recognize and adhere to state law applicable to emergency planning and response, such as first-aid and automated external defibrillator (AED) laws.

4. Describe court rulings and analysis in AED-related negligence cases that originated in fitness facilities.

5. Adhere to various published standards of practice applicable

to emergency action planning and response (1).

6. Appreciate the benefits of communicating with local emergency professionals and the facility's risk management advisory committee to mitigate emergency-related risks in fitness facilities.

7. Develop and implement a written, comprehensive Emergency Action Plan (EAP) for (a) medical emergencies and (b) evacuation emergencies.

8. List and describe the material components of an effective EAP, such as staff member credentials, internal and external communication systems, and proper maintenance of first-aid kits and AEDs (1).

9. Describe the roles and responsibilities of the facility manager/owner, EAP coordinator, manager on duty, and other staff members in the development and implementation of the facility's EAP.

10. From a legal liability perspective, understand the importance of providing EAP staff training which includes regular drills and rehearsals (1).

11. Describe the legal significance of developing and implementing proper post-emergency procedures, including the preparation and retention of Injury Reports (1).

12. Implement 10 risk management strategies to minimize legal liability exposures related to emergency planning and response.

INTRODUCTION

This chapter discusses the most common emergencies that occur in fitness facilities and explains how fitness facility managers/owners can prepare. Fitness managers and exercise professionals should begin by assessing legal requirements; forming at least a general understanding of applicable federal and state laws, administrative regulations, and court rulings. Next, exercise professionals can look to standards of practice published by professional organizations for guidance in structuring effective policies and procedures. After reviewing applicable laws and professional standards, it is time to put knowledge into action. This chapter will discuss how to develop and implement effective **Emergency Action Plans** (EAPs) that reflect laws, regulations, and standards of practice. Toward the end of the chapter, 10 risk management strategies are described that can minimize legal liability exposures related to emergency planning and response.

Chapter 11 addresses two categories of emergencies: (a) medical emergencies, resulting from **sudden cardiac arrest** (SCA) and other major physical injuries, and (b) emergencies requiring evacuation, including natural disasters, inclement weather, fires, and active shooters or bomb threats. To minimize liability, having a contingency plan for each type of emergency is essential. Staff training programs and practice drills can be used to improve execution of a facility contingency plan and employee response. Recalling loss prevention and loss reduction described in Chapter 2; strategies used to prevent injuries reflect loss *prevention* strategies (such as providing protective equipment to employees) while strategies focusing on emergency response reflect loss *reduction* strategies.

In an emergency situation, potential harm increases when bystanders do not know how to respond. Without a plan, crucial decisions must be made under tremendous pressure. Legal liability can arise when mistakes are made. Fitness facility managers/owners have an opportunity to mitigate legal risk by anticipating potential emergencies and preparing how to respond. As described throughout this textbook, legal threats are mounting for fitness facilities for a variety of reasons. This chapter focuses on reducing injuries, saving lives, and mitigating liability through preparing comprehensive EAPs. For both legal and moral reasons, this should be a top priority of fitness managers and exercise professionals.

ASSESSMENT OF LEGAL LIABILITY EXPOSURES

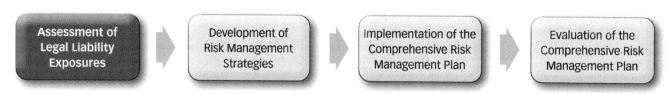

Legal liability can be categorized into (a) penalties handed down by federal, state and/or regulatory bodies, and (b) damages awarded through civil litigation. To identify areas of exposure, it is necessary to first understand the laws and regulations applicable to the industry. This section details primary legal sources written by government legislatures, administrative organizations, and judicial directives. Federal regulations are addressed first, followed by state laws and the courts' interpretations of those statutes. As secondary guidance, professional organizations like the NSCA and ACSM publish standards, guidelines and policy statements often used in civil disputes to demonstrate satisfaction of, or failure to meet, the applicable standard of care.

Federal Laws

As described in Chapter 1, administrative organizations are created by legislatures at all levels of government to regulate specific activities and/or industries (1). As detailed in Chapter 3, the Occupational Safety and Health Administration (OSHA) is responsible for ensuring employers provide reasonably safe and healthful workplaces for U.S. employees (2). OSHA standards set minimum safety and health requirements; they do not prohibit employers nor states from adopting more stringent requirements. Accordingly, employers must be particularly diligent in understanding and complying with unique, and often stricter state requirements. Beyond ethical obligations to protect employees from harm, there are serious financial risks for failing to comply with OSHA regulations including significant fines, termination of business operations, and possible jail time for blatant, repeated offenses.

This section describes OSHA's General Industry Standards, which regulate facility design, therapeutic services, proper ventilation, hazardous chemicals, and medical treatment. This section will also discuss **OSHA's Bloodborne Pathogens (BBP) Standard**. OSHA classifies fitness facilities under Industry Group 799, defining the class as "establishments primarily engaged in operating reducing and other health clubs, spas, and similar facilities featuring exercise and other active physical fitness conditioning, whether or not on a membership basis" (3, p.1). Additional OSHA requirements are described in this textbook as follows:

- **Chapter 3**: General Duty Clause and Hazard Communication Standard
- **Chapter 10**: Specifications for Accident Prevention Signs/Tags and Occupational Noise Exposure Standard

OSHA has broad enforcement powers. The agency may conduct random inspections and investigate any type of accident involving an employee. Employees are encouraged to report unsafe working conditions or violations of the BBP Standard and enjoy protection from retaliation for doing so under Sec. 11(c) of the OSH Act (4). According to OSHA Office of Management Systems, the most expensive violations of the BBP Standard cost employers an average of nearly $5,000 (5). Common violations include incomplete exposure control plans and failing to make testing results available to exposed employees (5). In 2014, fines totaling nearly $200,000 were upheld against an employer for failing to conduct proper training and provide Hepatitis B vaccinations to workers who handled potentially contaminated laundry (6).

OSHA's General Industry Regulations

The following information is offered to summarize federal regulations most directly affecting fitness facilities and should be supplemented by further research if necessary. OSHA General Industry regulations can be found online (7). To help ensure compliance, facility managers/owners should consider OSHA-authorized training courses which are available in multiple levels of comprehensiveness (8).

Facility Design for Exit Routes

Fitness facility owners have a legal and ethical duty to provide a reasonably safe environment for employees and participants. This includes facilitating unburdened entry and departure. OSHA requires adequate routes of egress based on the size of the building, occupancy, and arrangement. Exits must meet size requirements, should be designed to reduce exposure to high-risk areas, and must allow for unimpeded departure. Fire-retardant properties of paints and solutions used in and around exits must be periodically re-applied. As discussed in Chapter 10, clear evacuation signage should be utilized to direct occupants to a safe area. In addition, an outdoor space serving as a safe environment during an emergency must be large enough to hold all occupants.

Failure to ensure appropriate routes of egress can result in criminal penalties or substantial civil damages. After an investigation in 2009, OSHA proposed fines of nearly $250,000 against a Home Goods located in New York (9). The store was accused of blocking exit routes with stock and equipment. In comments regarding the Home Goods investigation, Former Assistant Secretary of Labor for OSHA, Dr. David Michaels, stated, "there can be no delay in exiting a workplace during a fire or other emergency when the difference between escape and injury or death can be measured in seconds…employers must ensure exit routes are unobstructed at all locations" (9, p. 2). The National Fire Protection Association (NFPA) estimates more than 13,000 fires occur in mercantile properties each year, accounting for 12 deaths, 300 injuries and over $600 million in property damage (10).

Causes of emergency evacuation can include fire, substantial weather hazards or threats of violence. Fitness managers, particularly in facilities with lots of equipment, should evaluate their facilities to ensure exit routes remain accessible. If facilities offer kitchens to members or staff, owners should collaborate with local fire departments to implement policies for preventing and responding to cooking fires. For additional information regarding facility design requirements, refer to Life Safety Code NFPA 101, compiled by the NFPA (11).

Specialty Therapies—Cryotherapy and Sauna

The safeguards necessary to maintain a reasonably safe environment for employees can depend on the services offered by each facility. Potential health benefits from exposure to extreme temperatures has popularized cryotherapy and more extreme methods of sauna (12). If a fitness facility offers potentially dangerous therapeutic services which require personal protective equipment, facility employees must be properly trained in safe maintenance and use (13). In these facilities, maintaining a reasonably safe environment might include instructing employees how to recognize medical warning signs, providing appropriate protective equipment or implementing procedures to prevent prolonged exposure.

In 2014, a New Jersey spa was cited by OSHA for exposing employees to excessive heat (14). At this bulhavjeungmok sauna, in which temperatures could reach 700° F, lapses were found regarding procedures to limit employee exposure, protective equipment provided to workers, and in communications warning workers of hazards. The company was forced to settle with OSHA after facing penalties amounting to an estimated $25,000. In 2015, a 24-year-old spa manager in Nevada died just minutes after entering a cryotherapy chamber at the center where she worked (15). Had the woman been using the chamber during business hours, Nevada OSHA would have had jurisdiction to analyze the training policies and safety measures utilized by the wellness center. These events demonstrate how important it is to document safety policies and train employees whose work includes using or maintaining potentially dangerous services.

Hazardous Chemicals

Facility owners and management must protect workers from exposure to hazardous chemicals by providing necessary equipment and adequately warning employees of the risks. Similar to specialty therapies discussed above, the potential for chemical exposure depends on services provided by a fitness facility. Facilities with pools or steam rooms may use cleaning products which contain toxic chemicals, triggering a need to comply with applicable OSHA regulations.

OSHA's broad definition of "hazardous chemical" encompasses any toxic chemical, irritant or sensitizer. Employers must implement a written program providing for worker training, warning labels, and access to Safety Data Sheets (SDSs). SDSs are a standard way to convey information about the proper handling of chemicals. Information may include instructions for the safe use, potential hazards associated with a particular material, and procedures for handling spills. Regulations for using common, household consumer products in commercial facilities are less stringent. Failing to communicate hazards to employees is the second-most common citation issued by OSHA. More information on SDSs is available at: https://www.osha.gov/Publications/OSHA3514.html.

On the final day of 2012, OSHA levied fines totaling more than $60,000 against a fitness facility which repeatedly failed to provide eye, face and hand protection for workers using liquid and other hazardous chemicals (16). The Illinois gym was further cited for failing to develop a hazardous communication program and neglecting SDSs for on-site chemicals. Employers have a responsibility to know the hazards that exist in their workplace and to provide employees with appropriate protective equipment.

Proper Ventilation

Facility managers/owners should prioritize the air quality of their facilities in order to provide a healthier environment for members and gain a marketing advantage over competitors. Air quality is particularly important in facilities promoting high intensity training. Hard breathing brings air deep into the lungs, exacerbating harm caused by pollutants. A 2012 evaluation of Portuguese fitness facilities exposed widespread air quality deficiencies in the industry (17). In a majority of locations, researchers recorded unacceptable concentrations of carbon dioxide, volatile organic compounds, and formaldehyde. Examiners expressed the greatest concern for concentrations of dust and formaldehyde, substances which can lead to respiratory concerns including asthma.

Heavy breathing, especially in smaller workout rooms such as aerobic studios or indoor cycle rooms, can result in disproportionate levels of carbon dioxide as related to oxygen. Inadequate oxygen can produce a suffocating effect, causing health concerns escalating from increased fatigue, headaches and sweating to cardiac arrest or stroke. OSHA has established a Permissible Exposure Limit for CO_2 of 5,000 parts per million (0.5% CO_2 in air) averaged over an 8-hour work day (18). Ensuring appropriate airflow is key for maintaining appropriate CO_2 balance, as outdoor air typically ranges from 300 to 400 ppm (0.03% to 0.04%). OSHA recommends taking the following measures to ensure appropriate air ventilation and quality for workers: install local exhaust ventilation systems to remove contaminants; facilitate natural ventilation; properly place air inlets and exhausts; use filtration or electric cleaners; control humidity in the range of 20%-60%; and control temperature between 68-76° F (19).

Although not typically the cause of acute medical emergencies, airborne bacteria and viruses can cause infections and allergic reactions leading to more severe medical concerns. These contaminants are especially prevalent in humid environments which cater to mold and mildew. The International Building Code requires moist air to be vented outside the building to prevent recirculation (20). Accordingly, fitness facilities must ensure proper ventilation and sanitation of locker rooms, steam rooms, saunas, and pool/wet areas. Additional information pertaining specifically to indoor air quality is provided by OSHA (21).

Medical Treatment Plans/Supplies

To encourage businesses to prepare for workplace injuries, federal regulations require first-aid kits to be properly stocked and conveniently located. Given the high potential for physical injuries in fitness facilities, a comprehensive first-aid kit and emergency response equipment must be accessible and operational at all times. The extent of preparation required depends primarily on the likelihood of injury within a business. Employers are tasked with conducting internal evaluations of their environment, considering the risks of the work and the likelihood and severity of injury.

OSHA's General Industry Standards require employers to ensure medical treatment is in near proximity or that a person at the workplace is adequately trained to render first aid (22). Qualified providers of first-aid training include the American Heart Association (AHA) American Red Cross (ARC), National Safety Council (NSC), and private institutions. OSHA has interpreted "near proximity" as 3-4 minute response time in cases of serious injuries, such as cardiac arrest or uncontrolled breathing. Employers must prepare accordingly, depending on the types of injuries reasonably expected to occur within their business. Relevant considerations include location of workplace, availability of/access to emergency medical personnel, travel distance to medical care and availability of transportation.

Fitness facilities must maintain a "Class A" first-aid kit, but due to the likelihood of injury in such an active environment, managers/owners should consider including more comprehensive first-aid equipment. Each first-aid kit should include small and large sterile gauze pads, adhesive bandages, gauze roller bandages, triangular bandages, wound cleaner, scissors, a blanket, adhesive tape, latex gloves, resuscitation equipment, elastic wraps, a splint, and clear directions for obtaining emergency assistance. The number of first-aid kits maintained on site will depend on the size of the club and number of occupants.

OSHA regulations require businesses to record all workplace injuries when an employee receives medical treatment beyond first aid (23). A business is exempt from these recording requirements if it employs 10 or fewer employees or is involved in a low-hazard industry. Owners should contact their local OSHA compliance office for additional information regarding specific requirements and to request a compliance assessment. Facility owners should review OSHA's Best Practices publication when developing a first-aid program (24). See Table 11-1 for a summary of the General Industry Standards applicable to fitness facilities.

Table 11-1	Summary of Selected OSHA General Industry Standards*
Facility Design for Exit Routes	◗ Maintain unimpeded routes of access and egress ◗ Provide clear signage alerting occupants of exit routes ◗ Post informational graphics depicting emergency procedures
Specialty Therapies— Cryotherapy and Sauna	◗ Assess services offered for potential threats ◗ Train employees for safe use and maintenance ◗ Document training policies and sessions
Proper Ventilation	◗ Evaluate facility for areas of poor ventilation/high risk ◗ Install/Maintain a quality HVAC system ◗ Facilitate natural airflow ◗ Control temperature and humidity
Hazardous Chemicals	◗ Evaluate hazardous chemicals used for cleaning or maintenance ◗ Provide appropriate protective equipment to employees ◗ Implement a written program providing for worker training, warning labels, and access to Material Safety Data Sheets
Medical Treatment Plans/Supplies	◗ Conduct a workplace hazard analysis to evaluate foreseeable injuries ◗ Determine the type and quantity of first-aid materials to maintain at the facility ◗ Ensure compliance with applicable state laws ◗ Develop written first-aid policies and procedures ◗ Periodically monitor emergency medical supplies ◗ Record any workplace injuries or illnesses (25)

*Occupational Safety and Health Standards, 29 C.F.R. §§ 1910.1–1910.1499 (1974).

OSHA's Bloodborne Pathogens Standard

The regularity of minor injuries and cuts during physical exercise highlights the need for fitness facilities to comply with OSHA's Bloodborne Pathogens (BBP) Standard (26). OSHA's BBP Standard aims to protect employees from bloodborne pathogens, defined as "pathogenic microorganisms that are present in human blood and can cause disease in humans. These pathogens include, but are not limited to, hepatitis B virus (HBV) and human immunodeficiency virus (HIV)" (26, p. 1). The BBP Standard became effective in March 1992, at a time when AIDS represented the primary cause of death for U.S. men aged 25-44 (27). The purpose of the BBP Standard is to mitigate occupational exposure to blood and **other potentially infectious materials (OPIM)**. Occupational exposure broadly extends to employees whose duties may reasonably lead to contact with blood or OPIM. In the fitness setting, these employees can include maintenance workers or those tasked with responding to injuries. Certain fitness facility employees, like sales representatives or

front desk personnel, are not normally considered to have occupational exposure and, therefore, are not covered by the BBP Standard unless they are (a) trained in first aid and responsible for rendering first aid, or (b) likely to come in contact with blood or OPIM as part of their job duties (28). Generally, the BBP Standard would not apply to fitness facility employees whose duties would not avail them to come in contact with blood or OPIM.

Where applicable, OSHA's BBP Standard prescribes safeguards to protect workers against health hazards related to BBPs. Compliance with the BBP Standard can be categorized in three parts: (a) providing BBP training to all employees who have regular exposure to blood or other potentially infectious materials as part of their job, (b) implementing the required OSHA BBP documents and safety controls for the organization to protect staff from exposure, and (c) designating and training a compliance officer tasked with managing and operating the facility BBP safety program (29). OSHA's BBP documents and safety controls include a written **Exposure Control Plan (ECP)** including, but not necessarily limited to, the components addressed in Exhibit 11-1. OSHA emphasizes that the ECP should be an evolving policy, to be reviewed and updated annually (30).

Responsibility for adhering to the BBP Standard lies with the employer. To ensure compliance with the BBP Standard, employers should assess the responsibilities of each staff position and evaluate whether exposure to blood or OPIM can be reasonably anticipated. Positions which incorporate physical contact with members, child care or cleaning responsibilities are particularly vulnerable to exposure. OSHA has provided a number of publications to encourage and support compliance including a convenient Fact Sheet (31). Adhering to the BBP Standard offers an opportunity to mitigate legal risk and create a safer work environment for employees and fitness participants.

From 2011 to 2014, OSHA found more than 4,041 violations of the BBP Standard, the most common being inadequacies of ECPs (32). To ensure compliance, facility managers/owners should be diligent in developing a comprehensive ECP and reviewing OSHA's BBP Enforcement Procedures (33). Failure to comply with the BBP Standard can result in monetary penalties and increased exposure to litigation.

State Laws

States are free to create their own rules so long as they do not conflict with those established at the federal level (34). Taking advantage of this autonomy, some states have implemented specific rules and regulations regarding first aid, **automated external defibrillators (AEDs)**, Good Samaritan statutes, and Do Not Resuscitate (DNR) orders. Examples of these laws are provided below, along with how courts have interpreted state statutes pertaining to AEDs in fitness facilities. Several cases focus on whether a law which requires an AED to be available on site carries a legal duty to use that AED when warranted.

First-Aid Laws

First aid refers to the initial assistance provided to any person suffering from either a minor or serious illness or injury, with care provided to preserve life, prevent the condition from worsening, or to promote recovery.

Exhibit 11-1: Components of an Effective Exposure Control Plan (ECP)*

- **Program Administration.** Names and contact information for those responsible for ECP operations

- **Employee Exposure Determination.** Identification of employees reasonably expected to be protected under the BBP Standard

- **Implementation and Controls.** Detail how employees are protected, protective equipment provided, procedures which must be followed

- **Hepatitis B Vaccination.** Inform employees of their rights, provide who will train employees regarding Hepatitis B vaccinations

- **Post-Exposure Follow-up Evaluation & Administration.** Persons and procedures in place for post-exposure documentation and harm mitigation

- **Employee Training.** What information will be provided to employees

- **Recordkeeping.** Training records, medical records, incident reporting

*Occupational Safety and Health Administration. Model Plans and Programs for the OSHA Bloodborne Pathogens and Hazard Communications Standards. 2003. Available at: https://www.osha.gov/Publications/osha3186.pdf. Accessed January 17, 2020; 26. Occupational Safety and Health Standards, 29 C.FR. § 1910.1030 (2012).

States often impose additional requirements regarding on-site first-aid/safety equipment. Like federal obligations, violation of state law can result in fines, termination of business activities, civil damages, or even criminal penalties.

Wisconsin and California offer examples of state-specific rules regarding first-aid training and preparedness. Wisconsin's Department of Health Services requires each fitness center to have an employee with up-to-date first-aid and CPR certifications through either the AHA or ARC (35). In Wisconsin, first-aid training should consist of at least five hours of training in theory and practice, including classroom instruction, competency testing and a final written examination. If a fitness facility wishes to implement their own first-aid training course, a training plan must be submitted to, and approved by, the Wisconsin State Department. In California, employers are tasked with assessing the work environment and providing adequate first-aid materials (36). In addition, all first-aid kits must be approved in writing by a licensed physician (37). These state-specific first-aid policies demonstrate the need for employers to be diligent in understanding the applicable rules regarding safe work environments and emergency preparedness.

AED Laws—Overview

In order to understand laws governing AEDs in fitness facilities, it helps to recognize why AEDs are so important. **Sudden cardiac arrest (SCA)** occurs when irregularities in the heart's electrical system cause the heart to suddenly stop beating. When the heart stops, blood cannot reach the brain and other vital organs. The shock, or defibrillation, initiated by an AED is the only effective method for treating ventricular fibrillation (VF), the most common cause of SCA (38). According to the AHA, widespread use of defibrillators could save at least 20,000 lives annually in the U.S. (39).

It should be noted SCA is not a heart attack, which occurs when blood flow to the heart is restricted. Someone experiencing a heart attack may feel discomfort or tightness over a period of days, while the consequences of SCA are much more dramatic. Response time is crucial. The delivery speed of defibrillation is the primary determinant of success in resuscitative attempts for VF cardiac arrest. If treatment is not received within 4-5 minutes, a victim of SCA will likely suffer irreversible brain damage, stroke and/or death (40). Survival rates decrease 7% to 10% with every minute of delay in initiating defibrillation: "50% at 5 minutes, 30% at 7 minutes, 10% at 9 to 11

minutes, and 2% to 5% after 12 minutes" (40, p. 43). See Figure 11-1. To increase chance of survival, rescuers must immediately activate the EMS system, provide effective CPR, and administer early defibrillation.

Fitness facilities and other businesses of public assembly must be prepared to respond to all crises, including cardiac emergencies. Relying on data compiled by the Resuscitation Outcomes Consortium, the AHA estimates 350,000 people in the U.S. experience an out-of-hospital cardiac arrest every year (41). Cardiac emergencies are not limited to vulnerable, at-risk or symptomatic populations. According to the AHA, 25% of individuals experiencing an out-of-hospital cardiac arrest had no previous symptoms (41).

Studies regarding the risk of cardiovascular events from participation in vigorous exercise were described in Chapter 6. The general conclusions from these studies were: (a) the risk of SCA or sudden cardiac death (SCD) from vigorous exercise is quite rare, and (b) that the risk for a cardiovascular event "is higher during or immediately after vigorous exercise, especially in habitually sedentary individuals who have underlying cardiovascular disease" (40, p. 2). Although early research gave rise to the belief that vigorous exercise increased the risk of death by SCA (42), researchers have since established that vigorous exercise, in itself, does not increase the risk of SCA (43). For example, in a 2015 study analyzing SCAs in middle-aged populations, only 63 of nearly 1,300 SCA events occurred during exercise activities (44). A more recent study had similar results, showing SCA during exercise to be rare and suffered most often by middle-aged men (45). In an effort to correlate certain types of exercise with SCA, cycling and heavy labor emerged as the most common activities causing SCA (46). However, nearly an equal number of events occurred during moderate-to-vigorous exercise as at rest. For those with symptoms of heart disease who may be deconditioned, bouts of vigorous exertion are associated with a transient increase in the risk of SCA, but this risk is diminished by habitual vigorous exercise and the risk of SCA is not increased in kind with the frequency of exercise (47).

Even if exercise does not increase SCA threat, cardiac emergencies still occur in fitness facilities. It is important to maintain a properly functioning AED on site. A 2014 national study that surveyed ACSM

Figure 11-1: Survival Rates: Speed of Defibrillation*

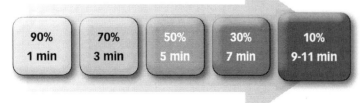

| 90%
1 min | 70%
3 min | 50%
5 min | 30%
7 min | 10%
9-11 min |

*Survival Rates Decrease 7%-10% with Every Minute of Delay. Response Time: Three to Five Minutes or Less (40)

KEY POINT

Several studies have investigated the relationship between vigorous intensity exercise and an increase risk of SCA. For an updated review on this topic, see the following 2020 AHA Scientific Statement that describes the "cardiovascular and health implications for moderate to vigorous physical activity, as well as high-volume, high intensity exercise regimens, based on current understanding of the associated risks and benefits" (p. e1). This statement has been endorsed by the ACSM and AACVPR.

Exercise-Related Acute Cardiovascular Events and Potential Deleterious Adaptations Following Long-Term Exercise Training: Placing the Risks Into Perspective—An Update (Franklin BA, Thompson PD, Al-Zaiti SS, et al.)

Circulation. 2020;141:e705-e736. Doi: 10.1161/CIR.0000000000000749. Available at: https://www.ahajournals.org/doi/10.1161/CIR.0000000000000749.

certified exercise physiologists found that 35% of fitness facilities had at least one cardiovascular emergency in the last five years (48). Several studies show AEDs save lives. In an 18-year study which reviewed over 250 sports facilities in Italy, facilities with AEDs on site (82%) were four minutes faster to administer shock treatment than facilities without (49). Of the 15 SCAs occurring in facilities with an AED, all but one patient survived without neurological damage. By contrast, only one of 11 patients survived if there was no AED on site. When considering passage of the Community Access to Emergency Defibrillation Act of 2002, Congress found communities that have established and implemented public access defibrillation programs have elevated the out-of-hospital SCA survival rate as high as 50% (50).

The simplicity of administering an AED has transformed the device from a treatment option to a mandated response tool in limited circumstances. Designed to be used by laypersons, devices earning FDA-approval (those legally marketed in the U.S.) provide directions both audibly and visually, and administer defibrillation when necessary (51). American Red Cross Training Services simplify AED administration into seven steps, comprising predominantly of

clearing the scene, ensuring a dry surface, applying the AED pads, and following directions provided by the device (52). Given the simplicity of AED use and the relationship of trust between fitness participants and some exercise professionals, a legal duty to administer an AED can arise depending on the circumstances and jurisdiction.

AED Laws—Examples

States must adhere to minimal standards established at the federal level. In 2000, Congress amended the Public Health Service Act with the Federal Cardiac Survival Act (53). The legislation was meant to provide an example for the private sector, creating guidelines for placing AEDs in federal buildings and making recommendations for training courses, maintenance and testing, and coordination with local **emergency medical services (EMS)**. The Act also offered protection from civil liability for emergency responders who used or acquired AEDs.

Various states have enacted laws specifically addressing AED availability, staff training and reporting obligations. A number of jurisdictions require fitness facilities to keep an AED on site and more have proposed legislation and are in the process of becoming law (54). In addition to the states discussed below, Iowa, Indiana, Louisiana, Massachusetts, Maryland, Nevada, New Jersey, Oregon, Pennsylvania, Rhode Island, and the District of Columbia require health clubs, sports clubs, and/or gyms to maintain an AED on site (55). Each of these statutes require employee CPR/AED training. Other states that do not have specific AED statutes for fitness facilities, may have other similar requirements. For example, fitness centers is Wisconsin must have at least one employee present on the premises who has successfully completed first-aid and CPR courses (56). AEDs may be recommended in other states, but not legally required. Some statutes also cover unstaffed facilities. In Pennsylvania, if fitness facilities offer services during unstaffed hours, they must have at least one AED available and instruct new members where it is located (57).

The applicability of AED requirements can depend on how "health club" or "fitness facility" is defined. For example, New York specifically enumerates an exhaustive list of activities falling under the definition of "health club" (58), while Colorado's terminology is broader, subjecting more fitness-related facilities to Colorado's requirements (59). Examples of state laws pertaining to AED availability in fitness facilities provided below are not exhaustive, but are meant to provide an overview of typical requirements, expectations, and consequences for violations among various jurisdictions.

Arkansas (60)

Arkansas defines "health spas" broadly to include any organization selling memberships in physical exercise programs or the right to use exercise equipment or therapeutic facilities. Health spas include martial arts studios, college fitness centers, country clubs, and certain weight control services. Arkansas "health spas" or fitness facilities must have at least one AED on site, located in the place most accessible to employees and guests. If a facility offers unstaffed service hours, that facility must provide signage indicating the location of the AED and directions for use. Arkansas expressly disaffirms a duty to use an AED, but legal liability may arise if an AED is used with gross negligence (recklessly disregarding the consequences). In addition, if a fitness facility fails to maintain an AED on site, any membership contract is voidable.

California (61)

California defines "health studio" as facilities offering access for any purpose relating to physical exercise on a membership basis, excluding hotels and similar businesses which offer fitness facilities. California courts have refused to reallocate to landlords the burden of ensuring AEDs are maintained on site, placing this responsibility solely on facility managers/owners (62). California expressly insulates facility employees and facility board of directors from civil liability from the use or nonuse of AEDs when rendering emergency care, provided the employee's conduct is not grossly negligent or willful misconduct (61). However, managers/owners of fitness facilities must satisfy certain requirements to earn similar treatment:

1) The AED must be maintained and regularly tested according to manufacturer guidelines;
2) The AED must be checked for readiness at least once every 30 days;
3) In the event of a cardiac emergency, the EMS system must be activated as soon as possible, and the use of the AED must be reported to the local EMS agency and the licensed physician associated with the facility EAP;
4) For every AED acquired by the facility (up to five), one employee must have completed a CPR/AED training course; and
5) A written plan must be developed detailing the procedures to be followed in the event of a cardiac emergency (61).

Given the specificity of California's requirements, fitness facility owners/managers face significantly higher legal risk if they are not proactive in Emergency Action Planning. Failure to adhere to the requirements above opens the door for civil liability if an agent of the facility negligently uses, attempts to use, or fails to use an AED to render emergency care or treatment.

Illinois (63)

Illinois broadly identifies "physical fitness facilities" as any athletic field, court, stadium or any indoor establishment focusing primarily on cardiovascular exertion or gaming where participants engage in relatively continuous physical activity. Excluded are facilities catering to less than 100 individuals per year, facilities in hospitals or hotels, and facilities where participants do not focus primarily on cardiovascular exertion, including driving ranges, bowling lanes and (somewhat surprisingly) yoga studios. Physical fitness facilities must have at least one working AED on site which is maintained and tested according to the manufacturer's guidelines. If the facility is outdoors, the AED must be in a building within 300 feet of the activity which provides unimpeded, open access to the housed AED during the outdoor event. Fitness facilities must ensure a trained AED user is available during all staffed business hours. The spotlight case described later, *Locke v. Life Time Fitness, Inc.,* demonstrates the legal consequences for failing to properly train employees in CPR/AED administration.

Michigan (64)

Michigan has a slightly narrower definition for fitness facilities subject to AED requirements. In Michigan, "health clubs" are establishments providing, as its primary purpose, services to assist patrons in physical exercise, weight control, or figure development. Excluded from the definition are hotels and similar businesses with a fitness facility for guests as well as organizations with facilities exclusively for an individual sport or a weight reduction center. Managers/owners of health clubs are obliged to (a) hire at least one individual who has completed a recognized CPR/AED training course; (b) maintain an AED in a manner which is obvious and readily accessible; and (c) develop and implement an EAP to respond to emergencies during hours of operation. Michigan expressly disaffirms, on behalf of fitness facility managers, owners and employees, a duty to use the on-site AED should a cardiac emergency arise. Violators of the act are subject to monetary penalties.

New York (65, 66)

New York "health clubs" with 500 members or more are classified as a "public access defibrillation provider" (PADP). These facilities must maintain an AED on site during business hours and employ, or otherwise maintain, at least one AED/CPR certified individual on site. In addition, PADPs must ensure AEDs are appropriately maintained and tested, notify the regional council of the existence, location, and type of AEDs it possesses, report any AED uses to local emergency medical services, and clearly identify the location of AEDs. In addition, the statute, New York General Business Law § 627-a(3), limits liability of employees administering AED treatment insofar as actions are not grossly negligent or willful and wanton (65).

New York offers particularly interesting case law on the issue of whether civil liability arises for merely negligent use or nonuse of an AED in the rendering of emergency care. As discussed in the following spotlight case, *Miglino v. Bally Total Fitness,* the statute insulates PADPs and agents of PADPs who respond to a cardiac emergency. However, in the more recent holding

in *Diniro v. Aspen Athletic Club,* the court refines this protection, holding that breach of duty may exist if the AED on site is non-operable.

State Law—Legal Risk

Failure to abide by state laws requiring on-site AEDs carries significant legal risk. In 2007, an Illinois circuit court ruled that failure to maintain an AED amounted to gross negligence, or reckless indifference for the safety of the fitness facility's members (67). This rationale opens the door for plaintiffs to seek punitive damages (damages beyond those actually incurred). Considering SCA survival rates, punitive damages carry potentially severe consequences for fitness facilities.

Each jurisdiction with AED-specific laws pertaining to fitness facilities requires at least one properly maintained device on site. In *Diniro v. Aspen Athletic Club* (68), a New York appellate court refused to grant Aspen Athletic Club's motion for summary judgment after not one, but *two* AED's failed during attempts to help a participant suffering SCA. In the court's opinion, Aspen's failure did not amount to gross negligence absent evidence of "spite or malice, or a fraudulent or evil motive . . . or such a conscious and deliberate disregard of the interests of others that the conduct may be called willful or wanton" (p. 1790). This case exemplifies how statutory requirements can give rise to an affirmative duty; here, to ensure a working AED is available on site. Although the ruling in *Diniro v. Aspen Athletic Club* ultimately limited plaintiff's recovery to actual damages, those damages arising from cardiac emergencies present substantial risk for fitness facilities if statutory mandates are neglected.

The court's ruling in *Miglino v Bally Total Fitness* (2011) represented the first court to find that an affirmative duty to use an AED exists. Although the 2013 New York appellate court overturned this ruling, *Miglino v Bally Total Fitness* may foreshadow the future of AED policy. The 2011 court referred to lifesaving statistics of AEDs described in the ACSM and AHA joint position statement, *Automated External Defibrillators in Health/Fitness Facilities* (99). This court also reviewed the legislative intent of the New York statute,

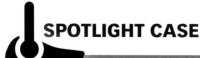

SPOTLIGHT CASE

Miglino v. Bally Total Fitness of Greater N.Y., Inc.
20 N.Y.3d 342 (N.Y. App., 2013)

FACTS

Historical Facts:

At about 7:00 a.m. on March 26, 2007, Gregory Miglino, Sr. suddenly collapsed while playing racquetball at his New York fitness club. Kenneth LaGrega, an AED/CPR certified personal fitness trainer was standing at the front desk with a receptionist when he learned of the emergency. The receptionist immediately dialed 911 and made an announcement requesting help from anyone with medical training. LaGrega rushed to assist Miglino. After checking Miglino's pulse and seeing he was breathing, LeGrega left to check the status of the 911 response. When he returned, other gym members, a medical doctor, and a medical student, had responded to the announcement and were administering CPR. An AED was brought to the room where Miglino was located but was never used. Emergency medical services (EMS) arrived at the gym at 7:07 a.m. EMS administered shocks to Miglino with an AED to no avail. The ambulance arrived at the hospital at 7:45 a.m. where Miglino was pronounced deceased.

Procedural Facts:

Gregory Miglino, Jr., as executor of the Miglino's estate, brought action against Bally's alleging the club was negligent in failing to use an AED on his father. Plaintiff alleged the New York statute (General Business Law § 627-a) implicitly required "public access defibrillation providers" (health clubs with 500 or more members) to use an AED if circumstances warranted. Bally filed a motion to dismiss, asserting plaintiff's complaint failed to state a claim upon which relief could be granted. The Suffolk County Supreme Court denied the defendant's motion, allowing the claim to be heard. On appeal, the Appellate Division in the Second Judicial Department affirmed the denial and went a step further, interpreting the New York statute to create a duty for health club employees to use AEDs if necessary. *Miglino v Bally Total Fitness of Greater N.Y., Inc.*, 92 A.D.3d 148 (N.Y. App. Div., 2011). Questioning this court's ruling and interpretation of the statute, Bally appealed.

ISSUE

Based on the New York statute, do health clubs in New York have a duty to use an AED if circumstances warrant their use?

COURT'S RULING

No. The appellate court ruled that statute does not create an affirmative duty to use an AED in the event of a cardiac emergency in a health club.

COURT'S REASONING

New York General Business Law § 627-a requires certain health clubs to have, during business hours, at least one AED on site during staffed hours and a person certified to use an AED and administer CPR. Because the statute does not specify whether using an AED is required, the crux of the court's debate was whether this responsibility was implied by the terms of law. The Court of Appeals held that the new duty would be too significant to imply. Lawmakers would have expressly stated an intent to impose such a responsibility on fitness club owners.

Opponents felt the Court of Appeals interpretation renders the statute meaningless. In the view of the appellate court in the 2011 *Miglino* case and Chief Judge Lippman, who entered a dissenting opinion in the Court of Appeals ruling, the purpose of the statute and protections included within the law suggest an implied "duty to use". Statements from

Miglino continued...

legislative hearings indicate the purpose of the law was to make life-saving devices available in high risk environments. To support this argument, the court referred to the American Heart Association's Position Statement—Automated External Defibrillators in Health/Fitness Facilities—published in *Circulation* in 2002.

In response to the dissenting opinion, the Court of Appeals stated that "such a duty would engender a whole new field of tort litigation, saddling health clubs with new costs and generating uncertainty. The legislature is unlikely to have imposed such a new duty absent an express statement..." (pp. 349-350).

Lessons Learned from *Miglino*

Legal
- In New York, fitness facility employees do not have a legal duty to use an AED if a SCA occurs. However, other legal duties do exist regarding AEDs based on the New York statute.

- The ruling in the 2011 *Miglino* case could have significantly expanded the responsibilities of fitness centers during emergencies, but it was overruled by this court.

Risk Management/Injury Prevention
- Fitness manager/owners need to be aware of and follow provisions within AED state statutes.

- Fitness facilities need to have medical emergency equipment (e.g., first-aid kit, AED) and staff members who possess current certification in first-aid, CPR, and AED.

- Facility staff members need to know how to properly carry out medical emergency procedures (e.g., practice the procedures in trainings and rehearsals).

- Mock emergency drills should be conducted at least on a quarterly basis if not more often; and some of these drills/rehearsals should be undertaken on an unannounced basis.

which was to make AEDs readily available for use in gyms and to save lives. The court stated

> *...inasmuch as there is no dispute that General Business Law § 627-a requires certain health club facilities to provide an AED on the premises, as well as a person trained to use such device, it is anomalous to conclude that there is no duty to use the device should the need arise. Stated differently, why statutorily mandate a health club facility to provide the device if there is no concomitant requirement to use it?* (Miglino, 2011, p. 157).

With an evolving understanding of how crucial it is to quickly administer defibrillation; future courts may conclude that failing to use an available AED is reckless disregard for the safety and welfare of the person in peril. Failing to use an AED may appear even more egregious if employees had prior CPR/AED training. In fitness facilities, the relationship between exercise professionals and participants could create a heightened responsibility of care. Clearly, whether an affirmative duty to use an AED exists depends on the totality of the circumstances. While proving gross negligence is a substantial hurdle for plaintiffs to overcome, AEDs have become widely available and easy to use, making it difficult for defendants to rationalize nonuse, especially in the fitness setting.

Following *Miglino v. Bally Total Fitness*, New York courts revisited AED use in fitness facilities in *Diniro v. Aspen Athletic Club* (68). As previously referenced, two AEDs were available on site and brought to the SCA victim, but neither AED functioned properly, critically delaying fibrillation. The participant never regained consciousness. In the subsequent proceeding, the court denied Aspen Athletic Club's motion for summary judgment. According to the court, failure to maintain an operable AED within the health club did not amount to gross negligence, but the question of whether reasonable care was used raised a triable issue for a jury to resolve. This ruling placed Aspen Athletic

Club in the precarious position of facing liability for compensatory damages. Surviving summary process also raises the question of whether Aspen's conduct amounts to **negligence per se**. Negligence per se is available when "the plaintiff is a member of the class intended to be benefited by the statute" and "the statute is intended to protect against the very hazard that caused the plaintiff's injury" (69, p. 5). Plaintiffs similarly situated to those in *Diniro v. Aspen Athletic Club* have a strong argument that both prongs of negligence per se have been satisfied. The effect of this determination would greatly reduce the plaintiff's burden, as it would raise a **rebuttable presumption** that the Defendant acted negligently.

KEY POINT

Compliance with state law will become a focal point in any relevant litigious dispute. Plaintiffs point to noncompliance as evidence of a breached duty of care, while adherence can support defendants' claims that reasonable care was provided under the circumstances. State laws governing AED maintenance and use in fitness facilities are jurisdictionally unique and continually evolving. Facility managers/owners need to consult with their attorney to ensure state and local laws applicable to emergency preparedness and response are understood and observed.

Good Samaritan Laws

In legal terms, a "Good Samaritan" is someone who renders aid in an emergency to an injured person on a voluntary basis. For example, an individual (volunteer) who witnesses an injury in a public setting can choose to render aid or not. If he/she chooses to render aid, Good Samaritan laws offer protection from ordinary negligence. However, in a fitness facility, some employees do not have an option to render aid to an injured participant—they have a duty to act because of the relationship that is formed, as described below and in many of the cases in this chapter. Sometimes, exercise professionals, while on the job, believe they have a choice to render aid to an injured participant because of Good Samaritan laws, which is not the case.

Good Samaritan laws are derived from public policy to encourage caregivers and rescuers to help others in emergency situations. All 50 states have enumerated some level of protection, but state laws differ in scope and applicability of protections afforded. In practice, Good Samaritan statutes insulate volunteers from legal liability for accidental errors which cause further injury. To apply, aid must be given at the scene of the emergency, and the volunteer must not be acting to receive an award or payment.

Generally, witnesses and bystanders have no legal obligation to assist anyone injured or in danger (70). However, if action is taken to provide assistance, help must be provided in a reasonable manner under the circumstances, or how a reasonable, prudent person would act in a similar situation. This is referred to as the "ordinary" standard of care. Failure to act in accordance with the ordinary standard of care can result in criminal charges or civil liability for damages if injury results. Good Samaritan laws protect volunteers if their actions accidentally cause further injury, unless the volunteer acted with gross negligence, or reckless disregard for the consequences.

PRACTICAL EXAMPLE

Good Samaritan Laws

Imagine you are at the gym walking on a treadmill when someone running next to you collapses. He is in his 50s, unresponsive, and upon checking his pulse, you feel nothing. You recently read this textbook and know the likelihood of survival diminishes every second the heart remains stagnant. Sensing an obligation to help, you begin chest compressions. The man ends up surviving, but your compressions slightly fractured two of his ribs. Without a Good Samaritan law in place, you may be liable to the man for fracturing his ribs even though your actions likely saved his life. Whether your conduct was "reasonable" under the circumstances is a question of fact a jury will determine retroactively. If your method of performing CPR was to jump on the man's chest, your conduct may be considered "gross" or "willful and wanton" negligence, in which case, you would be liable for fracturing the man's ribs.

All 50 states and the U.S. federal government have expanded Good Samaritan laws to limit the liability of AED users. These statutes protect authorized personnel from civil liability, as long as using an AED is warranted and the device is utilized without malice or reckless disregard for the victim's rights. A recent bill proposed at the federal level seeks to expand protections regardless of whether the person who used the AED complied with signage, received training, or was assisted or supervised by a licensed physician (71).

Many states have also expanded Good Samaritan protection to citizens who call emergency assistance in the event of a drug overdose. Prior to these expansions, those at the scene of the incident (who typically, were involved in the drug use) exposed themselves to drug-related charges by calling for help. While uncommon, drug overdoses can occur in any public setting, including fitness facilities. Protocols for responding to drug overdose within a fitness facility should be considered during Emergency Action Planning.

Duty to Act

As discussed in Chapters 1 and 4, each element of negligence: duty, breach, causation, and harm must be satisfied in order to raise a "prima facie" cause of action sufficient to survive summary judgment. There can be no liability for negligence without breach of a duty owed to the plaintiff. The question of whether there is a legal duty to administer an AED to save someone suffering from SCA has been extensively litigated. Deeply rooted in the common law, there is no legal duty to assist another who is in peril (70). Absent a special relationship, an affirmative "duty to act" must be imposed by law or regulation.

In some situations, a witness to an emergency will have a legal duty to act. One with a duty to act must do so as a reasonable, prudent person under the circumstances; also known as the ordinary standard of care. This duty arises when actor and victim have a special relationship and the threat of harm arises in the course of that relationship (70). Special relationships giving rise to a duty to act include parent/child, employer/employee, and landowner/occupier and

PRACTICAL EXAMPLE

Affirmative Duty to Act

Imagine an Olympic swimmer standing beside a lake bearing witness to a recreational swimmer struggling to stay above the water. No matter how vulnerable the victim or how easy it would be for the Olympian to save the day, the Olympian could not be held legally liable for choosing not to save the victim. However, upon jumping in the water (or taking alternative action), a rescuer accepts the duty to act reasonably, in accordance with the ordinary standard of care. If the Olympian jumped in the water to help, but unreasonably decided to give up and turn back before reaching the victim, the Olympian may be liable for damages caused by his/her decision.

invitee. As described in Chapter 10, an "invitee" is someone who enters the land of another for the purpose of business dealings. Property owners/occupiers have a legal duty to make their property reasonably safe and/or warn invitees of nonobvious or hidden dangers. Property owners/occupiers, including fitness facility owners/managers, must conduct reasonable inspections of their property to satisfy this obligation. The existence and scope of a property owner's duty to protect visitors against hazards is a question of law for the court to resolve on a case-by-case basis (72). See case law examples in Chapter 10 regarding duties toward invitees.

Courts have identified a special relationship between school officers and student-athletes creating a heightened duty of care. This heightened duty is exemplified by the following spotlight case, *Limones v. Sch. Dist.*, and is particularly applicable to fitness facilities accessible to minors and those located within high school and/or college campuses.

AED Case Law

Most disputes heard by courts revolve around the existence and scope of a fitness facility managers/owners' duty to reasonably protect participants. See Exhibit 11-2 for questions presented regarding a duty to act. Due to the fact-dependent nature of the existence of a legal duty, various jurisdictions employ different

SPOTLIGHT CASE

Limones v. Sch. Dist.
161 So.3d 384 (Fla., 2015)

FACTS

Historical Facts:

On Nov. 13, 2008, Abel Limones Jr., a high school athlete for East Lee County High School, was playing in a soccer match against Riverdale High. At about 7:40 p.m., Abel collapsed. Within three minutes his pulse was undetectable. Abel's coach, Thomas Busatta and two nurses, who were in attendance, rushed to perform CPR. No one responded to Coach Busatta's calls for an AED. Unbeknownst to coaches and bystanders, an AED was on a golf cart parked at the far end of the field. At or about 7:50 p.m., the Fire Department arrived on the scene and shocked Abel using an AED, but to no avail. Emergency medical services used their own machine to deliver four additional shocks. A series of intravenous medications were administered to finally resuscitate Abel at 8:06 p.m., twenty-three minutes after the 911 call. Abel survived the event but suffered severe disabilities requiring life-long, 24-hour care.

Procedural Facts:

The plaintiffs, Abel Limones Sr. and Sanjuana Castillo, filed this action on behalf of Abel alleging the School Board was negligent in failing to maintain an AED close enough to the field or failing to use an AED on Abel. Despite expert testimony that Abel would not have suffered brain damage had the AED been utilized sooner, the trial court granted summary judgment in favor of the School Board.

While acknowledging the school district's duty to supervise its students and prevent aggravation of an injury, the appellate court analogized the circumstances with another Florida case, *L.A. Fitness International, LLC v. Mayer.* In *L.A. Fitness,* the appellate court ruled that a commercial health club had a duty to summon emergency responders to a patron in cardiac distress but did not have duty to have an AED on the premises.

Accordingly, the appellate court affirmed the trial court's decision, holding that the school district did not have a duty to make available, diagnose the need for, or use an AED in the event of a sudden cardiac arrest (SCA) during a high school sporting event. In addition, the school district was afforded immunity under Florida's "Good Samaritan" statute, which protects "any person who acquired the device and makes it available for use" from civil liability. In doing so, the court found the school district qualified as a "person" as provided in the statute. By having an AED available on the field, the school district qualified for statutory protection, even though the AED was not accessed or used. Disagreeing with the ruling of the appellate court, the plaintiffs appealed to the Florida Supreme Court.

ISSUE

Did the Florida Supreme Court uphold the appellate court's ruling?

COURT'S RULING

No, the Florida Supreme Court quashed the appellate court's ruling and remanded the case for trial.

COURT'S REASONING

Regarding the duty the school district owed to Abel Limones Jr., the court referring to the Restatement (Second) of Torts, stated that "a party does not have a duty to take affirmative action to protect or aid another unless a special relationship exists which creates such a duty" (p. 390). Based on previous Florida court rulings, a special relationship exists between schools and their students because "a school functions at least partially in the place of

Limones continued...

parents during the school day and school-sponsored activities" (p, 390). Given this special relationship, a school is required to reasonably supervise students during all school-sponsored activities including those that occur beyond the boundaries of the school. Florida courts have recognized five specific duties of schools regarding the supervision of student athletes. The fifth duty states "schools must take appropriate measures after a student is injured to prevent aggravation of the injury" (p. 390). Because Abel was injured while participating in a school-sponsored soccer game, the Supreme Court concluded that the school district had "a duty of supervision and to act with reasonable care under the circumstances; specifically,...a duty to take responsibility to take appropriate post-injury effort to avoid or mitigate further aggravation of his injury" (p. 391).

The Supreme Court chose to distinguish *Limones* from *L.A. Fitness International, LLC.* According to the Court, the relationship between an adult customer and commercial health club is far different than that between a student athlete and a school. Although both are recognized as relationships, the former involves two adults whereas the latter involves a minor. In addition, Florida's legislature requires high schools that participate in interscholastic athletics to acquire an AED and train appropriate personnel in AED use. No such regulations have been enacted for health clubs, "even though the foreseeability for the need to use an AED may be similar in both contexts" (p. 392).

The Court then addressed whether the school district was statutorily immune from suit. The Court identified two classes protected from liability by Florida's Good Samaritan statute: (1) users or attempted users, and (2) acquirers. Acquirers are immune from harm that may result only when an AED is actually used or attempted to be used. Therefore, the school district was not entitled to immunity.

Lessons Learned from *Limones*

Legal

▶ Because of the special relationship that exists between schools and students, schools have a heightened duty to supervise and act to protect students from harm.

▶ The extent of what is required is subject to evolve with contemporary emergency protocols that may consider the student's age and activity, the extent of the injury, the available responders, and surrounding facts.

▶ States may have statutes specifying the supervision duties owed to student-athletes.

▶ Distinct special relationships create different standards of care (e.g., a business proprietor-customer relationship is different than a school district-student relationship).

▶ Good Samaritan laws provide immunity only when applied to the protected classes specified in state statutes. This immunity did not apply to the school district in *Limones*.

Risk Management/Injury Prevention

▶ School athletic programs need to have a comprehensive EAP that meets all of the requirements mandated in state statutes as well as published standards/guidelines regarding emergency planning for youth sport programs.

▶ Duty owed to students extends beyond school boundaries. If a school operates a fitness facility or requires its student-athletes to use an exercise facility, the school may be required to supervise and reasonably act to protect students from harm.

▶ Fitness facilities that provide programs/services for minors may require greater supervision and safeguards compared to adult programs/services.

methods to determine whether a duty exists, as described in the following AED cases in New Jersey, Texas, California, and Florida.

New Jersey

In *Stelluti v. Casapenn Enterprises, LLC* (73), the New Jersey Supreme Court held that private fitness facilities owe "a standard of care congruent with the nature of their business, which is to make available the specialized equipment and facility to their invitees who are there to exercise, train…That is . . . a duty not to engage in reckless or gross negligence." (p. 313). This standard reflects New Jersey's Good Samaritan statute, which immunizes actions taken in good faith while rendering care at the scene of an emergency (74). "Good faith" means "honesty of purpose and integrity of conduct, without knowledge . . .that the conduct is wrong" as defined by the court in *Desiervo v. Township of Elmwood Park* (75, p. 15). To establish reckless, willful or wanton injury, a plaintiff must show the defendant acted consciously and intentionally with knowledge of existing conditions, and that his conduct would likely produce an injurious result (75).

Desiervo v. Township of Elmwood Park (75) exemplifies the highly fact-dependent analysis New Jersey courts will employ when determining the duty of care in emergency scenarios. In *Desiervo v. Township of Elmwood Park,* plaintiffs alleged emergency response personnel (ERP) failed to properly administer necessary emergency assistance to the victim who was unresponsive following a prescription drug overdose. After considering expert testimony regarding the appropriateness of using an AED, the court found ERP acted reasonably in deciding not to perform CPR or use an AED because the victim had a pulse. The court was persuaded by AHA guidelines for lay rescuers and EMTs, which provide, "the use of an AED is limited to patients who do not have a pulse and are not breathing" (75, p. 11). Accordingly, summary judgment was granted in favor of the defendants. Notwithstanding the high burden placed upon plaintiffs to prove gross negligence, *Desiervo v. Township of Elmwood Park* supports the proposition that a duty to use an AED may be appropriate if a victim is without a pulse and the circumstances otherwise warrant AED administration.

Exhibit 11-2: Duty to Act: Questions Presented

- Does the relationship between facility manager/owner and participant raise a duty to provide first aid?

- Does "first aid" extend to use of an AED when a SCA occurs on site?

- Do state laws requiring AEDs to be on site imply a duty to act, or use the AED on a participant suffering SCA?

- Do court decisions requiring the availability of "specialized equipment" create a duty to use that equipment?

- Can published standards of practice create a legal responsibility to use an AED?

Texas

Texas courts consider several interrelated factors, including the risk, foreseeability, and likelihood of injury, weighed against the social utility of the actor's conduct, the magnitude of the burden of guarding against the injury, and the consequences of placing the burden on the defendant. In *Potter v. 24 Hour Fitness* (76), none of the defendant's employees responded when Charles Potter collapsed while exercising. Instead, another facility member administered CPR until emergency personnel arrived. Although Charles' heart was successfully defibrillated, he remained in a non-responsive state until his death four months later. Despite the apparent inaction of the fitness facility, the Texas court found the facility's legal duty had been satisfied by calling EMS and because CPR had been initiated. The court noted however, if the defendant had held itself out as prepared to administer an AED to participants, or hired personnel specially trained to respond to cardiovascular emergencies, the facility may not have been entitled to summary judgment.

In *Boggus obo Casey v. Texas Racquet & Spa, Inc*, 2018 WL 3911090 (Tex. App., 2018), John Casey suffered a cardiac arrest while participating in a cycling class. An employee called 911. About five minutes later, after Casey started to turn blue, another employee began CPR. An AED was located nearby, but no one used it. EMS personnel arrived and defibrillated Casey, but he suffered severe brain damage resulting in permanent disabilities. Casey's wife, Ginny Boggus, sued the club alleging, among other things, that the club failed to (a) properly train its employees on the use of the AED and, (b) comply with Chapter 779 of the Texas Health and Safety Code.

Under Chapter 779, entities that acquire an AED are required to ensure that users are trained. Requirements, in part, include:

1) each user of the automated external defibrillator receives training given or approved by the Department of State Health Services in:
   (A) cardiopulmonary resuscitation; and
   (B) use of the automated external defibrillator; and

2) a licensed physician is involved in the training program to ensure compliance with the requirements of this chapter (p. 4).

The trial court granted the defendant's motion for summary judgment, but the appellate court held that the "fitness club failed to meet its summary judgment burden to conclusively negate at least one essential element of the plaintiff's claim relating to the club's failure to train its employees on the use of an AED" (p. 1). The case was remanded for further proceedings. Fitness managers/owners need to realize that, even in states without a specific AED statute that applies to health clubs, other statutes may apply which need to be reviewed and followed.

Zihlman v. Wichita Falls YMCA (77) exemplifies the competing legal arguments for establishing an affirmative duty to act. The claim in *Zihlman v. Wichita Falls YMCA* arose when 56-year-old Elaine Thomas suffered a SCA while exercising at her local YMCA in September 2007. YMCA employees were immediately notified upon Elaine's collapse and an AED was retrieved, but employees did not begin CPR and the AED was not used. EMS arrived about 10 minutes after the 911 call was made. EMS initiated the first AED shock within about one minute of their arrival. Unfortunately, efforts to revive Elaine were unsuccessful. Elaine's survivors brought suit against the YMCA, claiming the fitness facility was grossly negligent in failing to properly and timely treat Elaine's cardiac arrest and in failing to properly train its employees. Plaintiffs sought punitive damages up to $3,000,000 per child for loss of the relationship and mental anguish.

In their complaint, the plaintiffs in *Zihlman* provided a historical review of AEDs beginning in 1986 when the AHA and the *Journal of the American Medical Association* "identified 'health club personnel' as capable first responders and recommended users of AEDs" (77, p. 76). This historical review also described the 2002 ACSM/AHA joint position statement (99) recommending AEDs in health clubs and listed several health clubs that followed this recommendation, establishing industry norms. The plaintiffs claimed the "YMCA knew, or should have known, of all these published standards and industry developments as they happened" (77, p. 77). The YMCA defended itself by disavowing a duty to care for Elaine. According to the defendants, Elaine's death was caused by pre-existing hypertension and heart problems. The YMCA pointed to common law principles which mandate only reasonable care under the circumstances (78). The defendants argued "reasonable care" for a fitness facility does not encompass training employees (or ensuring employees are trained) to provide life-saving aid (77). The case settled in August 2011, after nearly two years of litigation, soon after the defendants filed a motion for summary judgment.

California

California courts have held that Health and Safety Code § 1797.196 and Civil Code § 1714.21 do not impose a duty to activate an AED upon the occurrence of a medical emergency. However, facility managers/owners must not increase the risks to participants above those inherent in the sport. In *Jabo v. YMCA of San Diego County* (79), the court classified a property owner's duty to protect visitors against hazards as a question of law for the court to resolve on a case-by-case basis. In *Jabo*, a 43-year-old man collapsed from SCA while playing soccer at his local YMCA. The YMCA staff member on duty failed to bring an AED to the field as a precautionary measure, although five were available within the facility. The court held that under these circumstances, the facility owners had acted reasonably in maintaining readily available AEDs. However, the court reiterated their previous position, stated in *Verdugo v. Target Corp.* (80), that California's AED statutes do not preclude courts from finding business owners may owe customers additional duties of care when medical emergencies arise. The *Jabo v. YMCA San Diego County* ruling allows California courts to find facility owners negligent if

AEDs are unavailable or if conduct for which a facility is responsible otherwise enhances risks beyond those inherent in physical exercise.

Florida

Due care in Florida centers on how "first aid" is defined. In *L.A. Fitness International, Inc. v. Mayer* (81), a participant, Alessio Tringali, collapsed while using a step machine in April 2003. The facility did not have an AED on site and facility employees chose not to administer CPR, fearing a stroke or seizure had been suffered. Despite best efforts, EMS were unable to resuscitate the participant. The daughter of deceased, Julianna Tringali Mayer, claimed that L.A. Fitness:

> *"(1) failed to properly screen the deceased's health condition at or about the time he joined the health club; (2) failed to administer cardiopulmonary resuscitation (CPR) to him; (3) failed to have an automatic external defibrillator (AED) on its premises and to use it on the deceased; and (4) failed to properly train its employees and agents for handling medical emergencies"* (p. 552).

The jury found the defendant negligent and awarded Mayer $619,650 in damages. Dr. Anthony Abbott served as an expert witness for the plaintiff. In his testimony, Dr. Abbott discussed the health club industry's standards of care in April 2003. He stated:

> *"L.A. Fitness violated the industry's standards of care by failing to have a written emergency plan and to employ qualified personnel for handling emergencies. He said that the standards promulgated by the industry's authorities, including the International Health and Racquet Sports Club Association (IHRSCA) [sic] and the American College of Sports Medicine, are directed at responding to cardiopulmonary emergencies..." and that "L.A. Fitness' plan was inadequate; an emergency plan "is designed to assign various roles to individuals and how they carry those roles out"* (p. 554).

L.A. Fitness appealed claiming it "satisfied its duty to render assistance to the deceased as a matter of law when it promptly summoned professional medical assistance for him" (81, p. 552). The appellate court agreed and reversed the trial court's ruling. In its analysis of duty, the appellate court held fitness facilities do not have a duty to administer "skilled treatment" to patrons who suffer a medical emergency. The only duty owed is to provide "first aid," a duty that "does not encompass . . . skilled treatment, such as CPR" (81, p. 559). The court explained, there is no statutory duty in Florida which requires a business have an AED on its premises. Further, industry custom and practice can help define a standard of care, but "do not give rise to an independent legal duty" (81, pp. 556-557).

The *L.A. Fitness International, Inc. v. Mayer* analysis was consistently applied to facilities located within hotels in *De La Flor v. Ritz-Carlton Hotel* (82). While the duty owed by fitness facilities in Florida appears consistent, the court's reasoning raises a question; given the increasing simplicity of using an AED, when does AED use fall from classification of "skilled treatment?" To avoid the consequences of this inevitable transition, facility owners should ensure AEDs are available and appropriately maintained on site and train employees to administer AEDs when warranted.

KEY POINT

As demonstrated in the AED spotlight case *Limones* and other cases described in this chapter, courts have employed different methods to determine whether there is a legal duty to have and use an AED. However, to save lives and avoid lawsuits, facility owners/managers and exercise professionals need to have at least one AED on site and should use it when necessary.

Do Not Resuscitate (DNR) Orders in Out-of-Hospital Settings

A do-not-resuscitate order, or DNR order, is a medical order written by a physician which instructs health care providers not to perform CPR or other advanced life support techniques if a patient's heart stops beating. Typically, DNR orders or similar advance directives are completed on behalf of individuals in healthcare settings who are terminally ill or elderly and frail. DNR orders and other forms of advance directives are particularly applicable to fitness facilities offering services to elderly populations, including programs within assisted living facilities. The scope and applicability of DNR orders are governed by state law. Generally, fitness facilities are not obligated to follow DNR orders, as decisions about stopping life-saving efforts should be made by licensed medical professionals. Most states, including New York and Texas as described next, provide for special DNR orders that are effective outside hospitals, wherever the person may be in the community.

In 1991, New York implemented non-hospital DNR orders covering first responders and emergency medical technicians called to the scene of an emergency (83). The statute insulates EMS personnel from liability for honoring the DNR order reasonably and in good faith. EMS personnel must honor the order unless they reasonably believe it is invalid or if objecting family members arrive at the scene and confrontation appears likely. An individual need not be terminally ill to obtain a DNR order in New York. The Court of Appeals has held the right to refuse life-sustaining treatment is not dependent upon a medical condition (84).

In Texas, a properly issued out-of-hospital DNR order is valid and must be honored by responding healthcare professionals who have discovered the order and confirmed the identity of the patient (85). Health care professionals responding to the scene of an emergency are not required to accept an out-of-hospital DNR order that does not meet statutory requirements, which include responses provided in the places designated and a properly dated signature. Texas gives DNR orders significant weight, requiring adherence unless the patient or patient's representative at the scene requests life-sustaining treatment be initiated or continued.

As for fitness facility managers/owners, if a participant presents a DNR order or out-of-hospital equivalent directive, contact your legal counsel to ensure compliance with applicable state laws. Should this scenario arise, industry professionals recommend adhering to the emergency response policy and providing reasonable care under the circumstances until emergency personnel arrive (86). Responding medical professionals should be informed of the DNR order and deferred to in deciding whether life-supporting care should continue.

Published Standards of Practice

As discussed in Chapter 4, it is the responsibility of fitness managers and exercise professionals to be familiar with published standards of practice. Like state laws, these standards may be employed by either side of litigation disputing whether due care was provided as they were in *Miglino v. Bally Total Fitness, Zihlman v. Wichita Falls YMCA*, and *L.A. Fitness International, Inc. v. Mayer*. If properly adopted and applied, published standards of practice demonstrate a fitness facility's diligence in caring for the safety of its members. If deviated from or ignored, professional standards can support claims of breach of duty. Independent organizations like the American National Standards Institute (ANSI) and professional organizations such as the ACSM and NSCA have issued standards or guidelines relating to emergency response planning. Fitness managers and exercise professionals should review published standards of practice with the goal of satisfying the core principles reflected.

Independent Organizations

The ANSI operates to design and safeguard fair standards and quality conformity assessment systems across all U.S. industries. In 2015, ANSI collaborated with the International Safety Equipment Association (ISEA) to revise their minimum performance and supplies standards for workplace first-aid kits (87). The updated voluntary consensus standard classifies first-aid kits based on the anticipated number of users, the complexity of the work environment, and the level of hazards. Class A kits represent minimum workplace requirements while Class B kits must be maintained where the risk of severe injury is high, like shipyards, construction, or logging businesses. First-aid kits designated Class B possess all the items found in Class A kits, but in greater quantities, and with the inclusion of a splint and tourniquet. Minimum quantities and volumes of first-aid kits contents can be found on ANSI's website (88).

When deciding the class and type of kit that may be most appropriate, facility managers should consider present risks, potential severity, and likelihood of an incident. After assessing the number of employees, physical layout of the facility and remoteness to emergency services, employers should consider whether multiple first-aid kits are needed and whether kits need to be supplemented with additional supplies. The selection of these items should be based on the recommendation of a person competent in first aid who is aware of the hazards faced and the number of employees at the worksite. Fitness facilities must maintain a "Class A" first-aid kit, but due to the likelihood of injuries (see Table 2-3 in Chapter 2) where physical activity is performed, more comprehensive first-aid equipment may be warranted (89).

Professional Organizations

A general description of the standards and guidelines published by eight different professional organizations was provided in Chapter 4. The following describes emergency planning and response standards and guidelines published by these organizations as well as the ACOEM Position Statement and ACSM/AHA Joint Position Statement regarding AEDs. Fitness managers should obtain these publications to review the standards and guidelines in their entirety.

1) *ACSM's Health/Fitness Facility Standards and Guidelines,* 5th edition, 2019 (90)
   This publication contains eight standards and two guidelines pertaining to emergency planning and policies. The standards describe several requirements, such as having (a) written emergency response policies and procedures, (b) an adequate number of AEDs located in the facility to allow a time from collapse to defibrillation of three-five minutes, (c) practice sessions at least every six months, and (d) a staff member on duty during all operating hours who is trained and certified in CPR and AED. Other standards address compliance with AED laws and OSHA standards (e.g., hazardous chemicals, bodily fluids). Guidelines recommend fitness facilities extend opportunities for emergency training to each employee and implementing an incident reporting system for documenting all medical incidents, including emergency situations.

2) *ACSM's Guidelines for Exercise Testing and Prescription,* 10th edition, 2018 (91)
   This publication includes an appendix titled Emergency Risk Management. This appendix provides a brief overview of emergency guidelines for fitness facilities, including clinical settings. It also provides recommendations for implementing an AED program as well as a list of related Internet resources.

3) *NSCA Strength & Conditioning Professional Standards & Guidelines,* 2017 (92)
   This publication provides two standards and one guideline addressing emergency action planning and response. The standards provide for the training of fitness professionals in emergency response (e.g., universal precautions, CPR, and first aid), the development of a written, comprehensive EAP and posting it within the facility, and practicing the EAP at least quarterly. Components of an effective EAP are also described.

   The NSCA offers recommendations for EAPs specific to high school and collegiate sporting events, which can be reflected in the EAPs of fitness facilities. For example, NSCA recommends athletic administrators establish an emergency contact and collect information about unique health factors for all student-athletes. Similarly, fitness facilities should document and maintain emergency information for all members. This information may be used reactively to prevent further harm in the event of an emergency, or proactively, to provide precautionary advice to high-risk participants.

   The NSCA gives particular consideration to lightning-related hazards and natural emergencies. According to the National Oceanic and Atmospheric Administration, lightning strikes cause about 26 fatalities during sporting events each year. A lighting safety plan should be implemented by fitness facilities offering outdoor exercise classes or activities.

4) *IHRSA (International Health, Racquet & Sportsclub Association) Club Membership Standards in IHRSA's Guide to Club Membership & Conduct,* 3rd edition, 2005 (93)
   The IHRSA requires facilities conforming to its standards to develop and execute an effective

EAP that includes "three critical components: (1) a timely response; (2) an appropriate plan; and (3) qualified personnel" (93, p. 4). A staff member with CPR certification should be available at all times.

5) ***Medical Fitness Association's Standards and Guidelines for Medical Fitness Center Facilities,*** 2nd edition, 2013 (94)

Standards and guidelines published by the Medical Fitness Association provide a road map for medically integrated fitness facilities seeking to enhance the quality of their services. They also distinguish "medical fitness centers" from traditional health and fitness facilities. Fitness facilities collaborating with medical professionals may market their services as safer and better suited for dealing with emergency situations. Key factors identified which set medical fitness centers apart are: (a) active and regular medical oversight, (b) staff qualifications including all staff members maintaining AED and CPR certifications, and (c) written policies and procedures concerning emergency response.

The chapter titled Risk Management and Emergency Response contains five standards and 22 guidelines. The standards require, among other policies and procedures, a written emergency response plan, an appropriate number of AEDs, signage including (a) hazardous chemicals and blood-borne pathogens, and (b) fire and related emergencies. Guideline #6 recommends holding emergency drills at least four times each year.

6) ***Exercise Standards & Guidelines Reference Manual,*** 5th edition, 2010, published by Aerobics and Fitness Association of America (AFAA) (95)

The AFAA recommends that all facilities develop and implement a written emergency response plan. The emergency plan should be rehearsed and practiced four times per year as recommended by other authorities. In addition, steps are described that should be followed when an emergency occurs including calling EMS (i.e., 911 in most areas) and providing appropriate care until EMS arrives. Fitness instructors should maintain CPR and AED certifications. First-aid training is also recommended.

7) ***Safeguarding Health and Well-Being, Medical Advisory Committee Recommendations: A Resource Guide for YMCAs,*** 2011 (96)

This publication strongly recommends YMCA facilities maintain an on-site AED, accessible within a 90-second walk from anywhere in the facility to reduce response time in the event of a cardiac emergency. This publication also recommends that YMCAs follow published standards of practice such as the ACSM/AHA joint position statement (99) regarding the use and accessibility of AEDs and the ACSM's Standards and Guidelines (90). Several other recommendations are addressed, such as having (a) staff members certified in CPR/AED, (b) operating guidelines regarding HIV/AIDS, and (c) a medical advisory committee that establishes emergency response procedures consistent with state and local laws. The YMCA encourages branch facilities to have certain AED equipment specifically designed to deliver lower energy levels for pediatric victims. In addition, guidelines and staff requirements are provided regarding the use of supplemental oxygen.

8) ***American Association for Cardiovascular and Pulmonary Rehabilitation (AACVPR), Guidelines for Cardiac Rehabilitation and Secondary Prevention Programs,*** 5th edition, 2013 (97)

The AACVPR provides eight guidelines regarding emergencies with each guideline describing several recommendations. Examples of these guidelines include emergency equipment and maintenance, professional staff and emergency care, and personnel requirements related to emergency care. For example, regularly scheduled and documented emergency procedure in-services (trainings) should occur at least four times per year. The appendix includes related documents such as daily emergency cart checklist, emergency equipment maintenance log, and mock code (i.e., SCA) and emergency in-service log.

9) ***American College of Occupational and Environmental Medicine (ACOEM)—AEDs*** (98)

The ACOEM recommends creating a complete AED program with clearly defined managerial responsibilities to address the prevention of SCA mortality among working age adults. A qualified professional should be assigned to manage all medical aspects of the program. The AED program should represent a component of a more general emergency response plan and should include: awareness and placement of AEDs to ensure easy and timely access; efficient communication procedures in the event of a cardiac emergency; assessment of scene and patient; CPR and AED response protocols; clinically appropriate transportation to a medical facility; equipment maintenance and replacement protocols; and methods of post-incident documentation and follow-up care. The ACOEM emphasizes that acquiring an AED is but one aspect of an AED program. An effective program should be continuously managed and refined.

10) *ACSM/AHA Joint Position Statement—AEDs* (99)

The ACSM and AHA released an updated Joint Statement in 2002 specifically addressing AEDs in health/fitness facilities. The organizations premised their recommendations by explaining, the time from collapse to defibrillation represents the single greatest determinant of survival in the event of cardiac arrest. ACSM/AHA statistics suggest an increase in adverse cardiovascular events caused by the steadily increasing membership of populations over the age of 35 (the group most affected by cardiovascular disease and cardiac arrest). In light of growing threats, this ACSM/AHA publication includes four standards directly applicable to emergency planning. Every fitness facility is encouraged to document and implement an EAP in coordination with local EMS. The Joint Statement highlights the importance of conducting bi-annual practice drills with an AED to help ensure efficiency of the facility EAP and practice documenting AED events while respecting protected personal information.

KEY POINT

Emergency equipment (e.g., AEDs, first-aid kits) alone does not save lives—rather, it is the cumulative efforts of planning and proper response by well-trained staff members. Almost all of the published standards of practice recommended regular staff trainings (rehearsals, drills) to help ensure the facility's written medical EAP will be carried out properly and efficiently when an injury occurs. The spotlight case, *Locke v. Life Time Fitness, Inc.*, demonstrates the importance of staff training from a legal liability perspective.

SPOTLIGHT CASE

Locke v. Life Time Fitness, Inc.
20 F. Supp. 3d 669 (D. Ill., N.D., 2014)

FACTS

Historical Facts:

Antowine Locke, a member of Life Time health and fitness club, collapsed while playing basketball at the club due to an apparent cardiac arrest. Employees at the club allegedly failed to retrieve an AED available at the club. EMS personnel arrived at the scene within six minutes but were unable to save Locke. When Locke became a member of the club, he was required to sign a member agreement that included an exculpatory clause which included, in part:

ASSUMPTION OF RISK AND WAIVER OF LIABILITY

I understand that there is an inherent risk of injury, whether caused by me or someone else, in the use of or presence at a Life Time Fitness center, the use of equipment and services at a Life Time Fitness center, and participation in Life Time Fitness' programs. This risk includes, but is not limited to:

Locke continued...

1. Injuries arising from the use of any Life Time Fitness' centers or equipment, including any accidental or 'slip and fall' injuries;

2. *Injuries arising from participation in supervised or unsupervised activities and programs within a Life Time Fitness center or outside a Life Time Fitness center,* to the extent sponsored or endorsed by Life Time Fitness;

3. *Injuries or medical disorders resulting from exercise at a Life Time Fitness center, including,* but not limited to, heart attacks, strokes, heart stress, sprains, broken bones and torn muscles or ligaments; and

4. *Injuries resulting from the actions taken or decisions made regarding medical or survival procedures.*

I understand and voluntarily accept this risk. I agree to specifically assume all risk of injury, whether physical or mental, as well as all risk of loss, theft or damage of personal property for me, any person that is a part of this membership and any guest under this membership while such persons are using or present at any Life Time Fitness center, using any lockers, equipment, or services at any Life Time Fitness center or participating in Life Time Fitness' programs, whether such programs take place inside or outside of a Life Time Fitness center. I waive any and all claims or actions that may arise against Life Time Fitness, Inc., its affiliates, subsidiaries, successors or assigns (collectively, 'Life Time Fitness') as well as each party's owners, directors, employees or volunteers as a result of any such injury, loss, theft, or damage to any such person, including and without limitation, personal bodily or mental injury, economic loss or any damage to me, my spouse, my children, or guests resulting from the negligence of Life Time Fitness or anyone else using a Life Time Fitness center. If there is any claim by anyone based on any injury, loss, theft or damage that involves me, any person that is a part of my membership, or any guest under this membership, I agree to defend Life Time Fitness against such claims and pay Life Time Fitness for all expenses relating to the claim, and indemnify Life Time Fitness for all obligations resulting from such claims (p. 672).

Procedural Facts:

The wife of the decedent, Tracy Locke, filed a wrongful death claim against Life Time Fitness due to the negligence of the employees. Locke alleged Life Time Fitness failed to: (a) use the AED on a club member, (b) adopt an emergency response plan, (c) train employees to properly identify and respond to health emergencies, (d) have such trained employees present during business hours, and (e) provide proper crowd control following the collapse of member. Additionally, Locke alleged Life Time Fitness employees had negligently and incorrectly informed the 911 operator that Antowine Locke was suffering from an asthma attack.

Life Time Fitness contested the plaintiff, Tracy Locke, should be barred from pursuing her wrongful death claim based on the terms set forth in the assumption of risk and waiver of liability provisions included in the membership agreement her husband signed. Accordingly, Life Time Fitness asked the court for summary judgment.

ISSUE

Did the assumption of risk and waiver of liability in the member agreement, signed by the decedent, bar the wrongful death claim made by the plaintiff, the decedent's wife?

COURT'S RULING

No, the plaintiff was not barred to pursue her wrongful death claim based on one of the negligent claims made against the defendant (i.e., the failure to properly train Life Time employees regarding health emergencies). Therefore, summary judgment was denied on this claim.

COURT'S REASONING

Referring to previous case law, the court stated that a valid exculpatory clause "must spell out the intention of the parties with great particularity" and "contain clear, explicit, and unequivocal language referencing the types of activities…

Locke continued...

it encompasses for which the plaintiff agrees to relieve the defendant from a duty of care" (p. 673). Although the exculpatory clause covers injuries resulting from a heart attack, the exculpatory clause is silent on the issue of improper training of Life Time employees relating to responding to medical emergencies. The court stated that Life Time Fitness could have added "inadequate training" to the exculpatory clause but chose not to do so.

The defendant also argued that Antowine assumed the inherent risk of injury and that improper training of Life Time employees was an inherent risk, addressed in the assumption of risk and waiver of liability provisions, by the following statement: *Injuries resulting from the actions taken or decisions made regarding medical or survival procedures.* According to the court, this statement "does not specifically encompass the training of Life Time Fitness employees to respond to health emergencies" and thus "Life Time has not shown that the parties contemplated that Antowine would assume the risk for injuries resulting from the inadequate training of Life Time employees as how to deal with health emergencies" (p. 674).

Lessons Learned from *Locke:*

Legal

▸ A wrongful death claim is a type of civil claim under tort law.

▸ Based on this court in Illinois, exculpatory clauses need to be explicit. Although the exculpatory clause absolved the defendant from liability for several negligent claims made by the decedent's wife in this case, it did not for improper training of employees regarding health emergencies because it was not included in the clause.

▸ How specifically exculpatory clauses need to be is based on state law and thus, competent legal counsel is needed to prepare such statements.

▸ The assumption of risk defense was ineffective because Antowine would not have assumed an inherent risk of improper training of employees.

Risk Management/Injury Prevention

▸ Fitness facilities need to have a well-written emergency action plan to cover all types of medical emergencies—minor, major, and life-threatening.

▸ Facility staff members need to know how to properly carry out medical emergency procedures (e.g., practice the procedures in trainings and rehearsals) and how to properly prepare an incident report form after each medical emergency for documentation purposes.

▸ Facilities need to have medical emergency equipment (e.g., first-aid kit, AED) and staff members who possess current certifications in first-aid, CPR, and AED.

DEVELOPMENT OF RISK MANAGEMENT STRATEGIES

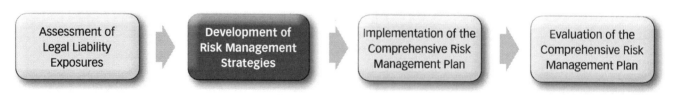

Assessment of Legal Liability Exposures ▸ Development of Risk Management Strategies ▸ Implementation of the Comprehensive Risk Management Plan ▸ Evaluation of the Comprehensive Risk Management Plan

Emergency Action Plans

Emergency planning begins with identifying potential threats. Facility management must prepare for emergencies beyond the more common medical scenarios. Every EAP should function to reasonably protect the health and safety of employees, members, and guests. By anticipating potential emergencies and working with professionals to create a systematic response, fitness managers/owners and exercise professionals can maximize opportunities to control the situation and mitigate harm when an emergency occurs.

EAPs need to address two major types of emergencies: (a) potential dangers which may trigger evacuation, such as inclement weather, fire, or an active shooter, and (b) medical emergencies such as a sudden cardiac arrest or a bone fracture. For each foreseeable scenario, fitness managers/owners are encouraged to follow the acronym DRI:

- *Develop* a written contingency plan;
- *Rehearse* procedures and implement staff training programs to maintain response readiness; and
- *Improve* effectiveness by measuring performance and getting feedback from emergency response and medical professionals.

The Department of Homeland Security provides a comprehensive resource entitled "Emergency Response Plan." It covers about every possible emergency situation that could arise in the workplace and includes a helpful section (Ten Steps to Developing an Emergency Response Plan) as well as links to many resources. It is available at: https://www.ready.gov/business/implementation/emergency.

OSHA offers an interactive online program (Evacuation Plans and Procedures eTool) that can assist small to mid-sized organizations to develop and implement an OSHA-compliant EAP (100). Fitness facility managers/owners can utilize this easy-to-use system to create a foundational EAP. Elements of an effective EAP should incorporate methods of reporting emergencies, escape routes and evacuation procedures, delegation of employee responsibilities, post-emergency documentation and managerial contact information.

EAP—Evacuation Plans

Congregation of large groups presents public safety and environmental risks. As a component of an effective EAP, every fitness facility must have a practiced plan for evacuating all participants and employees. According to OSHA, those responsible for developing the EAP need to determine: (a) conditions when evacuation is necessary, (b) designation of the person(s) authorized to initiate evacuation, (c) specific evacuation procedures, (d) methods for accounting for employees after

an evacuation, and (e) provide appropriate protective equipment and/or respirators to ensure a reasonably safe environment (101). To comply with OSHA regulations, fitness facilities must ensure unobstructed access to exit routes and have appropriate exit and evacuation signage to direct participants and employees to safety. See Figure 11-2 for an example evacuation floor plan that can be posted.

Fitness facility managers/owners must also account for the specific needs of their participants. Under the Americans with Disabilities Act, both public and private entities must ensure equal access to programs and services for people with disabilities (102). The Act "applies with equal force to facially neutral policies that discriminate against individuals with disabilities" (103, p. 1061). This includes policies which disparately impact people with disabilities by, for example, requiring the use of stairs for evacuation. A recent article exploring emergency response procedures of academic institutions identified weaknesses in egress routes, especially in older buildings, which presented risks for individuals with disabilities (104).

Figure 11-2: OSHA's Interactive Floorplan Example*

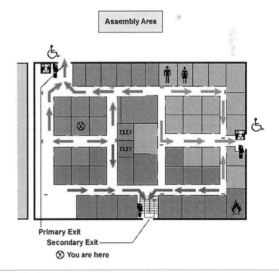

*From: https://www.osha.gov/SLTC/etools/evacuation/floorplan_demo.html. Accessed February 23, 2020.

Natural Disasters

Depending on geographical location, natural disasters including tornadoes, hurricanes, flooding and/or earthquakes may require independent response planning. The impact of a disaster can be moderated by establishing and practicing a plan for evacuation, securing, and reevaluating complete insurance coverage, and communicating with facility members, neighboring businesses and agencies involved in disaster response. Evacuation to a designated safety zone or bunker may be necessary. Designating staff responsibilities beforehand and conducting mock evacuations demonstrate a fitness facility's commitment to staff and participant safety. OSHA recommends identifying a place to take shelter, monitoring local weather warning systems, and establishing procedures to account for individuals in the building (105).

Fire

Fires can be caused by faulty electrical wiring of exercise equipment, faulty outlets, cooking accidents, gas leaks, or set intentionally. Under common law principles of premises liability, business owners are responsible for maintaining their properties in order to prevent hazardous situations that may result in a fire (106). OSHA regulations require each EAP to include procedures addressing evacuation due to a fire, highlighting the importance of communicating with local fire departments and emergency response professionals (107). Although OSHA does not specifically require fire maps to be posted within facilities, clearly informing members of the location of secondary exits and emergency equipment is encouraged and may be required by insurance carriers or local agencies. Facility owners should review and implement state and local requirements to demonstrate prioritization of staff and participant safety.

According to the U.S. Fire Administration, the number of fires in the U.S. has been steadily declining since 2008 (108). However, the severity of occurrences has caused a recent spike in monetary damages and destruction. In 2018, over 1.3 million fires resulted in an estimated $25.6 billion in direct property loss, including $12.4 billion in losses from major California wildfires (109). In 2015 and 2017, wildfires accounted for the destruction of over 10 million acres of land. In March 2019, a fire broke out in the utility closet of a Costa Mesa, California gym, requiring patrons to

evacuate (110). In February 2019, fire erupted after an aerosol can fell on a malfunctioning transformer within the maintenance closet of a New York Gold's Gym. Two employees were transported to the hospital for treatment, but staff members were able to control the fire by using extinguishers and contacting emergency responders in accordance with the facility's EAP (111).

Active Shooter

An effective EAP should consider how to respond to an active shooter. Active shooter incidents have occurred in at least seven fitness facilities since 2009 (112). In May 2019, four men and a boy were shot at a recreation center in Washington, D.C. (113). According to the FBI, active shooter prevention requires an active commitment by facility managers/owners to mitigate harm. When faced with an active shooter emergency, three options are presented: run, fight, or hide. Fitness managers/owners should consider the circumstances which dictate the appropriate response. Similar to OSHA's virtual EAP program, the U.S. Department of Homeland Security offers a virtual training tool designed to help organizations develop their active shooter emergency action plan (114). Effective active shooter EAPs, like other components of the more general facility EAP, include developing methods of communication, delegation of responsibility, employee training and post-event accounting and follow-up procedures. Fitness facilities managers/owners should collaborate with local law enforcement in the development of an effective active shooter EAP and employee training program.

Threats of violence can come in many forms. According to the Department of Justice, bomb threats to assembly locations, where people gather for recreational, educational, or social purposes, increased by 30% from 2016 to 2017 (115). A Planet Fitness located in Michigan initiated emergency protocols when a member's WIFI network was labeled "remote detonator," and made available through the network (116). In Connecticut, a training grenade was found in a trash can outside an LA Fitness, resulting in evacuation of the facility (117).

If there is suspicion of an explosive device in the vicinity, law enforcement should be contacted and the facility should be immediately evacuated in a practiced manner. Facility staff should be trained how to respond to bomb threats or suspicious packages. As an aspect of this training, employees answering phones should be taught how to gather and record evidentiary information from threatening callers in a calm and concerned manner.

After an evacuation (or a threat of violence or violent act) has taken place, the incident needs to be documented. An evacuation report, similar to the sample Injury Report in the appendix, can be developed. Documentation is essential for legal liability reasons as well as to comply with any applicable laws and OSHA regulations. See the OSHA websites (100, 101) for more information on documentation. Local first responders have their own documentation that is completed after responding to an emergency. First responders and staff members at regional OHSA offices offer a useful resource for fitness facilities developing evacuation plans and employee training programs.

EAP—Medical Emergency Plans

Many fitness facilities are unprepared to handle an emergency. Since the AHA and the ACSM initially collaborated in 1998 to publish recommendations for emergency response planning, various surveys have been conducted to evaluate industry compliance. As

discussed, the AHA/ACSM jointly believe every fitness center should have a written EAP and practice established procedures at least twice per year. Four other professional organizations recommended rehearsals or drills at least four times per year. Fitness facilities should maintain as many AEDs as needed to keep SCA response time under five minutes (40).

A study of Ohio fitness facilities revealed that the majority of the facilities (53%) had no written emergency response plan and 92% failed to conduct emergency response drills as described in published national standards (118). A national study found that only 61% of facilities had taken steps to ensure that staff members fully understood how to implement the facility's written EAP (119). A 2008 survey of Washington fitness facilities found just 68% of the survey respondents indicated their facility utilized a written emergency response plan for sudden cardiac arrest (SCA) (120). Of the clubs with more than 1,500 members, 71% maintained an on-site AED (120).

The gap between AHA/ACSM and other professional organizations' recommendations and practical application shows that many fitness facilities either (a) have not created a medical EAP, or (b) are not providing adequate staff training. These deficiencies can easily result in uncertainty, panic and/or wasted time when an emergency occurs. Given the frequency of

Table 11-2	Spotlight Cases in Previous Chapters: Improper Emergency Care		
SPOTLIGHT CASE (CHAPTER)	**INITIAL INJURY**	**IMPROPER ACTION OF EXERCISE PROFESSIONAL(S)**	**RESULTING INJURY OR DEATH**
Howard v. Missouri Bone and Joint Center (6)	Athlete felt pop/sharp pain in lower back while performing squat lifts (pain level of 6)	Instructed the plaintiff to complete the set of lifts versus stopping and seeking medical care (pain level of 10)	Herniated disc requiring surgery and permanent damage to spine
Bartlett v. Push to Walk (7)	While performing a new exercise, individual with spinal cord injury became symptomatic	Instructed/encouraged the plaintiff to perform an exercise again versus stopping and seeking medical care—serious symptoms/pain resulted	Fractured leg that could not be repaired due to his spinal cord injury and unable to continue with exercise therapy
UCF Athletics Association v. Plancher (8)	Athlete collapsed after experiencing signs/symptoms of overexertion during intense workout	Instructed the athlete to continue with the drills versus addressing the signs and symptoms and seeking medical care	Collapsed again resulting in death
Miller v. YMCA of Central Massachusetts, et al. (10)	A Silver Sneakers participant found unconscious in steam room	Employees unable to access the steam room to shut off the steam vent and administer emergency care	Multiple surgeries for second degree burns; Death resulted three weeks later

SCA occurrences, coupled with increased popularity of recreational exercise and the growing prevalence of hypertension and obesity, facilities not following professional recommendations avail themselves to significant legal risk.

Supplementing cases discussed in this chapter; previous chapters have described cases involving improper emergency actions by fitness facility employees which may have aggravated harm. See Table 11-2 (previous page) for spotlight cases described in other chapters. As demonstrated in these cases, serious injuries or death may have been prevented if appropriate emergency care had been promptly provided.

Developing Effective EAPs

EAPs should correspond to the type of facility and the risk level of each facility's participants and personnel. Staff training and preparedness as part of a medical EAP is always important, but becomes particularly crucial if a facility markets its services to populations with a greater propensity for certain medical conditions. "At-risk" populations include men aged 35-45 who, according to the Cleveland Clinic, are affected by SCA twice as often as their female counterparts (121). It is important to remember that 60% of adults in the U.S. have one chronic disease and 40% have two or more chronic diseases, as described in Chapter 6.

Developing effective EAPs is one of the most important investments fitness facilities can make to reduce liability arising from evacuation situations or medical emergencies. The burdens of a lawsuit extend beyond attorney's fees, expert witnesses, and the energy spent defending against claims of negligent care. A public dispute can portray lack of care for participant health and safety. By contrast, maintaining readiness to respond to emergency scenarios helps participants feel safe, which can encourage consumer loyalty. Committing assets to the development of effective EAPs not only has the potential to save lives, it is an essential component of a strong organization.

Anticipating variables which arise during an emergency is a key component of the planning process. Prior to an emergency, management can establish codes to alert staff without creating panic, delegate responsibilities, consider the availability and accessibility of

equipment, communicate with professional services, receive feedback, and refine procedures. No single plan can accommodate all fitness facilities. Facility design, location, the type of emergency, location of the emergency and specific needs of participants must be considered. EAPs must be comprehensive but easy to execute. The role of facility managers/owners is to place staff in the best position to respond in an appropriate manner when an emergency occurs. This includes making sure appropriate equipment is available and well-maintained. In addition, effective communication and training will enable staff to know their responsibilities and remain calm while executing their role. Emergencies must be handled as a team in a prompt, intentional manner.

Putting an EAP into Action

An effective EAP requires multiple layers of effective communication. Facility employees trained in emergency medical response techniques need to be alerted where the incident has occurred without causing panic in the facility. To alert employees, an EAP may designate code words which trigger an appropriate response. Most hospitals use codes blue, red and black to alert staff to emergencies within the building. "Blue" signifies a patient is suffering cardiac arrest, "Red" constitutes a fire alarm and "black" triggers evacuation due to a bomb threat. Since a number of people may be aware of these codes, fitness facilities may choose alternative codes to avoid creating panic. However, facility managers should consider that citizens familiar with common emergency codes may be medical professionals who have received emergency response training and may be able to provide assistance.

In addition to alerting staff, local EMS may need to be contacted. An EAP should include how to determine whether it is necessary to call EMS (e.g., 911), which staff members are responsible for making this call and what information to provide. An EAP should include how to identify the participant needing medical assistance. Once identified, the participant's emergency information should be recovered and provided to EMS upon their arrival. Personal information regarding each participant should include an emergency contact and unique health factors. As described in

Chapter 6, obtaining medical and emergency contact information should be obtained upon joining the facility, or prior to participation in facility programs, and kept on file for quick access when needed. An EAP should provide for when to contact this person and what information to provide. Implementing mock scenarios can support providing communication in a calm, practiced manner.

Execution of Responsibilities

Perfectly written EAPs are useless without employees capable of executing their roles. Facility managers/owners need to take a proactive approach to training their employees and requiring necessary AED/CPR and first-aid certifications. Emergencies are innately chaotic. Facility employees, typically focused on providing members with an enjoyable fitness experience, may react unexpectedly during an emergency. To remind employees of their roles during an emergency, abbreviated EAPs should be posted in various areas within the facility for quick reference.

Conducting mock training scenarios is an essential preparation tool. These drills may incorporate the participation of EMS or professional medical providers. At its conclusion, each training drill should be reflected upon to sharpen the response and anticipate additional variables. Practicing the EAPs can expose flaws in a response plan before lives are at risk. Facility owners/managers should remember that juries may not be sympathetic to the pressures of real-life emergency scenarios.

After an Emergency Occurs

An emergency event does not conclude after first responders (e.g., police, firefighters) or EMS take control of the scene. From a legal perspective, documenting the event and fulfilling the appropriate reporting requirements are as important as actions taken during the emergency. Post-incident forms should be created for use after an evacuation or violent threat, as described above, and after a medical emergency such as the Injury Report shown in the appendix. Information collected in an Injury Report includes: location of the incident, member information, names of staff who responded, response measures, witness information, and creating a timetable of the event (i.e., when the collapse occurred, when staff responded, when an AED was brought to the scene/administered, when EMS arrived, etc.).

Most states that require fitness facilities to maintain AEDs also require reporting their use to local EMS and/or state health departments. For example, Arizona requires each trained responder who uses an AED on a person to submit a written report to the bureau of EMS and trauma systems in the Department of Health Services (122). Additional information regarding state AED requirements can be found earlier in this chapter.

RISK MANAGEMENT STRATEGIES

The following strategies highlight foundational components of effective EAPs. As previously discussed, each facility is unique and demands individualized emergency response planning. Factors to consider include the types of programs or services offered by the facility, membership size and demographics, staff size and experience, local EMS availability, and facility size and layout. Legal risk can never be completely absolved, but implementing the following strategies will help to reduce litigation costs and demonstrate attentiveness and care for the health and safety of fitness participants.

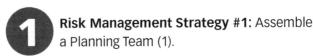 **Risk Management Strategy #1:** Assemble a Planning Team (1).

For fitness facility manager/owners, the first step in implementing effective EAPs is to decide who will participate in developing the written EAPs. The planning team may consist of professional staff members, management, and members of the facility's risk management advisory committee (e.g., legal counsel, insurance representatives, medical professionals) as well as local first responders including EMS personnel. An EAP coordinator (e.g., a full-time professional staff member) should be identified at this stage in accordance with industry best practices. This role carries significant responsibility. The EAP coordinator needs to be made aware of their duties and the position should be formalized with an official job title. The EAP coordinator should possess excellent teaching skills that are needed to properly train staff members who serve as **manager on duty (MOD)** and other staff members regarding their EAP duties while on the job. MOD is described under Risk Management Strategy #4. With the assistance of legal counsel, the EAP planning team should first assess all applicable state and local rules and regulations pertaining to emergencies within businesses and places of public assembly. After gaining an understanding of statutory and regulatory requirements, the team should assess the types of emergencies most likely to occur and establish EAP priorities accordingly. This assessment should consider how professional guidance and incident trends relate to the fitness facility's unique characteristics.

 Risk Management Strategy #2: Comply with Federal Laws, State Laws, and Published Standards of Practice.

At the federal level, OSHA has enacted a number of regulations applicable to fitness facility emergency preparedness and response planning, such as the General Industry Standards and Bloodborne Pathogen Standard. These two OSHA standards were briefly described earlier in this chapter. It is essential that fitness manager/owners consult with legal counsel to help ensure they are compliant with all OSHA regulations included in these two standards plus additional OSHA regulations briefly discussed in other chapters as well as other federal and state OSHA regulations not covered in this textbook. As a reminder from Chapter 3, any business with one or more employees needs to comply with federal OSHA regulations. Also, as stated earlier, OSHA requires employee training that includes hazardous substances, bloodborne pathogens, and emergency situations including how to exit the building. Training is required so that employees know what to do if an OSHA inspector arrives to inspect the premises (123).

OSHA inspections can occur anytime, both scheduled and unannounced. Fitness managers/owners seeking exemption from OSHA inspections may consider applying for OSHA's Voluntary Protection Program (VPP). Participating private employers must undergo a rigorous on-site evaluation by a team of safety and health professionals. More information about applying for OSHA's VPP can be found on OSHA's webpage (124). Additional information regarding compliance with federal regulations is offered by OSHA Regional Offices (125). Each of the ten OSHA Regional Offices has a BBP coordinator available to help with BBP-specific compliance questions.

In addition to federal requirements, it is essential for fitness facility managers/owners to understand and adhere to OSHA state laws and other state laws applicable to their EAPs. As presented earlier, these include without limitation: first-aid, AED, Good Samaritan, and DNR statutes. As with federal laws, it is essential that fitness managers/owners seek counsel from a licensed attorney who is familiar with their state laws.

EAPs should reflect published standards of practice. Various publications were summarized above describing standards and guidelines such as CPR/AED certifications of employees, having and using AEDs, and practicing the EAP. As demonstrated in the *Miglino*, *Zihlman*, and *Mayer* cases, these publications may be introduced by plaintiffs as evidence that the courts may consider when determining duty in negligence cases.

3 **Risk Management Strategy #3:** Develop Evacuation and Medical Emergency EAPs.

Fitness facilities should have written EAPs for staff members to follow as previously described—one EAP that covers evacuation plans (including violent threats/acts) and one that covers medical emergencies. These written plans can be included in the facility's Risk Management Policies and Procedures Manual (RMPP) and used in staff training programs. The facility EAP team should take time to proactively consider ideal evacuation routes, plan for contingencies, and coordinate with local emergency response professionals to collect input from as many qualified sources as possible.

Most of this chapter's discussion of medical emergency planning has been directed toward sudden cardiac arrest. As previously stated, every minute which passes without an effective heartbeat reduces the chances of survival by 10%. Responding to a SCA with speed and efficiency should be the facility's top priority. Facility managers/owners need to realize that their level of preparation will dictate the extent to which a medical emergency affects their organization.

Beyond SCAs, injuries within fitness facilities can come in multiple varieties. Medical issues can be classified into four categories: (a) minor injuries, including small lacerations or a sprained joint, (b) serious injuries, like severe vertebrae issues or bone fractures, (c) injuries which cause major bleeding, and (d) life-threatening events. A written contingency plan should be established for each category including appropriate first-aid/CPR/AED procedures and staff responsibilities. To make responsibilities easier to understand, these contingency plans can be summarized in a flowchart clearly depicting steps staff should follow in the event of an emergency. See Figure 11-3 for an example of a flowchart that summarizes a medical emergency contingency plan for a "serious injury" scenario. The employee in this scenario would be the employee first on the scene (first responder) and the supervisor would likely be the MOD. Both have several responsibilities including the provision of proper first aid to the victim until EMS arrives.

Risk Management Strategy #4: Determine Staff Credentials and Allocate Responsibilities (1).

All staff members who may be called upon to respond to a medical emergency should be trained and certified in first aid, CPR, and AED. Various organizations offer these certifications but it is best to consider organizations such as the AHA and American Red Cross. The certifications selected should meet the qualifications specified by certifying organizations such as ACSM (e.g., the CPR certification cannot be obtained online—there must be a hands-on practical component). Fitness managers/owners may want to consider AHA Training Centers which are independent businesses that have entered into an agreement with AHA to provide CPR and first-aid training based on AHA curriculum and products.

Facility employees typically requiring EAP training and first-aid, CPR, and AED certifications include, but not limited to, managers/supervisors, personal fitness

Figure 11-3: Flowchart: Example Contingency Plan for a "Serious Injury"

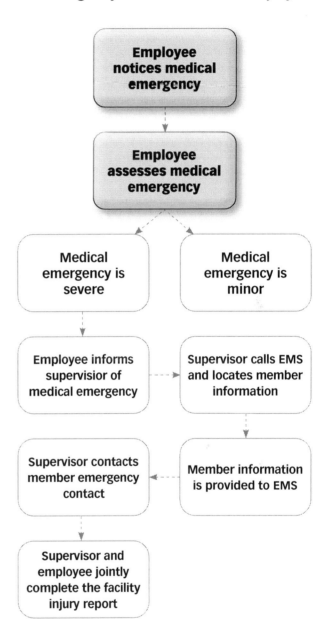

trainers, group exercise instructors, independent contractors, child care personnel, and front desk receptionists (1). Facility managers/owners should consider having the EAP coordinator, and perhaps other professional staff members, obtain instructor certifications in first aid, CPR, and AED. These staff members could provide periodic in-service staff trainings so employees can conveniently re-certify when needed. The fitness manager or EAP coordinator should keep employee certification records to ensure employees maintain current certifications. It is important that new employees receive EAP training and obtain their certifications in a timely fashion such as during the probationary phase of their employment.

At all times during facility operation, a professional staff member should be designated as the MOD (1). The MOD will likely be in the best position to determine the appropriate classification of a medical incident, assist EMS if necessary, and lead the execution of a facility's EAP. The MOD assumes the responsibility for completing post-incident documentation such as an Injury Report. A sample Injury Report is provided in the appendix.

 Risk Management Strategy #5: Establish an Effective Communications System (1).

A well-developed EAP should include a system of communication which cultivates organization and structure during emergency situations. The best time for planning appropriate communication is before an emergency occurs. Relevant questions to answer include:

1) How will the first staff member responding to the scene inform other staff members and the MOD of the emergency?

2) How do procedures differ based on the location of the emergency?

3) Who will contact EMS, if necessary, and what will be said?

4) If the first responder (or MOD) on the scene determines the need for an AED or first-aid kit, how and to whom is this communicated so that the AED is delivered in a timely fashion?

An effective internal communications system is essential. The facility's written EAP should address these questions as well as provide protocols for all anticipated scenarios. Some facilities may consider developing coded language in order to maintain control of an emergency situation. Using "code blue" procedures similar to common hospital EAPs may alert qualified medical professionals present in the facility who may be able to offer support. Some facilities implement panic buttons, similar to banks, which alert the front desk and/or other staff of the location of an emergency.

Some fitness facilities also have emergency phones located throughout the facility.

Emergency signage throughout the facility should be included as a component of the EAP. For example, each facility should provide signs clearly depicting where AED(s) are located. Each AED should include instructions for use on the device's storage container. Fitness facility managers or EAP coordinators need to post, in high-traffic areas, abbreviated versions of EAP protocols or flowcharts for responding to the most serious threats, such as fire or SCA. This way, staff members are constantly reminded of the emergency response procedures and fitness participants know their health and safety is a facility priority. As described in Chapter 10, pointing out all facility safety signage should be done during an orientation for new participants.

In the development phase of each EAP, external communication with local emergency response professionals is essential. These professionals can provide guidance and assistance to help ensure EAPs are properly developed and effective communication procedures with local emergency agencies have been addressed and incorporated. The contact information for these local emergency agencies should be posted at the front desk. EAPs should designate who will meet emergency response professionals when they arrive and direct them to the specific location of the emergency.

Note: *The above risk management strategies (#1 through #5) reflect the facility's Evacuation EAP and Medical Emergency EAP. Risk Management Strategies #6 through #8 primarily reflect the facility's Medical Emergency EAP. Risk Management Strategies #9 and #10 reflect both. However, if a medical emergency occurs when an evacuation or violent act occurs, the medical emergency EAP also needs to be followed.*

 Risk Management Strategy #6: Provide and Maintain AED(s) and First-Aid Kits (1).

All fitness facilities should maintain at least one comprehensive first-aid kit and an operable AED, even if not required by state law. The number of AEDs a facility needs, and their placement, should be determined based on the size and layout of the facility. AEDs should be situated in a manner permitting administration to a victim in under five minutes (40), regardless of the victim's location within the facility. AEDs should be easy to access. Directions for use should be provided on the housing compartment. As described in Chapter 10, signage indicating the locations of all first-aid kits and AEDs should be posted. These locations should be included in the facility's written EAP and reviewed in staff trainings. Facilities electing to provide additional emergency equipment may consider making supplemental oxygen available and training staff members in the appropriate use of such equipment.

The *Diniro v. Aspen Athletic Club, LLC* case, previously described, demonstrates the importance of performing regular inspections of AEDs to help ensure they are operating properly. In this case, the fitness facility had two AEDs but neither were operable. Regular maintenance of all first-aid kits and AEDs is essential. The maintenance specifications provided in the AED owner's manual must be followed just as maintenance specifications in the owner's manuals for all exercise equipment need to be followed, as described in Chapter 9. Fitness managers or EAP coordinators should accept the responsibility to frequently check and re-stock first-aid kits with appropriate supplies. Information about what a first-aid kit should contain is provided by the American Red Cross (126). OSHA regulations also need to be followed for medical emergency equipment as described above. AEDs must be inspected and maintained regularly as specified in a minority of state statutes.

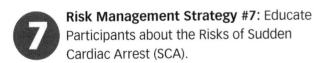

Risk Management Strategy #7: Educate Participants about the Risks of Sudden Cardiac Arrest (SCA).

As previously discussed, SCA is a failure of the heart's electrical system which subsequently diminishes or ceases blood flow to the brain and other vital organs. During exercise, muscles consume more oxygen, creating a greater demand from other biological systems. In response, hearts increase the rate at which blood is pumped throughout the cardiovascular system. This enhanced output causes variations in blood pressure

as vessels dilate to allow blood flow. Failure to properly warm up or cool down after exercise can cause imbalances in oxygen requirements or blood flow for which the body is not prepared. This can cause SCA in someone with documented or latent cardiovascular disease.

By understanding common causes for SCA, fitness facility managers/owners can create policies and procedures to educate participants how to properly prepare for exercise and transition from a vigorous workout. As described in Chapter 10, one of the educational topics to cover in the facility orientation for new participants addresses basic principles of safe exercise (e.g., warm-up, cool-down, progression, monitoring intensity, and signs/symptoms of overexertion). It is important for exercise professionals to educate participants how to exercise safely as well as how to design a training program appropriate for their personal health and fitness level. Dr. Anthony Abbott, Founder and President of Fitness Institute International, Inc., believes exercise professionals can help prevent the occurrence of SCAs and other injuries by following STEPS, an acronym for screening, testing, evaluating, programming, and supervising (127). These STEPS are further detailed in Chapters 6-8.

Risk Management Strategy #8: Develop and Implement Post-Emergency Procedures (1).

It is essential that professional staff members serving in MOD roles receive comprehensive training on how to properly carry out their responsibilities, including all post-emergency procedures. After a medical emergency, these procedures include interviewing eyewitnesses, taking photographs, and properly completing an Injury Report. In the event of an evacuation or violent threat, an Evacuation Report should be properly completed. These responsibilities should be included in the MOD's job description.

From a legal perspective, preparing for what to do after an emergency is as important as actions during the emergency itself. Facility employees should be trained regarding what to say and, more importantly, what not to say to an injured participant or others. Employees should express sympathy for the participant's situation, but should not verbally accept responsibility for the injury or say that the facility's insurance will cover medical costs. These comments may be used against the club in court proceedings should the event result in litigation. If the injured participant is cognizant and responsive, the MOD or first staff member to respond to the scene should ask the participant to describe what happened. The participant's explanation should be recorded into an Injury Report, providing as much detail as possible about any surrounding circumstances. If the member is unresponsive, details about the incident should be requested from any participants who witnessed the injury immediately after the injury. Contact information from any eyewitnesses should be recorded as well as their responses to questions asked by the MOD or other designated staff member regarding the incident. Relevant inquiries include: what happened, how did it happen, and when did it happen as well as if the witness observed any unusual behavior of the victim (e.g., misusing the equipment) prior to the injury. It is best to consult with legal counsel as to additional types of interview questions for witnesses.

After a medical emergency scene is cleared, the facility's EAP may require the MOD to take photographs of the area where the incident occurred (e.g., surface conditions, nearby signage, exercise equipment involved in the emergency). If equipment was involved, the MOD should record the name of the manufacturer and serial number of the equipment. A product defect may supersede facility liability if the defect caused the injury. Of course, if a piece of equipment is damaged, other participants need to be notified that the equipment is out-of-service until repaired. See Chapter 9 for such notification procedures.

Once all evidence is obtained, the Injury Report should be promptly completed. See Appendix 11 for a sample form. The facility's manager/owner and the EAP coordinator should seek advice from legal counsel and insurance professionals in the development of the Injury Report. A copy of the Injury Report should be retained at least until the applicable state statute of limitations comes to an end and in accordance with the advice of legal counsel. Most states require personal injury claims to be brought within two or three years. However Maine, for example, permits a claimant to file suit for up to six years. In some injury cases, the facility's EAP may require the facility's manager to immediately send a copy of the Injury Report to the facility's legal counsel and/or insurance provider.

After a serious medical emergency, staff members may be asked to comment about the incident by participants, media, lawyers, and/or insurance providers representing the injured victim. Staff members should be trained how to properly respond to such inquiries and how their comments could be detrimental to the facility if they do not follow facility policies. For example, a proper response might be, "please contact our designated spokesperson or the facility's manager for details about the incident" and to not offer any other information.

After a medical emergency, the MOD or manager should contact the injured party or one of the victim's emergency contacts. This follow-up shows sympathy for the situation and provides an opportunity to receive a status report of the injury. This can be useful to anticipate the potential for future legal action, allowing ownership to plan accordingly. Any information obtained should be added to the Injury Report.

The final step of post-emergency procedures should be to evaluate the execution of the EAP. For example, the facility manager, EAP coordinator, and the MOD completing the Injury Report should determine if all EAP procedures were carried out properly. If not, there may be a need for re-training of staff members. The facility's EAPs should be continually updated as new scenarios and variables are considered as well as any changes in laws and published standards of practice. After updates are made to the facility EAPs, staff training will be necessary to inform staff members of the changes.

 Risk Management Strategy #9: Conduct Training Drills and Refine the Facility's EAPs.

It is essential to continually test the facility's EAPs by conducting regular training drills and working with staff members to improve response procedures. Having a team that knows how to promptly handle an emergency, with control and confidence in their abilities, can mean the difference between life and death. Each version of the EAP should be considered a working draft which can always be improved. Training drills can be announced or initiated without notice. They should include practicing the EAPs for both evacuation scenarios/violent threats and for various categories of medical emergencies from different locations throughout the facility. Each trial should include post-incident procedures, including completion of an Injury Report or Evacuation Report. Documentation of rehearsals should be carefully retained to demonstrate diligence in the facility's commitment to participant safety. Some administrators suggest videotaping rehearsals for documentation and review. Once drafted, each revised EAP should be approved by the EAP planning team, the risk management advisory committee or legal counsel, and medical professionals providing consultation as well as EMS and the local fire/police departments. As described previously, EAP practice drills or rehearsals should occur two-four times per year according to published standards of practice.

Different types of emergency preparedness exercises can broadly be combined into two major groups and test different aspects of an organization and/or systems' emergency preparedness: (a) discussion-based exercises (often referred to by different names, including tabletop or desktop exercises, workshops or seminar-based exercises) and, (b) operation-based exercises (such as drills, functional exercises/ command post exercises, and field exercises) (128). Operation-based exercises are more difficult to conduct and they demand significantly more resources than discussion-based exercises. However, they allow the testing of equipment, plans, procedures, and communication under conditions similar to a real emergency event. Also, see Figure 2-4 in Chapter 2—the Four Ps of Staff Training.

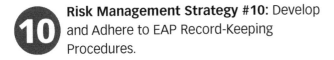

Risk Management Strategy #10: Develop and Adhere to EAP Record-Keeping Procedures.

All components of the facility's EAPs should be formalized in writing and appropriately stored. Injury Reports, Evacuation Reports, and any other relevant documentation, as determined by legal counsel, need

KEY POINT

Although professional organizations have indicated practice drills be conducted two-four times per year, the actual number needed is based on whether facility employees have acquired "competence" (knowledge and skills) to properly carry out the EAPs. More than four may be needed. Facility managers and EAP coordinators should *formally assess* the competence of staff members after EAP trainings and drills. As demonstrated in the cases described in this and other chapters, negligence claims regarding the failure to provide EAP training of staff members are common. In addition, state laws may require such training, such as the state of Texas that requires AED training as described in the *Boggus obo Casey* case.

to be kept secure for a period of time at least as long as the state's statute of limitations. Should legal action arise, these documents will be useful for demonstrating that the facility's personnel properly carried out their duties and responsibilities in accordance with any laws and published standards of practice. The following are examples of documents and components of the facility's EAPs that need to be maintained and kept in a secure location:

a) Medical EAP and Evacuation EAP
b) A written ECP applicable to OSHA's BBP Standard
c) Dates of staff trainings and EAP rehearsals, list of staff members attending trainings/rehearsals, and formal "competence" assessments of staff as well as any medical experts participating in an advisory capacity
d) The name of the EAP coordinator or individual who conducted staff trainings/rehearsals, their credentials, and the content of the training
e) Certification (first aid, CPR, AED) records of all staff members responsible for carrying out the EAPs
f) Inspections of first-aid kits and AEDs
g) Injury and Evacuation Reports and any related evidence gathered post-incident (Note: these reports need to be kept private, confidential, and secure)

RISK MANAGEMENT AUDIT Emergency Planning and Response		
RISK MANAGEMENT (RM) STRATEGY*	**YES ✓**	**NO ✓**
1. Assemble a Planning Team.		
2. Comply with Federal Laws, State Laws, and Published Standards of Practice.		
3. Develop Evacuation and Medical Emergency EAPs.		
4. Determine Staff Credentials and Allocate Responsibilities.		
5. Establish an Effective Communications System.		
6. Provide and Maintain AED(s) and First-Aid Kits.		
7. Educate Participants about the Risks of Sudden Cardiac Arrest (SCA).		
8. Develop and Implement Post-Emergency Procedures.		
9. Conduct Training Drills and Refine the Facility's EAPs.		
10. Develop and Adhere to EAP Record-Keeping Procedures.		

*See the section above—Development of Risk Management Strategies — for the recommendations associated with each risk management strategy and then, for each RM Strategy marked NO, create a list of action steps that need to be completed to meet the recommendations described in that RM strategy.

KEY TERMS

- Automated External Defibrillators (AEDs)
- Emergency Action Plans (EAPs)
- Emergency Medical Services (EMS)
- Exposure Control Plan (ECP)
- Manager on Duty (MOD)

- Negligence per se
- OSHA's Bloodborne Pathogens (BBP) Standard
- Other Potentially Infectious Materials (OPIM)
- Rebuttable Presumption
- Sudden Cardiac Arrest (SCA)

STUDY QUESTIONS

The Study Questions for Chapter 11 can be found on the Fitness Law Academy website (www.fitnesslawacademy.com) under Textbook. They are provided in a fillable format for convenience.

APPENDIX

This chapter's appendix follows the References.

REFERENCES

1. Eickhoff-Shemek JM, Herbert DL, Connaughton, DP. *Risk Management for Health/Fitness Professionals: Legal Issues and Strategies.* Baltimore, MD: Lippincott Williams & Wilkins, 2009.

2. Occupational Safety and Health Standards, 29 C.F.R. § 1910 (1974).

3. Description for 7991: Physical Fitness Facilities. U.S. Department of Labor OSHA. Available at: https://www.osha.gov/pls/imis/sic_manual.display?id=183&tab=description. Accessed December 20, 2019.

4. Occupational Safety and Health Act, 29 U.S.C. §660(c) (1984).

5. BBP Violations Carry Hefty OSHA Fines, OSHA Office of Management Systems. October 2010. Available at: http://blogs.hcpro.com/osha/wp-content/uploads/2010/10/BOIC-p_5-OSHA.pdf. Accessed January 28, 2020.

6. OSHA News Release—Region 2. U.S. Department of Labor OSHA. October 23, 2014. Available at: https://www.osha.gov/news/newsreleases/region2/10232014. Accessed December 17, 2019.

7. Regulations (Standards—29 CFR). U.S. Department of Labor OSHA. Available at: https://www.osha.gov/laws-regs/regulations/standardnumber/1910. Accessed December 17, 2019.

8. OSHA-Authorized Outreach Training Online. OSHA Education Center. Available at: https://www.oshaeducationcenter.com/. Accessed December 17, 2019.

9. OSHA News Release—Region 2. U.S. Department of Labor OSHA. January 14, 2010. Available at: https://www.osha.gov/news/newsreleases/region2/01142010. Accessed December 20, 2019.

10. Campbell R. NFPA's Structure Fires in Stores and Other Mercantile Properties. December 2015. Available at: https://www.nfpa.org/News-and-Research/Data-research-and-tools/Building-and-Life-Safety/Stores-and-other-mercantile-properties. Accessed December 20, 2019.

11. Codes and Standards. National Fire Protection Association. Available at: https://www.nfpa.org/codes-and-standards/all-codes-and-standards/list-of-codes-and-standards/detail?code=101. Accessed December 21, 2019.

12. Chatterjee S, Burns TF. Targeting Heat Shock Proteins in Cancer: A Promising Therapeutic Approach. *International Journal of Molecular Sciences,* 18(9), 2017.

13. Training Requirements in OSHA Standards. Occupational Safety and Health Administration. Available at: https://www.osha.gov/Publications/osha2254.pdf. Accessed December 22, 2019.

14. Citation and Notification of Penalty. U.S. Department of Labor OSHA. January 24, 2014. Available at: https://www.osha.gov/ooc/citations/SuperKingSaunaNJLLC_928086_and_923424_0124_14.pdf. Accessed December 22, 2019.

15. McGee K, Turkewitz J. Death of Woman in Tank at a Nevada Cryotherapy Center Raises Questions About Safety. *The New York Times.* October 26, 2015. Available at: https://www.nytimes.com/2015/10/27/us/death-of-woman-in-tank-at-a-nevada-cryo-therapy-center-raises-questions-about-safety.html. Accessed December 22, 2019.

16. OSHA News Release—Region 5. U.S. Department of Labor OSHA. December 31, 2012. Available at: https://www.osha.gov/news/newsreleases/region5/12312012. Accessed November 22, 2019.

17. Ramos CA, Wolterbeek HT, Almeida SM. Exposure to Indoor Air Pollutants During Physical Activity in Fitness Centers. *Building and Environment,* 82, 349-360, 2014.

18. Carbon Dioxide Health Hazard Information Sheet. U.S. Department of Agriculture, Food Safety and Inspection Service Environmental, Safety and Health Group. Available at: https://www.fsis.usda.gov/wps/wcm/connect/bf97edac-77be-4442-aea4-9d2615f376e0/Carbon-Dioxide.pdf?MOD=AJPERES. Accessed December 22, 2019.

19. OSHA Technical Manual. Indoor Air Quality Investigation. U.S. Department of Labor. Available at: https://www.osha.gov/dts/osta/otm/otm_iii/otm_iii_2.html. Accessed December 22, 2019.

20. 2018 International Mechanical Code. International Code Council. August 2017. Available at: https://www.ci.independence.mo.us/userdocs/ComDev/2018%20INTL%20MECH%20CODE.pdf. Accessed December 22, 2019.

21. Indoor Air Quality. U.S. Department of Labor OSHA. Available at: https://www.osha.gov/SLTC/indoorairquality/. Accessed December 22, 2019.

22. Occupational Safety and Health Standards, 29 C.F.R. § 1910.151(b) (2011).

23. Recording and Reporting Occupational Injuries and Illnesses, 29 C.F.R. § 1904.7(b) (2001).

24. Best Practices Guide: Fundamentals of a Workplace First-Aid Program. U.S. Department of Labor OSHA. 2006. Available at: https://www.osha.gov/Publications/OSHA3317first-aid.pdf. Accessed January 17, 2020.

25. OSHA's Form 300. U.S. Department of Labor OSHA. Available at: https://www.osha.gov/recordkeeping/new-osha-300form1-1-04-FormsOnly.pdf. Accessed December 22, 2019.

26. Occupational Safety and Health Standards, 29 C.F.R. § 1910.1030 (2012).

27. Update: Mortality Attributable to HIV Infection Among Persons Aged 25-44 Years — United States, 1991 and 1992. Centers for Disease Control and Prevention. *Morbidity and Mortality Weekly Report,* 42(45), 869-872, 1993.

28. Standard Interpretations. U.S. Department of Labor OSHA. September 17, 2004. Available at: https://www.osha.gov/laws-regs/standardinterpretations/2004-09-17-0. Accessed January 17, 2020.

29. OSHA Bloodborne Pathogen Compliance. BloodbornePathogenTraining. 2019. Available at: https://www.bloodbornepathogen-training.com/Content/brochures/BloodbornePathogenComplianceOverview.pdf. Accessed January 17, 2020.

30. Model Plans and Programs for the OSHA Bloodborne Pathogens and Hazard Communications Standards. U.S. Department of Labor OSHA. 2003. Available at: https://www.osha.gov/Publications/osha3186.pdf. Accessed January 17, 2020.

31. OSHA Fact Sheet. U.S. Department of Labor OSHA. 2011. Available at: https://www.osha.gov/OshDoc/data_BloodborneFacts/bbfact01.pdf. Accessed January 17, 2020.

32. Bloodborne Pathogens Compliance Still a Concern. Occupational Health & Safety. May 29, 2018. Available at: https://ohsonline.

References continued...

    com/articles/2018/05/29/bloodborne-pathogens-compliance-still-a-concern.aspx. Accessed Dec. 22, 2019.

33. Occupational Exposure to Bloodborne Pathogens OSHA Instruction CPL 2.103, Field Inspection Reference Manual. U.S. Department of Labor OSHA. November 27, 2001. Available at: https://www.osha.gov/pls/oshaweb/owadisp.show_document?p_table=directives&p_id=2570#XIII. Accessed January 17, 2020.

34. U.S. Const. Art. VI, Cl. 2.

35. First Aid and CPR Training for Employees of Fitness Centers, Wis. DHS § 174.04 (1999).

36. Medical Services and First Aid, Cal. Code Regs. tit. 8, § 3400(c) (2019).

37. Cal/OSHA Workplace First-Aid Kit Requirements. SoCal First Aid. Available at: https://www.socalfirstaid.com/blog/calosha-workplace-first-aid-kit-requirements/. Accessed January 17, 2020.

38. Sudden Cardiac Arrest & Early Defibrillation. AED Authority. Available at: https://www.aedauthority.com/cardiac-arrest/. Accessed January 17, 2020.

39. Facts, Every Second Counts, Rural and Community Access to Emergency Devices. American Heart Association. 2013. Available at: https://www.heart.org/idc/groups/heart-public/@wcm/@adv/documents/downloadable/ucm_301646.pdf. Accessed January 18, 2020.

40. *ACSM's Health/Fitness Facility Standards and Guidelines.* Sanders ME. (ed). 5th Ed. Champaign, IL: Human Kinetics, 2019.

41. Benjamin EJ, Virani SS, Callaway CW, et al. Heart Disease and Stroke Statistics—2018 Update: A Report From the American Heart Association. *Circulation*, 137(12), 355-373, 2018.

42. Koplan JP. Cardiovascular Deaths While Running. *Journal of the American Medical Association*, 242(23), 2578-2579, 1979.

43. Don't Worry About Sudden Cardiac Arrest During Exercise. Harvard Health Publishing. July 17, 2015. Available at: https://www.health.harvard.edu/heart-health/dont-worry-about-sudden-cardiac-arrest-during-exercise. Accessed January 31, 2020.

44. Marijon E, Uy-Evanado A, Reinier K, et al. Sudden Cardiac Arrest During Sports Activity in Middle Age. *Circulation*, 131(16), 1384–1391, 2015.

45. Allan KS, Grunau BE, Haines M, et al. Sudden Cardiac Arrest During Exercise Occurs Infrequently and With Few Warning Symptoms. *Circulation,* 140, A227, 2019.

46. Toukola TM, Kauppila JP, Pakanen L, et al. Characteristics and Prognosis of Exercise-Related Sudden Cardiac Arrest. *Frontiers in Cardiovascular Medicine*, 26(5), 102, 2018.

47. Albert CM, Mittleman MA, Chae CU, et al. Triggering of Sudden Death from Cardiac Causes by Vigorous Exertion. *The New England Journal of Medicine*, 343(19), 1355-1361, 2000.

48. Craig AC, Eickhoff-Shemek JM. Adherence to ACSM's Pre-Activity Screening Procedures in Fitness Facilities: A National Investigation. *Journal of Physical Education and Sports Management,* 2(2), 120-137, 2015.

49. Penela D, Aschieri D, Pelizzoni V, et al. Impact of Automated External Defibrillator Background in Amateur Sportive Centres: 18 Years Experience, *European Heart Journal*, 38(1), 528, 2017.

50. Community Access to Emergency Defibrillation Act of 2002, 42 U.S.C. § 244 (2002).

51. Automated External Defibrillators (AEDs). Food and Drug Administration. November 18, 2019. Available at: https://www.fda.gov/medical-devices/cardiovascular-devices/automated-external-defibrillators-aeds. Accessed January 18, 2020.

52. AED Steps. American Red Cross. Available at: https://www.redcross.org/take-a-class/aed/using-an-aed/aed-steps. Accessed January 18, 2020.

53. Cardiac Arrest Survival Act, 42 U.S.C. § 238p (2000).

54. AED State Laws. AED Brands. Available at: https://www.aedbrands.com/resource-center/choose/aed-state-laws/. Accessed January 18, 2020.

55. State Laws on Cardiac Arrest and Defibrillators. National Conference of State Legislatures. Available at: http://www.ncsl.org/research/health/laws-on-cardiac-arrest-and-defibrillators-aeds.aspx#Health_Clubs. Accessed December 22, 2019.

56. Fitness Center Staff Requirements. Wis. Stat. § 100.178 (2008).

57. Employee Available to Administer CPR, c.1 Exception. 73 Pa Stat. § 2174 (2012).

58. N.Y. Gen. Bus. Law § 621 (2005).

59. Colo. Rev. Stat. § 6-1-102 (2019); Werner AD. Compliance with Health and Fitness State Laws: Background, Best Practices and Key Takeaways for Health and Fitness Club Owners. *The National Law Review.* August 2, 2016. Available at: https://www.natlawreview.com/article/compliance-health-and-fitness-state-laws-background-best-practices-and-key-takeaways. Accessed December 22, 2019.

60. Health Spas. Ark. Code Ann. § 20-13-1306 (2007).

61. Health Studios; Acquisition, Maintenance, Training, and Use of Automated External Defibrillators; Civil Liability for Emergency Care or Treatment; Public Safety Requirements; Waiver. Cal. Health & Safety Code § 104113 (2020).

62. *Day v. Lupo Vine Street L.P.*, 22 Cal. App. 5th 62 (Cal. App., 2018).

63. Physical Fitness Facility Medical Emergency Preparedness Code, 77 Ill. Adm. Code §§ 527.100—527.1100 (2014).

64. Act 23 of 2006, Mich. Comp. Laws Serv. §§ 333.26311—333.26314 (2006).

65. Automated External Defibrillator Requirements. N.Y. Gen Bus Law § 627-a (2010).

66. Automated External Defibrillators: Public Access Providers. N.Y. Public Health Law § 3000-b (2015).

67. *Fowler v. Bally Total Fitness Corp.*, 2007 Ill. Cir. LEXIS 2 (Ill. Cir. Ct., 2007).

68. *Diniro v. Aspen Athletic Club, LLC*, 173 A.D.3d 1789 (N.Y. App. 4th, 2019)

69. *Coene v. 3M Co. ex rel. Minnesota Min. & Mfg. Co.*, 2015 WL 5773578 (W.D.N.Y., 2015).

70. Restatement (Second) of Torts, §§ 314-320 (1965).

71. H.R. 1227: Cardiac Arrest Survival Act of 2019. Govtrack. Available at: https://www.congress.gov/bill/116th-congress/house-bill/1227/text.

72. Radel FR, Labbe AA. The Law of Premises Liability—An Overview. Groelle & Salmon. Available at: https://www.gspalaw.com/the-law-of-premises-liability-an-overview/. Accessed January 19, 2020.

73. *Stelluti v. Casapenn Enterprises, LLC*, 203 N.J. 286 (N.J., 2010).

74. Emergency Care. N.J. Stat. § 2A:62A-1 (1987).

75. *Desiervo v. Township of Elmwood Park*, 2016 N.J. Super. Unpub. LEXIS 945 (Super. Ct. App. Div., 2016).

76. *Potter v. 24 Hour Fitness United States Inc.*, 2014 U.S. Dist. LEXIS 188132 (N.D. Tex., 2014).

References continued...

77. *Zihlman v. Wichita Falls YMCA*, In: Herbert DL. New AED Case Filed Against YMCA in Texas. *The Exercise Standards and Malpractice Reporter*, 24(5), 74-79, 2010.
78. Restatement (Second) of Torts § 282 (1965).
79. *Jabo v. YMCA of San Diego County*, 27 Cal. App. 5th 853 (Cal. App. 4th 2018).
80. *Verdugo v. Target Corp.*, 59 Cal. 4th 312 (Cal., 2014).
81. *L.A. Fitness International, LLC v. Mayer*, 980 So. 2d 550 (Fla. Dist. Ct. App., 2008)
82. *De La Flor v. Ritz-Carlton Hotel Co., L.L.C.*, 930 F. Supp. 2d 1325, 1330 (S.D. Fla., 2013).
83. N.Y. Pub. Health Law, §§ 2994-AA—2994-GG (2020).
84. *Fosmire v. Nicoleau*, 75 N.Y.2d 218 (N.Y. App., 1990).
85. Tex. Health & Safety Code Ann. §§ 166.081—166.102 (2020).
86. Eggert K. Do Not Resuscitate Orders at the Gym? West Bend. Aug. 28, 2017. Available at https://cultureofsafety.thesilverlining.com/safety-blog/do-not-resuscitate-orders-at-the-gym. Accessed January 4, 2020.
87. American National Standard— Minimum Requirements for Workplace First Aid Kits and Supplies. ANSI/ISEA. June 17, 2015.
88. Kelechava B. Workplace First Aid Kits—ANSI/ISEA Z308-2015— Classes, Types, and the Standard. ANSI. June 29, 2018. Available at https://blog.ansi.org/2018/06/workplace-first-aid-kits-ansi-isea-z308-2015/#gref. Accessed January 5, 2020.
89. Occupational Safety and Health Standards, 29 C.F.R. § 1910.151 App A (2011).
90. *ACSM's Health/Fitness Facility Standards and Guidelines.* Sanders ME. (ed). 5th Ed. Champaign, IL: Human Kinetics, 2019.
91. *ACSM's Guidelines for Exercise Testing and Prescription.* Riebe D. (ed). 10th Ed. Philadelphia, PA: Lippincott Williams & Wilkins, 2018.
92. NSCA Strength and Conditioning Professional Standards and Guidelines. *Strength and Conditioning Journal*, 39(6), 1-24, 2017. Available at: https://www.nsca.com/education/articles/nsca-strength-and-conditioning-professional-standards-and-guidelines/. Accessed November 5, 2018.
93. IHRSA Club Membership Standards. In: *IHRSA's Guide to Club Membership & Conduct.* 3rd Ed. Boston, MA: International Health, Racquet & Sportsclub Association, 2005. Available at: http://download.ihrsa.org/pubs/club_membership_conduct.pdf. Accessed November 5, 2018.
94. *Medical Fitness Association's Standards & Guidelines for Medical Fitness Center Facilities*, Roy B. (ed.). 2nd Ed. Monterey, CA: Healthy Learning, 2013.
95. *Exercise Standards & Guidelines Reference Manual.* 5th Ed. Sherman Oaks, CA: Aerobics and Fitness Association of America, 2010.
96. *Safeguarding Health and Well-Being, Medical Advisory Committee Recommendations: A Resource Guide for YMCAs.* Chicago, IL: YMCA of the USA, February 2011. Available at: http://safewise.com/downloads/MAC_2010a_Collection.pdf. Accessed November 5, 2018.
97. American Association for Cardiovascular and Pulmonary Rehabilitation (AACVPR). *Guidelines for Cardiac Rehabilitation and Secondary Prevention Programs.* Williams MA, Roitman JL (eds). 5th Ed. Champaign, IL: Human Kinetics, 2013.
98. Starr LM. ACOEM Position Statement. Automated External Defibrillation in the Occupational Setting. *Journal of Occupational and Environmental Medicine,* 54(9), 1170-1176, 2012.
99. American College of Sports Medicine and American Heart Association Joint Position Statement. Automated External Defibrillators in Health/Fitness Facilities. *Medicine and Science in Sports and Exercise*, 34(3), 561-564, 2002.
100. Evacuation Plans and Procedures eTool. U.S. Department of Labor OSHA. Available at: https://www.osha.gov/SLTC/etools/evacuation/expertsystem/default.htm. Accessed January 26, 2020.
101. Evacuation Elements. U.S. Department of Labor OSHA. Available at: https://www.osha.gov/SLTC/etools/evacuation/evac.html. Accessed January 26, 2020.
102. Title II of the Americans with Disabilities Act of 1990, 42 U.S.C. § 12131 et seq. (1990).
103. *California Foundation for Independent Living Centers v. County of Sacramento*, 142 F. Supp. 3d 1035 (E.D. Cal., 2015).
104. Lee B. Accessible Evacuation Plans in Higher Education: Equal Egress and the Americans with Disabilities Act. *Florida Coastal Law Review*, 18, 393, 2017.
105. Evacuation & Shelter-in-Place. U.S. Department of Labor OSHA. Available at: https://www.osha.gov/SLTC/emergencypreparedness/gettingstarted_evacuation.html. Accessed January 26, 2020.
106. Restatement (Second) of Torts, § 343 (1965).
107. Occupational Safety and Health Standards, 29 C.F.R. § 1910.157 (2002).
108. U.S. Fire Statistics. U.S. Fire Administration. Available at: https://www.usfa.fema.gov/data/statistics/#tab-1. Accessed February 2, 2020.
109. Evarts B. Fire Loss in the United States During 2018. National Fire Protection Association. October 2019. Available at: https://www.nfpa.org/~/media/FD0144A044C84FC5BAF90C05C04890B7.ashx. Accessed January 28, 2020.
110. Sclafani J. Fire Causes Evacuation of 24 Hour Fitness in Costa Mesa. Daily Pilot. March 13, 2019. Available at: https://www.latimes.com/socal/daily-pilot/news/tn-dpt-me-gym-fire-20190313-story.html. Accessed January 28, 2020.
111. Howland J. 2 Taken to Hospital After Flash Fire at Gold's Gym Caused by Aerosol Can, Transformer: Chief. *Poughkeepsie Journal*. February 24, 2019. https://www.poughkeepsiejournal.com/story/news/local/2019/02/24/flash-fire-golds-gym-caused-aerosol-can-transformer/2972425002/. Accessed January 28, 2020.
112. Vogler S. New Resource Helps Gyms Prepare for an Active Shooter Incident. IHRSA. October 12, 2018. Available at: https://www.ihrsa.org/about/media-center/press-releases/new-resource-helps-gyms-prepare-for-an-active-shooter-incident. Accessed January 26, 2020.
113. Berg A. Five Shot at Washington, D.C., Recreation Center. *Athletic Business E-Newsletter*. May 2019. Available at: https://www.athleticbusiness.com/facility-security/five-shot-in-washington-d-c-rec-center-shooting.html. Accessed January 26, 2020.
114. Active Shooter Emergency Action Plan Guide and Template. U.S. Department of Homeland Security. Available at: https://www.cisa.gov/publication/active-shooter-emergency-action-plan-guide. Accessed January 26, 2020.
115. Explosives Incident Report 2017. U.S. Department of Justice United States Bomb Data Center. Available at: https://www.atf.gov/file/128106/download. Accessed January 26, 2020.
116. Edevane G. WIFI named 'Remote Detonator' Triggers Mass Evacuation and Bomb Scare at Planet Fitness. *Newsweek*. April 16, 2018. Available at: https://www.newsweek.com/planet-fitness-evacuated-wifi-name-michigan-888088. Accessed January 26, 2020.

References continued...

117. Dempsey C, McWilliams K. Training Grenade Found Outside Connecticut LA Fitness. *N.Y. Daily News*. January 10, 2019. Available at: https://www.nydailynews.com/news/national/ny-bomb-found-la-fitness-connecitcut-20190110-story.html. Accessed January 26, 2020.

118. McInnis K, Herbert W, Herbert D, et al. Low Compliance With National Standards for Cardiovascular Emergency Preparedness at Health Clubs. *Chest Journal*. 120(1), 283-88, 2001.

119. Eickhoff-Shemek J, Deja K. Are Health/Fitness Facilities Complying with ACSM Standards? Part I. *ACSM's Health & Fitness Journal*, 6(2), 16-21, 2002.

120. Drezner JA, Irfan AM, Harmon KG. Automated External Defibrillators in Health and Fitness Facilities. *The Physician and Sportsmedicine*, 39(2), 114-118, 2011.

121. Sudden Cardiac Death (Sudden Cardiac Arrest). Cleveland Clinic. Available at: https://my.clevelandclinic.org/health/diseases/17522-sudden-cardiac-death-sudden-cardiac-arrest. Accessed January 26, 2020.

122. Automated External Defibrillators; Use; Requirements. Ariz. Rev. Stat. § 36-2262 (2020).

123. Murry J. What Employers Need to Know About OSHA. June 25, 2019. The Balance Small Business. Available at: https://www.thebalancesmb.com/what-is-osha-what-do-employers-need-to-know-about-it-398385. Accessed February 24, 2020.

124. Voluntary Protection Programs. U.S. Department of Labor OSHA Available at: https://www.osha.gov/vpp. Accessed January 26, 2020.

125. OSHA Offices by State. U.S. Department of Labor OSHA Available at: https://www.osha.gov/contactus/bystate. Accessed January 26, 2020.

126. Make a First Aid Kit. American Red Cross. Available at: https://www.redcross.org/get-help/how-to-prepare-for-emergencies/anatomy-of-a-first-aid-kit.html. Accessed January 27, 2020.

127. Abbott A. Professional Competency and Risk Management for Personal Trainers, Part I. *ACSM's Health & Fitness Journal*, 21(1), 38-40, 2007.

128. Skryabina, E, Reedy G, Amlot R, et al. What is the Value of Health Emergency Preparedness Exercises? A Scoping Review Study. *International Journal of Disaster Risk Reduction*, 21, 274-283, 2017.

This appendix includes a sample of an Injury Report. As stated in the text, the development of an Injury Report (and Evacuation Report) should be developed by the EAP planning team, the risk management advisory committee (e.g., legal counsel, insurance experts/provider), and medical professionals providing consultation.

SAMPLE: FACILITY INJURY REPORT

BASIC INFORMATION
Today's Date:
Facility (Name and Location):
Employee's Name (completing report):
Position:
Phone number:
Email:

INJURY INFORMATION
Date:
Time:
Location:
Body part(s) injured:
Description of injury:
Cause of injury:
Care provided:
Were emergency medical services contacted?

If yes, include EMS personnel and/or police name and contact information	
Name	**Contact Information**
1.	
2.	
3.	

INJURED PARTY
Name:
Address:
Phone Number:
Email:
Date of Birth (if known):
Relationship to Facility (Member/Participant/Spectator/Staff):

WITNESS INFORMATION		
(If eye-witnesses were interviewed, attach their written statements)		
Name	**Address**	**Contact**
1.		
2.		
3.		
4.		
5.		

Additional comments such as the following that are relevant to the Injury:

a) Comments from victim, if available:

b) Comments of staff member (first responder) and MOD:

c) Description of photos (attached to this report) taken, if applicable:

d) Other:

Signature: _____   Date: _____
                 (MOD)

Signature: _____   Date: _____
                 (Facility Manager)

Follow-up with Victim or Victim's Emergency Contact:

Employee Conducting Follow-Up: _____   Date: _____

Victim's Name/Emergency Contact's Name: _____

Comments:

LIST OF ABBREVIATIONS

AACVPR	American Association of Cardiovascular and Pulmonary Rehabilitation
AARP	American Association of Retired Persons
ACA	Affordable Care Act
ACE	American Council on Exercise
ACOEM	American College of Occupational and Environmental Medicine
ACOG	American College of Obstetricians and Gynecologists
ACSM	American College of Sports Medicine
ACSM's GETP	ACSM's Guidelines for Exercise Testing and Prescription
ADA	Americans with Disabilities Act
ADAAA	Americans with Disabilities Act Amendments Act
ADEA	Age Discrimination in Employment Act
AED	Automated External Defibrillator
AFAA	Athletics and Fitness Association of America
AGREE II	Appraisal of Guidelines for Research & Evaluation
AHA	American Heart Association
ALR	American Law Reports
AMI	Acute Myocardial Infarction
ANSI	American National Standards Institute
ANSI/ISO	ANSI/International Organization for Standardization
ARC	American Red Cross
ASEP	American Society of Exercise Physiologists
ASHRAE	American Society of Heating, Refrigeration, and Air-Conditioning Engineers
ASTM	American Society of Testing and Materials
BAA	Business Associate Agreement
BBP	Bloodborne Pathogens Standard
BIPA	Biometric Information Privacy Act
BOC	Board of Certification
BP	Blood Pressure
CAAHEP	Commission on the Accreditation of Allied Health Education Programs
CAATE	Commission on Accreditation of Athletic Training Education
CAD	Coronary Artery Disease
CBA	Collective Bargaining Agreement
CDC	Centers for Disease Control and Prevention
CE	Continuing Education
CECs	Continuing Education Credits
CEP	Clinical Exercise Physiologist
CEPA	Clinical Exercise Physiologist Association
CEUs	Continuing Education Units
CFR	Code of Federal Regulations
CFUs	Colony-Forming Units
CGL	Commercial General Liability
CHD	Coronary Heart Disease
CHEA	Council for Higher Education Accreditation
CIFT	Certified Inclusive Fitness Trainer
CLIA	Clinical Laboratory Improvement Amendments
COVID-19	Coronavirus Disease 2019
CPCS	Consumer Product Safety Commission
CPK	Creatine Phosphokinase
CPR	Cardiopulmonary Resuscitation
CPSC	Consumer Product Safety Commission
CPT	Certified Personal Trainer
CRF	Cardiorespiratory Fitness
CSCCa	College Strength and Conditioning Coaches Association
CSCS	Certified Strength and Conditioning Specialist
CUTPA	Connecticut Unfair Trade Practices Act
CV	Cardiovascular
CVD	Cardiovascular Disease
DAT	Direct Access Testing
dBA	Decibels
DNR	Do-Not-Resuscitate order
DOL	Department of Labor
e-PHI	Electronic Protected Health Information
EAPs	Emergency Action Plans
ECP	Exposure Control Plan
ECPs	Extreme Conditioning Programs
EEOC	Equal Employment Opportunity Commission
EHRs	Electronic Health Records
EIM	Exercise is Medicine®
EMRs	Electronic Medical Records
EMS	Emergency Medical Services
EMT	Emergency Medical Technician
EPA	Environmental Protection Agency
EPA	Equal Pay Act
ER	Exertional Rhabdomyolysis
ERP	Emergency Response Personnel
EU	European Union
FBI	Federal Bureau of Investigation
FCRA	Fair Credit Reporting Act
FDA	Food and Drug Administration

FDCA	Food, Drug, and Cosmetic Act	NCSL	National Conference of State Legislatures
FERPA	Family Educational Rights and Privacy Act	NEISS	National Electronic Injury Surveillance System
FITT-VP	Frequency, Intensity, Time, Type--Volume, Progression	NETA	National Exercise Trainers Association
		NFL	National Football League
FLSA	Fair Labor Standards Act	NFPA	National Fire Protection Association
FMLA	Family Medical Leave Act	NIOSH	National Institute for Occupational Safety and Health
FTC	Federal Trade Commission		
FTCA	Federal Tort Claims Act	NSC	National Safety Council
FTCA	Federal Trade Commission Act	NSCA	National Strength and Conditioning Association
GDPR	General Data Protection Regulation	NSPF	National Swimming Pool Foundation
GEI	Group Exercise Instructor	OCR	Obstacle Course Racing
GEL	Group Exercise Leader	OCR	Office of Civil Rights
GFI	Group Fitness Instructor	OPIM	Other Potentially Infectious Materials
GXT	Graded Exercise Test	OSHA	Occupational Health and Safety Administration
HBV	Hepatitis B Virus	OTJ	On-The-Job
HDL	High Density Lipoprotein	PA	Physical Activity
HHS	Health and Human Services	PADP	Public Access Defibrillation Provider
HHSOIG	Health and Human Services, Office of the Inspector General	PAR-Q+	Physical Activity Readiness Questionnaire for Everyone
HIIT	High Intensity Interval Training	PASQ	Pre-Activity Screening Questionnaire
HIPAA	Health Insurance Portability and Accountability Act	PAT	Performance Appraisal Tool
		PAVS	Physical Activity Vital Sign
HIT	High Intensity Training	PCP	Primary Care Physician
HITECH	Health Information Technology for Economic and Clinical Act	PEL	Permissible Exposure Limit
		PHI	Protected Health Information
HIV	Human Immunodeficiency Virus	PI	Principal Investigator
HR	Human Resources	PII	Personally Identifiable Information
HVAC	Heating, Ventilation, and Air Conditioning	RD	Registered Dietitian
IHRSA	International Health, Racquet & Sportsclub Association	RDN	Registered Dietitian Nutritionist
		RE-AIM	Reach, Efficacy, Adoption, Implementation, Maintenance
IRB	Institutional Review Board		
IRS	Internal Revenue Service	RMAC	Risk Management Advisory Committee
ISEA	International Safety Equipment Association	RMPPM	Risk Management Policies and Procedures Manual
ISSA	International Sports Science Association	RPE	Rating of Perceived Exertion
JCAHO	Joint Commission on Accreditation of Healthcare Organizations	RT	Resistance Training
		RT+V	Resistance Training and Valsalva
JCC	Jewish Community Center	SAH	Subarachnoid Hemorrhage
JTA	Job Task Analysis	SCA	Sudden Cardiac Arrest
LDL	Low Density Lipoprotein	SCCC	Strength and Conditioning Coach Certified
MCPA	Michigan Consumer Protection Act	SCD	Sudden Cardiac Death
MFA	Medical Fitness Association	SDSs	Safety Data Sheets
MOD	Manager On Duty	SOD	Supervisor on Duty
MRSA	Methicillin-resistant Staphylococcus aureus	SSI	Sport Science Institute
MSCC	Master Strength & Conditioning Coach	STEPS	Screening, Testing, Evaluating, Programming, and Supervising
NASM	National Academy of Sports Medicine		
NATA	National Athletic Trainers' Association	UCC	Uniform Commercial Code
NBC-HWC	National Board Certified Health & Wellness Coach	UGD	Universal Global Design
NBFE	National Board of Fitness Examiners	USDE	U.S. Department of Education
NBHWC	National Board for Health & Wellness Coaching	USF	University of South Florida
NCAA	National Collegiate Athletic Association	USPTO	U.S. Patent and Trademark Office
NCCA	National Commission for Certifying Agencies	VF	Ventricular Fibrillation
NCHPAD	National Center on Health, Physical Activity and Disability	VMS	Vitamins, Minerals and Supplements
		VPP	Voluntary Protection Program
NCSF	National Council on Strength & Fitness	YMCA	Young Men's Christian Association

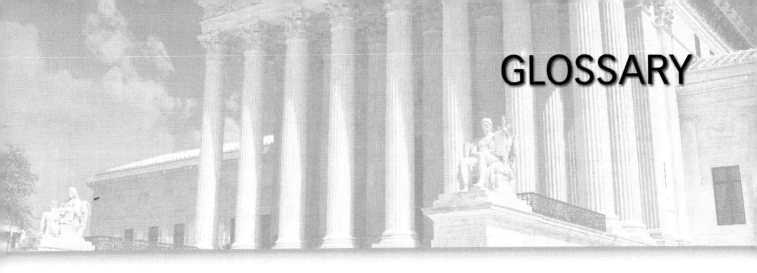

GLOSSARY

A

Accreditation A third-party designation requiring evidence that certain standards have been met. Examples in the exercise profession are academic programs (e.g., CAAHEP accreditation) and certification programs (e.g., NCCA accreditation).

Actual Cause Cause in fact determined by the "but for" test which states that an act is a factual cause of an outcome if, in the absence of the act, the outcome would not have occurred. For example, but for the contraindicated exercise that was prescribed, the injury would not have happened.

Acute Emergent Injuries In reference to strength training injuries, the types of injuries that are rare and need immediate emergency care such as musculoskeletal (e.g., fractures, dislocations), neurologic (e.g., stroke), and cardiovascular (e.g., aortic dissection).

Acute Non-Emergent Injuries In reference to strength training injuries, the types of injuries that are the most common and do not require immediate emergency care (e.g., muscular strains and ligamentous strains).

Administrative Law Rules and regulations that have the force and effect of law, and resolve disputes, similar to court trials, to determine if rules of administrative agencies have been violated and, if so, what sanctions should be imposed. For example, fitness facilities have had to pay financial penalties for violations of OSHA and IRS regulations.

Answer A response to a summons, prepared by the defendant's lawyer within a specified timeframe, that normally denies some or all of the allegations found in the complaint.

Assumption of Risk A legal doctrine in which a plaintiff cannot recover damages for a personal injury or wrongful death action. The defendant claims that no duty, whatsoever, was owed to the injured party, meaning no duty existed to protect the plaintiff from injuries due to risks inherent in the activity. To be an effective defense, the plaintiff must (a) possess full understanding of the risks inherent in the activity, and (b) voluntarily agree to participate in the activity.

Attractive Nuisance A legal doctrine that states that if land owners/occupiers maintain a condition on their land that attracts children, there are children around, and the condition poses a possible danger, there is not only a duty to warn but also a duty to take reasonable steps to protect the child's safety.

Automated External Defibrillators (AEDs) Portable devices that can (a) automatically diagnose a life-threatening cardiac arrhythmia such as ventricular fibrillation, and (b) deliver an electric shock through the chest to the heart to potentially allow a normal cardiac rhythm to resume following sudden cardiac arrest (SCA).

B

Beyond a Reasonable Doubt In a criminal case, the standard of proof (i.e. 100% certainty, no doubt) that is necessary to find a defendant guilty based on the evidence.

Biometric Data Information collected and used that can identify individuals such as fingerprint scans, body composition scans, iris scans/facial recognition, and biological data collected via wearable technology. Privacy issues need to be addressed by fitness/athletic facilities and programs that collect and use biometric data.

Biometric Information Privacy Act (BIPA) A law that regulates the collection and use of biometric data to help ensure one's privacy. Some states have biometric information privacy acts and other states are considering such statutes. Compliance with such laws may require fitness/athletic facilities and programs to give notice and obtain consent prior to collecting such data.

Biometric Screening The measurement of physical characteristics, such as height, weight, Body Mass Index (BMI), blood pressure, blood cholesterol, blood glucose, and fitness levels often taken and used as part of a workplace health assessment to benchmark and evaluate changes in employee health status over time.

Breach of Contract Occurs when one party does not fulfill its promises specified in the contract. Typically, it is not a crime or a tort, except in unusual cases. If litigation becomes necessary, the breaching party may be obligated by a court to pay compensatory damages or complete the specific performance stated in the contract.

Breach of Duty An act (i.e., the behavior or conduct that reflects negligent omission or commission), that caused the harm to the plaintiff. In determining if the defendant breached any duties, the court decides if the defendant met a certain standard of care (e.g., the level of care that an exercise professional owed to a plaintiff to help protect the plaintiff from harm).

Business Associates Persons who are not employees of a HIPAA covered entity but provide services to a covered entity that requires use or disclosure of protected health information (PHI). Business associates are often vendors of health care providers or health plans that provide services to the providers or plans involving the use of individual health information. HIPAA requires fitness facilities and exercise professionals who are "business associates" to protect the privacy and security of that individual's health information. 45 CFR § 160.103.

C

Case Law Court decisions that come from the judicial branch of the U.S., state, or local government. An aggregate of reported court cases that form a body of law, distinct from other primary sources of law (statutory and administrative law).

Causation An important element in proving negligence. The fact that the breach of duty, the negligent act, was what caused the injury. Courts often use the "but for" or "substantial-factor" tests to satisfy the causation requirement.

Cause of Action An appropriate legal basis for suing or the facts that give one person a right to seek relief against another person.

Chronic-Type Injuries In reference to strength training injuries, the types of injuries due to overuse, such as tendonitis.

Civil Law The body of law that pertains to civil or private rights and remedies. Civil law deals with disputes between two parties (plaintiff and defendant) and includes disputes involving tort, contract, and employment law.

Civil Liability A potential responsibility to pay damages (e.g., compensatory and punitive damages) or other court-enforcement for committing a civil wrong. It is distinct from criminal liability in which the at-fault party is subject to criminal punishment.

Clinical Exercise Testing A type of exercise test, often referred to as a graded exercise text (GXT), that is prescribed by a health care provider and conducted in a clinical setting. The major purpose is to diagnose coronary artery disease (CAD) or abnormal physiological responses.

Common Law A system that originated in medieval England when opinions and court rulings began to be recorded. This system was adopted by the U.S. at the time of the American Revolution. U.S. common law (or case law) is often referred to as judge-made law.

Comparative Negligence Fault that is measured in terms of percentages. Damages are allocated in proportion to the amount of fault (negligence) attributable to the plaintiff and the defendant. Most states have adopted "pure" or "modified" comparative fault systems.

Compartment Syndrome Severe muscle damage due to a swelling of muscle tissue that can lead to muscle necrosis (death)—a possible consequence of exertional rhabdomyolysis.

Compensatory Damages Actual damages or money awarded to the plaintiff for a real loss or injury which includes two types: (a) special or economic such as medical expenses and lost wages, and (b) general or non-economic such as pain and suffering and loss of consortium.

Competence The knowledge and skills that fitness managers and exercise professionals need to properly perform their job tasks and responsibilities. Courts will, perhaps, review the credentials of the defendant, but more importantly, courts will judge the "competence" of the defendant (i.e., did his/her conduct or actions/inactions breach any legal duties owed to the plaintiff).

Competent and Reliable Evidence According to the Federal Trade Commission (FTC), competent and reliable evidence includes tests, analyses, research, studies, or other evidence based on the expertise of professionals in the relevant area, that have been conducted and evaluated in an objective manner by persons qualified to do so, using procedures generally accepted in the profession to yield accurate and reliable results.

Complaint A formal document that initiates a civil lawsuit. In a negligence lawsuit, it will likely include allegations related to the plaintiff's harm, such as the negligent conduct of the defendant, and claims or theories of relief the plaintiff is seeking (e.g., monetary damages).

Comprehensive Risk Management Plan A plan that involves two major functions: (a) developing a Risk Management Policies and Procedures Manual, and (b) conducting staff training. The manual should reflect applicable laws and published standards of practice. Staff training is essential to help ensure that the policies and procedures in the manual are properly implemented.

Confidentiality The practice of permitting only certain authorized individuals to access information such as protected health information (PHI).

Contract An agreement that can be enforceable in court. Generally, contracts involve two or more parties who exchange binding promises. In a promise, each party declares that they will, or will not, take a specified action in the future.

Contractual Transfer of Risks A risk management strategy that utilizes a contract (e.g., waiver/release of liability and liability insurance) to pass along (or transfer) to others what would otherwise be one's own risk of loss.

Contributory Negligence Fault (negligence) on the part of the person claiming damages (plaintiff). If the plaintiff is even slightly negligent (e.g., 1% at fault), he/she is barred from recovering any damages. Because this is harsh rule, only a minority of states have adopted it.

Copyright Protects original works of authorship for many years. They include literary, dramatic, musical, and artistic works, such as poetry, novels, movies, songs, computer software, and architecture. Individuals can register their copyright with the U.S. Copyright Office.

Covered Entities A term defined by the HIPAA privacy and security rules that means health plans, health care clearinghouses, and health care providers that transmit any health information in electronic form in connection with a covered transaction. Fitness facilities and exercise professionals would not be considered a covered entity and, thus, subject to HIPAA privacy and security rules unless they are designated as a business associate. 45 CFR § 160.103.

Criminal Law The body of law that declares what conduct is criminal and dictates penalties for its commission. Criminal law deals with crimes against society and involves two parties: (a) the defendant who is the individual accused of a crime against society (the people), (b) and the people who are represented by the government, a district attorney.

D

Damages A loss due to physical and/or emotional injury to a person or property damage. Compensatory damages cover economic and non-economic losses and punitive damages can be awarded in addition to compensatory damages to punish the wrongdoer.

Defendant In a civil case, the party or parties the plaintiff is suing and, in a criminal case, the individual accused of a crime.

Depositions Examinations of witnesses during the pre-trial phase of a civil lawsuit that includes oral questioning of witnesses (or adverse parties) by the opposing attorney, under oath and in the presence of a court stenographer and the other party's attorney. Transcripts of depositions can serve as evidence at trial.

Design Defect A type of product defect that occurs when the design renders the product unreasonably safe and when the foreseeable risks of harm posed by the product could have been reduced or avoided by the adoption of an alternative design.

Desirable Operating Practices Standards of practice (e.g., standards, guidelines, and position statements) published by professional organizations that provide benchmarks (or best practices) of fitness facility staff functions (e.g., conducting screening, inspecting equipment, providing emergency care). It cannot be assumed they cover all major legal liability exposures facing fitness facilities and programs. Following laws (statutory, administrative, and case law) is also necessary.

Developmentally Appropriate Programs A safe and effective approach to teaching physical activity (or coaching sports) to children that respects the age and individual needs of each child (e.g., emotional/social health and physical health such as health risks and disabilities).

Direct Liability A type of employer liability to a third party due to negligent hiring, training, supervising and/or retention of an employee whose conduct harmed the third party. Employers can also be directly liable for failing to use reasonable care to select competent independent contractors who are hired to perform an activity that can create a risk of harm to others.

Discovery An often lengthy, pre-trial phase that continues until a civil lawsuit is settled or goes to trial. It involves various methods to learn about the facts in the dispute including interrogatories, depositions, and motions to produce.

Discretionary Function An exception specified in the Federal Tort Claims Act to which the government is not subject to liability even though a private employer could be under the same circumstances. For example, government employees who lead exercise programs for military personnel would, likely, not be found liable for injuries to recruits participating in those workout routines. The decisions regarding the workout routines reflect the discretionary function of those leading the training programs.

Dissenting Opinion A written opinion of a judge(s) that explains his/her arguments for disagreeing with the majority's opinion. Dissenting opinions may be relevant because they may provide the basis of arguments for overruling a majority opinion in the future.

Duplication The provision of a second set of important documents (written and/or electronic) stored at another location to serve as a back-up procedure in case the primary documents are ever lost or destroyed. Documents help demonstrate adherence to the law and/or the standard of care.

Duty An obligation that is formed from three primary origins (a) inherent in the situation, (b) voluntary assumption, and (c) mandated by statute. Courts determine duty by examining relationships formed (e.g., those inherent in the situation such as the relationships formed between exercise professionals and fitness participants). Because of these relationships, exercise professionals have a duty to provide *reasonably safe* programs for their participants by protecting them from exposure to unreasonable risks that may cause harm.

E

Emergency Action Plans (EAPs) Written plans that address two major types of emergencies: (a) potential dangers which may trigger evacuation, such as inclement weather, fire, or an active shooter, and (b) medical emergencies such as a sudden cardiac arrest or a bone fracture. EAPs should reflect laws, regulations, and published standards of practice.

Emergency Medical Services (EMS) A system that provides emergency medical care. Once it is activated by an incident that causes serious illness or injury, the focus of EMS is emergency medical care of the patient(s). See www.ems.gov.

Emotional Support Animals Animals that are often used as part of a medical treatment plan to help individuals improve their physical, social, emotional, and/or cognitive functioning. They are not considered service animals under the ADA.

Evidence Everything the judge or jury is entitled to consider in order to determine the facts in the case. It must be relevant to the case. Evidence not related to the facts is inadmissible.

Exculpatory Clause A contract clause used in waivers/releases of liability that specifies the exculpation of another, which releases one of the parties from liability for his or her wrong doing.

Exercise is Medicine® A collaborative effort co-launched by the ACSM and the American Medical Association that began in the U.S. in 2007 and has expanded into a worldwide health initiative managed by ACSM. EIM encourages physicians and other health care providers to (a) assess and record physical activity (PA) as a vital sign during patient visits, and (b) provide brief advice/exercise prescription or referral to a certified exercise professional or allied health professional.

Exertional Rhabdomyolysis (ER) A serious condition occurring from strenuous exercise that leads to a breakdown of skeletal muscle resulting in a protein (myoglobin) being released into the bloodstream. Excess myoglobin can lead to kidney damage and, in severe cases, kidney failure. ER can also lead to compartment syndrome. See compartment syndrome.

Expert Testimony The opinions of expert witnesses to educate the court as to the standard of care (duty) the defendant owed to the plaintiff and whether or not the defendant met the standard of care. Often, as a part of their testimony, they describe published standards of practice. If the court accepts the published standards as admissible evidence, then the standards of practice can become the standard of care.

Expert Witnesses Individuals who are called to educate the triers of fact by sharing their specialized knowledge and/or training. For example, in a negligence lawsuit, they educate the court as to the standard of care (or duty) that the defendant owed to the plaintiff and if, in their opinion, the defendant breached that duty.

Exposure Avoidance A risk management strategy that eliminates the risk of injury such as not providing treadmills and not offering extreme conditioning programs.

Exposure Control Plan (ECP) A written plan required by OSHA to eliminate or reduce occupational exposure to bloodborne pathogens. Components of an ECP include: (a) determination of employee exposure, (b) implementation of various methods of exposure control, (c) hepatitis B vaccination, (d) post-exposure evaluation and follow-up, (e) communication of hazards to employees and training, (f) recordkeeping, and (g) procedures for evaluating circumstances surrounding exposure incidents. 29 CFR §1910.1030.

Express Assumption of Risk Arises when a plaintiff explicitly consents (signs a written contract prior to participation) to relieve the defendant of a duty owed by the defendant regarding specific known risks.

F

Fact Witnesses Individuals who are called to testify regarding the facts only. For example, in a negligence lawsuit, they describe what they observed, heard, or felt regarding a personal injury.

FITT-VP Principle Used when establishing an exercise prescription as follows: F = Frequency, I = Intensity, T = Time, and T = Type, V = Volume (the total volume or amount of exercise), and P = Progression (advancement of the exercise program).

Formative Evaluation A type of evaluation of the comprehensive risk management plan that is on-going throughout the year and helps identify changes/improvements needed in the plan (e.g., after an injury, was the emergency action plan properly carried out; after observing improper performance of an employee, what type of re-training is needed).

Frivolous Conduct Conduct of little weight or importance. For example, a claim made by the defendant that the plaintiff's complaint is completely without merit in law, undertaken primarily to delay resolution or to harass another, or asserts material facts that are false.

G

General Jurisdiction Jurisdiction, based on federal and state statutes, refers to the geographic area in which a court has authority and the types of cases it has the power to hear. A court with general jurisdiction can hear and decide almost any type of case.

General Supervision A type of supervision in which the supervisor has the responsibility for overseeing an activity (e.g., supervising the fitness floor and observing participants to help ensure they are using the exercise equipment/facilities properly and following the facility's policies and procedures).

Governmental Immunity Immunity is an exemption or protection against civil liability under certain circumstances. Governmental immunity is used to bar liability claims against governmental entities. However, since the passing of certain federal and state tort claims legislation, injured parties have been able to sue governmental entities under certain circumstances. Although there are some distinctions between sovereign immunity and governmental immunity, they are often used interchangeably.

Gross Negligence A voluntary act or omission that goes beyond carelessness (ordinary negligence) that is often referred to as reckless or willful/wanton conduct in which there is a conscious disregard of a legal duty and the consequences of such disregard toward another. A plaintiff may recover punitive damages for such conduct that courts often define as the defendant's failure to exercise even slight care/diligence or an extreme departure from the standard of care.

Group Health Plan Wellness Program A wellness program that is either part of an employer's "group health plan," or is a group health plan in and of itself. A group health plan is an employer-sponsored welfare benefit plan to the extent that the plan provides medical care to employees or their dependents directly or through insurance or otherwise. Group health plan wellness programs need to comply with certain federal laws.

Guilty A term used when a defendant in a criminal case was found to have committed a crime. The defendant is subject to fines, community service, probation, imprisonment or any combination of these.

H

Health-Related Fitness Testing Fitness tests commonly conducted in fitness facilities that include assessments of cardiovascular endurance, muscle strength/endurance, flexibility, and body composition. Data collected are used to develop an individualized exercise prescription and measure progress.

High Intensity Training (HIT) A form of exercise that involves high intensity (maximal or near-maximal) exercise routines that do not include rest or recovery intervals and, thus, can significantly increase the risk of all types of injuries. HIT programs are also referred to as extreme condition programs (ECPs).

High-Intensity Interval Training (HIIT) A form of exercise that involves interval training that consists of alternating short periods of maximal-effort exercise with less intense recovery periods. Although considered a safer approach to exercise than HIT, several precautions need to be considered prior to having individuals participate in HIIT programs.

HIPAA Breach Notification Rule Requires certain responses by covered entities and business associates when a breach of unsecured PHI occurs. A "breach" means the acquisition, access, use or disclosure of PHI in a manner not permitted under the HIPAA Privacy Rule which compromises the security or privacy of the PHI. 45 CFR § 164.402.

HIPAA Privacy Rule Requires covered entities to have safeguards in place to ensure the privacy of protected health information (PHI). This rule sets forth the circumstances under which covered entities may use or disclose an individual's PHI and gives individuals rights with respect to their PHI, including rights to examine and obtain a copy of their health records and to request corrections.

HIPAA Security Rule Establishes national standards to protect individuals' electronic personal health information that is created, received, used, or maintained by a covered entity.

I

Improper Exercise Prescription A potential cause of injury when an exercise professional has a participant (a) perform an unsafe exercise, or (b) perform exercise at an intensity level that the participant was unable to safely tolerate, given the participant's health/fitness status.

Incident Report A form completed by an authorized employee, such as the manager on duty, that documents various types of incidents that occur in fitness facilities and that can provide evidence to help defend the facility in future litigations.

Inclusive Exercise Equipment Exercise equipment that is designed to be used by individuals with and without functional limitations or impairments. Providing such equipment will help fitness facilities comply with the ADA. Fitness facilities who opt not to provide designated inclusive equipment still need to comply with the ADA by providing exercise equipment that can be used by those with disabilities and provide proper spacing so the equipment is accessible.

Indemnification A clause within a contract in which a participant agrees to reimburse the service provider for any monetary loss resulting from an injury to the participant or an injury or loss caused by the participant. Generally, indemnification clauses/agreements are between two businesses.

Independent Contractor A self-employed individual who renders service for an employer and follows the employer's desires only as to the results of the work as specified in an agreement or contract. The contractor controls the manner and method of the service delivery.

Inherent Risks See Risks Inherent in the Activity.

Injunction A court order that requires an individual or a property owner to do something or to refrain from doing something (e.g., an order to stop providing dietary counseling without a license to practice dietetics).

Intentional Tort An act in which an individual intends to cause harm or acts knowingly that his/her conduct is substantially certain to cause harm. Examples include defamation and invasion of privacy. Many intentional torts can also be considered criminal acts because they violate statutes.

Interrogatories Written questions that are directed to either party (e.g., a set of written questions sent by the plaintiff's lawyer to the other party). The questions must be answered by the other party under oath, with the guidance of legal counsel, and within a given time period. The questions and answers can serve as evidence at trial.

Invitee A person who goes on the premises of a land owner/occupier with the express or implied invitation of the land owner/occupier for their mutual advantage. The land owner/occupier owes a duty to act reasonably toward an invitee regarding the activities/conditions on their land which involves reasonable inspection of the property for dangers and to reasonably repair and/or warn of dangers.

J

Job Task Analysis An assessment of job tasks that is often required to obtain accreditation. For example, the NCCA requires a job task analysis (JTA) for fitness organizations who want to obtain accreditation of their certifications. The JTA survey, completed by fitness professionals, contains questions regarding each job task listed on the survey. The results are used to develop competencies (knowledge and skills) to be covered on the certification examinations.

Jurisdiction See "general" jurisdiction and "subject matter" jurisdiction.

Jury Instructions Instructions regarding applicable laws given to the jury by the judge after the closing statements made by attorneys in a jury trial. The jury deliberates and returns with a verdict (the jury's decision).

L

Laboratory A facility that performs certain testing on human specimens in order to obtain information that can be used for the diagnosis, prevention, or treatment of any disease or impairment of a human being; or the assessment of the health of a human being; or procedures to determine, measure or otherwise describe the presence or absence of various substances or organisms in a human body.

Legal Liability Exposures Situations that create a risk of an injury (e.g., medical emergency, threatening weather) or reflect noncompliance to federal, state, and/or local laws, (e.g., a fitness facility that does not comply with the Americans with Disabilities Act and Automated External Defibrillator state statutes).

Legal Scope of Practice The activities that a licensed individual is permitted to perform within a specific profession as established by the profession's state board and defined in state statutes.

Liable A term used when a defendant in a civil case was found responsible for the plaintiff's harm. The defendant must compensate the plaintiff (usually financial compensation) for injuries or damages and may be ordered to stop the practice causing the harm.

Licensee A person who enters the premises of a land owner/occupier with the express or implied permission of the land owner/occupier but only for his/her own purposes. The land owner/occupier owes a duty to warn a licensee of any dangerous conditions that exist on the premises if actually known by the land owner/occupier.

Licensure The granting or regulation of licenses. For example, the practice of certain professions is restricted to only those who have obtained state licensure. It helps ensure the public is receiving quality (safe and effective) services from individuals who have met minimum educational requirements, as specified by state licensing boards and statutes.

Loss of Consortium A cause of action, usually by a spouse or child, for interference by a third party with the relationship of that person with his/her spouse or parent, respectively.

Loss of Parental Consortium A cause of action for interference by a third party with the parent-child relationship.

Loss Prevention A risk management strategy that involves minimizing the risk of injury and/or reflects compliance with federal, state, and local laws.

Loss Reduction A risk management strategy that mitigates or reduces the severity of an injury after it occurs such as providing appropriate emergency care,

M

Majority Opinion Appellate courts prepare a written opinion for each case they review, which is published so that lower courts and others are informed of their decisions and interpretations. If all the appellate judges agree, it is called a unanimous opinion. If it is not unanimous, the majority of the justices that do agree publish a majority opinion.

Manager on Duty (MOD) A designated professional staff member who has supervisory responsibilities of all fitness facility's operations during the hours the facility is open. Each MOD needs to be well-trained on how to properly carry-out the facility's policies and procedures.

Manufacturing Defect A type of product defect that occurs when a product deviates from its intended design specifications during production resulting in a defect.

Marketing Defect A type of product defect that occurs because of inadequate instructions or warnings when the foreseeable risks of harm posed by the product could have been reduced or avoided by the provision of reasonable instructions or warnings.

Medical Clearance A step in the pre-activity health screening process that involves a physician (or other health care provider) completing and signing a medical clearance form regarding whether or not his/her patient is medically cleared to participate in an exercise program. The physician may also indicate restrictions/limitations on the form that the exercise professional must follow when designing/delivering the exercise program.

Medical History A process involving the collection of an individual's medical history that is completed prior to conducting fitness testing, preparing individualized prescriptions, or teaching exercise classes for clinical populations. The data obtained on a medical history questionnaire is more specific than on a pre-activity screening questionnaire. It is needed so the exercise professional can take the necessary precautions given the individual's medical condition(s).

Medical Malpractice Negligence of a licensed health care provider. In medical malpractice cases, state statutes specify requirements for expert medical testimony.

Medical Release An authorization for release of PHI, which a patient signs, allowing disclosure of his/her medical information to a third party. For example, if an exercise professional wants to obtain medical records of his/her client such as GXT or lipid profile data, the client's health care provider will first have his/her patient sign a HIPAA compliant medical release. If an exercise professional wants to send a client's health/fitness data (e.g., health screening data, fitness testing data, progress reports) directly to the client's health care provider or other third party, the exercise professional should first have the client sign a similar medical release.

Membership Contracts Enforceable agreements between an individual (e.g., new fitness facility member) and a membership business/organization (e.g., a fitness facility). Many states have health club membership contract laws and/or consumer protection acts. Fitness facility managers/owners need to follow the requirements specified in these laws.

Mobile App A software application for a mobile device over which the Food and Drug Administration (FDA) will exercise enforcement discretion.

Mobile Medical App A software application that can be run on a smart phone, tablet or other portable computer, or a web-based software platform tailored to a mobile platform but executed on a server, that meets the definition of device in § 201(h) of the Food, Drug, and Cosmetic Act (FDCA) and is intended to: (a) be used as an accessory to a regulated medical device, or (b) transform a mobile platform into a regulated medical device. The FDA applies regulatory oversight of these apps.

Motion to Dismiss After a summons is delivered to the defendant, the lawyer for the defendant needs to respond within a given timeframe with an answer. Instead of an answer, a motion to dismiss (or demurrer) may be filed claiming the complaint is legally insufficient on substantive grounds or that the action is barred, procedurally.

Motions to Produce A method used during the pre-trial discovery phase which involves requests by legal counsel to a judge to order the opposing party to provide certain evidence that may be relevant in the case.

N

Negligence Careless conduct that causes harm. It can be defined as failing to do something that a reasonable prudent person (or fitness manager/exercise professional) would have done (omission) or doing something that a reasonable prudent person (or fitness manager/exercise professional) would not have done (commission) given the same or similar circumstances.

Negligence per se A type of ordinary negligence that can result from the violation of a state statute. The plaintiff does not have to prove negligence as he/she would in an ordinary negligence case, but does have to show that the violation of the statute caused the harm that the statute was intended to prevent and that the victim was in a class of persons that the statute was designed to protect.

Non-Traditional Personal Fitness Training Personal fitness training that is conducted outside a fitness facility such as (a) Internet training, (b) home training in either the trainer's home or in the client's home, and (c) outdoor training in areas such as public parks. To address the many unique legal liability exposures associated with non-traditional personal training, it is essential that trainers obtain legal consultation to address the legal liability exposures.

O

Open and Obvious Doctrine A defense, often used in premise liability cases, that protects a land owner/occupier from liability when a person was injured due a hazard on the owner/occupier's premises that was open and obvious. Open and obvious hazards, by their nature, apprise the individual of a potential hazard, which he/she can then take reasonable measures to avoid.

Ordinances Laws passed by local governments (e.g., municipalities and counties) and include rules such as parking regulations, zoning regulations, and leash laws.

OSHA's Bloodborne Pathogens (BBP) Standard An OSHA standard that requires employers to protect employees from bloodborne pathogens such as hepatitis B virus (HBV) and human immunodeficiency virus (HIV). The purpose of the BBP Standard is to mitigate occupational exposure to blood and other potentially infectious materials (OPIM). Occupational exposure broadly extends to employees whose duties may reasonably lead to contact with blood or OPIM. In a fitness setting, these employees can include maintenance workers and those tasked with responding to injuries. 29 CFR 1910.1030.

Ostensible Agency Situations where it appears to a third party (e.g., fitness participant) that the person providing services (e.g., an independent contractor) is an employee of the facility. If the third party is harmed by the independent contractor's negligence, the employer may be subject to vicarious liability, just as the employer would be when an employee's negligence causes harm to a third party.

Other Potentially Infectious Materials (OPIM) Body fluids including, but not limited to, semen, vaginal secretions, cerebrospinal fluid, synovial fluid, pleural fluid, peritoneal fluid, pericardial fluid, amniotic fluid, saliva in dental procedures, and any other body fluid that is visibly contaminated with blood.

Out-of-Court Settlement A pre-trial settlement between the two parties (e.g. plaintiff and defendant). About 95% of personal injury cases end in a pre-trial settlement meaning that, approximately, one in 20 cases go to trial to be resolved by a judge or jury.

P

Patent A limited duration property right relating to an invention, granted by the U.S. Patent and Trademark Office, in exchange for public disclosure of the invention. Patentable materials include machines, manufactured articles, industrial processes, chemical compositions, exercise equipment, wearable technology, or weight loss product.

Pattern or Practice A type of accusation in race discrimination cases which can occur if a fitness facility has rules or practices that target, whether intentionally or unintentionally, members of a certain race or national origin.

Personally Identifiable Information (PII) Personal data that can include medical, biometric, and financial information as well as an individual's name, social security number, or driver's license number. Fitness facilities and programs that collect such data need to be aware of data breach notification laws that exist in each state. Violations of such laws can be costly.

Places of Public Accommodation Businesses that are generally open to the public and that fall into one of 12 categories listed in the Americans with Disabilities Act (ADA). Some of these categories include hotels, restaurants, schools, doctors' offices, movie theaters, and fitness facilities.

Plaintiff In a civil lawsuit, the party who is bringing the lawsuit.

Pleadings The summons (delivered to the defendant after a complaint is filed) and answer (response to the summons) together.

Policy A definite course or method of action selected from among alternatives, and in light of given conditions, to guide and determine present and future decisions.

Pre-Activity Health Screening A process that involves having all new fitness participants complete a screening questionnaire to identify those who may be at risk of an untoward event while participating in a fitness facility's activities and those who may need to obtain medical clearance prior to participation in the facility's activities.

Precedent A term referring to a rule or decision made by a court of law that is then followed by future courts in similar cases. See also stare decisis.

Predictive Asset Management Technologies An emerging technology that tracks exercise equipment usage data and contains alert systems to notify facility managers when the equipment needs maintenance. The statistics obtained are useful for decision-making and record-keeping.

Premise Liability Premise liability is a legal concept that typically applies when an injury was caused by some type of unsafe or defective condition on one's property. To prevail with a premise liability claim, the injured party needs to prove that the property owner/occupier knew or should have known that the premises were in an unsafe/defective condition and failed to take proper action to correct the condition.

Preponderance of the Evidence The standard of proof (i.e., more likely than not or 51% or greater) needed in a civil case to demonstrate that the defendant's conduct caused the harm to the plaintiff.

Preventive Law Similar to risk management in that it requires creative thinking, timely planning, and purposeful execution to minimize legal liability risks. Like preventive medicine that focuses on preventing disease, preventive law focuses on preventing lawsuits. Both preventive medicine and preventive law are *proactive* (preventing problems before they arise) versus *reactive* (responding to problems after they arise).

Prima Facie Case Prima facie is a Latin term meaning "on its face." For example, in a prima facie negligence case, the plaintiff has produced sufficient evidence to support his/her allegations. The plaintiff's evidence compels such a conclusion if the defendant is unable to produce evidence to rebut it.

Primary Assumption of Risk An asserted defense to a negligence claim or lawsuit that involves the plaintiff assuming well-known, inherent risks to participating in an activity. For example, it is implied that one who engages in sport activities assumes the reasonably foreseeable risks inherent in the activity. To the extent a risk inherent in the sport injures a plaintiff, the defendant has no duty and there is no negligence. To be an effective defense, the evidence must show the plaintiff possessed full subjective understanding of the presence and nature of the specific risk, and voluntarily chose to encounter the risks.

Primary Sources of Law Federal and state constitutional law as well as law created by the executive, judicial, and legislative branches of the federal, state, and local governments.

Privacy The right of an individual to enjoy freedom from intrusion and the right to maintain control over certain personal information such as protected health information (PHI).

Private Law A category of law that defines, regulates, enforces, and administers relationships among individuals, associations, and corporations.

Procedural Law A category of law that prescribes methods of enforcing substantive law such as the law of jurisdiction and law of evidence.

Procedure A particular way of accomplishing something or a series of steps followed in a regular definite order.

Product Defects Flaws or imperfections in the manufacturing, design, and/or warning of a product that may lead to an injury for which a manufacturer/distributor can be found liable.

Product Liability A form of strict liability imposed upon a manufacturer (and/or distributor) because the product is negligently manufactured, distributed, or sold. Liability is imposed upon the manufacturer for a defect (design, manufacturing and/or marketing) in a product that makes it unreasonably dangerous to the user. The manufacturer is liable for injuries as long as the product was being utilized in a foreseeable manner.

Professional Scope of Practice Applicable to all professions and vocations that require special knowledge, skills, and training – not only licensed professionals. All non-licensed professionals, such as exercise professionals, should practice within their education, training, experience, and practical skills to stay within their professional scope of practice.

Professional Standard of Care See Standard of Care of a Professional.

Professionally-Guided Screening After new fitness participants complete a screening questionnaire, the information on the questionnaire is interpreted by an exercise professional (e.g., an individual with a degree in exercise science and professional certification) who determines if medical clearance is needed based on pre-determined criteria. If needed, the exercise professional obtains medical clearance from the participant's health care provider.

Proper Referral Practices Precautionary steps taken, prior to making a referral, to help minimize legal liability. For example, physicians (or other health care providers) can be liable for medical malpractice if they knew (or should have known) that the health care provider to whom they referred their patients was incompetent. They may also face liability if the clinic or medical facility to which they referred their patients was unaccredited or improperly staffed. The expectation is to exercise due care (e.g., investigate health care providers and facilities) prior to making referrals. Improper referrals can apply to all professionals including exercise professionals.

Protected Health Information (PHI) Individually identifiable health information in any format to which the Health Insurance Portability and Accountability Act (HIPAA) privacy and security rules apply. Under HIPAA, PHI means individually identifiable health information that is transmitted by electronic media, maintained in electronic media, or transmitted or maintained in any other form or medium. 45 CFR § 160.103.

Proximate Cause That which, in a natural and continuous sequence, unbroken by any efficient intervening cause, produces injury, and without which the result would not have occurred. For example, in a negligence lawsuit, the injury to the plaintiff must be reasonably related to the negligent act of the defendant.

Public Law A category of law that defines rights and duties with either the operation of government or relationships between the government and individuals, associations, and corporations.

Public Policy A court determination about what is in the best interest of society (e.g., community common sense and common conscience, extended and applied regarding matters of public morals, health, safety, welfare, and the like). Public policy considerations are often used by courts to determine if waivers/releases of liability are against public policy.

Punitive Damages Damages that are awarded, in addition to compensatory damages (economic and non-economic), to punish the wrongdoer for gross negligence, reckless, or willful/wanton conduct.

R

Reasonable Accommodation An Americans with Disabilities Act (ADA) requirement in which employers provide employees with reasonable accommodations which may include modifications or adjustments to the work environment to allow an employee with a disability to enjoy equal benefits and privileges of employment as enjoyed by similarly situated employees without a disability.

Rebuttable Presumption An assumption of fact accepted by the court until evidence to the contrary is introduced to disprove it.

Regulations Administrative laws, often referred to as rules and regulations, enacted by government regulatory agencies such as the IRS and OSHA. These agencies have the power to investigate violations of their regulations, resolve disputes, and impose sanctions when violations have occurred.

Remand An appellate court's decision to send the case back to a lower court for a new trial in compliance with the appellate court's instructions.

Respondeat Superior A legal doctrine where an employer can be vicariously liable for the negligent acts of their employees while they are performing their jobs. Vicarious liability is a form of strict liability.

Risk Management A proactive administrative process requiring strategic planning that will help minimize legal liability exposures.

Risk Management Advisory Committee A committee made up of experts in areas such as risk management, law, insurance, and medicine who provide guidance and expertise in the development of a comprehensive risk management plan.

Risk Management Audit An assessment (checklist) that fitness managers and exercise professionals can complete to determine what risk management strategies are (a) developed or (b) not developed in their facility.

Risk Management Policies and Procedures Manual A major component of a comprehensive risk management plan that includes written descriptions of a fitness facility's policies and procedures that reflect adherence to laws and published standards of practice.

Risks Inherent in the Activity Causes of injuries that are inseparable from the activity and just happen because of participation in physical activity or sport. They are no one's fault. Also referred to as inherent risks.

S

Safe and Effective Exercise Prescription An individualized exercise program that is designed and delivered based on the individual's health/fitness status. Exercise prescriptions for clinical populations should be prepared by exercise professionals with advanced knowledge/skills in clinical exercise and in collaboration with the individual's health care provider.

Safety Culture A set of core values and behaviors that emphasize safety as an overriding priority and expressed through what is said and done—through behavior.

Scope of Practice The activities a professional engages in when carrying out his/her practice that are within the boundaries or limitations of that particular profession (e.g., non-licensed professionals should practice within the limitations of their education, training, experience, and practical skills; licensed individuals should practice within the activities specified by state boards and licensing statutes).

Secondary Sources of Law Legal sources that analyze, inform, or summarize various legal topics and issues. Secondary sources help provide insight and understanding of primary sources of law.

Security Refers to the safeguards used to control access and protect information, such as protected health information (PHI), from disclosure to an unauthorized person(s).

Self-Guided Screening New fitness participants are provided a screening questionnaire that they complete/interpret on their own and, decide on their own, to obtain medical clearance. Such questionnaires usually provide guidance regarding the need for medical clearance and/or consultation before engaging in an exercise program.

Separation of Powers A provision in the Constitution that allows each branch to check on the other two branches to help prevent any one branch from, illegally, exercising power.

Service Animals Dogs and miniature horses that have been trained to do work or perform tasks for people with disabilities. The ADA has requirements addressing service animals (e.g., fitness facility staff members can ask only two questions—is the service animal required because of a disability and what work or task has the service animal been trained to perform).

Service Marks A designation of intellectual property that protects words or symbols that identify services.

Sovereign Immunity See governmental immunity.

Specific Supervision A type of supervision in which the supervisor (e.g., a personal fitness trainer or group exercise leader) is directly with an individual or small group and involves an "instructional" format. Specific supervision should provide the participant an opportunity to gain knowledge of the activity, an understanding of one's own capabilities, and an appreciation of the potential injuries that can occur so that he/she can assume the inherent risks of the activity.

Spoliation of Evidence Occurs when evidence is hidden, withheld, changed, or destroyed during or before litigation. Certain jurisdictions have statutes against spoliation of evidence in which a defendant can face fines and prison time whereas other jurisdictions may rely on case law.

Standard of Care The duty (or degree of care) that is required of a reasonably prudent person acting in same or similar circumstances.

Standard of Care of a Professional The standard of care that exercise professionals will be held to in a court of law. For example, the question for the court is, did the exercise professional (defendant) act like a prudent exercise professional, given the circumstances. In other words, the standard of care describes the level of care that an exercise professional owed to a plaintiff to help protect the plaintiff from harm.

Stare Decisis A Latin term meaning "it stands decided" referring to a rule or decision made by a court of law that is then followed by future courts in similar cases. See also precedent.

Statute of Frauds A state statute that requires certain types of contracts to be in writing in order to be enforceable (e.g., contracts involving the sale of exercise equipment of $500 or more).

Statutes The laws enacted through the legislative process at both the federal and state level.

Statutes of Limitations The period of time within which a federal or state lawsuit must be filed. For personal injury cases (civil lawsuits), this time period varies among states. In most states, it is two-three years. Criminal statutes of limitations also vary by state.

Statutory Certification Refers to state statutes that provide title protections. For example, in some states, only those who possess certain credentials can use titles such as certified dietitian or certified nutritionist. Others, who do not have the certain credentials, can practice in the nutrition profession but cannot use the titles specified in the statute.

Statutory Law The body of law that has been enacted through the legislative process at the federal, state, and local levels and is often termed "written" law. Examples of federal statutes are the ADA and HIPAA. Examples at the state level are AED and waiver (release of liability) statutes.

Strategic Planning A decision-making process that is utilized in the development of a comprehensive risk management plan. To be effective, a strategic planning model should be adopted. Those leading the process need to possess strong strategic planning and leadership skills.

Strict Liability A type of tort liability that is not based on fault, but instead on public policy. In certain situations, the injured plaintiff does not need to prove intent or negligence. The defendant is liable even if not at fault. Examples include workers' compensation and vicarious liability.

Subject Matter Jurisdiction Jurisdiction, based on federal and state statutes, refers to the geographic area in which the court has authority and types of cases it has the power to hear. The types of cases that courts will hear will depend on the jurisdiction. A court with subject matter jurisdiction (e.g., limited jurisdiction) is limited to the types of cases it can hear.

Subpoena A writ ordering a person to appear in court and testify as a witness. Prior to trial, attorneys on both sides can ask the court for a subpoena.

Substantive Law A category of law that creates, defines, and regulates the duties of parties and includes tort, contract, employment, and criminal law.

Sudden Cardiac Arrest (SCA) A condition that occurs when irregularities in the heart's electrical system cause the heart to suddenly stop beating. When the heart stops, blood cannot reach the brain and other vital organs. Ventricular fibrillation (VF) is the most common cause of SCA.

Summary Judgment A procedural device in which the moving party, the one that requests summary judgment, argues that there are not any significant questions of fact and that the applicable case law requires that they be awarded judgment. This motion may be made when a party believes discovery has shown that there are no real disputes as to the facts. If the motion is granted by the court, a trial will not occur. However, the opposing party may appeal the court's decision to grant the motion.

Summative Evaluation A type of evaluation of the comprehensive risk management plan that is conducted on a formal, annual basis and includes: (a) making revisions to reflect any changes in laws and/or published standards of practice, and (b) measuring outcomes such as attainment of the plan's goals.

Summons A notice that is commonly delivered by a court officer, which informs the defendant that a lawsuit has been filed against him/her and the prescribed amount of time he/she has to prepare an answer or response to the summons.

T

Technical Physical Specifications Standards of practice primarily published by independent agencies such as the CPSC (Consumer Product Safety Commission), ASTM (American Society for Testing and Materials), and exercise equipment manufacturers that provide specifications on equipment and facilities.

Tort Conduct that reflects a legal wrong that causes harm – physical harm, emotional harm, or both, upon which the courts can impose civil liability.

Trademarks Designations of intellectual property that protects words or symbols that identify goods.

Transitional Supervision A type of supervision that involves changing from specific to general supervision or from general to specific supervision (e.g., fitness floor supervisors who provide general supervision may, at times, need to transition to specific supervision when they notice a participant misusing the equipment and need to provide individual instruction).

Trespasser A person who enters the premises of a land owner/occupier without the permission of the land owner/occupier or without a legal right to do so. The land owner/occupier has no duty, in most cases, except to refrain from intentionally or willfully injuring the trespasser.

Triers of Fact The jury and/or court (judge) whose purpose is to declare the truth based on evidence presented to them.

Two-Way Communication The communication that continues (after obtaining medical clearance and the appropriate medical releases) between an exercise professional and his/her participant's physician (or other health care providers) regarding the participant's exercise program. This strategy can be effective to help avoid exercise prescriptions that might be construed to be "treating" a medical condition.

U

Unanimous Opinion Appellate courts prepare a written opinion for each case they review, which is published so that lower courts and others are informed of their decisions and interpretations. If all the appellate judges agree, it is called a unanimous opinion.

Unenforceable Contract A type of contract that violates a statute or is contrary to public policy. For example, waiver contracts (releases of liability) have been ruled as unenforceable based on state statutes or because they were against public policy.

Unsecured PHI For purposes of HIPAA, electronic PHI that is not protected through encryption or hard copy of PHI that is not destroyed.

V

Valsalva Maneuver Occurs when individuals hold their breath against a closed glottis causing a rise in blood pressure. It occurs with daily activities such as straining during defecating or lifting a heavy object. A concern is that heavy resistance training (RT) causes significant increases in blood pressure as does the Valsalva maneuver. RT combined with the Valsalva maneuver may cause further increases in blood pressure. However, it is difficult to avoid Valsalva with heavy RT. Heavy RT, with or without Valsalva, can increase the risk of neurologic and cardiovascular injuries, especially in individuals with certain medical conditions. These individuals need to seek medical consultation before beginning a heavy RT program.

Vendor A seller of goods or services. There are thousands of vendors in the fitness and wellness profession who sell products and services. Several criteria need to be considered when selecting a fitness and/or wellness vendor.

Vicarious Liability A type of strict liability imposed upon an employer for injuries to third parties caused by the negligent acts of their employees while performing tasks within their scope of employment. See also respondeat superior.

Voidable Contract A type of contract when an essential element is missing. The contract is said to be voidable, and either party may withdraw without liability.

W

Wearable Technology Devices that collect all kinds of different personal information including fitness trackers, smart watches, heart rate monitors, and GPS tracking devices. Fitness facilities and exercise professionals who have access to such data need to be aware of and comply with state data breach notification and privacy laws that may be applicable.

Workers' Compensation A type of strict liability in which the employer is liable for injuries sustained by an employee which arise out of or are in the course of employment. No negligence is assumed on the part of the employer or employee and state laws establish fixed damages awarded to employees or their dependents.

Writ of Certiorari A request of case records, made by the U.S. Supreme Court, to a lower court (e.g., court of appeals or highest state court) for a case that the Court has decided to hear an appeal. The Court receives approximately 7,000-8,000 petitions for a writ of certiorari each year and grants and hears oral argument in about 80 cases. When the Court decides not to review a case, the decision of the lower court stands.

Written Law A term used to collectively describe federal statutes, state statutes, and laws (ordinances) passed by local governments (e.g., municipalities and counties).

Wrongful Death A civil claim/lawsuit filed by the beneficiaries of an individual whose death was caused by the negligence or willful act of another. Wrongful death statutes exist in each state that provide a cause of action in favor of the beneficiaries (e.g., close relatives such as spouse, parent, child).

Please Note: Citations for Key Terms listed in the Glossary are provided in the text where the terms are defined. To locate, see the Index for the page number.

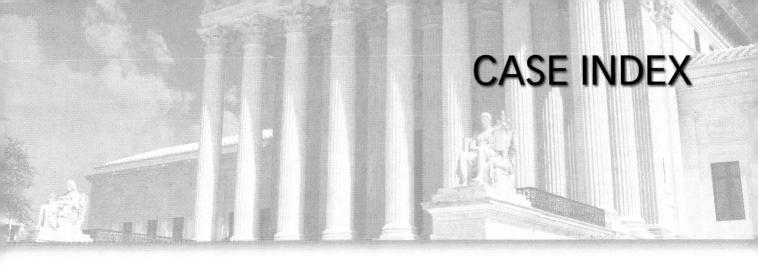

CASE INDEX

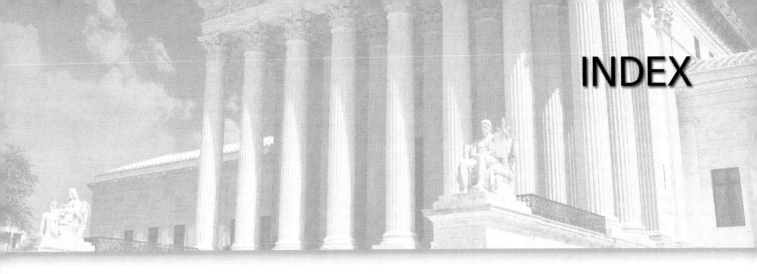

INDEX

A

AACVPR (American Association of Cardiovascular and Pulmonary Rehabilitation), 129, 171, 209

AARP (American Association of Retired Persons), 418

Aasa, U., et al., 350

Abbott, Anthony, 121, 172, 287, 294, 302, 352, 370–371, 410–411, 458

Academic programs, 161–164
    educational malpractice claims, 174
    future directions, 173–175
    gap between coursework and job responsibilities, 162–164
    marketing of, 185
    quality of, 173
    required academic courses, 162
    suggested courses to gain practical skills, 163

Accidental losses, 46

Accreditation, 164–166, 176–178

ACE (American Council on Exercise), 164, 170–171, 175

ACLS (Advanced Cardiac Life Support), 199

ACSM. *See* American College of Sports Medicine

ACSM/AHA Joint Position Statement, 295, 460–462

ACSM Exercise Professional Licensure Statement, 168

ACSM's Guidelines for Exercise Testing and Prescription, 128, 202, 208–212, 216, 226, 232–233, 235–237, 284–285, 460

ACSM's Health and Fitness Journal, 335

ACSM's Health/Fitness Facility Standards and Guidelines, 60, 127–128, 209, 374, 460

Active shooters, 466–467

Actual cause, 19

Acute injuries, emergent and non-emergent, 350

Acute myocardial infarction (AMI), 208, 295, 305

ADA. *See* Americans with Disabilities Act

ADA Standards for Accessible Design, 2010, 74

ADEA (Age Discrimination in Employment Act), 67, 80–81

Administrative law, 7

Admissibility of Evidence, on Issue of Negligence, of Codes or Standards of Safety Issued or Sponsored by Governmental Body of by Voluntary Association, 127

Advanced Cardiac Life Support (ACLS), 199

Advertising, 86–89, 184–187, 202

AEDs (Automated external defibrillators), 305, 445–449, 461–462, 471–472

Aerobics and Fitness Association of America (AFAA), 129, 170, 325

Age Discrimination in Employment Act (ADEA), 67, 80–81

AGREE (Appraisal of Guidelines for Research & Evaluation) II Instrument, 130, 211

Agreements, 27. *See also* Contract law

AHA. *See* American Heart Association

American Association of Cardiovascular and Pulmonary Rehabilitation (AACVPR), 129, 171, 209

American Association of Cardiovascular and Pulmonary Rehabilitation (AACVPR) Guidelines for Cardiac Rehabilitation and Secondary Prevention Programs, 461

American Association of Retired Persons (AARP), 418

American College of Occupational and Environmental Medicine (ACOEM)—AEDs, 461–462

American College of Sports Medicine (ACSM)
    academic programs, 161
    accreditation, 164
    ADA and, 260
    certifications, 170–171, 210, 236, 253, 274
    fitness facility orientations, standards for, 406
    Guidelines. *See ACSM's Guidelines for Exercise Testing and Prescription*
    licensure, 175

pre-activity health screening guidelines. *See* Pre-activity health screenings
    on wearable technology, 90

American Council on Exercise (ACE), 164, 170–171, 175

American Heart Association (AHA), 208–209, 295, 351, 446, 460–462

American Journal of Medicine, 304

American Kinesiotherapy Association, 175

American Law Reports (ALR), 127

American National Standards Institute (ANSI), 169, 459

American Red Cross (ARC), 443, 447, 473

American Senior Fitness Association, 283

American Society for Testing and Materials (ASTM)
    ADA and, 358–359
    equipment standards, 374, 378–380, 382–383
    New Practice for Standard Practice for Obstacle Course Events, 427
    signage specifications, 410
    spacing of equipment, 360
    unsupervised outdoor equipment, specs for, 419
    warning labels and signage for equipment, 363–364

American Society of Exercise Physiologists (ASEP), 161, 164, 175

Americans with Disabilities Act (ADA)
    accessible design and service animals, standards for, 398–399
    compliance with, 281–282
    disability discrimination, 72, 74–78
    exercise equipment safety and, 358–359, 378–379
    exercise prescriptions and, 259–260
    facility risks, management of, 398–399, 427–428
    federal employment law, 29
    fitness facility requirements under, 267
    inclusive exercise equipment, 359
    inclusive fitness symbol, 358f
    pre-activity questionnaires, 217–218
    resources to enhance compliance, 77

Made in the USA
Columbia, SC
25 October 2024

45032443R20293